OXFORD MEDICAL PUBLICATIONS

Critical care nursing
science and practice

Critical care nursing science and practice

SECOND EDITION

Sheila K. Adam
Nurse Consultant, Critical Care, University College Hospital, London, UK

and

Sue Osborne
Independent Nurse Consultant in Ciritical Care

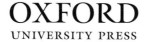
OXFORD
UNIVERSITY PRESS

OXFORD
UNIVERSITY PRESS

Great Clarendon Street, Oxford OX2 6DP

Oxford University Press is a department of the University of Oxford.
It furthers the University's objective of excellence in research, scholarship,
and education by publishing worldwide in

Oxford New York

Auckland Cape Town Dar es Salaam Hong Kong Karachi Kuala Lumpur
Madrid Melbourne Mexico City Nairobi New Delhi Shanghai Taipei Toronto

With offices in

Argentina Austria Brazil Chile Czech Republic France Greece
Guatemala Hungary Italy Japan South Korea Poland Portugal
Singapore Switzerland Thailand Turkey Ukraine Vietnam

Oxford is a registered trade mark of Oxford University Press
in the UK and in certain other countries

Published in the United States
by Oxford University Press Inc., New York

A catalogue record for the this title is available from the British Library

Library of Congress Cataloging in Publication Data attached

Typeset by EXPO Holdings Sdn Bhd., Malaysia
Printed in Great Britain
on acid-free paper
by Ashford Colour Press Ltd, Gosport, UK

ISBN 0-19-852587-7 (Pbk.: alk. paper) 978-0-19-852587-5 (Pbk.)

10 9 8 7 6 5 4 3 2 1

Preface

(The second edition of *Critical Care Nursing* is based on similar principles to the first, in that we have tried to combine the important clinical practice elements and knowledge with underlying and relevant theory. This powerful combination is aimed at nurses who wish to understand what is happening to their patients in order to deliver more effective, optimal, and appropriate nursing care. All the chapters that have been updated and in the case of the neurological chapter (Chapter 10), rewritten completely. The new chapters that have been added reflect the changing direction of critical care and the emphasis on prevention of critical illness itself as well as the complications and consequences of being critically ill. Critical care nurses are uniquely placed to address this, not only in terms of critical care outreach and post critical care follow up, but also by preventing complications such ventilator-associated pneumonia in their day-to-day care.

The emphasis on the importance of the highest quality nursing care for the critically ill patient and their family remains the cornerstone to every chapter.

Although primarily aimed at those becoming familiar with critical care, the book will also continue to provide a useful reminder and reference for many nurses who are already experienced in this complex field. Once again the underlying philosophy of this book is that of caring, competence, comprehensive knowledge, and clinical skills, underpinned by relevant research.

Sheila K. Adam
Sue Osborne

Acknowledgements

Chapter Authors

Chapter 10 – Neurological problems
Sandra Fairley – Clinical Nurse Specialist, Neurosurgical and Neuromedical Intensive Care, The National Hospital for Neurology and Neurosurgery, London

Siobhan McLernon – Senior Lecturer, South Bank University, London

Chapter Contributors

Chapter 3 – The patient within the critical care environment
Debbie Field – Weaning Nurse Specialist, Surreywide Critical Care Network

Chapter 8 – Cardiac surgery
Felicia Kwaku – Modern Matron, The Heart Hospital, UCLH Foundation Trust

Chapter 9 – Renal problems
Felicia Kwaku – Modern Matron, The Heart Hospital, UCLH Foundation Trust

Chapter 10 – Neurological problems
Jan Clarke – formerly Sister, Medical Intensive Therapy Unit, The National Hospital for Neurology and Neurosurgery, London (now Clinical Nurse Specialist for Motor Neurone Disease, The National Hospital for Neurology and Neurosurgery, London)
Judy Watkin – formerly Clinical Nurse Specialist for Acute Brain Injury, The National Hospital for Neurology and Neurosurgery, London (now at ICU/CCU Portiuncla Hospital, Ballinasloe, Co. Galway, Ireland)

Chapter Advisors

Chapter 10 – Neurological problems
Nick Hirsch – Consultant Neuroanaesthetist, The National Hospital for Neurology and Neurosurgery, London

Martin Smith – Consultant Neuroanaesthetist, The National Hospital for Neurology and Neurosurgery, London

Nicholas Davies – Specialist Registrar in Neurology, The National Hospital for Neurology and Neurosurgery, London

Chapter 16 – Endocrine, obstetric, and drug overdose emergencies
Deborah Wells – Senior Staff Nurse ITU/Midwife (formerly of St Georges Healthcare Trust)

Finally, Sheila Adam would like to thank her husband, David Fathers, and her two children, Florence and Alex, for their patience, encouragement, and enthusiasm, without which this book would not have been possible.

Contents

List of abbreviations

AA	arachidonic acid		CABG	coronary artery bypass graft
ABG	arterial blood gas		CAPD	continuous ambulatory peritoneal dialysis
ACE	angiotensin-converting enzyme		CAVH	continuous arteriovenous haemofiltration
ACh	acetylcholine		CBF	cerebral blood flow
AChE	acetylcholinesterase		CBV	cerebral blood volume
ACP			CCK	cholecystokinin
ACS	abdominal compartment syndrome		CCU	critical care unit/coronary care unit
ACT	activated clotting time		CI	cardiac index
ACTH	adrenocorticotrophic hormone		CIM	critical illness myopathy
ADH	antidiuretic hormone		CIMS	clinical information management system
ADP	adenosine diphosphate		CIP	critical illness polyneuropathy
AF	atrial fibrillation		CJD	Creutzfeldt–Jakob disease
AFE	amniotic fluid embolism		CK	creatine kinase
AFLP	acute fatty liver of pregnancy		CLL	chronic lymphatic leukaemia
ALI	acute lung injury		CML	chronic myeloid leukaemia
ALL	acute lymphatic leukaemia		$CMRO_2$	cerebral metabolic rate for oxygen consumption
AMI	acute myocardial infarction			
AML	acute myeloid leukaemia		CMV	controlled mechanical ventilation/cytomegalovirus
AP	airway pressure			
APACHE	Acute Physiology And Chronic Health Evaluation		CO	cardiac output
			COP	capillary oncotic pressure
APC	antigen-presenting cell		COPD	chronic obstructive pulmonary disease
APTT	activated partial thromboplastin time		CPAP	continuous positive airway pressure
ARDS	acute respiratory distress syndrome/adult respiratory distress syndrome		CPK	creatine phosphokinase
			CPP	Cerebral perfusion pressure
AS	aortic stenosis		CPR	cardiopulmonary resuscitation
AST	aspartate transaminase		CRIMYNE	critical illness myopathy and neuropathy
ATP	adenosine triphosphate		CSF	cerebrospinal fluid
AV	atrioventricular		CSU	catheter specimen of urine
			CSW	Cerebral salt wasting
BBB	blood–brain barrier		CT	computed tomography
BIS™	Bispectral Index monitoring		CVA	cerebrovascular accident
BiPAP	bilevel positive airway pressure		CVP	central venous pressure
BNP	brain (B)-type natriuretic peptide		CVR	cerebral vascular resistance
BP	blood pressure		CVVH	continuous venovenous haemofiltration
bpm	beats per minute		CVVHD	continuous venovenous haemodialysis
BSA	body surface area			

CVVHDF	continuous venovenous haemodiafiltration		HDU	high-dependency unit
CXR	chest X-ray		HFJV	high-frequency jet ventilation
			HHS	hyperosmolar, hyperglycaemic states
DAI	diffuse axonal injury		HITS	heparin-induced thrombocytopenia syndrome
DDAVP	l-deamino-8-D-arginine vasopressin (desmopressin)		HME	heat–moisture exchange
DI	diabetes insipidus		HOCM	hypertrophic obstructive cardiomyopathy
DIC	disseminated intravascular coagulation		HRS	hepatorenal syndrome
DID	delayed ischaemic deficit		HSE	herpes simplex encephalitis
DKA	diabetic ketoacidosis		5-HT	5-hydroxytryptamine
DO_2I	oxygen delivery index			
2,3-DPG	2,3-diphosphoglyceric acid		IABP	intra-aortic balloon pulsation/pump
DSA	digital subtraction angiography		IAH	intra-abdominal hypertension
DVT	deep vein thrombosis		IAP	intra-abdominal pressure
			ICH	intracerebral haematoma
ECC	external chest compressions		ICP	intracranial pressure
ECG	electrocardiogram		ICS	intracellular space
$ECCO_2R$	extracorporeal carbon dioxide removal		ICU	intensive care unit
ECMO	Extracorporeal membrane oxygenation		IDDM	insulin-dependent diabetes mellitus
EDH	extradural haematoma		IHD	intermittent haemodialysis
EDV	end diastolic volume		IM	intramuscular
EEG	electroencephalogram		IMA	internal mammary artery
EF	ejection fraction		IMV	intermittent mandatory ventilation
EMG	electromyography		INR	international normalized ratio
ESR	erythrocyte sedimentation rate		IPPB	intermittent positive pressure breathing
ESV	end systolic volume		IPPV	intermittent positive pressure ventilation
ET(T)	endotracheal (tube)		IPR	
$ETCO_2$	end tidal carbon dioxide monitoring		ISS	Injury Severity Score/interstitial space
			ITA	internal thoracic artery
FDPs	fibrin degradation products		ITP	idiopathic thrombocytopenic purpura
FES	fat embolism syndrome		IV	intravenous
FFP	fresh frozen plasma		IVC	inferior vena cava
F_iO_2	fractionated inspired oxygen		IVIg	intravenous immunoglobulin
FRC	functional residual capacity		IVS	intravascular space
FTc	corrected flow time			
FVC	forced vital capacity		JVP	jugular venous pressure
GBS	Guillain–Barré syndrome		KPTT	kaolin partial thromboplastin time
GCS	Glasgow Coma Score/Scale			
GFR	glomerular filtration rate		LAP	left atrial pressure
GH	growth hormone		LDH	lactic dehydrogenase
GI	gastrointestinal		LFPPV	low-frequency positive pressure ventilation
GIK	glucose–insulin–potassium		LiDCO™	lithium dilution cardiac output
GM-CSF	granulocyte–macrophage colony-stimulating factor		LMA	laryngeal mask airway
			LVEDP	left venticular end diastolic pressure
GTN	glyceryl trinitrate		LVEDV	left venticular end diastolic volume
HADS	Hospital Anxiety and Depression Scale		MAOI	monoamine oxidase inhibitor
Hb	haemoglobin		MAP	mean arterial pressure
Hct	haematocrit		MARS	molecular adsorption recycling system

MAST	military antishock trouser [suit]	PTH	parathyroid hormone
MET	medical emergency team	PV	peak velocity
MEWS	modified early warning score	PVR	pulmonary vascular resistance
MG	myasthenia gravis	PSVT	paroxysmal supraventricular tachycardias
MI	myocardial infarction		
MODS	multiple organ dysfunction syndrome	RAA	renin–angiotensin–aldosterone (pathway)
MRAP	mean right atrial pressure	RAP	right atrial pressure
MRB	manual resuscitation bag	RAS	reticular activating system
MRSA	methicillin-resistant *Staphylococcus aureus*	RIP	Riyadh intensive care program
MS	mitral stenosis	ROC	receiver operating characteristic
MUGA	multiple gated analysis (scan)	ROM	range of movement
MV	minute volume	ROS	reactive oxygen species
		RR	respiratory rate
NG	nasogastric	RRT	renal replacement therapy
NICE	National Institute for Clinical Excellence	RSBI	rapid shallow breathing index
NIDDM	non-insulin-dependent diabetes mellitus	rTPA	(recombinant) tissue plasminogen activator
NIV	non-invasive ventilation		
NPE	neurogenic pulmonary oedema	RTS	Revised Trauma Score
NS	not significant	RVDP	right ventricular diastolic pressure
NSAIDs	non-steroidal anti-inflammatory drugs	RVSP	right ventricular systolic pressure
O_2ER	oxygen extraction ratio	SA	sinoatrial
OGD	oesophagogastroduodenoscopy	SAH	subarachnoid haemorrhage
PA	pulmonary artery	SAPS	Simplified Acute Physiology Score
PACS	picture archiving and communication system	SBE	subacute bacterial endocarditis
		SBT	spontaneous breathing trials
P_aCO_2	partial pressure of arterial carbon dioxide	SCUF	slow continuous ultrafiltration
P_AO_2	partial pressure of alveolar oxygen	SD	standard deviation
PADP	pulmonary artery diastolic pressure	SDD	selective decontamination of the digestive tract
PAF	platelet-activating factor (PAF)		
PAOP	pulmonary artery occlusion pressure	SDH	subdural haematoma
PART	Patient At Risk Team (score)	SE	status epilepticus
PASP	pulmonary artery systolic pressure	SIADH	syndrome of inappropriate antidiuretic hormone
PAWP	pulmonary artery wedge pressure		
PCA	patient-controlled analgesia	SIMV	synchronized intermittent mandatory ventilation
PC-IRV	pressure-controlled inverse ratio ventilation		
PCP	*Pneumocystis carinii* pneumonia	SIRS	systemic inflammatory response syndrome
PCWP	pulmonary capillary wedge pressure	SLE	systemic lupus erythematosus
PD	peritoneal dialysis	S_aO_2	oxygen saturation of arterial blood
PE	pulmonary embolism/ plasma exchange	$S_{jv}O_2$	Jugular venous bulb oximetry
PEA	pulseless electrical activity	SpO_2	
PEEP	positive end expiratory pressure	SV	stroke volume
PERT	patient emergency response team	SVC	superior vena cava
pH_1	intramucosal pH	S_vO_2	mixed venous oxygen saturation
PMNLs	polymorphonuclear leucocytes	SVR	systemic vacular resistance
PP	pulse pressure	SVT	supraventricular tachycardia
ppm	parts per million		
PSV	pressure support ventilation	TBI	traumatic brain injury
PT	prothrombin time	TBG	thyroxine-binding globulin
PTFE	polytetrafluoroethylene	TCD	transcranial Doppler (ultrasonography)

TENS	transcutaneous electrical nerve stimulation	VAP	ventilator-associated pneumonia
TIPS	transjugular intrahepatic portal systemic shunt	VC-IRV	volume-controlled inverse ratio ventilation
TISS	Therapeutic Intervention Scoring System	VF	ventricular fibrillation
TMP	transmembrane pressure	VMA	vanillylmandelic acid
TNF	tumour necrosis factor	VO_2I	oxygen consumption index
tPA	tissue plasminogen activator	V/Q	ventilation/perfusion
TRH	thyrotrophin-releasing hormone	VSD	ventricular septal defect
TRISS	Trauma Score–Injury Severity Score	VT	ventricular tachycardia
TSH	thyroid-stimulating hormone	VZE	Varicella zoster encephalitis
TTP	thrombotic thrombocytopenic purpura		
TXA_2	thromboxane A_2	WBPTT	whole blood partial thromboplastin time
		WG	Wegener's granulomatosis
UPS	uninterrupted power supply	WPW	Wolff–Parkinson–White (syndrome)
UTI	urinary tract infection		

The critical care continuum

Introduction

The initial development of critical care as a speciality started with the grouping of patients into intensive care units (ICUs) in the 1960s according to their illness and dependence on the nurse (ICS 2003). Clearly identified separate geographical areas were established where patients could be cared for and which focused on respiratory and cardiovascular support. However, as

this separate speciality developed, a degree of segregation from other staff and wards also developed. Patients were admitted to critical care areas from the wards, cared for by a separate group of staff, and if they survived, returned to the wards with little or no ongoing follow-up from the critical care staff.

The impetus behind this development of separate ICUs evolved from the need for skilled personnel, specific resources (such as ventilators and electrocardiogram (ECG) monitors) and adequate facilities (piped gases, larger bed areas). As critical care became more sophisticated, training of skilled staff became formal and there was recognition of the need for competent, experienced and technically capable staff.

Once the requirement for critical care became established, there was a gradual shift in culture so that patients who required critical care (and this was often synonymous with mechanical ventilation) were considered only to be those patients within the boundary walls of the designated critical care areas.

As critical care has become more sophisticated, knowledge, skills, and expertise have grown. However, in spite of improvements in survival for many specific patient groups (such as those undergoing cardiac surgery), a high mortality rate remains for patients who develop sepsis and multiple organ failure.

In the last few years, a further shift in culture has occurred in critical care, predominantly in the UK, that encompasses:

- earlier involvement of critical care expertise in a bid to prevent patient deterioration;

- ongoing follow-up of patients discharged to the ward from critical care to prevent readmission.

This has been variously named 'critical care without walls', the 'critical care continuum', and 'critical care outreach'.

Redefining the limits of critical care

In spite of considerable effort, resource, and time, there has been little improvement over the years in outcome for patients admitted to critical care with sepsis and multiorgan failure. Sepsis is the leading cause of death in critical care with around 50% of patients dying within 6 months (Bernard *et al.* 2001). Some improvement may be possible with early accurate diagnosis and treatment, including appropriate antibiotics and resuscitation (Rivers *et al.* 2001, Lyseng-Williamson and Perry 2002). This early intervention needs to occur outside the critical care environment in ward areas or accident and emergency units (Rivers *et al.* 2001) in order to be most effective. This is a major factor in the need to expand the influence of critical care skills and responses outside the geographical area of the critical care environment itself.

The factors associated with the need for development of critical care outside the critical care unit are numerous. Many of them have come about due to changes in methods of managing and delivering care to

patients as well as changes to the education of nurses and doctors. These factors include:

1. Increasing number of acutely ill patients in hospital (increased primary care interventions, day surgery, reduced length of stay, etc.).

2. Increasing co-morbidity/multiple pathology and age of patients as well as increasing longevity of sufferers from chronic disease.

3. Decreased emphasis on acute illness in pre-registration education for nurses and increased emphasis on health education and prevention.

4. Decreased exposure to acutely ill patients during pre-registration education for nurses due to supernumerary practice and increased time in college.

5. Increased workload for medical teams with less time for supervision of junior staff.

6. An 'Ivory Tower' attitude from critical care staff resulting in decreased communication/sharing of knowledge and skills with ward staff.

7. Possible de-skilling of ward staff, particularly in early recognition of deterioration, as sick patients are more frequently cared for in critical care.

8. Transfer of routine observations such as temperature, heart rate, and blood pressure to healthcare assistants (untrained ward nursing staff), sometimes without proper supervision.

9. Decline of the monitoring of respiratory rate by wards staff as a sensitive but non-specific marker of deterioration (Odell *et al.* 2002)

In a study of quality of care of patients prior to critical care admission, McQuillan *et al.* (1998) identified six factors (Table 1.1) associated with suboptimal care of the acutely ill patient in the wards. Mortality in critical care was significantly higher ($p = 0.04$) in the group that received suboptimal care.

Some of these factors, particularly those requiring education, can be addressed by the development of critical care outreach services. Others, particularly cultural issues (such as 'coping' by junior staff without requesting senior help so as not to appear inadequate), require involvement and commitment for change from training bodies and professional groups as well as healthcare institutions themselves. The development of better levels of supervision and immediate access to skilled resources for critically ill patients needs to be met by a combination of organizational, critical care, and interprofessional initiatives.

TABLE 1.1 Causes of suboptimal care

Principal causes of suboptimal care*	1. Failure of organization
	2. Lack of knowledge
	3. Failure to appreciate clinical urgency
	4. Lack of experience
	5. Lack of supervision
	6. Failure to seek advice
Recategorized by system dysfunction	**Process:**
	1. Failure of organization
	5. Lack of supervision
	Education:
	2. Lack of knowledge
	3. Failure to appreciate clinical urgency
	Culture:
	4. Lack of experience
	6. Failure to seek advice

*From McQuillan et al. (1998).

Limitations of cardiopulmonary resuscitation

Although considerable education, resources, and effort have been put in to developing a fast and effective response to cardiac arrest, the outcome continues to be poor for patients who suffer a cardiac arrest.

In a study of 5505 patients, Herlitz *et al.* (2003) compared outcomes for patients who suffered an out-of-hospital cardiac arrest between 1980 and 1990 with out-of-hospital cardiac arrest outcomes between1990 and 2000. Survival to hospital was 24% in both decades; of these, only 37% survived to hospital discharge in 1980–1990, and only 35% survived to hospital discharge in 1990–2000 (p = not significant (NS)).

Overall survival to discharge from hospital was therefore approximately 8% and this had not improved over the 20 years studied. Factors which were identified as being associated with survival in out-of-hospital arrests included ventricular fibrillation/ventricular tachycardia (VF/VT) as first recorded rhythm, witnessed arrest, bystander initiated cardiopulmonary resuscitation (CPR), patient conscious at time of admission to hospital, and sinus rhythm on admission to hospital. Factors associated with decreased survival were chronic diuretic and oral hypoglycaemic medication.

Outcome for in-hospital arrests in an audit of 1368 patients was found to be around 17.6% (survival to hospital discharge) overall, increasing to 42.2% in VF/VT arrhythmias (Gwinnutt *et al.* 2000). This study also found an association with increased survival for VF/VT arrhyth-

mias, restoration of circulation in <3 min, and age <70 yr. Interestingly, the administration of any adrenaline was associated with decreased survival, probably because this is linked with longer periods of resuscitation.

Costs of CPR training programmes as determined by Lee *et al.* (1996) are estimated at $406,605 per life saved and $225,892 per quality adjusted life year. This is a huge outlay for such a poor outcome and suggests that other methods, primarily early detection and response, should be explored.

The aim of early warning scores and call criteria (collectively known as track and trigger mechanisms) is to help general ward staff to identify patients who are deteriorating and initiate a response before a terminal event occurs.

Early recognition of clinical deterioration in patients

Beginning in the early 1990s, work by Schein (1990), Franklin and Mathews (1994), and Rich (1999) found that many patients who subsequently suffered a cardiorespiratory arrest had evidence of physiological deterioration in the hours prior to this event. Rich (1999) also found some evidence that response times to patient deterioration are variable. Nurses took a mean of 21.4 min overall to notify doctors of physiological deterioration and resulting resuscitation survival was associated with a mean notification time of 14.3 min compared with 25.7 min for non-survivors. So the longer the response time to early indicators of deterioration, the less likely the patient was to survive (Tables 1.2 and 1.3).

In view of the poor outcome associated with cardiac arrest it makes sense to utilize the early indicators as

SIGNS OF DETERIORATION USED BY RICH (1999)

- New changes in systolic blood pressure—alteration (up or down) >20 mmHg
- New heart rate changes to <45 beats per min (bpm) or >125 bpm
- New ECG rhythm changes on the monitor
- New respiratory rate to <10 or >30 breaths/min
- New patient complaints of chest pain or dyspnoea
- New changes in patient's mental status
- New critical laboratory values

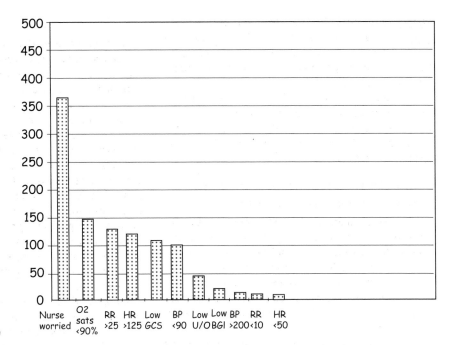

Fig. 1.1 Criteria triggering emergency calls to critical care outreach at UCLH Trust (2003)

an opportunity to intervene more quickly and attempt to prevent cardiac arrest occurring. This might then result in an improved outcome (Fig. 1.1).

Hillman *et al.* (2001) and McGloin *et al.* (1999) examined antecedents to sudden death or critical care admission. Hillman *et al.* (2001) found the most common physiological changes documented prior to deaths not preceded by cardiac arrest or critical care admission were systolic blood pressure (BP) <90 mmHg and respiratory rate (RR) >36 breaths/min. Concern was frequently documented, but not reasons why appropriate intervention did not occur. This was also found by McGloin *et al.* (1999) with tachypnoea (RR >25 breaths/

min), hypoxaemia (SpO_2 <90%) and hypotension (systolic BP <100 mmHg) most commonly associated with admission to critical care and death.

Hodgetts *et al.* (2002) used multivariate analysis of 118 cardiac arrest cases identified compared with 132 hospital in-patients and found three positive associations for cardiac arrest: (1) abnormal breathing indicator, (2) abnormal pulse and (3) abnormal systolic blood pressure. Risk factors were weighted and receiver oper-

TABLE 1.2 Time taken by nurses to notify physicians about physiological changes prior to cardiac arrest (Rich 1999)

Variable	Mean (min)	SD (min)
Overall mean time	21.4	32.9
Chest pain	7.3	6.8
Dyspnoea	10.5	8.4
ECG rhythm	22.3	34.8
Respirations	27.5	32.0
Blood pressure	28.4	42.7
Heart rate	31.0	40.2
Mental status	30.3	34.2

TABLE 1.3 Evidence of deterioration prior to cardiac arrest

Authors	No of patients	Results
Schein *et al.* (1990)	64	8% survival after cardiac arrest. 84% showed evidence of clinical deterioration
Franklin and Mathew (1994)	150	66% of patients had documented clinical deterioration prior to arrest
Rich (1999)	100	11% survival after cardiac arrest. Physiological change noted in 60% of patients up to 8 h prior to arrest

ating characteristic (ROC) analysis determined that a score of 4 had 89% sensitivity and 77% specificity for cardiac arrest while a score of 8 had 52% sensitivity and 99% specificity. All patients scoring greater than 10 suffered a cardiac arrest.

Parameters based on these findings have been developed into markers or indicators of acute deterioration for patients, accompanied by a dictated response usually requiring reaction within a set time frame from specified personnel.

Lack of skills in recognition and response to critical deterioration in ward patients

A study by Smith and Poplett (2002) found that knowledge about recognition and response to acute situations such as the recognition of complete airway obstruction or setting up of high-flow oxygen was poor in 108 junior medical staff. These are the group most likely to be called to deal with these situations by ward nursing staff, and it is vital that they can intervene effectively in order to prevent delays.

Similar gaps in knowledge are likely in nursing staff, and it is suggested that nurses use a degree of personal experience to assess the patient's state (Cioffi and Markham 1997). However, in an in-depth study of nurses' reasoning behind calling the medical emergency team (MET), Cioffi (2000) found there were four specific findings most likely to alert nurses to patients requiring urgent intervention (see box).

The combination of poor early recognition and lack of skill in responding to acute deterioration is likely to contribute to a poor patient outcome.

SPECIFIC FINDINGS ASSOCIATED WITH NURSES ACTIVATING THE MET FOR 'WORRIED OR CONCERNED'

- ◆ 'Not right' or 'unwell' declared by the patient or recognized by the nurse as a difference in the patient
- ◆ Colour, clamminess, and coldness with colour (quite pale, porcelain pale, pale dusky, and sort of grey) or draining colour
- ◆ Agitation
- ◆ Observations that were slightly abnormal or not unusual at all

Cioffi (2000)

Early intervention could improve outcome

It has been suggested that early recognition and aggressive intervention may be beneficial in preventing death and improving illness severity after the patient is admitted to critical care.

Studies in emergency care (Rivers et al. 2001) and in optimization prior to surgery (Wilson et al. 1999) have shown that patient outcome can be improved by early and aggressive intervention. Wilson et al. (1999) studied 138 patients and compared the effects of pre-operative enhancement of oxygen delivery against standard surgical practice. This required admission to critical care in the treatment group but not in the ward group. There was a significant ($p = 0.007$) improvement in survival in the treatment group as well as a reduction in length of stay. However, some of this improvement may simply have been due to admission to critical care pre-operatively.

Similarly Rivers et al. (2001) randomized patients in severe sepsis and septic shock admitted to emergency care (accident and emergency) to either receive standard care or optimization with a pulmonary artery catheter and fluid/inotropes following a protocol (Fig. 1.2). This early aggressive intervention reduced mortality from 46.5% to 30.5%.

The delay in responding to acute deterioration is also applicable to ward patients. In many cases although acute deterioration is recognized it may take some time either to access the correct level of support or to ensure transfer to a critical care unit. Rivers et al. (2001) suggest that the transition to multiorgan failure and critical illness can be denoted as 'golden hours' during which definitive recognition and treatment can be of maximal benefit and that these can occur when the patient is on the ward, in the accident and emergency department, or on the intensive care unit.

Lundberg et al. (1998) compared outcomes between 10 patients with onset of septic shock on the wards and 31 patients with onset in critical care. They found that ward onset of septic shock was associated with 5.5 times the risk of death, compared with critical care onset. Review of the clinical course suggested that there were delays in specific responses such as intravenous (IV) fluid resuscitation and inotropes in the ward patients. This was related to the need to transfer to critical care prior to delivery of inotropes.

Nursing staff are uniquely placed to recognize early deterioration and to activate an appropriate response from their colleagues, but because traditional hierarchical methods of doing this often resulted in delay, other forms of response have been set up.

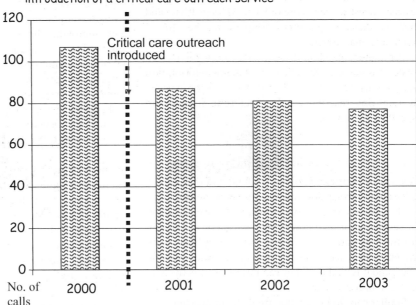

Fig. 1.2 In-patient cardiac arrest incidence following introduction of a critical care outreach service

Development of teams able to respond prior to cardiac arrest

Lee *et al.* (1995) in Liverpool, Australia, described the first team of this nature. The MET consists of critical care medical and nursing staff who respond to calls from ward staff based on a series of set criteria (Table 1.4). The team are based in the critical care unit and are trained in advanced resuscitation techniques.

Much of the literature supporting the development of these teams has come from studies undertaken by this group. There is excellent evidence showing a decrease in the incidence of cardiac arrest (Buist *et al.* 2002, Bellomo

TABLE 1.4 Criteria for calling the medical emergency team (Lee et al. 1995)

Cardiorespiratory arrest	
Threatened airway	
Respiratory rate	≤5 breaths/min, ≥36 breaths/min
Pulse rate	≤40 bpm, ≥140 bpm
Systolic blood pressure	≤90 mmHg
Repeated or prolonged seizures	
Fall in Glasgow Coma Score	>2 points
Concern about patient status not detailed above	

ESSENTIAL OBJECTIVES OF CRITICAL CARE OUTREACH

♦ To advert admissions (to the ICU) by identifying patients who are deteriorating and either helping to prevent admission or ensuring that admission to a critical care bed happens in a timely manner to ensure the best outcome.

♦ To enable discharges by supporting the continuing recovery of discharged patients on wards and post discharge from hospital and their relatives and friends.

♦ To share critical care skills with staff in wards and the community, ensuring enhancements for training opportunities and skills practice, and to use information gathered from the ward and community to improve critical care services for patients and relatives.

Comprehensive Critical Care (Department of Health 2000, pp. 14–15)

et al. 2003), some evidence for a reduction in unanticipated admissions to intensive care (Bristow *et al.* 2000), and minimal evidence for reductions in general hospital mortality (Bellomo *et al.* 2003). Furthermore, patients who do suffer a cardiac arrest whilst the team are present appear to have a better chance of survival (Bellomo *et al.* 2003).

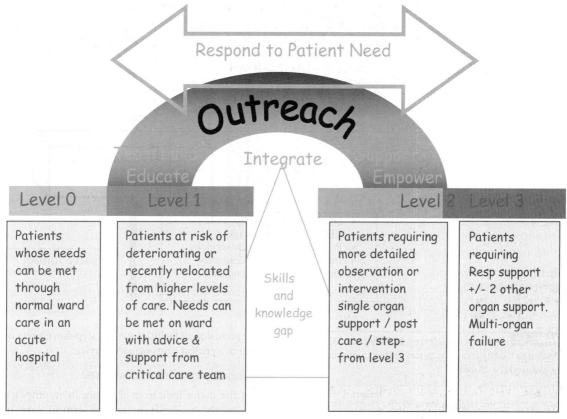

Fig. 1.3 Model of critical care outreach.

Development of critical care outreach services

In the United Kingdom the publication of two reports (*Critical to Success* (1999) and *Comprehensive Critical Care* (Department of Health 2000)) actively encouraged the establishment of critical care services that would respond to critically ill patients who were acutely ill outside the critical care unit. These are termed critical care outreach services and over 100 different forms of this service have been set up in hospitals throughout England.

Outreach services (Fig. 1.3) have an enormous variety of team personnel, hours of cover, responses, criteria or triggers used to call the service and level of education offered to other staff (Outreach Forum Report 2003). The difference between medical emergency teams and the critical care outreach service is that while the former concentrate solely on pre-critical care admission, the latter will cover both pre- and post-critical care admissions as well as enhanced training for ward staff.

The gap between survival in critical care and survival to discharge from hospital

Many studies have shown a considerable difference (up to 27%) between patient survival to discharge from critical care and patient survival to hospital discharge (Goldhill and Sumner 1998, Smith *et al.* 1999, Moreno and Agthé 1999). Smith *et al.* (1999) showed that mortality rate in a prospective study of 238 patients was associated with discharge TISS (Therapeutic Intervention Scoring System). Mortality in patients with TISS <10 was 3.7% compared with 21.4% when the TISS exceeded 20. Although a proportion of these deaths may be expected as part of a recognition that the patient is in the terminal phase of their illness, others are less obvious.

Goldhill and Sumner (1998) studied 12,762 critical care admissions from 15 critical care units and found over a quarter of all the deaths occurred after critical care discharge. The highest percentage of deaths after discharge occurred in patients admitted with respiratory problems.

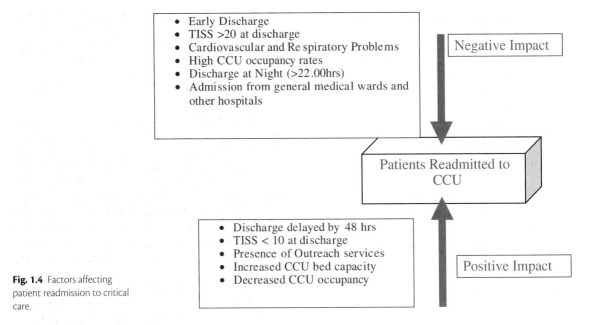

Fig. 1.4 Factors affecting patient readmission to critical care.

TABLE 1.5   Six variables selected by Daly *et al.* (2001) for discharge triage predictive model (either increased risk or reduced risk of dying)

Variable	Impact
Age	Positive
Chronic health points	Positive
Acute physiology points	Positive
Cardiac surgery	Negative
Length of ICU stay	Positive
Constant	Negative

Causes for this are difficult to determine. Moreno and Agthé (1999) suggest that early discharge (perhaps because of demand for beds) plays a role. This is supported by the work of Daly *et al.* (2001) who used a logistic regression model to identify those patients at risk of dying following discharge from critical care. Six variables were identified (see Table 1.5) and the model was applied to a validation data set. Those patients who stayed in the critical care unit (CCU) for more than 48 h after they were considered ready for discharge but who fell into a high risk group had a significantly reduced risk of dying.

It is therefore theoretically possible to identify high-risk patients at discharge and either prolong their stay in critical care or increase the level of support available to them after discharge. Unfortunately, in practice the demand for critical care beds often makes the former solution impossible and the latter solution will depend on the provision of facilities such as step-down units or the use of a critical care outreach service.

Readmission rates to critical care

One of the major indicators of failure in an outreach service is the readmission rate to critical care in patients during the same hospital stay. Readmission is associated with a five-fold increase in risk of mortality (Rosenberg *et al.* 2001), and the reduction of readmission rates should be one of the major goals for critical care outreach services. However, there are many factors which affect the likelihood of readmission (see Fig. 1.4).

Chen *et al.* (1998) reviewed the clinical features and outcomes of 236 patients readmitted to seven CCUs over a period of 13 months. They found that patients with cardiovascular and respiratory problems were most likely to be readmitted for the same illness. In addition, where patients developed new complications requiring readmission, 58% of them were respiratory in origin.

Post-critical care follow-up

The inclusion of ongoing advice and support from the critical care staff in the management of the patient's post-discharge care offers the patient, their family, and the ward staff an opportunity for continuity in terms of care. It also allows monitoring by critical care trained staff to continue into the ward area with the opportunity for an exchange of information and techniques for managing the highly dependent patient.

TABLE 1.6 Examples of physical problems after intensive care (Griffiths and Jones 2002)

Recovering organ failure (e.g. lung, kidney, liver, etc.)

Muscle wasting and weakness

    Reduced cough power

    Pharyngeal weakness

Joint pain and stiffness (particularly shoulders)

Numbness, paraesthesiae (peripheral neuropathy)

Taste changes resulting in favourite foods being unpalatable

Itching, dry skin

Disturbances of sleep rhythm and pattern

    Waking at night, poor sleep, not rested

Cardiac and circulatory decompensation

    Postural hypotension (autonomic neuropathy)

    Heart failure

Reduced pulmonary reserve

    Breathlessness on mild exertion

    Increased work of breathing

Disturbed sexual function

Iatrogenic

    Tracheal stenosis (e.g. repeated intubations)

    Nerve palsies (needle injuries)

    Scarring (needle and drain sites)

TABLE 1.7 Psychological problems following intensive care (Griffiths and Jones 2002)

Depression

    Anger and conflict with the family

Anxiety

    About recovery to normal state

    Panic attacks

    Fear of dying

Guilt

Recurrent nightmares

Post-traumatic stress disorder

The development of follow-up post-CCU discharge is an important factor in reducing the risk of readmission, but unless other issues are also addressed the service will be unable to make an impact on the rate of readmissions.

Probably the most important factor in reducing readmissions is the need to ensure that patients are physiologically ready to move to a reduced level of monitoring and intervention. While CCU bed capacity remains the deciding factor determining discharge it is unlikely that patients will be discharged appropriately. It is therefore vital that capacity is sufficient to prevent early discharge likely to reduce a patient's potential for survival.

Problems for patients recovering from critical care

Long-term physical and psychological effects are associated with an episode of critical illness. Although a greatly increased in-hospital mortality is associated with critical care admission, the long-term survival of critical care patients who are discharged home is not significantly different from that of patients following a general hospital admission (Keenan et al. 2002). The increased death rate seen initially after discharge is likely to be related to the precipitating disease for hospital admission rather than the intensive care stay itself.

There are many generic problems associated with the recovery from critical care illness. Examples of physical problems are listed in Table 1.6 and psychological problems in Table 1.7.

Follow-up clinics

Critical care follow-up clinics first started in 1990 in Whiston Hospital, Liverpool (Griffiths and Jones, 2002). The patients are seen at between 2 and 6 months after discharge from hospital allowing assessment of their physical and mental state.

Follow-up clinics allow intensive care staff a more complete understanding of the effects of critical illness and the ability to see the patient's experience of critical illness as a whole. These clinics also commonly afford the only opportunity for evaluating patients' responses

TABLE 1.8 Levels of patient need (Comprehensive Critical Care 2000)

Level 0	Patients whose needs can be met through normal ward care in an acute hospital
Level 1	Patients at risk of their condition deteriorating, or those recently relocated from higher levels of care whose needs can be met on an acute ward with additional advice and support from the critical care team
Level 2	Patients requiring more detailed observation or intervention including support for a single failing organ system or post-operative care, and those stepping down from higher levels of care
Level 3	Patients requiring advanced respiratory support alone or basic respiratory support together with support of at least two organ systems. This level includes all complex patients requiring support for multiorgan failure

TABLE 1.9 Intensive Care Society guidance on levels of care (2002)

Level	Criteria	Examples
Level 0	Requires hospitalization. Needs can be met through normal ward care	Bolus IV medication Oral medication Patient-controlled analgesia Observations required less frequently than 4 hourly
Level 1	Patient recently discharged from a higher level of care Patient in need of additional monitoring, clinical input, or advice	Observations required at least 4 hourly Physiotherapy or airway suctioning required at least 6 hourly, but not more than 2 hourly
	Patients requiring critical care outreach service support	Abnormal vital signs but not requiring a higher level of critical care
	Patients requiring staff with special expertise and/or additional facilities for at least one aspect of critical care delivered in a general ward environment	Renal replacement therapy (stable chronic renal failure) Epidural analgesia Tracheostomy care
Level 2	Patients needing single organ system monitoring and support (ACP definitions for patients already in receipt of single organ support are applicable to this group). Patients in need of advanced respiratory support as the only major organ system supported due to an acute illness would normally satisfy the criteria for level 3	Respiratory: needing more than 50% inspired oxygen; within 24 h of tracheostomy insertion; requiring non-invasive ventilation or CPAP; requiring physiotherapy or suctioning at least every 2 hours. Cardiovascular: unstable, requiring continuous ECG and invasive pressure monitoring; haemodynamic instability due to hypovolaemia/haemorrhage/sepsis; requiring single infusion of vasoactive drug with appropriate monitoring. Central nervous system: CNS depression sufficient to prejudice airway and protective reflexes; invasive neurological monitoring.

ACP – augmented care period; CPAP– continuous positive airway pressure

TABLE 1.9 Intensive Care Society guidance on levels of care (2002) *continued*

Level	Criteria	Examples
		Other: acute impairment of renal, electrolyte or metabolic function
	Patients needing pre-operative optimization. Requiring invasive monitoring and treatment to improve organ function	Haemodynamic/respiratory resuscitation or optimization. Insertion of invasive monitoring
	Patients needing extended post-operative care: extended post-operative observation is required either because of the nature of the procedure and/or the patient's condition. Included in this group would be patients needing short-term, i.e. less than 24 h, routine post-operative ventilation who are otherwise well with no other organ dysfunction, e.g. fast track cardiac surgery patients	Procedure: major elective surgery; emergency surgery in unstable or high-risk patient; increased risk of post-operative complications, interventions, or monitoring. Patient: intermediate surgery in patient >70 yr or ASA III or IV (severe system disease with functional limitation or worse)
	Patients needing a greater degree of observation and monitoring	Observation and monitoring that cannot be safely provided at level 1 or below, judged on the basis of clinical circumstances and ward resources
	Patient moving to step-down care	No longer need level 3, but not well enough to be classified as level 1 or 0
	Patient with major uncorrected physiological abnormalities: these physiological abnormalities, if uncorrected are likely to indicate a patient requiring at least level 2 care. Patients with lesser degree of abnormality or other physiological abnormalities may also require level 2 or 3 care	Respiratory rate >40 breaths/min or >30 breaths/min for >6 h. Heart rate >120 beats/min. Temperature <35°C for >1 h. Hypotension, e.g. systolic BP <80 mmHg for >1 h. Glasgow Coma Score (GCS) <10 and at risk of acute deterioration

ASA – American Society of Anaesthesiologists (physical status grades)

TABLE 1.9 Intensive Care Society guidance on levels of care (2002)   *continued*

Level	Criteria	Examples
Level 3	Patients needing advanced respiratory monitoring and support: excluded from invasive positive this group would be patients needing short-term, i.e. less than 24 h routine post-operative ventilationwho are otherwise well with no other organ dysfunction, e.g. fast track cardiac surgery patients. If ventilatory support exceeds 24 h, or other significant organ dysfunction develops, these patients now need level 3 care. ACP definitions for patients already in receipt of advanced respiratory support are applicable to this group	Respiratory failure from any cause that requires pressure mechanical ventilatory support BiPAP via any form of tracheal tube Extracorporeal respiratory support
	Patients needing monitoring and support for two or more organ systems, one of which may be basic or advanced respiratory support (note that this clarifies the apparent inconsistency between the suggested levels criteria in *Comprehensive Critical Care* (Department of Health 2000) and existing ACP definitions). ACP definitions for patients already in receipt of multiple organ support are applicable to this group	SIMV or CMV and continuous intravenous vasoactive drugs. SIMV or CMV and haemofiltration High-risk patients undergoing major surgery who are likely to require advanced respiratory support and monitoring/support of other organ systems Continuous IV medication to control seizures and supplementary oxygen/airway monitoring
	Patients with chronic impairment of one or more organ systems sufficient to restrict daily activities (co-morbidity) and who require support for an acute reversible failure of another organ system. ACP definitions for patients already in receipt of single organ support are applicable to this group	Severe ischaemic heart disease and major peri-operative haemorrhage COPD requiring home oxygen presenting with sepsis related to immunosuppression Angina on mild exercise and bronchopneumonia requiring CPAP

SIMV – synchronized intermittent mechanical ventilation; CMV – controlled mechanical ventilation; BiPAP – Bi-level positive airway pressure; CPAP – continuous positive airway pressure; COPD – chronic obstructive pulmonary disease

to their critical care stay and feedback to the staff about the effects of some of their interventions.

As with critical care itself, the patient should be assessed as a whole and the clinic should address both physical and psychological problems resulting from the critical illness.

Levels of patient need

In order to facilitate a more continuous view of critical care throughout the hospital, the national expert group report, *Comprehensive Critical Care* (Department of Health 2000) recommended that patients be categorized according to their level of need rather than a geographical location. These levels are defined in Table 1.8. More detailed explanation and definition have been published by the UK Intensive Care Society (ICS) in 2002 (Table 1.9). The ICS definitions allow the demand for different levels of care to be assessed and quantified throughout the hospital, removing geographical location from being the defining factor in the patient's access to critical care skills.

Changes to nursing on the ward as a result of outreach

Due to a number of different factors, the general level of skill for nursing acutely ill patients on the ward has been reduced over the years. These factors include:

- reduction in numbers of qualified nurses on the ward;

- expanding demands on nursing time from other components of the role;

- increasing dependence on unqualified staff to undertake patient observations;

- increasing use of automated BP and O_2 saturation monitors by untrained staff with accompanying reduction in awareness of their accuracy and use of alternative methods of patient assessment;

- decreased teaching on acute care skills within the pre-registration curriculum;

- increased numbers of intensive and high-dependency beds.

TABLE 1.10 (a) Example of track and trigger system: modified early warning score (MEWS) (Stenhouse 2000)

Score	Pulse (bpm)	Respiratory rate (breaths/ min)	Temp. (°C)	CNS level Patient response	GCS	Urine output	Systolic BP
3						Nil	>45% ↓
2	<40	≤8	≤35			<1 ml/kg/2 h	30% ↓
1	40–50					<1 ml/kg/1 h	15% ↓
0	51–100	9–14	35.0–38.4	Alert	15		Normal for patient
1	101–110	15–20		Voice	14	>3 ml/kg/2 h	15% ↑
2	111–129	21–29	≥38.5	Pain	9–13		30% ↑
3	≥130	≥30		Unresponsive	≤8		>45% ↑

TABLE 1.10 (b) Example of track and trigger system: patient emergency response team (PERT) call criteria

Please call the PERT nurse if:	RR >25 or <8 breaths/min
	Oxygen saturation <90% on ≥35% O_2
	Heart rate >125 or <50 bpm
	Systolic BP <90 or >200 mmHg
	Your patient looks unwell or you feel worried about their clinical state
Consider calling the PERT nurse and increase the frequency of monitoring if:	Oliguria (passing <30 ml urine/h)—discuss catheterization if not already catheterized, monitor urine output hourly, inform doctor if <30 ml for >2 h
	Repeated hypoglycaemia in spite of glucose support—monitor blood glucose hourly and post-bolus glucose therapy

In an attempt to reverse this trend outreach services from critical care have begun to deliberately accentuate increased education for ward staff and assistance/support for the care of the patient in the ward rather than early removal to a higher-dependency area. This aims to reduce the level of de-skilling in general nurses which is seen as responsible for some of the poor care delivery for dependent patients on the wards.

Alteration in behaviour is already evident, with increased use of respiratory rate monitoring in the wards, appropriate referral to outreach teams, and associated improved outcome (Odell *et al.* 2002, Priestley *et al.* 2004)

However, nurses do not care for patients on their own and there is also clear evidence that medical staff working in general hospital wards also have limitations which affect the acutely deteriorating patient on the ward (McQuillan *et al.* 1998).

Components of pre-ICU care

In order to reduce the level of acute illness associated with patients admitted from the general ward to critical care, there must be early recognition of deterioration in a patient's condition. Outreach services have attempted to use warning signs of early patient deterioration either in the form of unique indicators of physiological abnormality (e.g. RR >30 breaths/min) or as part of a scoring system (e.g. Patient At Risk Team (PART) score). These markers (known as track and trigger systems) alert the ward nursing and medical staff and require a directed response (Table 1.10).

Responses to the identification of a patient at risk on the general ward vary according to the way the outreach team is set up (Outreach Forum Report 2003). Many systems require a response within strictly defined time limits by the patient's own nursing and medical team. However, more commonly a designated person or team will respond to the call, providing immediate access to expert critical care assistance.

Probably the gold standard for this is the 24 h/day 7 day/week team which will provide round-the-clock support for critically ill patients on the ward. Only a third of outreach services in the UK provide this level of care (Outreach Forum Report 2003). However, it will be useful for the development of future services to compare the impact of different types of service set up in establishing how important it is to have 24-h cover.

Auditing the impact of pre-critical care intervention

All outreach services should incorporate data collection as part of their role. This allows evaluation of the impact of the service and provides a rich source of data to feed back to hospital staff and to improve services. In order to establish a global view of the effect of outreach, the following indicators should be considered:

1. Outreach team performance:

  ◆ Number of cardiac arrest calls (pre- and post-introduction of outreach) per 1000 hospital admissions.

  ◆ Number of critical care readmissions from the ward.

  ◆ The percentage of outreach calls requiring critical care admission.

  ◆ The length of stay, morbidity, and mortality associated with critical care admissions from general wards via outreach.

  ◆ The level of acute illness (using APACHE, and/or SAPS) in admissions to critical care via outreach.

  ◆ The number of facilitated appropriate 'Do not attempt resuscitation' orders.

  ◆ The number of averted critical care admissions and the impact on patient mortality and morbidity.

  ◆ Timing of critical care referral in relation to patient need and morbidity.

  ◆ The reduction in overall hospital mortality.

2. Ward staff performance:

  ◆ The number of cardiac arrest calls per ward with unremarked physiological deterioration in the hours prior to arrest.

  ◆ The number of inappropriate arrest calls to patient in terminal stages of illness.

  ◆ Incidence and frequency of observations recorded appropriately, e.g. respiratory rate.

  ◆ Assessed performance of specific skills such as suctioning of tracheostomies.

  ◆ Attendance at outreach calls for patients by the patient's own team (collaborative working).

Components of care post-critical care

Relocation or transfer from the critical care environment can be stressful for any patient. Relocation stress is defined as 'a state in which an individual experiences physiological and/or psychosocial disturbances as a result of transfer from one environment to another' (Carpenito 1997). Components likely to influence the patient's perception of the transfer have been identified from the literature by McKinney (2002) and are detailed in Fig. 1.5.

Conflicting evidence exists about how significant the impact of the transfer is to patients. Compton (1991) and Odell (2000) found that patients seemed to view the transfer from critical care in fairly neutral terms, with anxiety about the reduction in levels of care being tempered by the positive aspect of being well enough to move. However, Hall-Smith et al. (1997) found that some patients described the experience as 'highly traumatic'.

Suggested interventions which may improve the transfer experience and reduce relocation stress include:

◆ Pre-transfer preparation and teaching (Cutler and Garner 1995).

◆ Use of written information as a leaflet for both patients and families (McKinney 2002).

◆ Accentuation of the positive nature of transfer by critical care staff (McKinney 2002).

◆ Communication between ward staff and critical care staff with perhaps a visit from a member of the ward staff (Hall-Smith et al. 1997).

◆ Discharge planning and assessment.

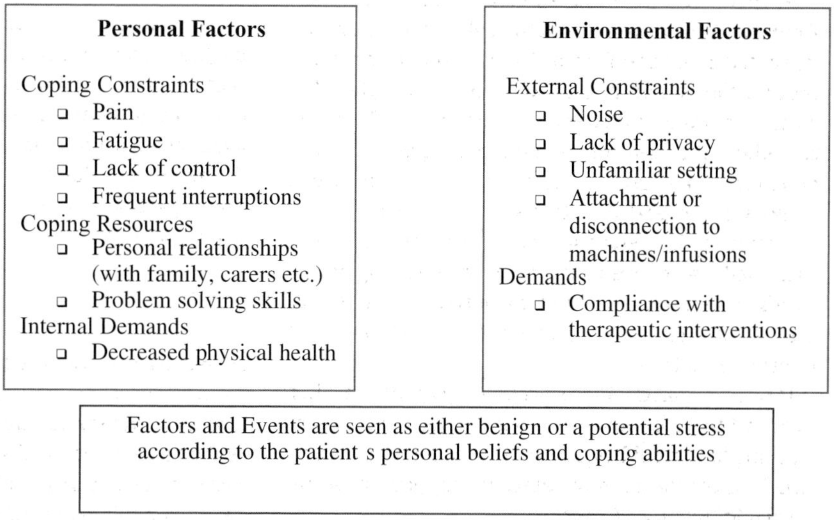

Personal Factors	**Environmental Factors**

Coping Constraints
  ❑ Pain
  ❑ Fatigue
  ❑ Lack of control
  ❑ Frequent interruptions
Coping Resources
  ❑ Personal relationships
     (with family, carers etc.)
  ❑ Problem solving skills
Internal Demands
  ❑ Decreased physical health
	External Constraints
	  ❑ Noise
	  ❑ Lack of privacy
	  ❑ Unfamiliar setting
	  ❑ Attachment or
	     disconnection to
	     machines/infusions
	Demands
	  ❑ Compliance with
	     therapeutic interventions

Factors and Events are seen as either benign or a potential stress according to the patient s personal beliefs and coping abilities

Fig. 1.5 Components likely to influence the patient's perception of transfer to the ward. (Adapted from McKinney (2002).)

Development of a post-critical care follow-up service will allow these issues to be addressed and progressed, ensuring that the physical and psychological recovery of the patient is not impeded.

Progressing the patient's recovery in the ward

The recovering critical care patient will face a large number of physical and psychological problems. These will include:

1. Muscle weakness and fatigue. Patients may lose up to 2% of their muscle mass per day during their illness due to the catabolic nature of the illness response. This may take up to a year to rebuild and patients will have severely limited muscle power for the first few months (Jones and Griffiths 2000). Ward staff are commonly unaware of this and may inappropriately label patients as lazy or unwilling to be independent unless this is explained.

2. The after effects of intubation/tracheostomy. Other common physical problems are associated with artificial airways such as endotracheal and tracheostomy tubes. Suspected tracheal stenosis related to long-term or repeated intubation and skin tethering related to percutaneous tracheostomies should be referred to ENT surgeons for early diagnosis and treatment.

3. Swallowing difficulties and taste alterations. Patients may experience swallowing difficulties or altered sensation when swallowing. The involvement of speech and language therapists at this point will make a difference to the patient's safe recovery and early recognition of a long-term problem such as tracheal stenosis. Taste alteration may also be common and can contribute to poor appetite.

4. Breathlessness on mild exertion. Poor respiratory reserve can be associated with residual fibrosis from pulmonary infection or from cardiovascular limitations

5. Altered sleeping patterns. Patients can have difficulty returning to their normal sleeping pattern and will often need naps during the day.

6. Poor memory and lack of concentration. The ability to remember recent events may be affected by benzodiazepine or other sedative administration during critical care but may also be related to the severity of illness. The ability to concentrate is similar and may take many months to recover. This can be very debilitating for patients, particularly if they have no memory of the severity of their illness (Griffiths *et al.* 1996). One proposed method of assisting with this has been the development of patient diaries (Bäckman and Walter 2001) which are used to record events (including photographs) on behalf of the patient either by staff or family.

DELUSIONAL MEMORY AND POST-TRAUMATIC STRESS DISORDER

Delusional memory—definitions

♦ A dream, nightmare, or hallucination experienced by the patient during their stay in critical care.

♦ A belief or memory of critical care that has been rejected as false by the patient.

♦ A belief or memory of events in critical care that is not shared by medical/nursing staff or family members present during the patient's stay.

Post-traumatic stress disorder—definition

Post-traumatic stress disorder (PTSD) is the development of characteristic symptoms after one or more traumatic events. Events that trigger PTSD involve experiencing a serious threat to one's own physical integrity, which is experienced with intense fear, horror, and helplessness. Diagnostic criteria for PTSD include a history of exposure to one or more traumatic events and symptoms from each of three symptom clusters: intrusive recollections, avoidant/numbing symptoms, and hyper arousal symptoms (Schelling *et al.* 1998).

7. Nightmares, hallucinations, delusional memories. Between 33% (Russell 1999) and 60% (Friedman *et al.* 1992) of patients will have no memory of critical care after 2 months. However, up to 73% may have some kind of delusional memory at 2 weeks (Jones *et al.* 2001), and where delusional memory is combined with no memory of factual events in the critical care environment there is a significant likelihood ($p = 0.02$) of development of post-traumatic stress disorder (Jones *et al.* 2001).

Instituting a rehabilitation programme of exercise, information, and contact, significantly improved SF-36 graded physical function scores ($p = 0.006$) in a randomized controlled trial of 150 patients after a period of critical care (Jones *et al.* 2003). The exercise programme formed part of a workbook given to the patients after discharge from critical care. However, giving the patients a discharge booklet alone did not affect the incidence of anxiety and depression (Jones and O'Donnell 1994). It would appear to be important for the patients to have ongoing follow-up with the opportunity to discuss issues relating to their illness as well as physical rehabilitation.

Components of a critical care follow-up clinic

It is clear that many patients who suffer a critical illness have severe ongoing physical and psychological

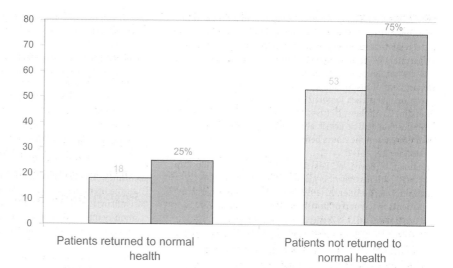

Fig. 1.6 Percentage of patients attending a critical care follow-up clinic who have returned to normal health by 3 months (figures from UCLH Trust critical care follow-up clinic).'

problems related directly to that illness and the time spent in the critical care environment. The roots of these problems sit firmly with critical care and should therefore be addressed by the same service; this not only allows the patient to have access to staff familiar with the environment and the patient's own experience but also allows the staff have access to understanding of the patient's ongoing issues and problems. The opportunity to research and learn about these issues can then be used to improve the way in which care is delivered and lessen the adverse effects associated with critical illness.

In general, it is unlikely that patients who are admitted for overnight stays post-operatively will need to attend a follow-up clinic, and most clinics will operate a cut-off system according to the length of time the patient has spent in critical care (commonly patients are included if they spend 2 days or more in a critical care environment). Although there is no evidence of a direct relationship between length of stay and incidence of problems, it would seem likely that the longer the stay, the greater the impact on the patient and their family.

Follow-up clinics should have a multidisciplinary approach—where possible a nurse, psychologist, physiotherapist and dietitian as well as a doctor should be involved.

Many patients will not have returned to full health until at least 6 months after their discharge from hospital (see Fig. 1.6).

Feedback to critical care staff

One of the most important aspects of the clinic role is to ensure that all staff are made aware of patients' experiences in the critical care environment. This can be both rewarding and educating for staff as they learn of patients' progress and return to health as well as developing an understanding of the way their actions are perceived or remembered by their patients.

References and bibliography

Audit Commision (1999). Critical to Success. Audit Commission (UK).

Bäckman, C., Walther, S. (2001) Use of a personal diary written on the ICU during critical illness. *Intensive Care Medicine* **27**, 426–9.

Bellomo, R., Goldsmith, D., Uchmo, S. *et al.* (2003). A prospective before-and-after trial of a medical emergency team. Medical Journal of Australia **179**, 283–7.

Bernard, G.R., Vincent, J.-L., Laterre, P.-F., *et al.* (2001). Efficacy and safety of recombinant human activated protein C for severe sepsis. *New England Journal of Medicine* **344**, 699–709.

Bristow, P.J., Hillman, K., Chey, T. *et al.* (2000). Rates of in-hospital arrests, deaths and intensive care admissions the effect of a medical emergency team. *Medical Journal of Australia* **173**, 236–40.

Buist, M.D., Moore, C.E., Bernard, S.A., *et al.* (2002). Effects of a medical emergency team on reduction of incidence of and mortality from unexpected cardiac arrests in hospital preliminary study. *British Medical Journal* **324**, 387–90.

Carpenito, L.J. (1997). *Handbook of Nursing Diagnosis*, p. 297. Lippincott, Philadelphia, PA.

Chen, L.M., Martin, C.M., Keenan, S.P. (1998). Patients readmitted to the intensive care unit during the same hospitalization. Clinical features and outcomes *Critical Care Medicine* **26**, 1834–41.

Cioffi, J., Markham, R. (1997). Clinical decision making: managing case complexity. *Journal of Advanced Nursing* **25**, 265–72.

Cioffi, J. (2000) Recognition of patients who require emergency assistance: A descriptive study, *Heart & Lung* **29**, 262–8.

Compton, P. (1991). Critical illness and Intensive care. What it means to the client . *Critical Care Nurse* **11**, 50–6.

Cutler, L., Garner, M. (1995). Reducing relocation stress after discharge from the intensive therapy unit. *Intensive and Critical Care Nursing* **11**, 333–5.

Daly, K., Beale, R. Chang, R. (2001). Reduction in mortality after inappropriate early discharge from intensive care unit logistic regression triage model. *British Miedical Journal* **322**, 1274–6.

Department of Health (2000). *Comprehensive Critical Care. A review of Critical Care Services*. Department of Health, London.

Department of Health and Modernisation Agency (2003). The National Outreach Report 2003. Department of Health (UK).

Franklin, C., Mathew, J. (1994). Developing strategies to prevent in-hospital cardiac arrest: analysing responses of physicians and nurses in the hours before the event. *Critical Care Medicine* **22**, 244–7.

Friedman, B., Boyee, W., Bekes, C. (1992) Long-term follow up of ICU patients. *American Journal of Critical Care* **1**, 115–17.

Goldhill, D.R., Sumner, A. (1998). Outcome of intensive care patients in a group of British intensive care units. *Critical Care Medicine* **26**, 1337–45.

Griffiths, R.D., Jones, C., Macmillan, R. (1996). Where is the harm in not knowing? Care after Intensive Care. *Clinical Intensive Care* **7**, 144–5.

Griffiths, R.D., Jones, C. (2002). Practical aspects after intensive care. In: *Outcomes in Critical Care* (ed. Ridley, S.), pp. 169–80. Butterworth-Heinemann, Oxford.

Gwinnutt, C.L., Columb, M., Harris, R (2000). Outcome after cardiac arrest in adults in UK hospitals: effect of the 1997 guidelines. *Resuscitation* **47**, 125–35.

Hall-Smith, J., Ball, C., Coakley, J. (1997). Follow-up services and the development of a clinical nurse specialist in intensive care. *Intensive and Critical Care Nursing* **13**(5), 243–8.

Herlitz, J., Bång, A., Gunnarsson, J., *et al.* (2003). Factors associated with survival to hospital discharge among patients hospitalised alive after out of hospital cardiac arrest: change in outcome over 20 years in the community of Goteborg, Sweden. *Heart* **89**, 25–30.

Hillman, K.M., Bristow, P.J., Chey, T. *et al.* (2001) Antecedents to hospital deaths. *Internal Medicine Journal* **31**, 343–8.

Hodgetts, T.J., Kenward, G., Vlachonikolis, I.G., *et al.* (2002). The identification of risk factors for cardiac arrest and formulation of activation criteria to alert a medical emergency team. *Resuscitation* **54**, 125–31.

ICS standards committee (2003). Evolution of Intensive Care in the UK Intensive Care Society, London, pp. 3–4.

Intensive Care Society (2002). Levels of critical care for adult patients. *Intensive Care Society*, London.

Jones, C., Griffiths, R.D. (2000). Identifying post intensive care patients who may need physical rehabilitation. *Clinical Intensive Care* **11**, 35–8.

Jones, C., Griffiths, R.D., Humphris, G., *et al.* (2001). Memory, delusions, and the development of acute posttraumatic stress disorder-related symptoms after intensive care. *Critical Care Medicine* **29**, 573–80.

Jones, C., O'Donnell, C. (1994). After Intensive Care, what then? *Intensive and Critical Care Nurse* **10**, 89–92.

Jones, C., Skirrow, P., Griffiths, R., *et al.* (2003). Rehabilitation after critical illness: A randomised controlled trial. *Critical Care Medicine* **31**, 2456–61.

Keenan, S.P., Dodek, A., Chan, K., *et al.* (2002). Intensive care unit admission has minimal impact on long-term mortality. *Critical Care Medicine* **30**, 501–7.

Lee, A., Bishop, G., Hillman, K., *et al.* (1995). The medical emergency team. *Anaesthesia and Intensive Care* **23**, 183–6.

Lee, K., Angus, D., Abramson, N. (1996). Cardiopulmonary resuscitation: what cost to cheat death? *Critical Care Medicine* **24**, 2046–52.

Lundberg, J.S., Perl, T.M., Wiblin, T., *et al.* (1998). Septic shock: An analysis of outcomes for patients with onset of hospital wards versus intensive care units. *Critical Care Medicine* **26**, 1020–4.

Lyseng-Williamson, K.A., Perry, C.M. (2002). Drotrecogin alfa (activated). *Drugs* **62**, 617–30.

McGlom, H., Adam, S., Singer, M. (1999). Unexpected deaths and referred to intensive care of patients on general wares. Are some cases potentially avoidable? *Journal of the Royal College of Physicians* **33**, 255–9.

McKinney, A. (2002). Relocation stress in critical care: a review of the literature. *Journal of Clinical Nursing* **11**, 149–57.

McQuillan, P., Pilkington, S., Allan, A., *et al.* (1998). Confidential inquiry into quality of care before admission to intensive care. *British Medical Journal* **316**, 1853–7.

Moreno, R., Agthé, D. (1999). ICU discharge decision-making: are we able to decrease post-ICU mortality? *Intensive Care Medicine* **25**, 1035–6.

Odell, M. (2000). The patient's thoughts and feelings about their transfer from intensive care to the general ward. *Journal of Advanced Nursing* **31**, 322–9.

Odell, M., Forster, A., Rudman, K., *et al.* (2002). The critical care outreach service and the early warning system on surgical wards. *Nursing in Critical Care* **7**, 132–5.

Priestley, G., Watson, W., Rashidian, A., *et al.* (2004). Introducing critical care outreach: a ward-randomised trial of phased introduction in a general hospital. *Intensive Care Medicine* **30**, 1398–404.

Rich, K. (1999). Inhospital cardiac arrest: pre-event variables and nursing response. *Clinical Nurse Specialist* **13**, 147–53.

Rivers, E., Nguyen, B., Havstad, S., *et al.* (2001) Early goal-directed therapy in the treatment of severe sepsis and septic shock. *New England Journal of Medicine* **345**, 1368–77.

Rosenberg, A.L., Hofer, T.P., Hayward, R.A., *et al.* (2001). Who bounces back? Physiologic and other predictors of intensive care unit readmission. *Critical Care Medicine* **29**, 511–18.

Russell, S. (1999). An exploratory study of patients' perceptions, memories and experiences of an intensive care unit. *Journal of Advanced Nursing* **29**, 783–91.

Schein, R.M., Hazday, N., Pena, M., *et al.* (1990). Clinical antecedents to in-hospital cardiopulmonary arrest. *Chest* **98**, 1388–92.

Schelling, G., Stoll, C., Haller, M., *et al.* (1998). Health-related quality of life and posttraumatic stress disorder in survivors of the acute respiratory distress syndrome. *Critical Care Medicine* **26**, 651–9.

Smith, G.B., Poplett, N. (2002). Knowledge of aspects of acute care in trainee doctors. *Postgraduate Medical Journal* **78**, 335–8.

Smith, L., Orts, C.M., O'Neil, I., *et al.* (1999). TISS and mortality after discharge from intensive care. *Intensive Care Medicine* **25**, 1061–5.

Stenhouse, C., Coates, S., Tivey, M., *et al.* (2000). Prospective evaluation of a modified early warning score to aid earlier detection of patients developing critical illness on a surgical ward. *British Journal of Anaesthesia* **84**, 663.

Wilson, J., Woods, I., Fawcett, J. *et al.* (1999) Reducing the risk of major elective surgery, randomised controlled trial of preoperative optimisation of oxygen delivery. *British Medical Journal* **318**, 1099–103.

The critical care environment

Introduction

Recognition of the need for critical care began in the 1950s. The subsequent development and proliferation of these specialized areas of patient care was due to the following factors:

- the general advances in healthcare technology which occurred following the Second World Wars and the Korean War;

- the advent of mechanical ventilation in response to the Copenhagen polio epidemic in 1952;

◆ the development of cardiac surgery with its requirement for intensive post-operative care.

As the speciality itself has progressed from these early beginnings, so too has the requirement for critical care units (CCUs), resulting in a demand that threatens to overwhelm provision.

The labour-intensive nature of the work and the need for specialist training has made the expansion of services both resource-consuming and very expensive. Thus, in the UK there are limited numbers of medical and nursing staff trained in critical care (Parker *et al.* 1998). This has resulted recently in the development of a slightly different approach, known as comprehensive critical care, which looks at responding to patient need in terms of their critical illness rather than their geographical location.

This approach embraces early recognition of patient deterioration in the ward area with supportive response from teams with critical care skills as well as providing continuation of support for patients who are discharged from the CCU. The specific goal is to prevent problems which might result in deterioration and readmission.

The patient therefore has access to appropriately skilled staff for the period of need rather than for the period of admission into critical care (Department of Health 2000). One of the aims of this approach is to reduce inappropriate admissions to CCUs and to facilitate discharge, thus making beds available for those patients who will benefit.

Defining critical care

There are numerous definitions of critical care. Most are brief statements of the types of patients who would be admitted to critical care and do not provide a comprehensive picture of the work that is undertaken or contribute to understanding of the service. However, there are useful common themes in determining the goals of critical care. Critical care exists to:

◆ provide care for severely ill patients with potentially reversible conditions;

◆ provide care for patients who require close observation and/or specialized treatments that cannot be provided in the general ward;

◆ provide care for patients with potential or established organ failure, most commonly the lungs;

◆ reduce avoidable morbidity and mortality in critically ill patients.

In a comprehensive critical care approach, levels of care are used to define the patient's needs regardless of location (see Chapter 1).

There is still a need for a clearly defined critical care (or level 2/3 care) area where the skills of specialist personnel and technology can be successfully combined in the management and care of critically ill patients.

Which patients benefit from critical care?

There are a number of reasons why critical care should only be offered to those patients who are likely to receive real benefit:

◆ Critical care can be physically distressing and potentially hazardous for patients.

◆ Critical care is potentially traumatic for patients in emotional, social and psychological terms and this combined cost should always be weighed against potential benefit.

◆ Critical care is an expensive resource which will clearly have an impact on other branches of healthcare when financial constraints are necessary.

◆ Critical care beds are limited. In 1999, 2.6% of hospital beds in the UK compared with 4.6% in Denmark and 10% in the United States were designated as critical care beds (Edbrooke *et al.* 1999).

Identifying patients who will benefit from critical care

Predicting which patients will benefit from critical care is extremely difficult. Many groups of patients in the past have only been given limited access to critical care but have turned out to have a similar (or occasionally better) outcome than groups with unlimited access. For instance, patients over the age of 60 are often seen as less likely to survive critical care, but one study of outcome showed only a modest increase in 6-month mortality from 44% at 55 yr, to 48% at 65 yr and 60% at 85yr. These results were adjusted for possibly less aggressive care in the older age groups (Hamel *et al.* 1999). Some disease-specific groups have also been shown to benefit, particularly from early aggressive CCU intervention, such as patients with haematological malignancies (Naik *et al.* 2001). Use of computerized prediction methods such as the Riyadh intensive care program (RIP) (Chang 1989) can only help to predict outcome rather than judge which patients should and should not be admitted.

The gradual broadening of groups likely to benefit from critical care has contributed to the increase in demand for these beds. Parker *et al.* (1998) suggest that simply increasing the number of available beds is not the answer and new ways of working must be investigated. Holcomb *et al.* (2001) suggest the use of protocols and managed care is likely to be one way of improving the efficiency of critical care without necessarily increasing bed numbers *per se*.

In different circumstances, some patients who are unlikely to benefit are admitted to critical care either as a consequence of medical/surgical intervention or in an emergency where diagnosis and cause of clinical deterioration is uncertain and refusal to admit to the CCU would be inappropriate. Once the patient is in CCU and treatment has been instigated then moral and ethical dilemmas can cloud the decision-making process in terms of continuing or escalating care. It is therefore appropriate where possible to utilize care conferences with the primary team as well as the critical care staff as a way of evaluating continued CCU care in a situation where survival is unlikely (this is discussed in more detail in Chapter 17).

Admission guidelines

In view of the need for appropriate referral and admission to critical care, many units have guidelines to direct appropriate utilization. A priority system model has been suggested by the American College of Critical Care Medicine (1999). This defines patients who will benefit from CCU admission and those who will not (Table 2.1). The dual purpose of this model is to support decisions on an individual patient need basis and to allow triage where bed availability is limited.

All admission guidelines require an identified clinical lead who has the responsibility of making decisions about admission and discharge of patients. This is usually the consultant responsible for critical care but could also be an experienced senior nurse. In the UK the guidelines for admission to critical care (Department of Health 1996) suggest the following factors should be considered prior to accepting a patient:

♦ Little or no potential to reverse the illness?

♦ Presence of significant co-morbidity?

♦ A stated or written preference against critical care?

If any of these factors are present then critical care should not be offered unless there are exceptional circumstances.

Local policies are usually based on these premises but will also include detail of process and individual

TABLE 2.1 Priorities for admission of patients to critical care

Priority	Description	Example
1	Critically ill, unstable patients in need of intensive treatment and monitoring that cannot be provided outside the CCU. Usually these treatments include ventilator support, continuous vasoactive drug infusions, etc.	Patients with acute respiratory failure. Haemodynamically unstable patients
2	Intensive monitoring is required and immediate intervention may be needed. No therapeutic limits are stipulated	Patients with chronic co-morbid conditions who develop acute severe illness which is potentially reversible
3	Critically ill patients with a reduced likelihood of recovery because of underlying disease or the nature of their acute illness	Patients with metastatic malignancy complicated by infection or airway obstruction
4	Patients who are either too well (i) or too sick (ii) for critical care and therefore generally not appropriate for CCU unless under highly specific circumstances. This may also apply to patients who have made a conscious decision not to undergo critical care	(i) Patients with low-level needs that can be met in the ward area with support, such as mild congestive heart failure, stable/conscious drug overdose. (ii) Patients with terminal, irreversible illness such as unresponsive metastatic cancer, severe, irreversible brain damage, or persistent vegetative state

responsibilities for CCU consultants, the nurse in charge of the unit, and bed managers.

Discharge guidelines

Discharge is considered in the following circumstances, but the final decision will depend on a number of associated factors such as level of care available on the wards, individual patient condition and needs, staffing, and expertise:

♦ The patient is stable and no longer requires active organ support.

♦ The patient is no longer benefiting from the treatment available.

◆ The patient (or family/partner) wish for transfer to palliative care facilities.

◆ A persistent/permanent vegetative state is confirmed.

Details about planning for discharge and supporting/ following up discharge are discussed in Chapter 1. Premature discharge from critical care is associated with increased morbidity (Goldfrad and Rowan 2000) which must be considered when discharge decisions are made. Ensuring communication about details of patient history and needs from CCU staff to ward staff is essential. Different methods of ensuring this include the use of transfer documentation, planned visits by ward staff to the CCU prior to transfer, and named links between CCU and ward nursing staff to facilitate queries. An outreach service will provide a link between the two areas.

The critical care unit as part of the hospital (Fig. 2.1)

The number of acutely ill patients in hospital has increased due to many factors both social and disease-related. This has had a considerable impact on the level of dependency of patients nursed in general wards as well as producing an increased demand for higher levels of care. The continuum of enhanced levels of care now includes such areas as post-anaesthesia care units (24-hour recovery units), high-dependency units, critical care units, step-down units, and progressive care units. None of these areas have been clearly defined

> **FACTORS INCREASING THE NUMBER OF ACUTELY ILL HOSPITAL IN-PATIENTS**
>
> ◆ Increasingly elderly population
>
> ◆ Increased survival in chronic disease
>
> ◆ Increased ability to treat and therefore survival in acute disease
>
> ◆ Increasing co-morbidity
>
> ◆ Hospice/community facilities for dying patients
>
> ◆ Increasing expectations from service users
>
> ◆ Moves to treat less acute interventions in the community or as day surgery

and it is perhaps easiest to use the levels of care distinction (see Chapter 1) rather than this ill-defined group of titles.

Clearly, not all hospitals will require level 3 CCUs and it is likely that level 2 will be the most commonly available level of critical care, with a requirement for all hospitals carrying out major surgery to have a minimum of level 2 facilities.

Geographical location of the critical care unit

Ideally, the CCU should be situated where it is in close proximity to the source of the patients and to the support services that are most frequently required (Hopkinson 1994) (Fig. 2.2).

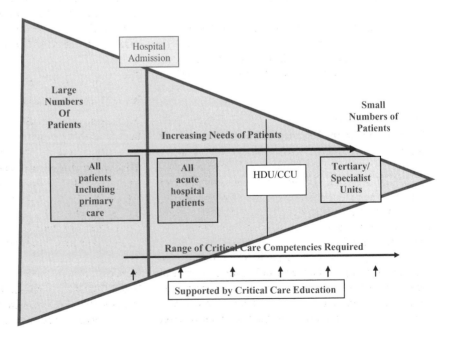

Fig. 2.1 Modelling the patient continuum through hospital and critical care admission.

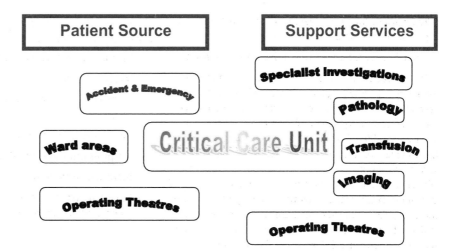

Fig. 2.2 Location of critical care with reference to patient sources and support services.

Any distance between the source of patients or support services and the CCU should be facilitated by the provision of dedicated lifts which are spacious enough to accommodate critically ill patients and the equipment and staff needed to accompany them.

Communications between these areas can be enhanced by direct telephone lines and/or intercom systems. The use of computerized results reporting systems has reduced many of the difficulties of obtaining information from blood tests, but until digital imaging (picture archiving and communication system (PACS)) is available for all hospitals, the difficulties of access to X-ray films in the clinical area without reporting will remain.

Movement of patients from one area of the hospital to another during the acute phase of critical care can be a high-risk procedure and staff and equipment must be appropriate to the task (see Chapter 3 for further details).

The critical care unit

Unfortunately, in the UK, many CCUs have been built either without clinician involvement in the planning stages or as a compromise situation in an inappropriate area of the hospital. This increases the difficulties of working in the CCU environment and may add to risks for the patient, for instance with poor access to bed areas, or insufficient space between beds adding to cross-infection risks.

It is no longer acceptable to build CCUs which do not conform to accepted standards of building for critical care such as the Health Building Note Requirements (HBN 57; Department of Health 2002). This comprehensive document gives clear guidelines as to size,

components, distribution and set -up of CCUs in the UK.

The planning of a unit which may take several years to build requires a good deal of foresight in terms of future equipment and service requirements. For example, the number and design of isolation cubicles may depend on the increase in multiresistant organisms or in changes in the way in which universal infection precautions are handled. Either may influence an increase or decrease in requirements and these kinds of elements are difficult to predict for several years ahead. The availability of new types of equipment may also mean either increased or decreased bed space requirements and the addition of such systems as computerized clinical information systems may require a very different layout for bed areas.

General requirements for the design of a critical care unit

It has been suggested that the optimum working number of CCU beds is eight or multiples thereof, based on the judgement that this is the number that can be successfully managed by one consultant and team (Ferdinande 1997). The average size unit in the UK in the late 1990s was six beds (Audit Commission 1999). It has been suggested that a unit with fewer than four beds, fewer than 200 admissions per year or a bed occupancy of less than 60% is not economical (AAGBI 1988).

Design

Most CCUs have a combination of open plan areas and cubicles, the recommended ratio is one or two cubicles per 10 beds (Ferdinande 1997). However, with the increasing number of resistant organisms and the increase in neutropenic patients, both source and protective isolation needs have grown and it is likely that one or two cubicles per six beds is nearer the requirement.

However, recent research suggests that automatic source isolation for methicillin-resistant *Staphylococcus aureus* (MRSA)—the most prevalent of a number of multiresistant organisms—may be unnecessary, as universal precautions are as effective in limiting its spread (Farr-Barry and Bellingan, 2004)

Size of bed areas in the CCU

Recommendations for the size of CCU bed areas vary. The ESICM guidelines (Ferdinande 1997) suggest a minimum of 20 m² for open plan areas and 25 m² for cubicles, but the Health Building Note from the UK Department of Health (2002) recommends 25 m² for open plan and 30 m² for cubicles. Sufficient room for the critical care team to move rapidly round the patient's bed as well as space for additional technology such as haemofiltration and intra-aortic balloon pumps is vital. In the rehabilitation phase, there must be space for the patient to sit out of bed and for family and friends to visit without feeling they are compromising care or are in the way.

Safety in the CCU

While it is imperative that safety measures are adhered to in all parts of the hospital, there are significant addi-

---

ADVANTAGES OF OPEN PLAN BED AREAS IN THE CCU

- Easier observation of patients
- Faster mobilization of staff and equipment
- More economic to maintain bed areas/more effective use of resources such as staffing
- Improved staff support and motivation
- Patients may find the open areas more stimulating in the rehabilitation phase

---

DISADVANTAGES OF OPEN PLAN BED AREAS IN THE CCU

- Less privacy for patients and relatives
- Increased cross-infection risks
- The environment can be noisier with increased sensory overload

---

REQUIREMENTS FOR SPECIFIC BED AREAS IN THE CCU

- Bed: mattress meeting needs of patients at high risk of developing pressure sores; electrically powered adjustment of patient position, bed height; tilt facility—trendelenberg and reverse trendelenberg; cot sides.
- Patient monitoring facilities allowing continuous measurement of ECG, up to three transduced pressures, core and skin temperatures, arterial oxygen saturation, respiratory rate.
- Ventilator, manual inflation bag with reservoir and oxygen supply, anaesthetic facemask, oropharyngeal airways, intubation equipment (if not on central trolley), humidifier or HME system.
- At least 24 electric sockets per bed, half of these to be designated sockets with uninterrupted power supply (UPS).
- At least three oxygen points, two compressed air points and two vacuum outlets situated 1.5 m above the floor on either a floor-, pendant-, or wall-mounted delivery system.
- Provision for manual charting or computerized information systems.
- Surfaces for preparation of infusions, drugs, and other interventions at an appropriate height.
- Storage space for linen, minimal disposables such as syringes, oral care packs, gauze, dressings, etc.
- Storage space for patient's possessions and hygiene requirements.

---

tional factors which require heightened awareness in the CCU. These are:

- A much greater abundance of electrical equipment, close to fluids and combustible gases.
- The ubiquitous use of oxygen (a highly combustible gas).
- The dependence of the patients on a variety of technology for life support.

These additional risks mean that all equipment should be checked prior to use for function and electrical safety and the following safety precautions followed:

- Any faults should be reported immediately and use of the equipment discontinued until the fault has been checked and repaired.

- All equipment should be regularly maintained.

- Accepted precautions for oxygen use should be vigorously adhered to (i.e. no naked flames, antistatic flooring and footwear, increased atmospheric humidity, care when defibrillating, etc.).

- All staff should be aware of and be regularly updated in health and safety procedures, including the action required in the event of fire.

- Equipment should be available at each bedside in the event of mechanical or power failure, e.g. manual resuscitation bags, back-up oxygen cylinders. Torches and battery-back up equipment should be available in the CCU.

- There should be facility to either turn off gas supplies and/or switch to a back-up system in each CCU.

- In the event of a fire, evacuation equipment should be available at each bedside and fire mattresses *in situ* and all staff should be trained in their use.

Responsibility for the safety of the patients rests equally with the organization and its employees. The organization is responsible for ensuring that procedures, equipment, and training are in place and the employees are responsible for adhering to procedures, carrying out safety checks, and attending training.

Cleanliness and infection control in the CCU

The most important and persistent source of cross-infection is unwashed hands (Reybrouck 1983, Gould 1991) and compared with the risks from poor hand-washing technique, the design of the CCU has less of an effect on the incidence of cross-infection. However, specific features will definitely assist in enhancing the likelihood of handwashing, such as the availability and design of hand-basins.

Hand-basins should be available both inside all single cubicles and just outside in the corridor for protective or source isolation. In open areas there should be no less than one hand-basin per two CCU beds . Each basin should have antiseptic scrub solutions, liquid soap, and alcohol gel. Towel dispensers should be kept supplied with towels as wet hands are even more likely to act as vectors of infection if they become contaminated. Ideally, all taps should be either elbow, foot, or sensor operated.

A storage space designated for all cleaning materials and equipment is essential in close proximity to the CCU. Floors should be swept and mopped at least daily and patient areas and equipment damp-dusted on a daily basis to reduce dust. There should be agreed protocols within the unit for the cleaning of bed areas following patient discharge. There should also be protocols to determine protective and source isolation procedures which every member of staff needs to be aware of.

Staff facilities

Critical care is a demanding working area and a rest room for staff which has facilities for making refreshments and snacks is essential. The consistently warm, air-conditioned environment can be very dehydrating and staff (as well as some patients) will need access to cooled water throughout their shifts. Staff facilities must be separate from any patient food preparation area.

Staff also require a changing area with showering facilities to ensure that uniforms are not worn to and from work thus transferring organisms to the home environment. Even with a daily change of uniform, home washing of uniforms is rarely adequate for all organisms and this may allow further cross-exposure for patients who are vulnerable.

Other necessary staff areas are an office for general use with computer and small library facilities, a teaching area and a bedroom for on-call medical staff. The extension of the European working time directive to doctors in training from 2003 and the ruling that 'on-call' time is counted as working hours has meant the introduction of shift systems for many medical staff. This has effectively ended the need for on-call rooms.

Visitors facilities in the CCU

Visitors to the CCU need a general waiting room, preferably slightly apart from the main unit to avoid observation of any potentially disturbing situations. The room should have toilets, telephones, and refreshment facilities and be decorated in a relaxed and informal style. In some cases, relatives require a room in which to stay overnight, and this should be available as near as possible to the unit.

An interview room for discussions with staff or as a quiet area after bad news or bereavement is also useful; this again should be decorated in a soothing and relaxed style.

General décor in the CCU

The decoration of a CCU should promote a relaxed and restful atmosphere for patients, staff, and visitors. It should be painted a colour that does not camouflage spillages and should be easily washable as well as being appropriate to a restful mood such as in cool or neutral colours. (Malkin 1992). Any paintwork, especially on the ceiling, should be of a matt as opposed to gloss finish to avoid reflection.

Wall-mounted clocks that are in easy view of the patient as well as staff should be placed in every bed area so that in the rehabilitation phase patients are able to orientate themselves to time.

All materials should be fire resistant.

Noise

Noise levels can be very high in the CCU, mainly due to the equipment alarms and constant activity. This can contribute significantly to sensory overload for the patient (see Chapter 3). Telephones must be in a position where they can be heard and answered by staff, but this can cause considerable disturbance to patients. Cordless phones are ideal if staff are not in the immediate vicinity of the telephone or to enable patients to speak to callers.

There has been considerable debate over the safety of mobile phones in the CCU area as the signal is thought to cause artefactual alarm conditions in some technology (Clifford *et al.* 1994). However, recent guidelines (MHRA 2004) have specified that only if the phone is very close (probably within 1 m) to medical equipment will the signal actually affect it.

One of the major contributors of noise are the equipment alarms and the safest way to reduce this is to ensure that alarm parameters are set appropriately and on the lowest possible safely audible setting. Encouraging prompt response to alarms will also reduce noise levels. The continuous or frequent alarm will become part of the general background noise and may not be responded to when indicating a real emergency. Use of noise-absorbent wall, floor, and ceiling materials can also help reduce the level of noise pollution.

Lighting

It is desirable for CCUs to have windows allowing in natural daylight. If the unit is situated on a lower floor with windows there must be the facility to ensure privacy and provide shade. This can be best achieved using blinds layered between glass or solar tinted glass, as blinds and curtains external to the glass can be a source of cross-infection unless removed and washed between each patient.

Good quality general lighting (recommended illumination 150 foot-candles) with either dimmer control or night lighting (recommended illumination 20–100 foot-candles) must be provided in all areas (Ferdinande 1997). Additional examination lights and theatre lights may be required for procedures.

Back-up emergency lighting in the event of mains power failure is essential.

Storage, utility, and technical areas

Many CCUs have inadequate storage space for the large volumes of equipment, disposables, fluids, and drugs which must be immediately available in the area. Top-up services restocking CCU two to three times per day are one way round the need to store large quantities of high-use, bulky items but this is labour-intensive and can be costly.

As the need for more readily available diagnostic/interventional equipment increases (e.g. trans-oesophageal echocardiography, bronchoscopy, ultrasound) more and more equipment is becoming situated in the CCU itself and this may take up a major amount of the available storage space.

Utility areas should be separated into clean (treatment, preparation and storage of drugs, IV and haemofiltration fluids, and equipment for procedures) and dirty (disposal of soiled linen and clinical waste, and sluice facilities). If possible, disposal of soiled linen and clinical waste from dirty utility areas should not pass through the unit.

Designated space is required for technical support, cleaning, repair, and maintenance of equipment within the CCU. Ideally, this should be situated close to the equipment storage areas.

Testing facilities near the patient should be available for arterial blood gases, electrolytes, and glucose. The need for other tests such as coagulation screens, lactate, troponin, and cardiac enzymes will depend on the nature of the patients in the individual CCU.

Emergency equipment

Defibrillator, drugs, and resuscitation equipment should be available in a central location in every CCU. They should be mobile and easily accessible. Intubation equipment may be kept either in a central location or at the bedside.

CCUs with cardiothoracic surgical patients should have equipment available for emergency thoracotomy (see Chapter 8) including diathermy and extra suction as well as a thoracotomy pack, internal defibrillation paddles, and drains (see Table 2.2).

Use of computerized clinical information management systems (CIMS)

The volume of data collected and interpreted by nurses in critical care has grown over the last 10 yrs and the level of monitoring now available for all aspects of

TABLE 2.2	Equipment requirements for a level 3 CCU
Monitoring and documentation	Cardiac monitors including 2–3 waveform, ECG, SpO$_2$, and respiratory rate, displays, and 12-lead ECG capability
	Cardiac output capability—either pulmonary artery catheter, Doppler, or pulse contour analysis
	Co-oximeter blood gas analyser with capability for electrolytes, lactate, and blood glucose
	End tidal CO$_2$ analyser
	BIS monitor
	Computerized clinical information system
Respiratory support	Patient-responsive third-generation ventilators
	CPAP and NIV machines
	Fibre-optic bronchoscope
Renal support	Haemofiltration machines
Radiology	Portable X-ray machine
	Digital X-Ray system or viewer
Cardiovascular support	Multiple infusion pumps
	Defibrillator and external pacing device
	Pacing boxes and flotation pacing catheters
Nutritional support	Enteral nutrition pumps
	Access to kitchen for snacks/oral diet
Miscellaneous	Range of electronic beds according to patient's pressure risk, equipped with bedside rails, and dripstands
	Warming/cooling mattresses
	Fans or air conditioning
	Blood warmers
	Blood fridge
	Hoists and support chairs
	Commodes/urinals and bedpans
	Dressing trolleys
	Storage for drugs, equipment, cleaning facilities, linen

BIS – bispectral index scale; NIV – non-invasive ventilation.

patient function has increased. The development of computerized systems to manage this level of information has become increasingly accepted as a logical method of releasing nursing time to allow increased patient care.

These systems are designed to collect information from any electronic equipment capable of exporting data in a digital format and then transposing the data into either graphical or numerical displays. These displays can be customized to suit the individual unit and then form an electronic patient record which includes demographic, physiological, biochemical, physical, and interventional information.

ADVANTAGES OF CIMS

- Direct collection of information from monitoring systems.
- Immediate access to CCU policies and protocols through an intranet.
- Development of prompts or reminders for care needs, e.g. 2 hourly mouth care.
- Sharing of information across the professions—use of a multiprofessional record.
- Reduction of repetitious note-recording. For example, diagnosis recorded in the physician assessment is automatically transferred to other records such as daily problem lists, physiotherapy assessments, etc.
- Immediate access to other electronic databases such as the hospital formulary and drug information.
- Direct transfer of laboratory results into current patient records via computerized results services.
- Audit and benchmarking of stored data is easier to access.

DISADVANTAGES OF CIMS

- Major amounts of training of both permanent and temporary staff is required.
- Confidentiality of patient records must be protected by a password system involving logging in and out of patient records. This must be managed by senior staff.
- Direct data collected must still be validated by staff otherwise erroneous readings will be collected as true. For example, if the arterial line transducer is on the floor the systolic reading will be much higher than in reality.
- Equipment must have the capacity to feed directly into the CIMS, e.g. ventilators and infusion pumps as well as monitors.
- Staff must be confident in the system and its reliability.

However, the use of a CIMS has many more potential advantages than simply releasing the nurse from charting observations. It is also possible for the system to provide failsafe mechanisms in terms of prompts and reminders as well as flagging up errors or triggering drug delivery.

Setting up a CIMS requires a huge investment of time and resource; however, some of the benefits identified, including rapid retrieval of data for audit, clinical decision support, and improved record-keeping for legal purposes (Harmworth and Still 2002), make it worth the outlay. It remains to be seen whether this will prove worthwhile but it does have tremendous potential.

The staffing of a critical care unit

The number, variety, and skills of the staff required in a CCU will reflect the level and activity of the unit. There are five main groups of staff:

- nursing (largest in number),
- medical,
- allied health professionals,
- administrative and clerical staff,
- cleaning and portering staff.

There are two models of staffing for CCUs in general. For many CCUs, the nurses, critical care consultants, and administrative staff will be the only group permanently attached to the CCU. Members of the various allied health professional groups will respond to referrals or provide a rotating cover service but will not be purely associated with the CCU itself. However, in larger units there will be designated members of the allied health professional groups who will also be permanently attached to the CCU. This has many advantages in terms of collaborative working and sharing of skills and competencies.

ALLIED HEALTH PROFESSIONALS

- Physiotherapists
- Pharmacists
- Radiographers
- Dietitians
- Speech and language therapists
- Medical physics technicians
- Occupational therapists
- Social workers

Nursing staff

There has been considerable debate over the numbers of nurses required to staff CCUs, and in particular over the ratio of nurses to critical care patients. While a full debate is not possible in this text, there are a number of issues which are worth considering:

1. The number of acutely ill patients in hospital is growing as methods of treatment change and the emphasis on primary healthcare increases. The number of patients surviving into old age, with an increasing likelihood of co-morbidity, and the number of chronically ill patients surviving past middle age have all dramatically increased the workload associated with in-hospital nursing care. This means that patients in general wards are sicker and require more care, as well as being more likely to require critical care.

2. The number of nurses available to deliver that care decreased during the 1990s as the effects of significant cuts in training places (28% of places were cut between 1992 and 1994; Department of Health 1999) were felt.

3. The average age of nurses is now 30, and more than 25% of the nursing population will reach retirement age in the next 10 years (UKCC 2002)

The implication of these issues is that there will be insufficient nurses available to maintain the current level of staffing in CCU, and the gold standard of one CCU nurse caring for one CCU patient may no longer be possible. However, with a flexible approach to working with patients at different levels of need it may be possible to continue to provide the highest quality of care within these limitations.

Nursing roles in the CCU

The vast majority of nurses in the CCU will be competent, critical care trained nurses, delivering direct care at the bedside to the patient and their family.

However, there is a need for a shift leader or coordinator (the nurse in charge), and frequently in larger units another nurse to act as general support to junior or newly appointed nurses, provide meal breaks without compromising patient safety, and facilitate other organizational issues. The nurse in charge is responsible for the care of the patients during his/her shift.

The continuing need for training in critical care skills means that a proportion of nurses will be novices or advanced beginners learning these skills while providing direct care as part of a structured critical care training course. They require supervision by the nurse in charge or other designated trained critical care nurse.

TABLE 2.3 Comparison of CCU manager, nurse consultant and clinical nurse specialist roles

CCU manager	Nurse consultant	Clinical nurse specialist
Responsibility for delivery of the service	Responsibility for leadership and development of the nursing service	Responsibility for delivery of high-quality nursing care
Responsibility for the budget	Responsibility for overall direction of and participation in teaching and education	Responsibility for delivery of teaching and education
Responsibility for recruitment and retention process	Responsibility for strategies for recruitment and retention	Responsibility for delivery of strategies for recruitment and retention
Delivery of appraisal and IPR process	Ensures appraisal and IPR occurs appropriately	Participates in appraisal and IPR
Deals with complaints and manages risk issues	Ensures benchmarking, audit and standard setting occur	Carries out benchmarking, audit and standard setting
Manages staff	Leads on research	Carries out research, may lead on it
	Develops/trials new methods of delivering the service	
	Acts in a consultative role to the hospital trust on critical care nursing issues	

IPR – individual performance review

A number of CCUs employ healthcare assistants who are trained to assist registered nurses in the delivery of nursing care. They may also have a stocking and cleaning responsibility.

The overall direction and running of nursing in the CCU will require a nurse manager and a nursing leader. In small units, one person will fulfil the role but in larger units the size of the task will require a manager and a professional/clinical lead as separate roles (Table 2.3).

The nursing establishment comprises a significant proportion of the overall budget of the CCU and therefore must be managed efficiently and cost-effectively. Maintenance of standards of nursing care must be balanced with staffing requirements and the dependency of the patients admitted.

Education of nursing staff in the CCU

A balance is necessary in the nursing establishment between the number of critical care nurses and those who are training in critical care. There are a range of different proposals for this percentage, but units who train students on the post-registration general critical care course will require at least 50% of their staff to have undertaken the course in order to provide an adequate number of supervisors and facilitators for the students. The validation of training in post-registration courses is now under the auspices of higher education providers.

Collaborative working in the CCU

One of the few organizational features clearly shown to have benefit for patient outcome and staff satisfaction in the CCU is the process of collaborative working (Baggs et al. 1992). This is described by Baggs et al. (1997) as 'nurses and physicians cooperatively working together, sharing responsibility for solving problems and making decisions to formulate and carry out plans for patient care'. It depends on a multiprofessional approach to the patient's problems and needs which is coordinated (usually by the medical consultant) on the ward rounds.

This type of working is supported by a multiprofessional patient record which is contributed to by all staff. The separation of medical, nursing, physiotherapy and other health professionals notes leads to duplication, confusion and decreased communication. If the written record cannot be completed as a common document, then there is a strong need for regular handover and meetings to enhance verbal communication between professions. The larger the unit, the more important this becomes.

Medical staff

The number of critically ill patients a single medical team is able to manage is about eight (Department of Health 2000). Each team should be led by a consultant trained in critical care medicine (Department of Health 2000) who will provide overall direction and supervision of care as well as teaching for junior medical staff, management, and leadership. It has been suggested that a full-time intensivist can reduce mortality rates and improve efficiency (Pollock et al. 1988, Pronovost et al. 2002). The Intensive Care Society (ICS) recommends that the CCU be consultant-led at all times (Intensive Care Society 1997). For units consisting of more than eight critical care beds, the number of teams should be increased pro-rata. There should be a member of the medical team resident or immediately available to the patients in the critical care unit 24 hours a day.

The 1997 ICS recommendations are that training in critical care should be at the higher professional training level for those wishing to make a career in critical care medicine. In the UK there are relatively few training programmes for medical staff wishing to specialize in critical care medicine. This has a historical cause, due to the slow acceptance of critical care as a speciality in its own right before the establishment of the Intercollegiate Board on Training for Critical Care Medicine in 1996.

A significant proportion of junior doctors should undertake a 3-month training period in CCU to allow development of basic resuscitation and acute management skills (ICS 1997). The European Society of Intensive Care Medicine (ESICM) has issued guidelines for training programmes in critical care medicine (ESICM 1996). The competencies associated with successful completion of the programme are:

1. Comprehensive theoretical knowledge of the field of critical care.

2. Adequate clinical experience of a wide variety of clinical problems and diseases commonly encountered in the CCU.

3. The ability to apply the most appropriate diagnostic procedures and treatment modalities in critical care patients.

4. Mastery of the medical–technical procedures commonly applied in the CCU.

5. The ability to implement ethical standards.

6. The ability to bear full responsibility for critically ill patients.

The ESICM also offers a remote access training programme (PACT) and a European Diploma of Intensive Care Medicine. Doctors who have trained for at least 2 years in critical care and 4 to 5 years in their basic speciality are eligible to apply.

References and bibliography

AAGBI (Association of Anaesthetists of Great Britain and Ireland) (1988). *Intensive Care Services—Provision for the Future.* AAGBI, London.

American College of Critical Care Medicine, Society of Critical Care Medicine (1999). Guidelines for ICU admission, discharge and triage. *Critical Care Medicine* **27**, 633–8.

Audit Commission (1999). *Critical to Success: The Place of Efficient and Effective Critical Care Services Within the Acute Hospital.* Audit Commission, London.

Angus, D., Kelley, M.A., Schmitz, F.J., *et al.* (2000). Current and projected workforce requirements for care of the critically ill and patients with pulmonary disease: can we meet the requirements of an aging population? *Journal of the American Medical Association* **284**, 2762–70.

Baggs, J.G., Ryan, S.A., Phelps, C.E., *et al.* (1992). The association between interdisciplinary collaboration and patient outcomes in a medical intensive care unit. *Heart and Lung* **21**, 18–24.

Baggs, J.G., Schmitt, M.H., Mushlin, A.I., *et al.* (1997) Nurse-physician collaboration and satisfaction with the decision-making process in three critical care units. *American Journal of Critical Care* **6**, 393–9.

Chang, R.W.S. (1989). Individual outcome prediction models for intensive care units. *Lancet* **ii**, 143–6.

Clifford, K.J., Joyner, K.H., Stroud, D.B., *et al.* (1994). Mobile telephones interfere with medical electrical equipment. *Australasian Physics, Engineering Science and Medicine* **17**, 23–7.

Department of Health (1996). *Guidelines on Admission to and Discharge from Intensive Care and High Dependency Units.* Department of Health, London.

Department of Health (1999). *Making a Difference.* Department of Health, London.

Department of Health (2000). *Comprehensive Critical Care: A Review of Adult Critical Care Services,* p. 10. Department of Health, London.

Department of Health (2002). *Intensive Care Units,* Health Building Note (HBN) 57. Department of Health, London.

Edbrooke, D., Hibbert, C., Corcoran, M. (1999). *An International Perspective: Review for the NHS Executive of Adult Critical Care Services.* Medical Economics and Research Centre (MERCS), Sheffield/DOH, London.

ESICM (European Society of Intensive Care Medicine) (1996). Guidelines for a training programme in intensive care medicine. *Intensive Care Medicine* **22**, 166–72.

Farr-Barry, M., Bellingan, G. (2004). Pro/con clinical debate: isolation precautions for all intensive care unit patients with methicillin-resistant *Staphylococcus aureus* colonization are essential. *Critical Care* **8**, 153–6.

Ferdinande, P. and ESICM Task Force (1997). Recommendations on minimal requirements for intensive care departments. *Intensive Care Medicine* **23**, 226–32.

Goldfrad, C., Rowan, K. (2000). Consequences of discharge from intensive care at night. *Lancet* **355**, 1138–42.

Gould, D. (1991). Nurses' hands as vectors of hospital-acquired infection : a review. *Journal of Advanced Nursing* **16**, 1216–25.

Hamel, M.B., Davis, R.B., Teno, J.M., *et al.* (1999). Older age, aggressiveness of care, and survival for seriously ill, hospitalized adults. *Annals of Internal Medicine* **131**, 721–8.

Harmworth, A., Still, B. (2002). Procurement and implementation of a clinical information system within an intensive care unit. *Care of the Critically Ill* **18**, 11–13.

Holcomb, B.W., Wheeler, A.P., Ely, E., *et al.* (2001). New ways to reduce unnecessary variation and improve outcomes in the intensive care unit. *Current Opinion in Critical Care* **7**, 304–11.

Hopkinson, R.B. (1994). How to plan an ICU. *Care of the Critically Ill* **10**, 57–62.

Intensive Care Society (1997). *Standards for Intensive Care Units.* Intensive Care Society. London.

Malkin, J. (1992). *Hospital Interior Architecture*. Van Nostrand Reinhold, New York (available from the Healthcare Design Research Alliance).

MHRA (Medicines and Health Care Regulatory Agency) (2004). *Guidelines For Mobile Communications Systems*. Department of Health, London.

Naik, P., Morris, E., Mackinnon, S., *et al*. (2001). Do critically ill patients with haematological malignancy survive intensive care and beyond? *Proceedings of the ICS Conference, London*, p. 89. Intensive Care Societies, London.

Parker, A., Wyatt, R., Ridley, S. (1998). Intensive care services; a crisis of increased expressed demand. *Anaesthesia* **53**, 113–20.

Pollock, M.M., Katz, R.W., Ruttimann, U.E., *et al*. (1988). Improving the outcome and efficiency of intensive care: the impact of an intensivist. *Critical Care Medicine* **16**, 11–17.

Pronovost, P., Angus, D., Dorman, T., *et al*. (2002). Physician staffing patterns and clinical outcomes in critically ill patients: a systematic review. *Journal of the American Medical Association* **288**, 2151–62.

Reybrouck, G. (1983). Role of the hands in the spread of nosocomial infections. *Journal of Hospital Infection* **4**, 103–10.

UKCC (United Kingdom Central Council for Nursing and Midwifery) [now the Nursing and Midwifery Council] (2002). *Statistical Report 2001–2*. NMC, London.

CHAPTER 3

The patient within the critical care environment

Introduction

During illness, a patient's emotional condition is inextricably linked with their physical condition, a concept which dates back to ancient Greece. Whilst any illness produces stress, an illness severe enough to require critical care intensifies not only the physical but also the psychological factors with which the patient and family must cope. Thus, the value of a holistic approach to the critically ill patient cannot be overemphasized. Many of the patient's needs and problems will be forgotten or negated if he or she is simply viewed as a collection of organs with varying levels of dysfunction. The equipment and its numerical representations of the state of organ dysfunction can assume an inappropriate importance if the patient as an individual is disregarded. A considerable part of the skill attached to nursing these patients concerns the ability to relate all of the information available to the patient as a whole and to view any change in their condition in context rather than in isolation.

This chapter will address the priorities of caring for critically ill patients, including their common needs and problems, as well as those of their families. Two particular concepts are important to the understanding of the critically ill patient: homeostasis and stress.

Homeostasis

Homeostasis is a process of self-regulation and maintenance of uniformity (from the Greek *homoios*, similar and *sta*, stand). Homeostatic mechanisms are triggered by any change in the genetically determined normal value of a given physiological variable. The aim of the homeostatic mechanism is always to return the variable to a steady state. This is achieved by negative feedback. Most of the physiological variables of the body are governed by homeostasis and invoke numerous complex mechanisms in order to maintain them within usually very narrow limits. An example is the maintenance of blood pH (the negative logarithm to the base 10 of hydrogen ion concentration, see Chapters 4 and 9) between the limits of 7.35 and 7.45. Any deviation from this will trigger a series of mechanisms including respiratory changes, metabolic changes, and renal changes in order to compensate for the change and return the level to normal.

Many critically ill patients have reached the limits of their body's compensatory mechanisms; interventions are then necessary in order to return the variable to the physiological normal. Unfortunately, these external interventions have no governing negative feedback

mechanisms and can only be controlled by external monitoring of the variable involved. Adjustment of the variable is carried out by the nursing or medical staff who manipulate the supportive therapy.

An example is the infusion of potassium for hypokalaemia. Blood levels must be taken following infusion in order to monitor the response. Further potassium may be given according to the result. Limited as the possible manipulations are, the maintenance of homeostasis is one of the most important aspects of caring for the critically ill patient. This provision of support for failing systems allows time for the patient's organs to respond to treatment or to recover from the initial insult.

Stress

All critically ill patients are stressed to a greater or lesser degree during their time in critical care. There is a limit to the level of stress that each person can tolerate; while many stressors cannot be reduced or eliminated there are some inherent in the critical care environment that can be relieved by appropriate nursing intervention. An example of this is the delivery of sufficient, understandable information to patients so that they can make sense of their surroundings. A patient's physiological response to stress can cause considerable added strain on failing organs. Some nursing interventions may be able to reduce the patient's level of stress and attenuate some of its effects. The stressors identified in Table 3.1 have features which can be managed by nursing interventions.

Theories of stress, such as Selye's general adaptation syndrome and the transactional model of stress, allow nurses to understand the patient's response to coping with the critical care environment:

1. Selye's general adaptation syndrome states that there are three phases to the response to stressors:
   (a) Alarm reaction—a transient phase which cannot be sustained.
   (b) Resistance or adaptation—this produces either a successful adaptation to the stressor or entry to phase (c).
   (c) Exhaustion and death. Controlled stress or a degree of stimulation is essential to life and growth but excessive or maladapted levels of stress are harmful.

2. Transactional model of stress. This model is based on the individual's perceptions of the 'stressful situation' and their perceived capabilities of coping with it. Stress is only considered to be present when there is a mismatch between the perceived demand and

TABLE 3.1 Stressors reported by mechanically ventilated patients. Adapted from Thomas (2003)

Stressor groupings	No of studies reporting stressor
Dyspnoea/air hunger	14
Tension/anxiety/stress	10
Fear	9
Pain/discomfort	8
Agony/panic/frustration	6
Fatigue	5
Inability to talk	5
Confusion/bewilderment/ altered level of consciousness	4
Anger/hostility	3
Depression	3
Insecurity/uncertainty	3
Mastery alterations	3
Sleeplessness	3
Hope alterations	2
Negative mood	1
Secretions	1
Self-efficacy alterations	1
Suctioning	1

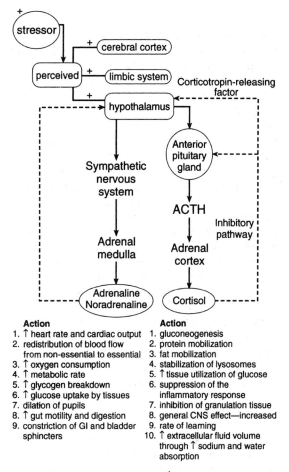

Action
1. ↑ heart rate and cardiac output
2. redistribution of blood flow from non-essential to essential
3. ↑ oxygen consumption
4. ↑ metabolic rate
5. ↑ glycogen breakdown
6. ↑ glucose uptake by tissues
7. dilation of pupils
8. ↑ gut motility and digestion
9. constriction of GI and bladder sphincters

Action
1. gluconeogenesis
2. protein mobilization
3. fat mobilization
4. stabilization of lysosomes
5. ↑ tissue utilization of glucose
6. suppression of the inflammatory response
7. inhibition of granulation tissue
8. general CNS effect—increased rate of learning
9. ↑ extracellular fluid volume through ↑ sodium and water absorption

Fig. 3.1 Stress, the hormonal response (↑ = increase).

the perceived ability to cope. The individual evaluates a situation based on their beliefs, experience and ability to respond (Lazarus, cited in Hibbert 2000). In this model, external factors (such as noise levels, bright light, etc.) and individual factors (such as fatigue and anxiety) are all components in the patient's ability to cope with the stressor.

Physical responses to stress

The limbic system (a rim of cortical tissue surrounding the hilum of the cerebral cortex and other associated deep structures) is involved in the relay of emotional states to the endocrine system. It has connections with the cerebral cortex for transmission of social and emotional influences, and connections with the hypothalamus for control of endocrine activity. Thus, hypothalamic activation of sympathetic nervous activity and adrenaline secretion is stimulated via the limbic system (Fig. 3.1).

Although the effects of the stress response are appropriate and useful in the short-term response to injury, in the long term the same effects are likely to be detrimental to recovery. The continued breakdown of protein stores will lead to muscle wasting and fatigue, the suppression of the inflammatory response will lead to

superinfection, the inhibition of tissue granulation will prevent healing and the increased extracellular fluid volume will produce oedema and altered fluid balance. A major nursing goal must be to reduce or eliminate extraneous stressors to allow the body to respond appropriately to injury but to prevent further complications associated with the stressed state.

Anxiety and fear

One of the most frequent non-physical stressors usually experienced by patients in the critical care environment is anxiety. In a recent study of 96 patients admitted to three critical care units, Rincon et al. (2001) used the Hospital Anxiety and Depression Scale (HADS) to determine the incidence of anxiety, depression, and delirium. They found that 24% of patients showed evidence of anxiety, 14% of depression, and 7.3% of delirium. Only half of these were identified and treated by the critical care staff.

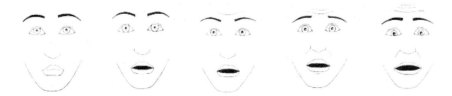

Fig. 3.2 The Faces Anxiety Scale. Reproduced from McKinley *et al.* (2003).

Anxiety is a state of disequilibrium or tension caused by apprehension of possible misfortune that prompts attempts at coping. To a greater or lesser degree it is an almost universal feature of patients admitted to the critical care environment. Most patients will respond using personal coping mechanisms if they are able to help themselves, or using the help and support of all members of the caring team and family if they are not.

Fear is a state of distress and apprehension causing sympathetic arousal. Anxiety or fear can occur as a result of any stress threatening personal security and self-determination.

Assessment of the level of anxiety a patient is feeling is very difficult, depending almost entirely on sub-jective clinical judgement. McKinley *et al.* (2003) have developed the Faces Anxiety Scale (Fig. 3.2) which achieves a 90% response rate for assessing a patient's anxiety in the critical care environment.

The response to fear and anxiety

The physiological response is that of sympathetic arousal, that is, increased circulating catecholamines, increased heart rate, blood pressure, and respiratory rate, dilated pupils, dry mouth (decreased saliva production), and peripheral and splanchnic vasoconstriction. The behavioural response depends on individual's background, culture, and social conditioning. All behaviours are aimed at coping with the stressor. Many of the stressors associated with being critically ill (fear of pain and death, isolation, loss of family support, physical discomfort) cannot be completely eliminated and patients frequently require help with coping. The following strategies can be used (see Table 3.2):

- ◆ Support and augment the patient's coping mechanisms.

- ◆ Communicate caring and understanding to the patient through attentiveness, tone of voice, touch, etc.

- ◆ Provide information repeatedly and in sufficient detail for the patient to understand and make sense of what is going on.

- ◆ Encourage and support relatives in reassuring patients and reiterating information. Allow the relatives as much time with the patient as is possible.

TABLE 3.2 Assisting coping mechanisms for anxiety. Adapted from Frazier *et al.* (2003)

Patients own mechanisms	Denial
	Rationalization
	Substitution of positive thoughts for negative
	Retention of control (often via the nurse) of aspects of care and the environment (e.g. position, lighting, personal hygiene)
Nursing interventions to reduce anxiety	Unrestricted family visiting
	Biofeedback
	Empathetic touch
	Encouragement to verbalize fears
	Ensure pain relief is adequate
	Increase the patient's sense of control of aspects of care/environment, e.g. lighting, temperature, timing of wash, meals, etc.
	Arrange for spiritual counselling
	Teach relaxation techniques
	Ameliorate environmental stressors
	Remain with the patient
	Offer meditation techniques
	Positive feedback for coping techniques
	Give appropriately worded and timed information
	Play music
	Therapeutic touch
	Speak calmly and slowly
	Administration of anxiolytic

- ◆ Consider the use of music therapy with slow flowing rhythms (Chlan 1998).

Sensory imbalance and disorientation

Sensory imbalance or disorientation occurs when the level of sensory stimuli received by the individual is either too great or too minimal to be meaningful or recognizable. A number of predisposing factors, including many of the drugs used, are associated with the critically ill patient (Gelling 1998).

There are five main types of sensory alteration according to Clifford (1985). All can apply to patients in critical care:

1. reduction of the amount and variety of stimuli;

2. monotony of indistinct, meaningless stimuli;

3. isolation, either physical or social;

4. confinement, immobilization, or restriction of movement;

5. increased sensory input.

Types 1 to 4 will cause sensory deprivation and type 5 will cause sensory overload. The causes of sensory alteration of types 1 to 4 are:

* loss of caring touch (although there may be an overload of procedural touch),

* increased confinement due to drains, IV lines, catheters, and sedation,

* isolation (either physical or social),

* limited visual stimuli.

The causes of type 5 sensory alteration are:

* continuous high noise levels due to equipment alarms, telephones, buzzers, staff conversation, etc. (Levels of noise in the critical care environment have been recorded that peak as high as 80 decibels and run continuously at a minimum of 50 decibels throughout the night (Topf and Davis 1993). Kahn *et al.* (1998) suggest that 51% of noise measured in the critical care environment is potentially modifiable and instituted noise abatement measures including staff education and feedback, and vibrate modes on bleeps. The highest recorded decibel level of noise came from talking, which can be modified by altering staff (and visitor) behaviour.)

* unfamiliar and frequently incomprehensible sounds;

* stressful environment with loss of meaningful sounds/environment from which the patient can orientate;

* frequent uninvited touch and invasion of personal space;

* constant lighting (i.e. lack of diurnal phasing of light levels).

The nurse has an important part to play in the prevention or alleviation of sensory imbalance. Many of the interventions controlled and initiated by nurses will have marked effects on the patient's sensory load.

PREDISPOSING FACTORS TO SENSORY IMBALANCE

* Alcohol/drug addiction

* Previous cerebral damage

* Psychological illness

* Chronic cardiovascular, respiratory, metabolic, or renal illness

* Increasing age

* Previous episodes of delirium

* Previous psychological stressors

PHARMACOLOGICAL AGENTS IMPLICATED IN SENSORY IMBALANCE

* Atropine and anticholinergics

* Aminocaproic acid

* Anticonvulsants

* Barbiturates

* Penicillin and cephalosporins

* Steroids

* Morphine

* Lidocaine

* Diazepam

* Digoxin

DEFINITIONS OF ALTERED PERCEPTION PRECIPITATED BY SENSORY IMBALANCE

* Illusion: a false interpretation of external (usually auditory or visual) stimuli.

* Hallucination: a false sensory perception occurring without external stimulus.

* Delusion: a fixed irrational belief not consistent with cultural mores. It may include persecutory, grandiose, nihilistic, or somatic ideas.

Strategies that will assist in optimizing the patient's response to sensory stimuli are to:

* Assess the patient for predisposing factors (see boxes).

* Provide pre-operative visits and information to elective admission patients to reduce anxiety associated with the unknown.

◆ Give repeated, frequent orientation to time, place, person, and events.

◆ Establish an appropriate day/night differentiation and accentuate markers of daily routine such as morning toilet, meals, etc.

◆ Make the patient comfortable for the night with attention to analgesia, sedation, positioning, warmth, and reduced light.

◆ Limit and cluster interventions during the night to allow periods of at least 90 min of uninterrupted sleep (Closs 1988a,b).

◆ Reduce unnecessary 'meaningless' noise.

◆ Use large clocks and calendars within the patient's sight.

◆ Introduce the patient to staff entering the patient's bed space.

◆ Have formal greeting and leavetaking from the nurse caring for them on each shift.

◆ Use family photos and familiar objects from home to create a less hostile environment.

◆ Encourage involvement of family members in conversation, obtain information about topics of interest to the patient, and include the patient in conversation,

◆ Ascertain the patient's likes and dislikes.

◆ Play music appropriate to the patient's taste (Chlan 1998).

◆ Use television, radio, newspapers, magazines, and conversation to provide meaningful stimulation.

◆ Include caring touch in communicating with the patient.

◆ Ensure that the patient can see out of windows and use natural light as much as possible.

◆ Provide explanations and information on the critical care environment to assist the patient in interpretation and understanding.

◆ Encourage autonomy in self-care where possible and provide explanations and information so that the patient may participate in decisions about daily care.

Every effort should be made to limit the impact of this technologically orientated environment with appropriate use of support from family and friends, alternative therapies, noise consideration, and therapeutic nursing interventions.

Disturbance of diurnal (circadian) rhythm

Humans possess a 24-hour cycle that is resistant to change. Extreme long-term disruption of this can be fatal. It is an unfortunate feature of the critical care environment that care and interventions must continue round the clock. This makes the patient vulnerable to disturbances of sleep and diurnal rhythm. However, recent work by Gabor *et al.* (2003) using polysomnography in seven mechanically ventilated patients found that only 20% of arousals and awakenings were due to noise and only 10% to patient care activities. They could not identify causes of 68% of awakenings.

In the critical care environment, disturbance is due to:

◆ the constant need for interventions to the patient throughout the 24-hour cycle and the high level of continuous noise (Topf and Davis 1993);

◆ loss of rapid eye movement (REM) sleep;

◆ loss of the regenerative phase (slow wave) of non-REM sleep;

◆ inappropriate nursing routine where morning baths may be carried out at a time when patients are at their lowest ebb (between 2 a.m. and 5 a.m.);

◆ inadequate pain relief; this is a major sleep-disturbing factor (Puntillo 1990, Rotondi *et al.* 2002).

The effects of sleep disturbance on the patient can include (Closs 1988a,b, Wallace *et al.* 1999, Jones *et al.* 2001, Parthasarathy and Tobin 2004):

◆ irritability and anxiety

◆ physical exhaustion and fatigue

◆ elevation of nocturnal blood pressure (during awakening)

FUNCTIONS OF SLEEP

◆ Mental restoration.

◆ Anabolic processes.

Protein synthesis is inhibited by cortisol, glucagon, and catecholamines which reach their highest level during the day.

During sleep, energy expenditure falls and energy is stored within cells. Levels of ATP rise high enough for protein synthesis to occur.

Growth hormone (which stimulates protein and RNA synthesis and amino acid uptake) reaches peak secretion rates during slow-wave sleep.

- disruption of immune function (decreased natural killer cell activity)
- reduced endurance of respiratory muscles and response to hypercapnoea
- increased energy expenditure and negative nitrogen balance
- cognitive dysfunction.

Once again, there are a number of interventions under the nurse's control which will limit the detrimental effects of 24-hour care:

- Assess the patient's sleep pattern by observing sleep/wake states overnight. Nurse observers' assessments were found to be accurate in 82% of cases allowing early recognition of potential problems (Edwards and Schuring 1993).
- Dim the lights and reduce environmental noise for the night period.
- Use earplugs and noise-cancellation headsets where patients are in open critical care areas (Wallace *et al.* 1999).
- Provide protected periods of uninterrupted sleep of at least 90 min.
- Carry out only vital observations and interventions at night.
- Institute 'quiet time' periods when the critical care environment as a whole reduces light and sound to as little as is safely possible, e.g. between 2 and 4 a.m. (Olson *et al.* 2001).
- Avoid procedures likely to add to patient stress between the hours of 2 a.m. and 5 a.m. (the lowest levels of cortisol and other stress-related hormones are secreted during this time).
- Ensure pain relief and other comfort needs such as warmth, comfortable position, reassurance, etc. are all addressed prior to sleep.

Although sedation from benzodiazepines, narcotic analgesics, and propofol commonly produce sleep-like behaviour in patients, the effect is not always that of true sleep. REM sleep and slow-wave sleep are suppressed by benzodiazepines and narcotics and may not provided the true physiological benefits associated with sleep (Parthasarathy and Tobin, 2004).

Critical care (ICU) delirium

Delirium is defined as an acute change or fluctuation in the course of a patient's mental status, plus inattention

and either disorganized thinking or an altered level of consciousness (Ely *et al.* 2001a,b). It can also be referred to as ICU syndrome or ICU psychosis but neither term has valid definitions and may detract from establishing the cause of delirium (Justic 2000).

Delirium has four essential elements Justic (2000):

- disordered attention or arousal
- cognitive dysfunction
- acute development of signs and symptoms (hours to a few days)
- a medical rather than psychiatric cause.

Recent research has shown a range of incidence of delirium in the critically ill ranging from 19% (Dubois *et al.* 2001) to 87% (Ely *et al.* 2001a,b). Overall, the elderly are more likely to develop delirium although Ely *et al.* (2001a,b) found other more frequent risk factors in the critically ill such as the use of benzodiazepine or narcotics. Significant under-recognition of delirium has been due to the lack of operational definitions and a valid and reliable method of assessment.

Risk factors extrapolated from the general hospital patient population have been applied to the critical care patient but Dubois *et al.* (2001) have identified a number of significant risk factors (see box) from a study of 216 patients admitted to the critical care area.

There are two subtypes of delirium, both of which are frequently seen in critically ill patients. Hypoactive

SIGNIFICANT RISK FACTORS ASSOCIATED WITH CRITICAL CARE DELIRIUM

- Morphine
- Epidural
- History of hypertension
- Smoking history
- Raised bilirubin level

Dubois *et al.* (2001)

PRE-EXISTING RISK FACTORS FOR CRITICAL CARE DELIRIUM IN ELDERLY (>70 YR) PATIENTS

- Dementia
- Severe illness
- Visual/hearing impairment
- Elevated urea-creatinine ratio

HOSPITAL-RELATED RISK FACTORS FOR CRITICAL CARE DELIRIUM

- Malnutrition
- Adding more than three medications during the hospital stay
- Presence of a urinary catheter
- Iatrogenic complications
- Use of physical restraint

Inouye and Charpentier (1996)

---

delirium is evident when the patient becomes withdrawn, lethargic, and apathetic, sometimes to the point of complete unresponsiveness. It is not commonly identified in the critical care patient. Hyperactive delirium is more typically thought of as critical care delirium. The patient exhibits extreme levels of agitation and emotional lability, often leading to refusal of care and disruptive behaviour such as shouting, violence, removal of catheters, and attempts to leave.

Delirium is associated with an increased length of stay in hospital (Ely *et al.* 2001*b*) and can be associated with increased levels of morbidity (self-extubation and removal of iv catheters). Use of assessment tools such as the Confusion Assessment Method—ICU (Ely *et al.* 2001*a*) can allow early identification of delirium and monitoring of progress.

Communication

Communication is a universal need and a universal problem in critical care. The normal processes are disrupted by sedation, opiates, endotracheal and tracheostomy tubes, fluctuating levels of consciousness, and fear. One of the greatest skills required by a critical care nurse is the ability to communicate. It requires patience, motivation, a perception of the patient as an individual, perseverance, and experience to provide the patient with an appropriate level of understanding and response. In a study of 100 patients who had been unconscious in the critical care environment, Lawrence (1995) showed clear evidence that patients heard, understood, and responded emotionally to what was being said to them, even when they were not thought to be aware. This strongly supports the need to remain acutely aware of what is said in front of patients in order to ensure that it is therapeutic communication. Elliott and Wright (1999) identified seven categories of verbal communication:

- procedural/task intentions
- orientational information

- reassurance
- apologies/recognition of discomfort
- efforts to elicit a response
- intentional and unintentional distraction (humour, singing, and light-hearted references)
- social conversation with colleagues while recognizing the patient's presence.

Most communication was short, reflecting the difficulties of ongoing communication for both patients and staff.

Barriers to communication experienced by critical care patients have been identified by Borsig and Steinacker (1982):

1. Psychical and psychological conditioned causes—previous psychiatric illness, psychiatric disturbance related to the critical care environment.

2. Socially conditioned causes—hospitalization and unfamiliarity of the environment, use of jargon, ethnic differences, social isolation.

3. Chemically conditioned causes—drugs such as sedatives, narcotics, and muscle relaxants.

4. Environmental causes—sensory deprivation, sensory overload, isolation, loss of familiar environment, and contact with the outside world.

5. Organic and therapeutic causes—fatigue, breathlessness, presence of endotracheal or tracheostomy tube, neuropathy, head injury, and other aspects of illness or treatment.

Effective and therapeutic communication is a vital aspect of nursing intervention. Insufficient communication can invoke feelings of isolation, frustration, anxiety, and fear (Bergbom-Engberg and Haljamäe 1993). There are a wide variety of alternative methods and aids which should be utilized to assist the patient in communicating (see box and Table 3.3).

An important adjunct to finding and using an appropriate method of communication is the need to record and pass on this information to other members of the caring team. Effective patient-orientated documentation is essential. The patient's feelings of isolation, alienation, and fear can and should be reduced by the promotion of effective communication from all members of staff (Ashworth 1980).

Patients' perceptions of their critical illness

Much can be gained in understanding the problems facing the critically ill by listening to survivors' accounts of their experience in critical care. There are a number of problems which affect the patient's ability to per-

TABLE 3.3	Communication devices
Passy–Muir valve	
Possum Portascan (uses the ability to suck or press to alter indicators on a screen)	
Pen/pencil and paper	
Lip-reading	
Alphabet board	
Touch	
Symbol board/book	
Mime/gesture/facial expression	
Computer	
Eye contact	
Magic writer	
Electronic communicator, e.g. Lightwriter	

ceive and make sense of what is going on around them. Their ability to communicate these problems is often seriously limited (see above) and staff may only become aware of them when the patient finally becomes well

---

STRATEGIES FOR COMMUNICATING EFFECTIVELY WITH CRITICALLY ILL PATIENTS: SPEECH, WRITING, SYMBOLS, MIME, TOUCH

- Assess the patient's ability to see, hear, touch, respond, understand, use sign language, speak.

- Identify the most appropriate communication device(s) according to patient ability (see Table 3.3).

- In pre-operative visits prepare the patient for communication difficulties, agree gestures for minimal communication, and document them.

- Use positive feedback such as smiling, nodding attentively, giving the patient full attention.

- Use touch as a means of communicating to the patient that they have attention and empathy (Verity 1996).

- Orientate the patient to time and place, and identify who is speaking to them.

- Use appropriate questions: open questions for the patient who is able to speak/communicate more fully; closed questions for patients who can only gesture and nod.

- Include the patient's visitors and family in planning methods of communication.

---

enough to describe them. Personal accounts of experiences in critical care by former patients are a valuable source of information about the sort of problems that occur (Griffiths and Jones 2002).

Follow-up studies have shown that 33–63% of patients have little or no recollection of their stay in the CCU (Friedman *et al.* 1992, Russell 1999, Rotondi *et al.* 2002). However, those who do remember their stay have several important points to make (Heath 1989, Russell 1999, Griffiths and Jones 2002, Rotondi *et al.* 2002). The main themes from research are outlined below, followed by suggestions for limiting the specific problems identified.

Presence of endotracheal tube and discomfort

Patients describe the presence of the endotracheal tube as very uncomfortable, particularly during turning or movement. Oral tubes are felt to cause a continuous gagging sensation but keep the mouth moist by stimulating saliva. Nasal tubes are felt to be less uncomfortable although the degree of discomfort is related to the level of trauma on intubation:

- Mouth care is important.

- Support of the tube during movement or turning is essential to prevent further discomfort.

- Use specific commercially available methods of securing tubes or pad areas of friction/pressure if standard tape is used.

Disconnection from the ventilator

Patients who undergo long-term ventilation develop considerable psychological dependence on the ventilator. They describe the situation of disconnection from the ventilator as terrifying and feel that it seems an intolerable length of time before they are reconnected. These feelings are bound up with the level of confidence they have in the staff caring for them.

The ventilator alarms are also a source of distress as patients are often unable to identify if they emanate from their ventilator or that of another patient. If the alarm is allowed to continue for any length of time it can cause considerable stress to the patient listening to it:

- A level of trust and confidence must be developed between the patient and his/her nurse.

- Disconnection from the ventilator should only be carried out after full explanation to the patient and reassurance that it will not continue any longer than necessary.

- Ventilator alarms should be cancelled as quickly as possible and their cause and its remedy explained to the patient.

Communication

Patients express great frustration at their inability to speak and are warmly appreciative of patient and persistent efforts by nursing staff to understand them. In particular, lip-reading is mentioned as an important factor in relieving the patient's distress at being unable to speak:

- Communication by the patient should be given a high priority by the nurse.

- Patient, persistent attempts at understanding are valued by patients.

- Perfecting the ability to lip-read (in orally intubated patients) is an essential achievement (Drane 1986).

- Use adjuncts for communication such as spell boards, wipe clean boards, and communication devices

The importance of touch

Patients describe the comfort of human touch, and hand-holding in particular. It is an important indicator to the patient that they are cared for (Estabrooks 1989, Verity 1996):

- Use hand-holding and touch to communicate caring and comfort.

Staff noise and talking at the bedside

The high noise levels associated with the critical care environment have already been discussed. While some patients find a level of background noise comforting, many found difficulty in sleeping and felt generally disturbed by high levels of noise. In particular, 'radios played at high volumes', 'staff chatter', and 'nurses who raise their voices unnecessarily when talking to patients' were mentioned:

- Aim to keep background noise levels low.

- Use normal level of speech when talking to patients.

- Do not play radios loudly unless it is music played specifically for the patient.

- Reduce levels of noise during night hours (see above).

Sensory deprivation and temporal disorientation

Many patients report an inability to distinguish the passage of time. They find high levels of fluorescent light unpleasant and appreciate natural daylight where possible:

- Where possible, long-term patients should be nursed where natural light is available.

- Methods of marking the time and the day should be used (see above).

Dreams and hallucinations

Patients frequently refer to dreams and/or hallucinations that they have experienced during their critical illness. Many of them have a prison, depersonalization, or torture theme (Daffurn *et al.* 1994, Skirrow 2002). This sounds a reasonable rationalization of some of the events which they have experienced. However, they provide a frightening and distressing perception of the situation:

- It is difficult to help the patient in these situations.

- Touch, verbal reassurance, comfort, and communication may help.

- Having factual memories or awareness of the critical care environment may help the patient to understand or deal with them (Jones *et al.* 2001).

Transition to the ward

Many patients who have spent a lengthy period in critical care express great fear of transfer to the ward (Jones and O'Donnell 1994, McKinney and Melby 2002). They feel that the loss of an individual nurse caring for them means a period of neglect while they are still unable to perform most of their care needs themselves:

- Use of a step-down care facility, such as a high-dependency unit, may be of help.

- High levels of liaison and communication between ward and unit staff may smooth the transition. A visit from key ward staff to the patient on the unit prior to transfer may also benefit.

- Appropriately timed discharge (i.e. not as an emergency to make way for a new admission) is also important (see Chapter 1).

Pain experience

Patients identify pain as one of the biggest stressors associated with critical care. Many indicate that analgesia did not bring total relief (Puntillo 1990, Tittle and McMillan 1994) and that communicating their pain was difficult:

- Make a regular assessment of pain using visual analogues (see below).

- Evaluate the efficacy of analgesia following administration.

- Use alternative methods of pain relief such as warmth, massage, imagery, etc. (see later for further details).

Supporting and maintaining patient/family relationships

The term 'family' includes all those who provide the patient's intimate social support structure. Problems affecting family relationships when a member is critically ill are due to:

- Loss of normal communication and interaction.

- Increased levels of stress related to the patient's illness.

- Family anxiety about outcome.

- In emergency admissions, the shock of the sudden critical illness and removal of the patient from his/her family role.

- The threat to family stability and loss of normal family rituals and day-to-day routine.

Jamerson et al. (1996) identified four phases that families experience when a relative is in critical care. These are hovering, information seeking, tracking, and garnering resources (see Table 3.4). The main response to these is active seeking of information by the family members.

Family needs have been identified by a body of research using Molter's (1979) Critical Care Family Needs Inventory (Forrester et al. 1990, Rukholm et al. 1991, Price et al. 1991, Leske 1991, Wilkinson 1995). Leske's (1991) meta-analysis of the research identified five common factors:

1. The need for support.

2. The need for comfort.

3. The need for information.

4. The need for proximity.

5. The need for assurance.

It may not be possible to fulfill all these needs, particularly with regard to patient prognosis, but an

---

FAMILY SUPPORT NETWORK

- Nursing staff
- Medical staff
- Social work department
- Spiritual support
- Extended family, friends, neighbours
- Specialist support groups
- Community workers (e.g. family doctor, district nurse)

TABLE 3.4 A model of families' experiences in critical care. Adapted from Jamerson et al. (1996)

Category	Definition	Possible nursing interventions
Hovering	Initial stress, confusion and uncertainty in family members	Individual: Anticipate need for information and provide. Orientate families to critical care environment /routine. Assess any previous experiences in critical care. Provide empathy and advocacy for the family. Organizational: Provide volunteers, pastoral care, or ancillary staff to provide information on patient status
Information seeking	Active gathering of information about the patient	Individual: Anticipate information needs and supply updates. Include the family in discharge planning. Organizational: Provide message board for exchange of information. Provide printed orientation booklet and distribute. Post visiting hours
Tracking	A process of observing, analysing and evaluating the patient's care	Individual: Provide basic as well as high-tech nursing care. Treat families with respect and dignity. Maintain flexible open communication. Assign consistent caregiver. Organizational: Provide privacy through facilities/environment. Provide in-service training to maintain nursing skill/ knowledge
Garnering resources	The acquisition of resources to meet the family's perceived needs	Individual: Allow individualized flexible visiting. Assess the need for a family gatekeeper. Provide open honest communication.

TABLE 3.4 A model of families' experiences in critical care. Adapted from Jamerson *et al.* (1996) – *continued*

Category	Definition	Possible nursing interventions
		Collaborate with family regarding treatment and discharge plans.
		Allow families to assist with non-technical care
		Organizational:
		Provide a waiting environment with comfort items and diversionary activities.
		Supply phones.
		Identify areas for solitude

awareness of them will direct efforts to support the family and to meet them as far as is possible.

Research into interventions to meet family needs is not extensive but Appleyard *et al.* (2000) have trialled the use of a volunteer programme to provide comfort and support as well as liaison to families in the CCU waiting room. Results showed a significant increase in the level of comfort reported by families using the family needs inventory.

Other suggested strategies based on experience and on suggestions made by researchers are listed below:

♦ care of the family should be a multidisciplinary responsibility, preferably coordinated by the nursing staff as they are the point of continuity.

♦ The family should be given repeated, detailed updates of the patient's condition, progress, and, where possible, prognosis (Leske 1991, Jamerson 1996).

♦ A common approach must be sought from all support staff, and particularly between medical and nursing staff with constant intercommunication about contacts with the family.

♦ A common record should be kept of all approaches by support staff to the family (Wilkinson 1995).

♦ Questions should be answered honestly.

♦ Where possible, the family should be included in planning and carrying out the patient's non-therapeutic care.

♦ The family should have encouragement and education in communicating, touching, and caring for the patient.

♦ The strengths and weaknesses within the family coping mechanisms should be identified. Support should be aimed at accentuating strengths and moderating or diminishing weaknesses (De Jong and Beatty 2000).

♦ The family should have open access to the patient but be encouraged to take time away from the patient in order to rest when necessary and have time to themselves (Dracup 1993).

♦ In the longer-term critically ill patient the family may need encouragement and assistance to resume a modified form of daily life.

♦ The support team should monitor family members closely for signs of failure to cope, overwhelming stress, and exhaustion.

Overall, the aim should be to establish a positive, supportive relationship with the family. Family support can be time-consuming and emotionally draining but is an essential part of maintaining the patient's coping mechanisms and morale. It should be considered to be one of the most important aspects of nursing the critically ill patient.

Models for delivery of nursing care

Conceptual nursing models or frameworks are designed to guide the application of nursing practice. The utility of nursing models has been questioned and has been the subject of recent published debate (Tierney 1998, Heath 1998). There is no doubt, however, that conceptual frameworks (Fawcett 1989) can be beneficial in developing and understanding the process of delivering nursing care. Riehl and Roy (1980) define a nursing model as 'a systematically constructed, scientifically based, and logically related set of concepts which identify the essential components of nursing practice, together with the theoretical basis of the concepts and values required for their use by the practitioner'.

The proliferation of different models in recent years has illustrated one fundamental point: no single model of nursing will reflect all areas of nursing practice. It is appropriate to use different models for different types of patients, and even for different periods during the patient's course of illness. The use of a nursing model should be viewed as an enhancement of nursing practice rather than a theoretical outline to be applied without thought or alteration to all types of patients.

Similarly, the use of the medical model in some circumstances should not be dismissed out of hand. It can

TABLE 3.5 Examples of models used in critical care

Model	Characteristics
Mead	Activities of Daily Living (adapted from Roper–Logan–Tierney)
Synergy	Dimensions of nursing
Roy	Adaptation

be particularly useful for refining priorities in acute situations where the patient's physiological problems require urgent action.

It is not appropriate to include an exhaustive description of nursing models currently used in critical care in this chapter (see Table 3.5). However, the process of identifying a model or framework of care will be described.

Nursing philosophy

The primary step in development of nursing theory is to establish a philosophy for the unit. The philosophy should contain:

* the values, ideals and goals of the nursing staff,

* a synopsis of how the staff view the patient and his/her needs,

* the environment in which care is delivered, and

* any other significant external issues which will affect the delivery of care.

The key issues that need consideration in forming a philosophy are:

1. The nature of care—caring is seen as the foundation of nursing practice.

2. Social viability—does the philosophy meet the expectations of society, is it seen as important by society, and does it have value for the profession of nursing?

3. The extrinsic environment of care—the philosophy should reflect the nature of the environment in which it is carried out (i.e. a critical care philosophy will bear different hallmarks to a community care philosophy).

4. The intrinsic environment of care—this refers to the way nursing or the delivery of care is organized within the environment.

Multidisciplinary philosophy

Many critical care units work primarily as multidisciplinary teams and it is important that the philosophy reflects the whole team's approach and not simply that of the nursing staff. If it does not, then it

NURSING METAPARADIGM CONCEPTS (FAWCETT 1989)

* Person—the recipient of nursing actions.

* Environment—the recipient's significant others and surroundings.

* Health—the wellness or illness state of the recipient.

* Nursing—the actions taken by nurses either on behalf of or which the recipient requests.

is likely that the values and views expressed within the philosophy will remain an abstract rather than a real exercise.

Nursing models

The key points of the philosophy should be reviewed and used as a basis either for matching a published nursing model or for building a new model. Certain concepts are central to nursing as a discipline and are the foundation stones for building any model. They are known as metaparadigm concepts and include: person, environment, health, and nursing (as an activity).

Application of these concepts to critical care can imply problems which require special consideration:

1. The barriers to communication involved in critical care mean that the patient as a person may be difficult to know and assess. Information regarding aspects other than physical state may be obtainable only second-hand through relatives or friends. Similar problems relate to the patient's environment. These aspects must be taken into account and the nursing model chosen should neither discount them completely nor place too heavy an emphasis on them.

2. Critical care nursing accentuates the importance of the physical state of the patient as this forms the basis for admission. The nurse is frequently working in critical situations where other aspects must take second place. However, these priorities will change in different circumstances and it is important that physical aspects give way to psychological or social needs where it is appropriate and beneficial to the patient to do so. One of the real values of a well-considered framework of care is the ability to switch emphasis appropriately without diminishing the patient's physical and psychological well-being.

3. The complexity of the physical and physiological problems of the critically ill patient requires a framework which will allow a clear and succinct approach

to assessment, intervention, and evaluation. One of the reasons the medical model has been so useful to critical care nurses is its clarity of structure and suitability to physical and physiological problems.

The key components of nursing models (Aggleton and Chalmers 1986) are the:

- nature of people (people and their needs),
- causes of problems likely to require nursing intervention,
- nature of the assessment process,
- nature of the planning and goal-setting process,
- focus of intervention during the implementation of the care plan,
- nature of the process of evaluating the quality and effects of nursing care given.
- role of the nurse.

The influence of the model on the delivery of care

The emphasis of the model chosen will have an influence on the care given. If the model is chosen to reflect the philosophy of the unit then that emphasis will be in accordance with the values and ideals encompassed in the philosophy. However, it is not the only factor influencing care, and although important it must take its place amongst numerous others such as medical interventions and values, education, research, new therapies, nursing staffing, and skill mix.

Priorities of care

While the importance of psychological and social support for patients in critical care cannot be underestimated, the hierarchy of human need must assign priority to those things which will cause death or extensive harm to the patient.

Good critical care practice seeks to prevent emergency situations, where possible, by employing close observation and monitoring of the patient and skilled interpretation of the information obtained. Early warning of impending problems and appropriate treatment based on this can prevent some emergencies. There will always be a proportion of sudden overwhelming disasters but many potentially life-threatening events can be circumvented by the skill and knowledge of the nurse who identifies these early signs. By the nature of their critical illness, patients in the critical care environment are more likely to develop life-threatening problems and emergency situations.

Bedside emergency equipment

A major priority for the nurse taking over the care of the patient must be to ensure that emergency equipment at the bedside is both functioning and available. Unit-wide emergency equipment, such as defibrillators, intubation equipment, and pacing systems, should be checked by a designated nurse during each shift.

The following equipment/skills provide a minimum basic standard of safety for emergency events and will at least allow the nurse to maintain a patient's vital functions until help arrives.

1. Equipment for airway protection:
   - Check that the suction is functioning by occluding the end of the suction tubing and ensuring a vacuum pressure builds up (see Chapter 4 for details).
   - Ensure that the correct size suction catheters are available for the size of the patient's endotracheal or tracheostomy tube (see Chapter 4).
   - If closed suction systems are used, check connections and the entire length of the plastic sleeve for patency, then clear the catheter with normal saline injected through the irrigation port to ensure function.
   - An oropharyngeal (Guedel) airway of a size appropriate to the patient (usually 2 for women and 3 for men) and a Yankauer sucker should also be available.

2. Equipment for support of the patient's breathing:
   - Check that the manual resuscitation or rebreathe bag is functioning and leak-free by occluding the end of the valve outlet with the valve screwed tight. The bag should inflate to a taut pressure without air escaping.
   - Any nurse responsible for a ventilated patient should be competent to ventilate them with a manual resuscitation bag. It is the only method of ensuring adequate ventilation and oxygenation if the ventilator or gas supply fails. It may also be necessary to manually ventilate the patient in the event of emergency evacuation.
   - Check that the bag has the correct attachment to allow ventilation, and that it is attached to an oxygen (not air) delivery system. There should be a catheter mount if the patient is intubated, and an anaesthetic facemask if not.
   - An anaesthetic facemask should be available at the bedside at all times in case of accidental extubation.
   - Check any portable oxygen cylinders to ensure they are at least half full.

3. Equipment for support of the patient's circulation:

- ◆ Check that the arterial or non-invasive blood pressure monitoring system is functional and accurate. Ensure transducers are placed at the correct height (see Chapter 5).
- ◆ Every nurse caring for a patient should be competent in performing external cardiac compressions (see Chapter 7). The cardiac arrest call button should be functioning, or help should be within easy calling distance.
- ◆ In almost all critical care patients some form of IV access should be available and patent.
- ◆ As a basic precaution, every nurse should run through these checks at the beginning of each shift and whenever they take over the care of a patient.

Other additional checks of drug infusions and fluids to ensure that the patient is receiving what is prescribed will also be necessary. Checks specific to therapy such as renal replacement therapy (see Chapter 9) should also be carried out.

Common core problems for patients in the critical care environment

Many of a patient's problems are present as a result of the body's response to critical illness and the nature of the critical care environment. There are, therefore, a number of problems which are experienced by the majority of critically ill patients. These are listed in Table 3.6. These common core problems are discussed in this chapter if they constitute a global problem or in the chapters listed if they refer specifically to a system.

Pain relief and sedation

The experience of pain is a complex phenomenon involving social, cultural, emotional, psychological, and physiological components.

Pain is aggravated in the ICU by:

- ◆ anxiety and fear,
- ◆ difficulty in communicating pain,
- ◆ life-saving priorities may displace the importance of pain relief (e.g. limiting opioid doses when blood pressure is low).

Pain contributes to the patient's stress and can increase confusion, paranoia, and delirium, as well as decreasing the resistance of the patient to other stressors. Patients' recollections of critical care show that their greatest worries were pain and the inability to lie

TABLE 3.6 Common core problems for intensive care patients	
Problem	**Chapter**
Airway maintenance	Respiratory problems (Chapter 4)
Support of ventilation	Respiratory problems (Chapter 4)
Support of circulation	Cardiovascular problems (Chapter 6)
Fluid balance	Renal problems (Chapter 9)
Nutrition	Gastrointestinal and nutrition problems (Chapter 11)
Elimination	Gastrointestinal and nutrition problems (Chapter 11)
Pain relief and sedation	This chapter
Communication	This chapter
Anxiety/fear	This chapter
Maintenance of sensory balance	This chapter
Support of the family	This chapter
Alterations in diurnal rhythm	This chapter
Prevention of the effects of limited mobility	This chapter
Personal hygiene	This chapter

comfortably. Pain was also the leading cause of sleeplessness (Thomas 2003).

Puntillo (1990) suggests that pain is often inadequately assessed in the critically ill patient due to the patient's inability to communicate verbally and that nurses frequently underestimate the patient's analgesic requirements as a result.

Physiology of pain

The feeling of pain is caused by a noxious stimulus generated by release of products from tissue damage or nerve terminal damage. The products known to induce a noxious stimulus include bradykinins, histamines, prostaglandins, and hydrogen ions. They act by binding to nerve receptors and depolarizing the nerve membrane thus initiating an action potential and impulse generation in the nociceptive fibres. This impulse will produce both a spinal (reflex) and central response (see Fig. 3.3 for pain pathways).

Pain is perceived at thalamic and forebrain levels and constitutes both sensory and reactive components. The thermal threshold is used as a determinant of sensory pain threshold and is remarkably constant between one person and another (44–45 °C). However, an individual's reaction to that sensation is greatly varied. The

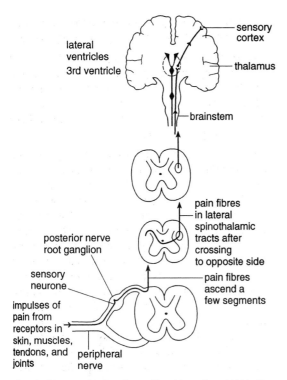

Fig. 3.3 Diagram of pain pathways (from Verran B. and Aisbitt P. (1988) *Neurological and Neurosurgical Nursing*, Edward Arnold, reprinted with permission).

perception of pain by an individual may be altered according to other factors such as environment, experience, culture, mood, and pathology. Thus, the meaning any individual attaches to the pain they perceive will affect his or her response.

As a further factor in individual response to pain, the endogenous opioid (endorphin release) system will allow varying degrees of modulation of perceived pain. It is suggested that endorphin release occurs in response to pain, elevated blood pressure, fear, stress, restraint, and hypoglycaemia. Many of these factors are present in the critically ill and may allow for at least some reduction in perceived pain. Unfortunately, it is not possible to assess the level of endogenous opioid available or even to manipulate it, and the patient's response to pain is the only method currently available to indicate requirements for analgesia.

There are a number of theories of pain perception reflecting the complexity of the phenomenon. One of the most accepted and applicable of the current theories is Melzack and Wall's (1965) gate control theory.

The perception of pain transmitted by small-diameter nerve fibres (these carry pain stimuli) can be inhibited by stimulation of large-diameter nerve fibres (these carry innocuous information). The mechanism is postulated as follows:

1. The small-diameter fibres inhibit modulation by specialized tissue and excite cells which act as activators of central transmission of sensory and emotional aspects of pain. They therefore 'open the gate'.

2. The large-diameter fibres inhibit the excitatory cell activity and 'close the gate' to pain.

3. Higher central nervous system processes can influence the gate control via inhibitory messages to the spinal cord.

The gate control theory explains the effects of many alternative pain therapies. Thus, rubbing, use of transcutaneous electrical nerve stimulation (TENS), and massage, preferentially stimulate large-diameter fibres which inhibits, to a varying degree, central transmission of pain stimuli.

Assessment of a patient's pain

Nurses' assessment of a patient's pain has been shown to be influenced by a number of variables including ventilatory status, length of time after surgery (Gujol 1994), and the patient's ability to communicate (Puntillo 1990). Assessment within an ICU setting is extremely difficult, particularly in situations where the patient is unable to communicate verbally. Where nonverbal communication is impossible the nurse must rely on physiological variables, such as tachycardia, raised blood pressure, and physical responses (e.g. sweating and lacrimation). Unfortunately, these responses are subject to an enormous range of contributory factors which limit their interpretation.

Even when patients are able to express pain verbally their response is frequently underestimated and analgesia withheld. Puntillo (1994) found that only 48% of a sample of 35 patients had analgesia administered in the hour prior to chest drain removal. The mean visual analogue score for the intensity of pain of the procedure was 6.6; and it was described by patients as 'tender', 'sharp', and 'heavy' pain.

Tittle and McMillan (1994) studied 44 patients in both an ICU and a surgical unit and found that patients continued to experience pain even following pain management interventions. An average of only 30% of the maximum possible prescription for opiate analgesia was administered to the ICU patients. Documentation was also minimal giving little idea of the patient's response to the dose administered or the intensity of the pain experienced. In addition, although most nursing responses to patients' pain are pharmacological in nature (combining the use of analgesia and sedation), a small number use alternative methods of pain relief such as repositioning, massage, reassurance, and providing information (Gélinas *et al.* 2004). More worryingly, in a study of 183 pain episodes, Gélinas *et al.* (2004) found that 40% of pain episodes were not reassessed after interventions to verify their effectiveness. Puntillo (2002) found that the use of a pain chart or tool for adequate recording was associated with improved levels of pain management.

Methods of pain relief

1. Analgesia. Opiates and synthetic opioids are the mainstay of pain relief for critical care patients. In the ventilated patient the added advantage of blunting of the respiratory drive is useful in managing modes of ventilation which are not physiological. Intravenous infusions produce a more consistent analgesia which can be titrated to patient response. Dose will depend on age, weight, haemodynamic status, and clinical effect. Use of IV boluses (small dose, delivered slowly) prior to any unpleasant procedure will provide increased analgesic effect over the short term.

2. Regional analgesia. Epidural analgesia is most advantageous following upper abdominal and chest surgery, when coughing, deep breathing, and mobility are facilitated. The epidural catheter is inserted between T7 and T10 for abdominal and thoracic pain or at Ll–2 or L2–3 for lower abdominal and pelvic pain. Analgesia may be delivered either as a constant infusion or boluses.

3. TENS. Large-diameter afferent nerve fibres are stimulated by a low-level electric current thus selectively inhibiting transmission of pain signals via small-diameter nerve fibres. The effect on ICU patients seems to be limited and may only reduce pharmacological analgesic requirements, rather than providing complete pain relief.

4. Nitrous oxide. Inhalation of a gas consisting of 50 per cent nitrous oxide and 50 per cent oxygen (Entonox) can provide good analgesic effect. It can only be used for short-term pain relief as bone marrow depression can occur after 36 hours. Its primary use at present is to provide pain relief to spontaneously ventilating patients who are able to use the demand valve system of delivery for analgesia during unpleasant procedures. It can also be delivered via a rigid oxygen mask but at a reduced percentage of nitrous oxide, due to entrainment. It is possible to deliver the gas through a positive pressure ventilator but this requires special adaptation of the gas delivery system.

5. Localized warmth and/or cooling. Application of local warmth using warming pads or warmed bags of fluid can help relieve aching or muscular spasm pain. Alternatively, topical cooling using permeable gel dressing or cool (but not iced) dressings can relieve some of the pain associated with burns.

6. Relaxation techniques and massage therapy. Relaxation techniques may be useful in relieving anxiety-related distress in patients who are able to cooperate or who can be taught prior to admission about the techniques used. Miller and Perry (1990) studied the effectiveness of slow, deep-breathing relaxation in relieving post-operative pain after cardiac surgery. The study group of 15 patients showed significant decreases in blood pressure, respiratory rate, and descriptive report of pain compared with the control group. However, there was no significant difference in requirement for analgesia. The effect of foot massage with and without aromatherapy on patients' anxiety following cardiac surgery has been evaluated (Stevensen 1994). Patients were significantly less anxious in the group treated with aromatherapy, although there was minimal difference in the reported level of pain.

7. The importance of communication. Attention to factors identified by the patient and his/her increasing anxiety (e.g. regarding pain, anxiety, and fear, need for information) is essential. Interventions such as these may assist in decreasing the 'distress' factor associated with pain perception and therefore increase the patient's ability to tolerate pain.

8. Patient-controlled analgesia (PCA). A small group of critically ill patients will be able to control their own pain management using a PCA infusion pump. The pump is set to deliver a specific dose of analgesia with a pre-set period of time which must elapse before the next dose can be delivered. Most PCA pumps record the number of actual patient demands for a dose of analgesia against the number of delivered doses of analgesia. This allows assessment of the efficacy of the set dose of analgesia.

Sedation in the critically ill

The goals of sedation in the critically ill patient are to:

- allay anxiety
- relieve discomfort
- aid sleep.

The achievement of these goals will depend on appropriate pain relief (see above).

Indications for sedation have been described by Oh (1990):

1. facilitation of mechanical ventilation.

2. Relief of anxiety.

3. Management of acute confusional states.

4. Implementation of treatment or diagnostic procedures.

5. Obtundation of the physiological response to stress to reduce tachycardia, hypertension, or raised intracranial pressure.

A sixth major indication is to prevent the patient being aware during paralysis. Opiate drugs are frequently given not only for their analgesic effect but also for anxiolytic and euphoric effects. They are often used in conjunction with sedative drugs to provide a combination of pain relief, drowsiness, and, when necessary, respiratory depression.

Assessment of the patient's level of sedation should be carried out at regular intervals using a sedation score (e.g. the UCLH Sedation Score, see Table 3.7). The aim is to maintain a score of between 0 and 1, unless the patient is particularly unstable or requires a mode of ventilation which is difficult to tolerate.

Types of sedative drugs

1. Benzodiazepines. These are sedative anxiolytics that promote amnesia. Used in combination with opiates, they can significantly reduce recall of unpleasant events and potentiate analgesic efficacy thus reducing analgesic requirements (Table 3.8). Benzodiazepines also act as anticonvulsants, muscle relaxants, and in prophylaxis of alcohol withdrawal. Reversal of benzodiazepine respiratory and central depressant effects can be accomplished in up to 80% of patients using flumazenil, a competitive benzodiazepine re-

TABLE 3.7   The UCLH Sedation Score

Score	State of patient
3	Agitated and restless
2	Awake and uncomfortable
1	Aware but calm
0	Roused by voice, remains calm
−1	Roused by movement
−2	Roused by noxious or painful stimuli
−3	Unrousable
A	Natural sleep

ceptor antagonist. Care must be taken to continue to observe the patient following administration due to the short half-life of flumazenil and the danger of re-sedation.

2. Propofol. Developed as an anaesthetic induction agent, propofol is now used as an infusion for short-term sedation in the critically ill (Table 3.8). It should be administered with caution in patients suspected of hypovolaemia or poor cardiovascular function as it has vasodilator and potent negative inotropic properties and can cause large falls in blood pressure. It is not licensed for use in children and should not be administered to anyone aged under 12 years.

3. Chlormethiazole. Chlormethiazole has sedative, anti-convulsant, and anti-emetic actions. It is useful for patients suffering from delirium tremens, acute agitation, confusional states, status epilepticus, and eclampsia (Table 3.8). Its cumulative effect may result in respiratory depression even when the dose remains unchanged. The relatively large fluid (electrolyte-free water) volume required for infusion can cause problems in patients who are fluid-restricted. Hyponatraemia can also result. Infusion concentrations higher than 0.8% have been associated with haemolysis. Care should be taken if the infusion is administered for more than 2–3 days as there is a recognized degeneration, associated with chlormethiaole, of certain plastics used in the manufacture of venous cannulae.

4. Ketamine. This is an anaesthetic and sedative agent with potent analgesic properties. It directly stimulates the myocardium and sympathetic nervous system but has little effect on respiration although it reduces airway resistance by its action on β-receptors (Table 3.8). It can be used in unstable, critically ill patients, and particularly in asthmatics, who will benefit from its bronchodilator effects. Its use is associated with distressing and unpleasant nightmares which may be stimulated by external irritation such as noise, touch, etc. It should thus be used with benzodiazepines to provide an amnesic effect.

5. Isoflurane (desflurane, sevoflurane). Isoflurane, desflurane and sevoflurane are inhalational anaesthetic agents used for short-term sedation in critically ill patients. Isoflurane has been shown to have a shorter time to extubation than midazolam but no difference in quality of sedation, haemodynamics, or duration of ICU stay. There are technical difficulties with their use due to the need for adapted ventilator circuits and scavenging equipment (Ostermann *et al.* 2000)

TABLE 3.8 Sedative drugs

Drug	Bolus dose	Infusion rate	Elimination half-life	Cautions
Diazepam	0.15–0.2 mg/kg slowly	Not recommended	20–90 h	Respiratory depression especially in the elderly. Hepatic and renal dysfunction prolongs action. Potentiates other CNS depressants. Active metabolites may prolong action. Paradoxical confusion/agitation with withdrawal symptoms in long-term use
Lorazepam	4 mg 4–6-hourly	Not recommended		Respiratory depression especially in the elderly. Slower onset, longer duration of action
Midazolam	50 µg/kg slowly	50–100 µg/kg/h titrated to response	2–4 h extended after infusion due to accumulation in fat	Respiratory depression especially in elderly. Hepatic and renal dysfunction prolongs action. Potentiated by cimetidine. 10% of patients are slow metabolizers. ↓SVR, ↑HR, and ↓BP increased in volume depletion, the elderly, and cardiac disease. Paradoxical confusion/agitation with withdrawal symptoms in long-term use
Propofol	1.0–2.0 mg/kg slowly	1.0–3.0 mg/kg/h	3–6 h	Negative inotropic effect. Large ↓ in BP especially with hypovolaemia or poor CVS function. Decreased clearance may occur in renal insufficiency and in the elderly. Seizures have been reported
Chlormethiazole	0.1–0.2 ml/kg/min	0.5–1.0 ml/min	8 h: may be extended after prolonged infusion	Metabolized in the liver. Increased bronchial secretions. Fluid overload possible. Causes haemolysis (?in higher concentrations). Tachycardia. Respiratory and cardiac depression
Ketamine	1.0–2.0 mg/kg added doses of 0.5 mg/kg	3.0–10.0 µg/kg/min	3–6 h	Tachycardia and ↑catecholamine stimulation. Minimal depression of respiration unless really large doses. Nightmares and hallucinations

Muscle relaxants (paralysing agents, neuromuscular blockers)

There are four major indications for the use of muscle relaxants (Table 3.9):

1. Facilitation of endotracheal intubation.

2. Assisting the use of certain ventilatory modes (e.g. inverse ratio ventilation).

3. Prevention of activity associated with high levels of oxygen consumption (e.g. shivering) in patients with very poor respiratory function and high fractionated inspired oxygen (F_iO_2).

4. Reducing muscle spasm associated with tetany.

Muscle relaxants should only be given to patients who are either intubated or about to be intubated. They should also only be used in conjunction with adequate sedation to avoid the terror of conscious paralysis. Levels of sedation should be assessed regularly by reducing or discontinuing the paralysing agent to allow assessment. Atracurium and vecuronium are least likely to be associated with adverse cardiovascular effects and should be considered for haemodynamically unstable patients (Table 3.9).

Malignant hyperthermia is a rare genetic disorder which can be precipitated by the use of muscle relaxants (mostly suxamethonium) but usually in combination with an inhalational anaesthetic. The patient becomes rapidly pyrexial and develops severe muscle rigidity. There are gross metabolic derangements as a result of abnormal cellular calcium metabolism. Treatment consists of stopping the muscle relaxant,

TABLE 3.9	Muscle relaxants			
Drug	**Bolus dose**	**Infusion rate**	**Elimination half-life**	**Cautions**
Atracurium	0.6 mg/kg		Short	Anaphylaxis has been reported. Adequate sedation required. Accumulation of a metabolite may cause seizures after some days. Breakdown is delayed in hypothermia and acidosis
Vecuronium	0.08–0.1 mg/kg	50–80 µg/kg/h (intermittent injection preferred)	Short	Anaphylaxis and prolonged effects reported. Renally excreted—use with caution in renal insufficiency
Pancuronium			Long	Renally excreted. Metabolized in liver to active metabolites: should not be used in hepatic failure. May cause tachycardia and hypotension due to vagal blockade

aggressive cooling, and administering intravenous dantrolene.

The key to successful sedation of critically ill patients is constant assessment of their responsiveness and comfort. This should be carried out using a sedation score or structured format to allow comparison between different staff members. Adjustment of sedative doses should then be carried out according to agreed unit protocols. Kress *et al.* (2000) found that daily inter-ruption of sedation until the patient is awake was associated with a significant reduction in length of ICU stay and duration of mechanical ventilation.

Bispectral Index monitoring (BIS™)

Bispectral Index monitoring is an objective method of monitoring awareness using a processed signal electroencephalogram (EEG) which is measured on a scale of 0–100, where 0 is a flat line EEG and 100 is fully

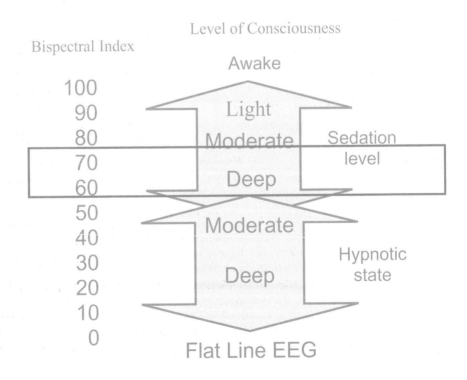

Fig. 3.4 Bispectral Index monitoring (BIS™) scale indicating level of consciousness.

awake (Fig. 3.4). It has mainly been used in the operating theatre but may potentially be useful in critical care, particularly when assessing underlying sedation levels in patients receiving muscle relaxants. There are some problems with monitoring as there may be spurious values with muscle movement and in encephalopathic patients.

Personal hygiene

Mouth care

The healthy mouth has rapidly proliferating squamous epithelial cells lining from the inside of the lips to the oropharynx. These cells are highly vulnerable to the effects of poor blood flow, malnutrition, and drug toxicity and are therefore particularly at risk in the critically ill patient.

The risk is increased by the loss of normal cleaning mechanisms, increased vulnerability of the patient to infection, and the presence of an oral endotracheal (ET) tube which causes pressure on the mucosa. Other contributory factors include:

- A decreased or absent oral fluid intake.

- Dehydration of the buccal mucosa related to inhaling dry gases, systemic dehydration, stress, and tachypnoea (which increases mouth breathing).

- Decreased salivary stimulation due to loss of food as a stimulating factor and increased sympathetic arousal.

- An increased likelihood of specific factors such as antibiotics, renal failure, vitamin deficiency, xerostomic drugs (e.g. atropine and catecholamines).

- Decreased host defence mechanisms giving rise to an increased risk of mouth infection, particularly *Candida*, herpes simplex virus, and *Streptococcus viridans*.

MOUTH CARE: DEFINITIONS

- Stomatitis: an inflammatory and ulcerative reaction of the oral cavity.

- Xerostomia: the subjective sensation of dryness in the mouth.

- Glossitis: inflammation of the tongue.

- Gingivitis: inflammation of the gums.

- Inability to maintain own oral hygiene.

- Continued formation of plaque and debris on teeth whether the patient is eating or drinking or not.

- presence of plaque will cause gingivitis.

- The oral ET tube can cause pressure problems and impede full assessment of and access to the oral cavity.

Little research has been performed on mouth care problems in the critically ill and even less on the efficacy of different mouth care procedures (Roth and Creason 1986). However, work in the dental and periodontal fields can be extrapolated in some cases to identify the correct tools and cleansing agents, and the few studies that do exist can provide some guidelines for oral hygiene in the critically ill (Howarth 1977, Miller and Kearney 2001, Pearson 2002). (See Table 3.10 for how to assess the condition of the mouth.)

Management of oral hygiene and preventive care

The frequency and type of hygiene intervention should be based on an assessment of the oral cavity (see Table 3.10) rather than routine care:

- A small, soft toothbrush moistened in water to provide a neutral pH (Gooch 1985) and used in a circular

---

| TABLE 3.10 | Assessment of the oral cavity. Adapted from Richardson (1987) and Crosby (1989) |

Oral cavity	Normal	Abnormal	Intervention
Mucosa	Pink, moist, intact, smooth	Reddening, ulceration, other lesions	Hydration, use of neutral mouthwash, pain-relieving anaesthetic gels for ulceration
Tongue	Pink, moist, intact, papillae present	Coated, absence of papillae with smooth shiny appearance, debris, lesions, crusted, cracks, blackened	Hydration, frequent neutral mouthwashes, use of a debriding agent such as sodium bicarbonate for blackened areas
Lips	Clean, intact, pink	Dry skin, cracks, reddened, encrusted, ulcerated, bleeding	Hydration, protection using petroleum jelly or KY jelly
Saliva	Watery, white, or clear	Thick, viscous, absent, blood-stained	Hydration, use of artificial salivas
Gingiva (gums)	Pink, moist, firm	Receding, overgrowing, oedematous, reddened, bleeding	Tooth brushing 2–3 times daily with small, soft brush. Chlorhexidine 10% mouthwash
Teeth	White, firm in sockets, no debris, no decay	Discoloured, decayed, debris present, wobbly	Tooth brushing 2–3 times daily with small, soft brush. Dental assessment

motion, or with short horizontal strokes, has been shown to be more effective than foam sticks or swabs in removing debris/plaque (DeWalt 1975, Pearson 2002).

◆ Dilute hydrogen peroxide (20% vol. solution diluted 1:4 with water) or sodium bicarbonate (half a teaspoon to 500 ml water) can be used for removing debris and dissolving tenacious mucus.

◆ If there is evidence of infection, such as stomatitis or gingivitis, use of an antimicrobial mouthwash or toothpaste such as chlorhexidine gluconate 10% may help (De Riso *et al.* 2001) but the major intervention is preventive removal of plaque (Kite and Pearson 1995, Pearson 2002).

◆ Lips should be protected from drying out with either Vaseline or KY jelly.

◆ A neutral mouthwash solution (non-hygroscopic) may be used for patient comfort but has not be shown to have any effect on maintenance of mucosal integrity.

◆ Limited use (two to three times a day) of lemon and glycerin hygroscopic mouthwash may help stimulate salivary production (Warner 1986), but artificial saliva sprays are probably more effective.

◆ If the mouth is very dry and fluids are limited or difficult to swallow artificial saliva spray may be of help.

◆ Dentures should be removed overnight—cleaning and soaking should be performed during this period.

◆ Adequate fluid hydration of the patient will help with xerostomia.

◆ Oral candida should be treated with nystatin mouthwash.

Severe oral problems can cause considerable distress to patients as well as providing a reservoir of organisms such as *Candida albicans* which can lead to systemic infection.

Altering nursing practice has been slow. Grap *et al.* (2003) reported that nurses were still much more likely to use a sponge (foam swab) than a small, soft toothbrush for oral care in intubated patients. An evidence-based protocol may help reduce the incidence of problems (Fitch *et al.* 1999).

Eye care

The healthy eye is protected from dehydration and infection by the production of tears. The tear film is made up of three layers, the outer lipid layer, the middle water-based layer, and the inner mucilaginous layer. Each layer has a specific purpose. The outer layer retards fluid evaporation and prevents overflow of tear film. The middle layer contains oxygen, electrolytes, and proteins including antibacterial agents. The inner layer aids wetting of the cornea. The normal rate of production of tears by the lacrimal gland is about 1–2 μl/min and these are spread over the surface of the cornea by the blink reflex.

As many as 60% of critically ill patients who are sedated and on muscle relaxants may develop corneal ulceration (Imanaka *et al.* 1997). Ventilated and sedated patients are particularly susceptible to eye care problems due to:

1. A reduced or absent ability to blink.

2. Incomplete lid closure.

3. Decreased tear production as a side-effect of certain drugs including atropine, phenothiazines, and tricyclic antidepressants.

4. Decreased resistance to infection and increased likelihood of cross-infection from respiratory pathogens (Hilton *et al.* 1983, Parkin *et al.* 1997). This is related to poor suction technique where the catheter is removed from the ET tube over the top of the eye, disseminating droplets containing organisms into the cornea (Ommeslag *et al.* 1987, Parkin *et al.* 1997).

5. An increased likelihood of orbital oedema due to the high intrathoracic pressures produced by positive pressure ventilation reducing venous return. This is exacerbated if the patient is nursed flat during periods of instability or if the tapes securing tracheostomy or endotracheal tubes are tied too tightly. The dependent areas are affected and fluid is forced into the periocular tissues and the conjunctival membrane.

6. Dehydration reduces tear production.

There are two common eye care problems associated with the ventilated or unconscious patient: *dry eyes* and *exposure keratopathy*. The problem of dry eyes is due to any, or all, of the above factors (1)–(6) as well as incorrect positioning of high-flow oxygen or a CPAP mask. This can quickly dry corneal surfaces even when the blink reflex is intact. Exposure keratopathy is caused by exposure of the corneal surface due to incomplete lid closure which leads to drying, epithelial erosions, and, ultimately, corneal ulceration. The risk of infection is also increased.

Management of the eyes and eye problems

1. Assess the following aspects to determine the required frequency of intervention:

♦ the patient's ability to close the eyelid voluntarily or involuntarily,

♦ patient position,

♦ the patient's hydration status,

♦ the condition of the cornea—look for evidence of infection (purulent or crusting exudate), clouding, haemorrhage, etc.,

♦ evidence of discharge,

♦ drugs.

2. Use sterile water for cleansing (saline has been found to disrupt the normal tear film structure and increase the rate of evaporation).

3. If corneal wetting is inadequate use artificial tears (methylcellulose drops) up to half-hourly.

4. If the corneal surface is constantly exposed, close the lids using hydrogel pads, paraffin gauze, or eye shields. Taping eyes is traumatic to the eyelid and can be unsightly for the patient's family, although some experts feel that this is the only secure method of keeping the patient's eyes shut (Suresh *et al.* 2000). Recently, use of a moisture chamber (a layer of polyethylene film ('cling film') that covers the eyes, extending beyond the orbits and eyebrows and which is taped to the face) has been shown to preserve the corneal epithelium significantly more effectively that the use of artificial tears(Cortese *et al.* 1995). It is as effective as lacrilube ointment and artificial tears (Koroloff *et al.* 2004),

5. Care should be taken when withdrawing suction catheters to avoid droplet transference of respiratory organisms to the corneal surface (Ommeslag *et al.* 1987). Bacterial keratopathy is associated with poor suction technique and the use of open suction systems (Parkin *et al.* 1997)

6. If the eye is discharging or obviously infected take a swab for microbial culture and sensitivity and apply appropriate topical antibiotic drops or ointment as prescribed.

Prevention of problems associated with urinary catheterization

Most critically ill patients are catheterized to allow close monitoring of urinary output. However, the presence of a urinary catheter has a number of problems associated with it. These are discussed below.

Problems to be addressed
Increased risk of urinary tract infection

According to the EPIC study (Vincent et al 1995), urinary tract infections are the second most common nosocomial infection in critical care patients. The incidence of bacteriuria in catheterized critical care patients is between 11 and 14% (Leone *et al.* 2001). This is due to:

♦ Trauma associated with insertion of the catheter which creates breaks in mucosal integrity allowing bacterial colonization.

♦ Contamination during insertion and afterwards due to poor hand-washing/hygiene procedures.

♦ Bypassing of the normal defence mechanisms of the urethra.

♦ Use of larger than necessary catheters which cause pressure on the urethral wall and ischaemia.

♦ Use of larger than necessary balloons which cause pressure on the bladder wall and an increase in residual urine.

♦ Obliteration of the natural urethral mucosal cleansing which occurs during voiding. The flow of urine in the normal condition discourages migration of pathogens.

♦ Susceptibility of the patient to infection is increased due to any serious underlying pathology.

♦ The critical care environment has an increased level of pathogenic bacteria (see section below on infection risks in critical care). Note that 55% of catheterized patients develop bacteriuria within 48 hours.

Trauma and discomfort associated with the presence of the catheter

This is due to :

♦ Use of catheters which are larger than necessary.

♦ Movement/dragging of the catheter.

♦ Use of balloons which are larger than necessary (Lowthian 1989).

Blockage of the catheter from debris or blood

This is due to:

♦ Poor urinary flow allowing debris to collect in the bladder.

♦ Urinary tract infection producing large amount of debris.

Management of problems associated with urinary catheterization

There should be strict asepsis for catheter insertion.

♦ Hand-washing must take place prior to any manipulation of the catheter.

◆ A closed urinary drainage system should be maintained with minimal manipulation of any part (Platt *et al.* 1983).

◆ Unimpeded urinary flow should be maintained with no reflux (positioning of the drainage bag is all important to ensure gravity-aided flow) (Mulhall *et al.* 1988).

◆ There must be strict asepsis for collection of a catheter specimen of urine (CSU) through the specimen port. (Note: the drainage system should never be disconnected for this.)

◆ Avoid bladder irrigation unless absolutely necessary. If possible, irrigate through the specimen port using a needle rather than disconnecting the drainage system (Burgener 1987).

◆ Use the smallest size catheter that will drain adequately. This is usually 12–14 Ch (= 4–4.5 mm external diameter) (Robinson 2001).

◆ Only use a 5–10 ml balloon catheter, unless immediately following bladder or prostatic surgery when a larger balloon may be necessary for haemostatic purposes (Belfield 1988).

◆ Attach the catheter to the inner aspect of the thigh using a specifically designed device to prevent drag (Hanchett 2002).

◆ Carry out daily, or more frequently if necessary, meatal cleansing with soap and water or saline. There is no evidence to support the use of antiseptic solutions for cleansing (Mulhall *et al.* 1988)

◆ Ensure that the catheter used is appropriate to the likely length of catheterization (PTFE, polytetrafluoroethylene) for medium-term use up to 4 weeks, hydrogel or silicone elastomer for up to 12 weeks' use. Patients with a latex allergy should only have a pure silicone catheter (Robinson 2001).

◆ Ensure that the foreskin does not remain retracted, which can cause a painful phimosis.

Prevention of the effects of restricted mobility

Most critically ill patients are either unable to move themselves or have only limited movement of their limbs. They remain in one position unless moved by their nurses, and when unstable are frequently nursed flat. Even in the recovery phase they are often too weak to move themselves and may remain in one position for much longer than normal. The effects of immobility are a major problem to the critically ill patient and prevention of problems can make the difference between recovery and death. The quality of life of any surviving patient may also be reduced if these problems are ignored.

The effects of restricted mobility
Increased risk of chest infection
The increased risk of chest infection is due to:

◆ basal collapse,

◆ increased secretions,

◆ decreased sputum clearance, and

◆ ventilation to perfusion (V/Q) mismatch secondary to atelectasis, dependent lung oedema, and alterations due to positioning.

Lung volumes (functional residual capacity (FRC) and residual volumes) are reduced when lying supine due to the rise in the diaphragm associated with the change in position of the abdominal contents. Impaired ability to cough, decreased ciliary movement, and weak thoracic muscles cause stasis and pooling of secretions. Production of alveolar surfactant may be impaired during periods when the patient is flat and the ratio of ventilation to perfusion is also altered by the supine, lateral, and prone position.

Increased risk of deep vein thrombosis and peripheral oedema
The increased risk of deep vein thrombosis and peripheral oedema during immobilization is due to:

◆ decreased venous return,

◆ venous stasis, and

◆ increased coagulability associated with loss of muscle pumps.

Loss of muscle movement means that the normal pumping mechanism returning venous blood to the heart is reduced. Pooling occurs which increases intracapillary hydrostatic pressure. This rise increases the movement of fluid through the capillary membrane into the interstitial tissues. The extracapillary shift of fluid increases the viscosity of the blood causing further stasis and increased risk of platelet aggregation and coagulation.

Muscle atrophy due to disuse
The rate of muscle atrophy is rapid in the early immobilization phase and is often accelerated by the catabolic nature of the patient's illness. The muscles of the thigh and calf usually exhibit the greatest reduction and lead to weakness and fatigue requiring long periods of convalescence to rebuild (Griffiths and Jones 2002).

Joint stiffness and contractures

The particular risk lies with flexion, as the flexor muscles are stronger than the extensors. If exercises to maintain the normal range of movement do not occur, the muscle becomes permanently shortened resulting in limb contractures. Common sites include plantar flexor, shoulder, hand, hip, and knee joints (Adam and Forrest 1999).

Demineralization and loss of density in the long bones

Loss of weight-bearing pressure within the long bones results in decreased osteoblastic (bone forming and repair) activity. Osteoclastic (bone destruction) activity continues, resulting in a loss of bone density and, ultimately, osteoporosis. Hypercalcaemia and hypercalciuria are seen within 1 to 2 days of immobility and have been associated with prolonged immobility in all age groups in spite of adequate calcium intake.

Peripheral nerve injury

The particular risk is ulnar nerve injury due to incorrect positioning. Pronation of the forearm in the supine position traps the ulnar nerve in the cubital tunnel and flexion of the elbow in this position will add further pressure on the ulnar nerve. Risk factors include diabetes mellitus, bed rest for more than 22 hours a day, age of patient >50 yr, and alcoholism (Chuman 1985).

Increased risk of pressure sores

This is due to pressure on dependent areas and an inability to change position as required.

Development of pressure sores is dependent on the product of the level of pressure exerted and the time it is exerted for. The higher the pressure, the less time is required for a sore to develop. The most vulnerable areas are the tissues over bony prominences (see Fig. 3.5).

Critically ill patients are particularly vulnerable to pressure sores due to a number of factors (see box). Studies show the development of pressure ulcers in between 12 and 56% of critical care patients (Jiricka et al. 1995, Carlson et al. 1999, Fife et al. 2001), most commonly on the sacrum or heels.

NICE (National Institute for Clinical Excellence) clinical guidelines (2001) identified risk factors for a general hospital population including:

♦ reduced mobility or immobility,

♦ sensory impairment,

Pressure points (see diagram)

(1) occiput	(7) sacrum
(2) acromion processes	(8) ischial tuberosities
(3) scapulae	(9) coccyx
(4) spinous processes	(10) medial epicondyles
(5) olecranon processes	(11) medial and lateral malleoli
(6) iliac crests	(12) calcaneus

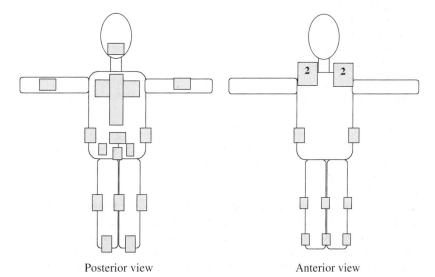

Fig. 3.5 Pressure points: 1, occiput; 2, acromion processes; 3, scapulae; 4, spinous processes; 5, olecranon processes; 6, iliac crests; 7, sacrum; 8, ischial tuberosities; 9, coccyx; 10, medial epicondyles; 11, medial and lateral malleoli; 12, calcaneus.

Posterior view   Anterior view

> ### PRESSURE SORE RISK FACTORS IN THE CRITICALLY ILL
>
> - Immobility
> - Emaciation and muscle wasting
> - Altered sensory function (often due to sedation) but also to decreased conscious level as part of multiorgan failure
> - Decreased cardiac output and tissue hypoperfusion
> - Increased vasoconstriction
> - Reduced venous return

- acute illness,
- level of consciousness,
- extremes of age,
- vascular disease,
- severe chronic or terminal illness,
- previous history of pressure damage,
- malnutrition and dehydration.

Critically ill patients generally exhibit at least three of these risk factors (see box) and therefore further more sensitive indicators may be required to differentiate high risk in the critically ill patient population. Batson *et al.* (1993) found five factors in a critically ill population which were specifically related to the development of pressure sores:

- diabetes,
- infusion of norepinephrine,
- infusion of epinephrine,
- restricted movement (e.g. traction, continuous venovenous haemofiltration intra-aortic balloon pump),
- patient too unstable to turn.

Relief of pressure simply by a 2-hourly change of position can be inadequate in the acutely ill and other methods of support may be required, such as special low-pressure or alternating-pressure support surfaces.

Increased risk of urinary tract infection

Increased risk of urinary tract infection in the critically ill patient is due to (Lauplan *et al.* 2002):

- urinary stasis,
- bladder distension,
- increase in urinary pH,
- decreased immune function,
- presence of a urinary catheter,
- length of stay,
- female gender.

The supine position results in the renal pelvis filling with urine before drainage via the ureter occurs. This urinary stasis acts as a focus for bacterial growth and the formation of renal calculi. There will also be an accumulation of urine in the bladder in the supine position due to filling of the dependent portion of the bladder prior to drainage via the urethra. This may be relieved by the presence of a urinary catheter. There may be an increase in urinary pH due to increased calcium and phosphate excretion which will increase the infection risk.

Increased incidence of nephrolithiasis (kidney stones)

This is due to increased urinary calcium excretion related to bone degeneration. Hypercalcaemia occurs as a result of degeneration of bone from disuse (see above) and this produces an increase in renal excretion of calcium and phosphate in the first week of bed rest. This can continue for up to 5 weeks.

Decreased gut motility and constipation

Muscle wasting and loss may include the muscles controlling excretion (diaphragm, abdominal muscles, and levator ani). Reduced gut motility may occur as a result of loss of stimuli such as the presence of food passing through the oesophagus.

The degree of immobility relates to the severity of illness, the need for sedation and paralysis, haemodynamic instability, spinal injuries, as a direct result of the illness, such as acute polyneuropathy (Guillain–Barré) syndrome, and loss of muscle function due to muscle wasting.

Management of problems due to restricted mobility

Central to the prevention of problems associated with immobility is the need to alter patient position frequently. This cannot always happen for reasons such as haemodynamic instability, changes in ventilation/ perfusion ratios due to shunting in certain positions, and spinal or pelvic trauma. In these situations other goals take priority but an awareness of the problems caused by periods of immobility will allow interventions to support and limit the effects during the rehabilitation phase. The following points are important in management:

- Regular turning and repositioning of the patient. Knowledge of the correct alignment and positioning of limbs to prevent joint injury.

- Use of specialist beds and mattresses which relieve pressure over susceptible points and spread the pressure load.

- Regular full inspection of skin integrity, with particular attention to the high-risk dependent areas.

- Passive limb movements and full range of movement (ROM) exercises for joints to maintain joint mobility.

- Where possible, active, isotonic limb and ROM exercises will maintain muscle strength and as well as joint mobility.

- Active chest physiotherapy, use of adequate humidification, etc. (see Chapter 4).

- Close observation of bowel function.

- Early commencement of feeding (especially enteral).

- Scrupulous attention to infection control measures.

- Early and frequent mobilization.

Prevention of the complications associated with immobility is unlikely to alter the patient outcome but may contribute significantly to the rate of rehabilitation and the degree of morbidity following discharge.

Infection risks in intensive care

Critically ill patients have a high incidence (between 10 and 15%) of nosocomial infection (EPIC study; Vincent *et al.* 1995). Richards *et al.* (1999) found that 31% of nosocomial infections in medical ICUs were due to urinary tract infections, 27% to pneumonia, and 19% to primary bloodstream infections. Almost all urinary tract infections (95%) were associated with urinary catheters, 87% of bacteraemias were associated with central lines, and 86% of nosocomial pneumonias were associated with mechanical ventilation. A large proportion of patient infection is therefore due to the invasive therapies required to support critically ill patients in the critical care environment. Invasive devices will facilitate colonization by nosocomial organisms and greatly increase vulnerability to infection.

As well as the high level of susceptibility, the increased incidence of antibiotic usage in the critical care environment creates resistant strains which can be transmitted from patient to patient (Bion *et al.* 2001).

Opportunistic and fungal infections can also occur as a result of compromised host defence mechanisms and the use of antibiotics, which reduce indigenous bacterial flora, allowing overgrowth of other organisms (Humphreys 2001).

The high risk of infection in the critically ill patient is due to both *patient-related problems*:

SIGNIFICANT RISK FACTORS FOR INFECTIONS IN CRITICALLY ILL PATIENTS
Presence of urinary catheter>10 days → 3.2-fold increase in risk
Stay in ICU> 3 days → 2.5-fold increase in risk
Intracranial pressure monitor *in situ* → 2.5-fold increase in risk
Arterial line → 1.5-fold increase in risk
Shock → 2.5-fold increase in risk
(Craven *et al.* 1988)

- invasive procedures and monitoring,

- supine body position and enteral feed (Drakulovic *et al.* 1999)

- abnormal humoral immunity,

- abnormal phagocytic function,

- abnormal antibody function,

- possible genetic factors (Bion *et al.* 2001),

and *environment-related problems*:

- high numbers of high-risk patients in one area,

- high usage of antibiotics encourages growth of resistant bacteria,

- if staffing levels fall to less than 1:1, cross-infection may be increased (Fridkin *et al.* 1996).

Intravascular devices

These comprise central venous catheters, arterial and peripheral venous cannulae, and pulmonary artery flotation catheters.

Any intravascular cannula left *in situ* will provide a direct portal of entry for microorganisms into the circulation. Local and systemic infections can occur even with peripheral cannulae, particularly if they are plastic, inserted as an emergency, or by cut-down technique, and left *in situ* for more than 72 hours (Maki 1989).

Patients with central venous catheters are likely to have a 9.2-fold increase in risk of infection if there is cutaneous colonization of the site. The most common site of origin of organisms causing catheter tip infections and bacteraemia is the catheter hub (Linares *et al.* 1985). There is conflicting evidence as to the infection rates associated with multilumen as opposed to single-lumen central venous catheters, with some studies reporting no difference in rates and some reporting a

ROUTES OF INFECTION IN INTRAVASCULAR DEVICES

- Hub contamination leading to transfer of organisms down the cannula
- Connections between the giving set and cannula such as three-way taps
- Site contamination
- Thrombosis of the cannula providing a medium for organism growth

significant difference (Dezfulian *et al.* 2003). The variation may be related to the heterogeneity involved in the study populations, with some studies using non-randomized samples. When higher-quality studies were examined in a meta-analysis by Dezfulian *et al.* (2003), there was no significant difference in catheter-related bloodstream infection. This is thought to be due to other advantages of multiple lumens such as decreased need for manipulation and use of multiple connection devices, and the reduction in the number of invasive procedures required with their use.

Use of needle-less systems, to allow access to central and peripheral venous catheters without breaking the circuit, may well reduce infection rates but current research in this area is limited.

Ventilator-associated pneumonia (VAP)

Ventilator-associated pneumonia refers to a new occurrence of pneumonia in intubated or acutely tracheostomized patients receiving mechanical ventilation (Rello and Diaz 2003).

Relevant risk factors involved in the development of this type of nosocomial pneumonia are frequently present in critically ill patients and include:

- presence of an endotracheal tube (risk is increased 21-fold),
- chronic ill health, particularly chronic pulmonary disease,
- malnutrition,
- use of H_2 (histamine receptor) antagonists to prevent stress ulceration (see Chapter 10),
- use of antibiotics,
- smoking,
- prolonged upper abdominal or thoracic surgery,
- impaired upper airway reflexes such as the cough reflex,

- advanced age and obesity,
- supine body position,
- enteral nutrition.

Mechanisms of infection include:

- contamination of inspired air (e.g. respiratory therapy equipment),
- spread from contiguous (neighbouring) infected tissue,
- blood-borne spread from distant infections on tricuspid valve vegetations,
- oropharyngeal and gastric colonization with transmission to the trachea probably by aspiration (Pingleton 1991).

Aspiration is the most frequent cause of infection in ventilated patients due to the presence of ET tubes. ET tubes provide protection from large volume aspiration but may actually facilitate transfer of tiny amounts of aspirate (microaspiration) by preventing closure of the vocal cords and bypassing the cough reflex. The presence of enteral feed in the stomach and the resultant rise in gastric pH may also be related to overgrowth of bacteria and an increase in aspiration pneumonia (Jacobs *et al.* 1990). Supine body position is also implicated in this; Drakulovic *et al.* (1999) have shown a significant decrease ($p < 0.003$) in the incidence of ventilator-associated pneumonia associated with nursing patients at 45° head up.

Most nosocomial pneumonias are due to Gram-negative organisms (Santamaria 1990, Richards *et al.* 1999). Prevention is the aim, as identification and treatment of the causative organism can be difficult and ineffective.

Preventative measures

1. Ventilator and circuits:
   - Use of HME humidifiers (with bacterial filters) rather than water bath humidifiers.
   - Regular change of ventilator circuits and manual ventilation systems at least every 48 hours if HME humidifiers are not used.
   - Scrupulous hand-washing and use of gloves prior to endotracheal suctioning.
   - Use of disposable nebulizers or scrupulous washing and drying of reusable nebulizers between use.
   - Use of closed suction catheter systems (Combes *et al.* 2000).

2. The patient:
   - Regular change of position allowing maximum basal lung expansion from semi-recumbent to left and right lateral.

- Regular chest physiotherapy (see Chapter 4).
- Maintain a semi-recumbent position (the patient's head is elevated to between 30 and 45°) (Drakulovic et al. 1999). This is associated with a reduction in the incidence of VAP from 34% to 8% in ventilated patients.

Urinary tract infections

Nosocomial urinary tract infections (UTIs) are the most frequent infections seen in critical care (Bihari 1992). Nearly all infections are related to the presence of an indwelling urinary catheter.

The most important preventative measure is to avoid urinary catheterization unless absolutely essential, although this will have little effect in the critically ill patient where monitoring of renal function and urine production is essential for managing most patients.. If catheterization is necessary, early removal should be a major goal, although this is frequently impractical in the critically ill patient

Catheter insertion should always be performed aseptically and thorough hand-washing carried out prior to any manipulation of the drainage system. Closed-circuit drainage systems should always be used. Use of topical antibiotics for irrigation and meatal cleansing have not been shown to have any effect,

Hand-washing

One of the major preventable routes of transmission of nosocomial infection is via the hands of unit personnel (20–40% of infections) and the single most important factor in preventing transmission is a scrupulous hand-washing technique (Turner 1993). Environmental factors, such as positioning of wash-basins with easy access from each bed area, and sufficient numbers of wash-basins to allow unrestricted access are important in supporting hand-washing. Education programmes may be effective in improving compliance (Butler 1998). The introduction of alcohol rubs, either in individual staff tubes which can be attached to uniforms or in bottles at the bedside, may be beneficial in increasing hand cleansing (Pittet et al. 1999).

Individual unit policy may vary on infection control procedures but the guidelines in Table 3.11 give a synopsis of the policies identified as reducing the level of nosocomial infection in intensive care.

Transfer of critically ill patients

Secondary transfer refers to transfer from or within a hospital setting. The transfer of critically ill patients requires thought, preparation, appropriate equipment, and a high level of expertise (ICS 2002). Unfortunately,

TABLE 3.11 Synopsis of measures for limiting infection in the critical care environment (Fridkin 1996, Pittet et al. 1999, Humphreys 2001)

Strict adherence to local infection control policies

Hand-washing/use of alcohol rub between patient contacts

Use of aprons and gloves for patient contact (universal precautions)

Maintaining a 30–45° semi-recumbent position to reduce aspiration

Maintaining staffing ratios appropriate to patient need/workload

Strict aseptic technique for dressings, line insertions, invasive procedures, etc.

Limitation of manipulation of IV lines, urinary catheters, dressings

Policy of immediate removal of IV lines if infection is suspected

Infection control standards/protocols for staff

Feedback from microbiology regarding infection rates

Avoidance of antacid ulcer prophylaxis and H_2 blockers in combination

Avoidance of endotracheal intubation wherever possible by use of CPAP (see Chapter 4) and other forms of non-invasive ventilation

Adherence to a locally defined antimicrobial policy

this is rarely seen when patients are rushed from one hospital to another as part of a desperate measure to find a critical care bed and may be a contributory factor in the increased morbidity associated with such moves. Bion et al. (1988) showed that most journeys are inadequately prepared for, hurriedly undertaken, noisy, traumatic, and frequently lead to a discontinuation of vital monitoring or therapy. Waddell (1975) found a high incidence of deterioration in the patient's condition directly accountable to being moved.

It is therefore imperative that the safest possible environment for transfer is created and the nurse should be responsible for ensuring that this is done before the journey starts. These journeys may constitute either accompanying a patient from one critical care unit to another, or going out from a specialist critical care unit to pick up a patient from another unit.

Suggested procedure

- Transfer should be handled by experienced, suitably qualified personnel.
- The equipment used should be designed for transport with reliable performance and battery back-up.
- Monitoring should consist of a minimum of ECG, pulse oximetry, invasive or non-invasive blood pressure, and end tidal CO_2 (Hope and Runcie 1993).

- Staff should be familiar with the equipment used.

- The patient should be stabilized prior to transfer.

- If it is likely that intubation or other therapeutic manoeuvres may be needed, these should be carried out prior to transfer.

- Ideally, mobile flying squads should be established to stabilize and then transfer patients.

- The patient's infective status should be checked in order that adequate precautions may be taken in the event of such problems as MRSA.

Care prior to and during transport

1. Ensure patient safety prior to and during transfer:
   - check all equipment for performance, battery life, and functioning alarm systems,
   - set up and use appropriate alarm settings,
   - ensure all staff transferring the patient are familiar with all equipment including emergency equipment.

2. Stabilize the patient prior to transfer and monitor the patient during transfer (Table 3.12). Any patient with respiratory problems should be assessed prior to the journey by an experienced intensivist or anaesthetist for possible intubation and elective ventilation prior to transfer. If the patient is not intubated he/she should be accompanied by someone experienced in intubation. Use of rebreathe bags over a long journey is likely to result in hypercapnia, but they are acceptable for short journeys.

3. Notification of relatives. Ensure relatives are aware of the reason for transfer, the approximate journey time, the details of the receiving hospital, and the name of the receiving consultant. If possible, provide a copy of the unit information booklet for patient's relatives and, if necessary, supply directions.

4. Collection of copies of documentation. The following are important: notes, X-rays, diagnostic reports, charts, nursing documentation, prescription chart. A synopsis of problems, incidents, and management as well as care given should be produced by the transferring hospital.

5. Arrangements for transfer:
   - These should be carried out only when the patient is virtually ready for transfer.

TABLE 3.12　Preparing the critically ill patient for transfer

Problem	Prior to transfer	During transfer
Airway and O_2 requirements	ABGs. CXR. Insert chest drains if necessary. Intubate if necessary. Chest physiotherapy and suction	Portable ventilator (ideally). Pulse oximetry. Portable suction and catheters. Oxygen supply with at least 1 h over calculated requirements. Rebreathe bag or Ambu bag
Cardiovascular support	Insert any central venous access/arterial lines. Correct any electrolyte or pH abnormality (as far as possible). Set up support drug infusions. Check temperature. Insert pacing wire if necessary	ECG and systemic BP monitoring. If possible, CVP monitoring facility. Continuous drug infusion via battery-operated pump. Portable defibrillator and emergency drugs to hand. Adequate bed linen for patient
Maintenance of fluid balance	Insert urinary catheter. Set up required infusions. Place nasogastric tube if necessary	Carry appropriate fluid for infusion plus extra colloid and crystalloid. Continue urinary and nasogastric drainage during transfer
Patient anxiety and fear of journey	Introduce transfer team to patient. Inform patient of reasons for transfer, location of receiving hospital, and approximate journey time. Reassure patient about relatives, visiting, and any other queries	Continue to reassure the patient and inform them of progress. Ensure the patient is secure and comfortable on the trolley
Pain control and sedation	Assess patient's pain. Ensure adequate supplies of analgesia for journey. Set up analgesic/sedative infusions if required	Reassess pain: sedation as necessary
Miscellaneous	Insert wound drains. Stabilize fractures. Assess pressure areas	Carry adequate drainage containers. Transfer on pressure-relieving mattress

- ◆ Notify ambulance control, and the police, if necessary.
- ◆ Inform the receiving hospital immediately prior to departure of an estimated time of arrival. (Note: Inter-hospital transfer by helicopter or aircraft is a specialized procedure which should only be carried out by trained teams.)

Elective versus emergency admissions to critical care

Most critical care units will admit a mixture of elective and emergency admissions. Preparation for these two types of patients is different and their needs and prognosis will also differ.

Elective patients

Admissions are usually post-operative but may occasionally be pre-operative if haemodynamic optimization is required:

1. The patient is usually prepared for admission, he/she may have visited the critical care area and will have been given information from nursing and medical staff as well as other healthcare professionals. It is likely that relatives will also be well informed and may have met critical care staff prior to admission. Thus, the elective patient has some defence or coping mechanisms to aid him/her in making sense of the environment.

2. The admission its usually only for a short period of time (frequently overnight) and the effects of ventilation, the critical care environment, close observation and monitoring, and sensory disturbance are likely to be minimal.

3. Recovery is usually swift unless complications develop and the patient may have only limited recollection of the time spent in the critical care unit due to a combination of anaesthesia and analgesia.

These factors make elective admission patients far less vulnerable to the problems associated with being in intensive care provided that care is taken to prepare them adequately and to prevent complications occurring.

Emergency admissions

1. By the nature of the crisis which precipitated admission, these patients are often sicker and have a poorer prognosis. Patient scoring systems, such as APACHE II (see Chapter 17), carry weighting which reflects this.

2. The lack of preparation increases fear and decreases the ability of the patient to cope with the stresses of the critical care environment. They are therefore highly vulnerable to the problems associated with an admission to critical care.

3. Recovery is frequently prolonged and less likely to occur, although this varies with the cause of admission.

4. The emergency produces shock and distress in both patient and relatives who must cope with this unexpected life-threatening event.

Strategies

1. Intensive and repeated information-giving is essential. People do not process information or retain it when distressed or shocked. It is therefore important to limit the amount of information given, but to repeat it frequently.

2. Support is often limited to the relatives when the patient is first admitted as the serious nature of the illness make it impossible to establish two-way communication. However, information-giving for the patient should continue, and reassurance that care and treatment are being carried accompanied by caring touch may help the patient.

3. Alternative support agencies for both relatives and patients should be considered and used where appropriate.

The dying ICU patient

Intensive care is associated with a high mortality rate which will vary from week to week but which is likely overall to be between 15 and 25% of patients (Rowan et al. 1993). In some cases, death will occur as a fairly immediate event following emergency admission to the unit and there will be little time to prepare either the patient or the family. In the majority of cases, death will occur after a period of several days on the unit and will be an expected outcome. In a small number of patients it will become evident that further intervention and the continuation of treatment is both distressing for the patient and futile. The ethics of decisions regarding withdrawal of treatment are discussed fully in Chapter 17; however, care of the dying patient and his/her family will be discussed here.

Withdrawal of treatment

It is generally accepted that once it has been decided that additional medical intervention will not assist the patient, the priorities change to those of care and comfort. It should be stressed to the family that this does not mean any reduction in the level of care the patient will receive.

Analgesia and sedation may have been carefully controlled to limit cardiovascular side-effects and important but uncomfortable treatment, such as physiotherapy and suction, may have been carried out on a frequent basis to assist the patient in achieving a cure. Once the decision is taken to withdraw or to limit further interventions then care as opposed to cure becomes the priority and the patient's physical and psychological needs should supersede any other considerations. Analgesia should be given at levels that ensure pain relief, and unnecessary interventions, such as suction, should be limited to the minimum required to maintain patient comfort.

Comfort, psychological care, and support are paramount, not only for the patient but also for the patient's family. Where the patient is able to respond, any decisions on pain relief, movement, personal hygiene, and comfort should be discussed with them.

Use of alternative methods of pain relief and dealing with anxiety should be considered. The patient may feel that they would prefer to be alert and able to communicate with their family as long as possible. In this case, they may negotiate a tolerable level of pain in order to avoid the drowsiness and disorientation associated with increased quantities of analgesia.

Supporting the family/friends of the dying patient

The phrase 'family/friends' will be used to cover all those with relationships of importance to the patient.

Kirchhoff *et al.* (2002) have identified six key points in the family/friends experiences with death in the intensive care unit:

1. Uncertainty pervades the end-of-life experience of patients' families in the critical care unit.

2. Family members are torn between technology and individual choice.

3. Family members experience a responsibility to protect the patient.

4. Families' information about the patient is often lacking or inadequate.

5. Effective communication with the staff is the best antidote for uncertainty among patients' family members.

6. Families need adequate opportunity to say good-bye.

The key messages to guide caring for family/friends of a dying patient are:

◆ There is an enormous need for effective provision of information (i.e. concrete and objective) and ongoing communication.

◆ Family/friends should be supported in letting go and saying goodbye to the patient.

◆ The patient's family/friends should be helped in managing the two alternating processes that occur in order to make sense of traumatic events—(1) intrusive experiencing and re-experiencing of the traumatic event and (2) protective denial (Kirchhoff *et al.* 2002).

Breaking the news of impending death

The family/friends should be told by a senior member of the medical staff who is familiar with the patient and family/friends. A member of the nursing staff should be present and, if appropriate, other professional support such as the chaplain or a counsellor.

The setting should be private, available for as long as necessary, and away from the hubbub of the unit (Dyer 1993).

Details may have to be repeated a number of times. The family/friends are usually distressed and may be able to take in only minimal information. They may need reassurance regarding concerns about the patient's level of suffering and discomfort and spiritual needs/values should be addressed. (Organ donation is dealt with in Chapter 10.)

Supporting the family in coping with death

The news that the patient is dying will usually destroy any hope that the family may have cherished for recovery. Having their deepest fears expressed as a certainty provides a trigger for a crisis point and it is often only then that they will break down. Responses range from grief to denial and anger. Some people use denial as a coping mechanism and will be unable to accept what is said to them. Their response may seem inappropriate to the gravity of the situation and staff may need to assess the individual to determine whether forcing them to face reality or retain their defence is appropriate.

Anger may also be expressed as a response to the situation and should be dealt with using understanding and tact.

Communication

Frequent communication and information within an open and honest relationship between staff and the family/friends are important aspects of support. Any conversation with the family/friends may include cues for help, information, and support, so listening is as vital as saying the right things at the right time. Use of non-verbal communication—touch, facial expression, sitting with the family—is comforting and expresses concern. Sometimes, it may be as helpful to sit in silence and it is useful for the nurse to become comfortable with this.

Participation in care of the patient

This should be discussed with the family/friends as well as the patient where possible, and areas of care which are appropriate should be defined. Support and encouragement as well as education and direction in the delivery of care should be given. Examples include:

- mouth care
- massage
- hair washing and brushing
- reading to the patient
- positioning limbs
- caressing and holding
- helping to take oral fluids.

Steinhauser et al. (2000) found that dying patients rated freedom from pain, being at peace with God, the presence of the family, being mentally aware, knowing treatment choices were followed, having their finances in order, feeling life was meaningful, able to resolve conflicts, and able to die at home as most important to them. This study importantly showed that patients ranked periods of lucidity as almost as important as the relief of pain, in order to make preparation for their death.

Continuity of care

The family/friends should not have to establish relationships with members of staff they do not know at this stage. It is important to provide continuity of care from a few nurses who are known to the family and who may express a sense of affinity to them. This will help the family to feel supported and relieve some of the stress they may feel. However, it is likely to increase the stress that these nurses experience and they may well require extra support from those in charge, or their peers.

Establishing delivery of care to suit the patient, family, and friends

The nurse should discuss with the family whether they prefer privacy with the patient or the company of the nurse and they should arrange their care accordingly. If the family prefer privacy the nurse should withdraw from the immediate area but reassure the family that he/ she is readily available should they or the patient need him/her.

The family/friends should also be approached as to whether they wish to be present at the patient's death and if there is anyone else they would wish to be there (e.g. the chaplain or their own minister). This information should be recorded and communicated clearly between all those looking after the patient so that whenever death occurs their wishes can be met.

If the family/friends have expressed the desire to be present at the patient's death every effort should be made to ensure that they are informed in time for them to reach the hospital, if they are not present. Many people experience guilt associated with bereavement and failing to arrive in time to be with their loved one at their death can only add to this.

The patients' family/friends should be supported in deciding how they wish to organize the interim time. All may wish to stay or they may take it in turns to remain with the patient until death is near.

After death has occurred

Interventions that will help the bereaved to eventually come to terms with the loss include:

- Viewing the body after death. This facilitates grief and ultimate acceptance of the loss.
- Avoidance of euphemisms for death.
- Providing opportunities to return to bereavement support groups either specific to the critical care unit or generically within the healthcare service.

If there is a follow-up counselling service available, offer this further help.

Give clear details of what is required for registering the death and arranging removal of the body by the undertakers. Ideally, there should be an information sheet with these details to give to the family, but if not, make sure they are written down.

The effect of caring for the dying patient on the nurse

There is no doubt that coping with the experience of death is stressful for anyone. The work of Glaser and Strauss (1965) showed that the majority of nurses at that time coped by avoidance of the dying patient. This is not a possible alternative for the critical care nurse and most will have to develop other coping mechanisms.

Support groups and networks available either within the unit itself or the hospital are a useful external release and have the added advantage of being confidential.

Peer group support can be important but can also work negatively for some individuals. Unit atmosphere is an important factor. An open, accepting environment where all staff feel able to express their feelings will help the majority to cope. Team feeling and concern for co-workers is also supportive.

Kincey *et al.* (2003) found that junior nursing (and medical) staff were far more likely to be stressed than more experienced senior staff and particular attention should be paid to strong mentorship, clinical supervision, and support for this group of staff. There will always be those who require more than this, however. Senior staff should be constantly aware and able to intervene if necessary to provide a safety net for those vulnerable to the stress of caring for the dying patient.

The quality of care the patient and family receive in the critical care unit will have a major impact on their lives, not only at the time but also for many years afterwards. It is a part of the caring aim of nursing to ensure that their experience is as benign as possible in the circumstances.

Test yourself

Questions

1. List 10 of the common psychological and physiological causes of stress in critically ill patients.

2. What would you assess/check as a first priority when taking over a patient's care at the bedside?

3. Your patient is intubated, ventilator-dependent, and sedated, with two chest drains *in situ*, and has been on the ICU for 10 days without nutrition. Review the care that they would require by first identifying their nursing problems and then planning (and prioritizing) your care (refer back to the chapter to validate your plan).

Answers

1. *Physiological causes of stress*: infection, organ failure, organ failure, hypoxia, hypo/hypervolaemia, pyrexia, malnutrition, electrolyte imbalance. *Psychological causes of stress*: anxiety and fear, sensory imbalance, hallucinations, lack of (REM) sleep, communication difficulties, loss of family interaction and support, nightmares, loss of autonomy/control of one's body

2. *Airway*: Function of suction equipment, suction setting, correct size of suction catheter, if closed suction

system check patency of sleeve and clear with saline to check function, presence of airway adjuncts such as a Guedel airway, and Yankauer sucker. If a tracheostomy tube in place check for dilators and replacement tubes, one the same size and one a size smaller. *Breathing*: Functioning manual resuscitation bag attached to oxygen. Spare catheter mount if intubated. Check any emergency oxygen cylinders to ensure they are at least half full.

Circulation: Check arterial line is functional and accurate (transducers at correct height). Ensure the position of the cardiac arrest call button is known. Check infusions (particularly vasoactive drugs) to ensure there is sufficient in the pump and they are compatible with the prescription.

References and bibliography

Adam, S., Forrest, S. (1999). Other supportive care. In: *ABC of Intensive Care* (ed. M. Singer, I. Grant), pp. 28–32 BMJ books, London.

Aggleton, P., Chalmers, H. (1986). *Nursing Models and the Nursing Process*. Macmillan, London.

Albarran, J. (1991). A review of communication with intubated patients and those with tracheostomies within an intensive care environment. *Intensive Care Nursing* **7**, 179–86.

Appleyard, M.E., Gavaghan, S.R., Gonzalez, G., *et al.* (2000). Nurse-coached interventions for the families of patients in critical care units. *Critical Care Nurse* **20**, 40–8.

Arnold, M. (2003). Pressure ulcer prevention and management: the current evidence for care. *AACN Clinical Issues* **14**, 411–28.

Ashworth, P. (1980). *Care to Communicate*. Royal College of Nursing, Research Series, London.

Barrie-Shevlin, P. (1987). Maintaining sensory balance for the critically ill patient. *Nursing* **3**, 597–601.

Batson, S., Adam, S., Hall, G., *et al.* (1993). The development of a pressure area scoring system for critically ill patients: a pilot study. *Intensive and Critical Care Nursing* **9**, 146–51.

Baun, M.M., Flones, M.J. (1984). Cumulative effects of three sequential endotracheal suctioning episodes in the dog model. *Heart and Lung* **13**, 148–54.

Belfield, P.W. (1988). Urinary catheters. *British Medical Journal* **296**, 836–7.

Bergbom-Engberg, I., Haljamäe, H. (1989). Assessment of patients' experience of discomforts during respirator therapy. *Critical Care Medicine* **17**, 1068–71.

Bihari, D.J. (1992). Nosocomial infections in the intensive care unit. *Hospital Update* 266–76.

Bion, J.F., Brun-Buisson, C. (2000). Introduction – infection and critical illness: genetic and environmental aspects of susceptibility and resistance. *Intensive care medicine* **26**, S1–2.

Bion, J.F., Wilson, I.H., Taylor, P.A. (1988). Transporting critically ill patient by ambulance: audit by sickness scoring. *British Medical Journal* **296**, 170.

Borsig, A., Steinacker, I. (1982). Communication with the patient in the intensive care unit. *Nursing Times Supplement* **78**, 2–11,

Burgener, S. (1987). Justification for closed intermittent urinary catheter irrigation/instillation: a review of current research and practice. *Journal of Advanced Nursing* **12**, 229–34.

Butler, K.J. (1998). Hand hygiene in Intensive care. *Care of the Critically Ill* **14**, 57–60.

Carlson, E.V., Kemp, M.G., Shott, S. (1999). Predicting the risk of pressure ulcers in the critically ill patient. *American Journal of Critical Care* **8**, 262–9.

Chlan, L.L. (1998). Effectiveness of a music therapy intervention on relaxation and anxiety for patients receiving ventilatory assistance. *Heart and Lung* **27**, 169–76.

Chuman, M.A. (1985). Risk factors associated with ulnar nerve compression in bed-ridden patients. *Journal of Neurosurgical Nursing* **17**, 338–42.

Clifford, C. (1985). Helplessness: a concept applied to nursing practice. *Intensive Care Nursing* **1**, 19–24.

Closs, J. (1988a). Patient's sleep-wake rhythms in hospital, part 1. *Nursing Times Occasional Papers* **84**, 48–50.

Closs, J. (1988b). Patient's sleep-wake rhythms in hospital, part 2. *Nursing Times Occasional Papers* **84**, 54–5.

Combes, P., Fauvage, B., Oleyer, C. (2000). Nosocomial pneumonia in mechanically ventilated patients, a prospective randomized evaluation of the Stericath closed suctioning system. *Intensive Care Medicine* **26**, 878–82.

Cooper, A.B., Thornley, K.S., Young, G.B. et al. (2000). Sleep in critically ill patients requiring mechanical ventilation. *Chest* **117**, 809–18.

Cortese, D., Capp, L., McKinley, S. (1995). Moisture chamber versus lubrication for the prevention of corneal epithelial breakdown. *American Journal of Critical Care* **4**, 425–8.

Cox, C., Hayes, I. (1999). Physiologic and psychodynamic response to the administration of therapeutic touch in critical care. *Intensive and Critical Care Nursing* **15**, 363–8.

Craven D.E., Kunches, L.M., Lichtenberg, D.A., et al. (1988). Nosocomial infection and fatality in medical and surgical intensive care unit patients. *Archives of Internal Medicine* **148**, 1161–8.

Crosby, C. (1989). Method in mouth care. *Nursing Times* **85**, 38–41.

Daffurn, K., Bishop, G.F., Hillman, K.M., et al. (1994). Problems following discharge after intensive care. *Intensive and Critical Care Nursing* **10**, 244–51.

De Jong, M.J., Beatty, D.S. (2000). Family perceptions of support interventions in the intensive care unit. *Dimensions of Critical Care Nursing* **19**, 40–7.

DeRiso, A. Ladowski, J., Dillon, T., et al. (1996). Chlorhexidine Gluconate 0.12% Oral Rinse Reduces the Incidence of Total Nosocomial Respiratory Infection and Nonprophylactic Systemic Antibiotic Use in Patients Undergoing Heart Surgery. *Chest* **109**, 1556–61.

DeWalt, E. (1975). Effect of timed hygienic measures on oral mucosa in a group of elderly subjects. *Nursing Research* **24**, 104–8.

Dezfulian, C., Lavelle, J., Nallamothu, B.K., et al. (2003). Rates of infection for single-lumen versus multilumen central venous catheters: a meta-analysis. *Critical Care Medicine* **31**, 2385–90.

Dracup, K. (1993). Challenges in critical care nursing. Helping patients and families cope. *Critical Care Nurse* (Suppl.), August.

Drakulovic M., Torres, A., Bauer T. et al. (1999). Supine body position as a risk factor for nosocomial pneumonia in mechanically ventilated patients: a randomised trial. *Lancet* **354**, 1851–8.

Drane, L. (1986). Watch my lips. *Nursing Times* **82**, 52.

Dyer, I.D. (1993). Breaking the news: informing visitors that a patient has died. *Intensive and Critical Care Nursing* **9**, 2–10.

Dyer, L.L. (1989). Training and development of the ICU nurse for critical care transport. *Critical Care Nurse* **9**, 74–80.

Dubois, M.J., Bergeron, N., Dumont, M., et al. (2001). Delirium in the intensive care unit: a study of risk factors. *Intensive Care Medicine* **27**, 1297–304.

Easton, C.E., Mackenzie, F. (1988). Sensory-perceptual alterations: delirium in the intensive care unit. *Heart and Lung* **17**, 229–37.

Edwards, G.B., Schuring, L.M. (1993). Pilot study: validating staff nurses' observations of sleep and wake states among critically ill patients using polysomnography. *American Journal of Critical Care* **2**, 125–31.

Elliott, R. (1999). Verbal communication: what do critical care nurses say to their unconscious or sedated patients? *Journal of Advanced Nursing* **29**, 1412–20.

Elliott, R., Wright, L. (1999). Verbal communication: what do critical care nurses say to their unconscious or sedated patients? *Journal of Advanced Nursing* **29**, 1412–20.

Ely, E.W., Margolin, R., Francis, J., et al. (2001a). Evaluation of delirium in critically ill patients: validation of the confusion assessment method for the intensive care unit (CAM-ICU). *Critical Care Medicine* **29**, 1370–9.

Ely, E.W., Gautam, S., Margolin, R., et al. (2001b). The impact of delirium in the intensive care unit on hospital length of stay. *Intensive Care Medicine* **27**, 1892–900.

Estabrooks, C.A. (1989). Touch: a nursing strategy in the intensive care unit. *Heart and Lung* **18**, 392–401.

Fawcett, J. (1989). *Analysis and Evaluation of Conceptual Models of Nursing*, 2nd edn. F.A. Davis, Philadelphia, PA.

Fiddian-Green, R.G., Baker, S. (1991). Nosocomial pneumonia in the critically ill: product of aspiration or translocation? *Critical Care Medicine* **19**, 763–9.

Fife, C., Otto, G., Capsuto, E.G., Brandt, K., Lyssy, K., Murphy, K. et al. (2001). Incidence of pressure ulcers in a neurologic intensive care unit. *Critical Care Medicine* **29**, 283–90.

Fitch, J.A., Munro, C.L., Glass, C.A., (1999). Oral care in the adult intensive care unit. *American Journal of Critical Care* **8**, 314–18.

Forrester, D.A., Murphy, P.A., Price, D.M., (1990). Critical care family needs: nurse–family member confederate pairs. *Heart and Lung* **19**, 655–61.

Frazier, S.K., Moser, D.K., Daley, L.K., et al. (2003). Critical care nurses' beliefs about and reported management of anxiety. *American Journal of Critical Care* **12**, 19–27.

Fridkin, S.K., Pear, S.M., Williamson, T.H., (1996). The role of understaffing in central venous catheter associated bloodstream infections. *Infection Control and Hospital Epidemiology* **17**, 150–8.

Friedman, B.C., Boyce, W., Bekes, C.E. (1992). Long-term follow up of ICU patients. *American Journal of Critical Care* **1**, 115–17.

Gabor, J., Cooper, A., Crombach, S., *et al.* (2003). Contribution of the intensive care unit environment to sleep disruption in mechanically ventilated patients and healthy subjects. *American Journal of Respiratory and Critical Care Medicine* **167**, 708–15.

Gélinas, G., Fortier, M., Viens, C., (2004). Pain assessment and management in critically ill intubated patients: a retrospective study. *American Journal of Critical Care* **13**, 126–35.

Gelling, L. (1999). Causes of ICU psychosis: the environmental factors. *Nursing in Critical Care* **4**, 22–6.

Gil, K.T., Kruse, J.A., Thill-Baharozian, M.C., (1989). Triple- vs. single-lumen central venous catheters. *Archives of Internal Medicine* **149**, 1139—43.

Glaser, B.G., Strauss, A.L. (1965). *Awareness of Dying.* Aldine Press, Chicago, IL.

Gooch, J. (1985). Mouthcare. *Professional Nurse* **1**, 77–8.

Grap, M.J., Munro, C.L., Bryant, S. (2003). Oral care interventions in critical care: frequency and documentation. *American Journal of Critical Care* **12**, 113–19.

Griffiths, C. and Jones, R., (2002). Practical aspects after intensive care. In: *Outcomes in Critical Care* (S. Ridley), Butterworth-Heinemann, Oxford. pp. 169–80.

Gujol, M.C. (1994). A survey of pain assessment and management practices among critical care nurses. *American Journal of Critical Care* **3**, 123–8.

Hanchett, M. (2002). Techniques for stabilizing urinary catheters: tape may be the oldest method but it's not the only one. *American Journal of Nursing* **102**, 44–8.

Heath, H. (1998). Paradigm dialogues and dogma: finding a place for research, nursing models and reflective practice. *Journal of Advanced Nursing* **28**, 288–94.

Heath, J. (1989). What the patients say. *Intensive Care Nursing* **5**, 101–8.

Hibbert, A. (2000). Stress in surgical patients: a physiological perspective. In: *Surgical Nursing* (ed. K. Manley, L. Bellman), pp. 152–67. Churchill Livingstone, Edinburgh.

Hilton, E., Uliss, A., Samuels, S. *et al.* (1983). Nosocomial bacterial eye infections in intensive-care units. *Lancet* **i**, 1318–20.

Hope, A., Runcie, C.J. (1993). Inter-hospital transport in the critically ill adult. *British Journal of Intensive Care* **3**, 187–92.

Howarth, H. (1977). Mouth care procedures for the very ill. *Nursing Times* **73**, 354–5.

Humphreys, H. (2001). Infection control on the intensive care unit. In: *Critical Care Focus 5: Antibiotic Resistance and Infection Control* (ed. H. Galley), pp.12–18. BMJ Books, London.

Inouye, S.K., Charpentier, P.A. (1996). Precipitating factors for delirium in hospitalized elderly persons : predictive model and interrelationship with baseline vulnerability. *Journal of the American Medical Association* **275**, 852–7.

Imanaka, H., Taenaka, N., Nakamura, J.,*et al.* (1997). Ocular surface disorders in the critically ill. *Anaesthesia and Analgesia* **85**, 343–6.

Intensive Care Society (ICS). (2002). Guidelines for transport of the critically ill adult. Intensive Care Society, London.

Jacobs, S., Chang, R.W.S., Lee, B., *et al.* (1990). Continuous enteral feeding: a major cause of pneumonia among ventilated intensive care unit patients. *Journal of Parenteral and Enteral Nutrition* **14**, 353–6.

Jamerson, P.A., Scheibmeir, M., Bott, M.J., *et al.* (1996). The experiences of families with a relative in the intensive care unit. *Heart and Lung* **25**, 467–74.

Jiricka, M.K., Ryan, P., Caryalho, M.A., *et al.* (1995). Pressure ulcer risk factors in an ICU population. *American Journal of Critical Care* **4**, 361–7.

Jones, C., O'Donnell, C. (1994). After intensive care—what then? *Intensive and Critical Care Nursing* **10**, 89–92.

Jones, C., Griffiths, R.D., Humphris, G.,*et al..* (2001). Memory, delusions, and the development of acute posttraumatic stress disorder-related symptoms after intensive care. *Critical Care Medicine* **29**, 573–80.

Jones, J., Hoggart, B., Withoy, J., *et al.* (1979). What the patient's say: a study of reactions to an intensive care unit. *Intensive Care Medicine* **5**, 89–92.

Justic, M. (2000). Does 'ICU psychosis' really exist? *Critical Care Nurse* **20**, 28–37.

Kahn, D., Cook, T., Carlisle, C., *et al.* (1998). Identification and modification of environmental noise in an ICU setting. *Chest* **114**, 535–40.

Kincey, J., Pratt, D., Slater, R., *et al.* (2003). A survey of patterns and sources of stress among medical and nursing staff in an intensive care unit setting. *Care of the Critically Ill* **19**, 83–7.

Kirchhoff, K.T., Walker, L., Hutton, A., *et al.* (2002). The vortex: families' experiences with death in the intensive care unit. *American Journal of Critical Care* **11**, 200–9.

Kite, K., Pearson, L. (1995). A rationale for mouth care: the integration of theory and practice. *Intensive and Critical Care Nursing* **11**, 71–6.

Koroloff, N., Boots, R., Lipman, J., *et al.* (2004). A randomised controlled study of the efficacy of hypromellose and Lacri-Lube combination versus polyethylene/Cling wrap to prevent corneal epithelial breakdown in the semiconscious intensive care patient. *Intensive Care Medicine* **30**, 1122–6.

Kress J.P., Pohlman, A.S., O'Connor, M.F., *et al.* (2000). Daily interruption of sedative infusions in critically ill patients undergoing mechanical ventilation. *New England Journal of Medicine* **342**,1471–7.

Kuch, K. (1990). Anxiety disorder and the ICU. *Clinical Intensive Care* **1**, 7–11.

Larson, E. (1985). Infection control issues in critical care: an update. *Heart and Lung* **14**, 149–55.

Lauplan, K.B., Zygun, D.A., Davies, H.D. *et al.* (2002). Incidence and risk factors for acquiring nosocomial urinary tract infection in the critically ill. *Journal of Critical Care* **17**, 50–7.

Lawrence, M. (1995). The unconscious experience. *American Journal of Critical Care* **4**, 227–32.

Leone, M., Garnier, F., Dubuc, M., *et al.* (2001). Prevention of nosocomial urinary tract infection in ICU patients: Comparison of effectiveness of two urinary drainage systems. *Chest* **120**, 220–4.

Leske, J. (1991). Internal psychometric properties of the critical care family needs inventory. *Heart and Lung,* **20**, 236–44.

Linares, J., Sitges-Serra, A., Garau, J., *et al.* (1985). Pathogenesis of catheter sepsis: a prospective study with quantitative and semiquantitative cultures of catheter hub and segments. *Journal of Clinical Microbiology* **21**, 357–60.

Lloyd, F. (1990). Eye care for ventilated or unconscious patients. *Nursing Times* **86**, 36–7.

Lowthian, P. (1989). Preventing trauma. *Nursing Times* **85**, 73–5.

Mackeneth, P.A. (1987). Communication in critical care areas: competing for attention. *Nursing* **15**, 575–8.

Maki, D.G. (1989). Risk factors for nosocomial infection in intensive care. *Archives of Internal Medicine* **149**, 30–3.

McKinley, S., Coote, K., Stein-Parbury, J. (2003). Development and testing of a faces scale for the assessment of anxiety in critically ill patients. *Journal of Advanced Nursing* **41**, 73–9.

McKinney, A., Melby, V. (2002). Relocation stress in critical care: a review of the literature. *Journal of Clinical Nursing* **11**, 149–57.

Melzack, R., Wall, P.D., (1965). Pain mechanisms: a new theory. *Science* **150**, 971–8.

Miller, K.M., Perry, P.A. (1990). Relaxation technique and post-operative pain in patients undergoing cardiac surgery. *Heart & Lung* **19**, 136–46.

Miller, M., Kearney, N. (2001). Oral Care for Patients With Cancer: A Review of the Literature. *Cancer Nursing* **24**, 241–54.

Molter, N.C. (1979). Needs of relatives of critically ill patients: a descriptive study. *Heart and Lung* **8**, 332–9.

Moore, T. (1989). Sensory deprivation in the ICU. *Nursing* **3**, 44–7.

Mulhall, A., Chapman, R., Crow, R. (1988). The aquisition of bacteriuria and meatal cleansing. *Nursing Times* **84**, 66–9.

NICE (2001). Pressure ulcer risk assessment and prevention, p. 2. National Institute for Clinical Excellence, London.

Oh, T.E. (1990). Sedation in intensive care. In: *Intensive Care Manual* (ed. T.E. Oh), p. 313 Butterworth, Sydney.

Olson, D.M., Borel, C.O., Laskowitz, D.T., *et al.* (2001). Quiet time: a nursing intervention to promote sleep in neurocritical care units. *American Journal of Critical Care* **10**, 74–8.

Ommeslag, D., Colardyn, F., De Lacy, J. (1987). Eye infections caused by respiratory pathogens in mechanically ventilated patients. *Critical Care Medicine* **15**, 80–1.

Oser, D.K., Daley, L.K., McKinley, S., *et al.* (2003). Critical care nurses' beliefs about and reported management of anxiety. *American Journal of Critical Care* **12**, 19–27.

Ostermann, M.E., Keenan, S., Seiferling, R., *et al.* (2000). Sedation in the intensive care unit: a systematic review. *Journal of the American Medical Association* **283**, 1451–9.

Parkin, B., Turner, A., Moore, E., *et al.* (1997). Bacterial keratitis in the critically ill. *British Journal of Opthalmology* **81**, 1060–3.

Parthasarathy, S., Tobin M.J. (2004). Sleep in the intensive care unit. *Intensive Care Medicine* **30**, 197–206.

Pearson, L., Hutton, J. (2002). A controlled trial to compare the ability of foam swabs and toothbrushes to remove dental plaque. *Journal of Advanced Nursing* **39**, 480–9.

Pingleton, S.K. (1991). Enteral nutrition and infection: benefits and risks. In *Update in Intensive Care and Emergency Medicine*, Vol. 14, (ed. J.L. Vincent), pp. 581–9. Springer, Berlin.

Pittet, D., Mourouga, P., Perneger, T.V. (1999). Compliance with handwashing in a teaching hospital. *Annals of Internal Medicine* **130**, 126–30.

Platt, R., Murdock, B., Polk, F., *et al.* (1983). Reduction of mortality associated with nosocomial UTI, *Lancet* **i**, 893–6.

Powell, C., Fabri, P.J., Kudsk, K.A. (1988). Risk of infection accompanying the use of single-lumen vs. double-lumen subclavian catheters: a prospective randomized study. *Journal of Parenteral and Enteral Nutrition* **12**, 127–9.

Price, D.M., Forrester, D.A., Murphy, P.A., *et al.* (1991). Critical care family needs in an urban teaching medical center. *Heart and Lung* **20**, 183–8.

Puntillo, K. (1990). Pain experiences of intensive care unit patients. *Heart and Lung* **19**, 526–33.

Puntillo, K., Stannard, D., Miaskowski, C., *et al.* (2002). Use of a pain assessment and intervention notation (P.A.I.N.) tool in critical care nursing practice: nurses' evaluations. *Heart and Lung* **31**, 303–14.

Puntillo, K. A. (1994). Dimensions of procedural pain and its analgesic management in critically ill surgical patients. *American Journal of Critical Care* **3**, 116–22.

Puntillo, K.A. Stannard, D., Miaskowski, C., *et al.* (2002). Use of a pain assessment and intervention notation (P.A.I.N.) tool in critical care nursing practice: Nurses' evaluations. *Heart & Lung* **31**, 303–14.

Rees-Williams, C., Meyrick, M., Jones, M. (1988). Making sense of urinary catheters. *Nursing Times* **84**, 46–7.

Rello, J., Diaz, E. (2003). Pneumonia in intensive care. *Critical Care Medicine*

Richards, M.J., Edwards, J.R., Culver, D.J., *et al.* (1999). Nosocomial infections in medical intensive care units in the United States. National Nosocomial Infections Surveillance. *Critical Care Medicine* **27**, 887–92.

Richardson, A. (1987). A process standard for oral care. *Nursing Times* **83**, 38–40.

Riehl, J.P., Roy, C. (1980). *Conceptual Models for Nursing Practice*, 2nd edn. Appleton-Century-Crofts, New York.

Rincon, H.G., Granados, M., Unutzer, J., *et al.* (2001). Prevalence, detection and treatment of anxiety, depression and delirium in the adult critical care unit. *Psychosomatics* **42**, 391–6.

Robinson, J. (2001). Urethral catheter selection. *Nursing Standard* **15**, 39–42.

Roth, P.T. Creason, N. (1986). Nurse administered oral hygiene: is there a scientific basis? *Journal of Advanced Nursing* **11**, 323–31.

Rotondi, A.J., Chelluri L., Sirio, C., *et al.* (2002). Patients' recollections of stressful experiences while receiving prolonged mechanical ventilation in an intensive care unit. *Critical Care Medicine* **30**, 746–52.

Rowan, K.M., Kerr, J.H., Major, E., *et al.* (1993). Intensive Care Society's APACHE II study in Britain and Ireland II: outcome comparisons of intensive care units after adjustment for casemix by the American APACHE II method. *British Medical Journal* **307**, 977–81.

Rukholm, E., Bailey, P., Boutu-Wakulczyk, G., *et al.* (1991). Needs and anxiety levels in relatives of intensive care patients. *Journal of Advanced Nursing* **16**, 920–8.

Russell, M.T., McElwee, M.R. (1987). Compensating for xerostomia in the critically ill patient. *Critical Care Nurse* **7**, 98–103.

Russell, S. (1999). An exploratory study of patients' perceptions, memories and experiences of an intensive care unit *Journal of Advanced Nursing* **29**, 783–91.

Santamaria, J. (1990). Nosocomial infections. In: *Intensive Care Manual*, 3rd edn (ed. T.E. Oh), pp. 409–21. Butterworth, Sydney.

Simmons L.E., Riker, R.R., Prato, B.S., *et al.* (1999). Assessing sedation during intensive care unit mechanical ventilation with Bispectral Index and the sedation-agitation scale. *Critical Care Medicine* **27**, 1499–504.

Simpson, T.F., Armstrong, S., Mitchell, P. (1989). AACN demonstration project: patient's recollections of critical care. *Heart and Lung* **18**, 325–32.

Skirrow, P. (2002) Delusional memories of ICU. In: *Intensive Care Aftercare* (ed. R. Griffiths, C. Jones), pp. 27–35. Butterworth-Heinnemann, Oxford.

Steinhauser, K., Christakis, N., Clipp, E., *et al.* (2000). Factors considered important at the end of life by patients, family, physicians, and other care providers. *Journal of the American Medical Association* **284**, 2476–82.

Stevensen, C.J. (1994). The psychophysiological effects of an aromatherapy massage following cardiac surgery. *Complementary Therapies in Medicine* **2**, 27–35.

Stanton, D.J. (1991). The psychological impact of intensive therapy: the role of nurses. *Intensive Care Nursing* **7**, 230–5.

Suresh, P., Mercieca, F., Morton, A., *et al.* (2000). Eye care for the citically ill. *Intensive Care Medicine* **26**, 162–6.

Szaflanski, N.L. (1993). Immobility phenomena in critically ill adults. In: *Critical Care Nursing* (ed. J.M. Glochesy, C. Breo, S. Cardin, *et al.*), pp. 31–54. W.B. Saunders, Philadelphia, PA.

Thomas, L. (2003). Clinical management of stressors perceived by patients on mechanical ventilation. *AACN Clinical Issues* **14**, 73–81.

Tierney, A., (1998). Nursing models: extant or extinct? *Journal of Advanced Nursing* **28**, 77–85.

Tittle, M., McMillan, S. (1994). Pain and pain-related side effects in an ICU and on a surgical unit: Nurses management. *American Journal of Critical Care* **3**, 25–30.

Topf, M., Davis, J.E. (1993). Critical care unit noise and rapid eye movement (REM) sleep. *Heart and Lung* **22**, 252–8.

Turner, J. (1993). Hand-washing behavior versus hand-washing guidelines. *Heart and Lung* **22**, 275–7.

Verity, S. (1996). Communicating with sedated, ventilated patients in intensive care: focusing on the use of touch. *Intensive and Critical Care Nursing* **12**, 354–8.

Vincent, J.-L., Bihari, D.J., Suter, P. *et al.* (1995). The prevalence of nosocomial infection in intensive care units in Europe: results of the European Prevalence in Intensive Care (EPIC) study. *Journal of the American Medical Association* **274**, 639–44.

Waddell, G. (1975). Movement of critically ill patients within hospital. *British Medical Journal* **2**, 417–19.

Wallace, C.J., Robins, J., Alvord, L.S., *et al.* (1999). The effect of earplugs on sleep measures during exposure to simulated intensive care unit noise. *American Journal of Critical Care* **8**, 210–19.

Warner, L.A. (1986). Lemon-glycerine swabs should be used for routine oral care. *Critical Care Nurse* **6**, 82–3.

Wilkinson, P. (1995). A qualitative study to establish the self perceived needs of family members of patients in a general intensive care unit. *Intensive and Critical Care Nursing* **11**, 77–86.

Respiratory problems

Physiology and anatomy

The primary function of the respiratory system is to supply oxygen to the metabolically active tissues and remove the waste product, carbon dioxide. This function takes place in complete interdependence with the circulatory system's prime role of blood transport.

$$O_2 + Fuel = Energy + CO_2 + H_2O$$

Respiration can be divided into four components:

1. Mechanical movement of gases into and out of the lungs.

2. Exchange of these gases across a membrane.

3. Carriage of gases to and from the tissues.

4. Metabolic process in the cell to produce energy.

Movement of gases

This is usually referred to as ventilation and is the product of the movement of the chest wall and diaphragm. Movement of the gases is brought about by the creation of a pressure gradient between mouth and alveoli.

The trans-airway pressure (P_{ta}) is the difference between pressure at the mouth and that at the alveoli. It can be negative (as in normal breathing) or positive (as in positive pressure ventilation) and this gradient will initiate gas flow.

Transpulmonary pressure (P_{tp}) is the difference between alveolar pressure and pleural pressure. It is always negative and maintains lung expansion. The lungs are thus maintained in a neutral position by the slightly negative pressure (–5 mmHg) between the parietal pleura lining the chest wall and the visceral pleura covering the lung (Fig. 4.1).

Inspiration occurs when the diaphragm and the intercostal muscles contract, pulling the lungs downwards and outwards. This increases the volume within the lungs creating a negative pressure (–3 mmHg) which sucks air in. During deep inspiration it is possible for the negative pressure to reach –35 to –40 mmHg (Des Jardins 1988).

Expiration occurs when the inspiratory muscles relax and the elastic nature of the lung tissue forces a recoil to the neutral position. A slightly positive pressure is then exerted on the lung and air is forced out.

The elasticity of the lung is an important feature and depends on two factors. The first is the high surface tension of the alveoli which acts as a potent force pulling the alveoli closed and resisting expansion. The surface tension is decreased by the secretion of surfactant, a lipoprotein substance produced by the epithelial lining. A number of elements can affect the production of this substance with serious consequences for the ability to expand alveoli (see Table 4.1). The problems associated with neonatal respiratory distress syndrome are in part due to the inability of immature lungs to produce surfactant leading to poor elasticity and vastly increased work of breathing. The second factor affecting elasticity is the elastic fibres of the lung itself which tend to contract.

When breathing becomes difficult, or increased during exercise, other respiratory muscles may be used to increase ventilation. These are known as the accessory muscles of respiration. They consist of the neck, trapezius, pectoral, and external intercostal muscles in inspiration and the abdominal and internal intercostal muscles in expiration.

Work of breathing

The degree of effort involved in moving a specific volume of air into and out of the lungs is known as the work of breathing and can be affected by:

TABLE 4.1 Causes of pulmonary surfactant deficiency (after Des Jardins 1988)

General	Acidosis
	Hypoxia
	Hyperoxygenation
	Atelectasis
	Pulmonary vascular congestion
	Starvation
Specific	Acute respiratory distress syndrome (ARDS)
	Infant respiratory distress syndrome (IRDS)
	Pulmonary oedema
	Pulmonary embolus
	Excess pulmonary lavage/hydration
	Drowning
	Extracorporeal oxygenation

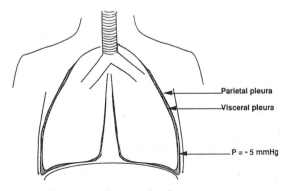

Parietal pleura
Visceral pleura
P = - 5 mmHg

Fig. 4.1 Maintenance of negative pleural pressure.

- the resistance of the airways to flow of air,
- the elasticity of the lung tissue,
- any obstruction to flow,
- chest wall compliance.

These factors comprise the compliance of the respiratory system, which is expressed as the change in volume of the lung over the change in pressure required to produce that change in volume ($\Delta V/\Delta P$, ml/cm H_2O). It is the inverse of the degree of stiffness of the lung (i.e. when a lung is compliant it will expand easily but when non-compliant it will be more resistant to expansion). The greatest compliance is where small changes in pressure reflect the greatest change in volume.

Lung compliance can be classified into static and dynamic compliance:

1. *Static compliance.* As the name suggests, static compliance refers to compliance of the lung measured under static conditions produced by occlusion of the airway for a brief period at the end of inspiration. This allows an assessment of compliance without the pressure associated with flow resistance. It is measured by occluding the airway at end inspiration for a minimum of 2 s to allow the plateau pressure to be reached:

$$Cst_{rs} = \frac{\Delta V}{\text{End inspiration occluded (plateau) pressure}}$$

where Cst_{rs} is the static compliance of the respiratory system and ΔV is tidal volume. The normal range is 60–100 ml/cm H_2O (Tobin 1991).

2. *Dynamic compliance*: Dynamic compliance refers to the change in pressure from end inspiration to end expiration:

$$Cdyn_{rs} = \frac{\Delta V}{\text{End inspiratory pressure (immediate) – end expiratory pressure}}$$

TABLE 4.2	Causes of alteration in lung compliance (Oh 1990)
Lung compliance is decreased by:	Pulmonary congestion
	Increased pulmonary smooth muscle tone
	Increased surface tension
	Pulmonary fibrosis, infiltration, or atelectasis
	Pleural fibrosis
Lung compliance is increased by:	Pulmonary oligaemia (deficient blood volume)
	Decreased pulmonary smooth muscle tone
	Augmented surfactant release
	Destruction of lung tissue (e.g. emphysema)

where $Cdyn_{rs}$ is the dynamic compliance of the respiratory system and ΔV is tidal volume.

In healthy lungs there is little difference between static and dynamic compliance at all respiratory rates. In patients with airway obstruction, the dynamic compliance decreases rapidly as the respiratory rate rises while there is little change in the static compliance (Table 4.2).

Gas exchange

Not all airways are available for gas exchange which only takes place in the respiratory lobule. Areas of the lung not available for gas exchange are known as dead space. There are three types of dead space.

1. *Anatomical dead space.* The volume of the airway in which gas exchange cannot take place is known as the anatomical dead space. It consists of the nose, pharynx, trachea, and bronchi and is usually about 150 ml in a normal-sized adult. This means that of any tidal volume inspired (~5–8 ml/kg for a normal

TABLE 4.3	Lung volumes	
Term	**Volume**	**Definition**
Tidal volume (V_T)	5–9 ml/kg (~500 ml)	Volume of gas/air that will move in or out of lungs in a normal quiet breath
Minute volume (MV)	5–9 ml/kg × 12 (= 5–6 litres) calculated by multiplying V_T by the respiratory rate	Volume of gas/air that will move in and out of lungs over the period of 1 min
Vital capacity (VC)	3000–4800 ml	Maximum volume of gas that can be exhaled after a maximum inspiration
Anatomical dead space	2 ml/kg (~150 ml)	Volume of gas filling conducting airways (nose down to lower airways but not bronchioles)
Functional residual capacity (FRC)	1800–2400 ml	Volume of air remaining in the lungs after normal exhalation

> - Effective alveolar ventilation per unit time (V_A) = Expired minute volume (V_E) – physiological dead space (V_D).
> - Physiological dead space = anatomical + alveolar dead space. It is variable depending on the ventilation and perfusion of alveoli thus a ratio of dead space to tidal volume is used (V_D/V_T).
> - The ratio of V_D to V_T is normally <0.3.

spontaneous breath), 150 ml is not able to either oxygenate or remove carbon dioxide.

2. *Alveolar dead space.* This refers to alveoli which are ventilated but not perfused with pulmonary blood. They are therefore unable to contribute to gas exchange.

3. *Physiological dead space.* This is the sum of the anatomical and alveolar dead space. It can be increased by old age, anaesthesia, controlled ventilation, and chronic lung disease. It can be increased acutely by pulmonary embolism. Hypoventilation will increase the ratio of dead space to tidal volume though not the actual dead space volume (Table 4.3).

Gas exchange only takes place in those areas where the barrier between gas contained within alveoli and blood passing through the alveolar capillaries is thin enough to allow movement across the pulmonary capillary membrane. An enormous surface area of approximately 70 m² is provided for the movement of gas. This area results from the convoluted surfaces of the alveoli and the distribution of a small volume of blood throughout the pulmonary membrane. The resulting close contact between individual red blood cells and the respiratory membrane enables diffusion of gases across the two membranes at a fast and efficient rate (Fig. 4.2).

Gas diffusion

Diffusion is defined as the movement of molecules from an area of high concentration towards an area of low concentration. The diffusion of gases across the respiratory membrane is affected by two laws governing the physical properties of gases: Dalton's law of partial pressures and Boyle's law.

Dalton's law of partial pressures

The first part of the law refers to pressure exerted by gases:

The pressure exerted by a mixture of gases is equal to the sum of the pressures which each would exert if it alone occupied the space.

The partial pressure of a gas is the force exerted by it when contained within a space and is a measure of the amount of gas.

Air is made up of three main gases, nitrogen (N_2, 79%), carbon dioxide (CO_2, 0.03%) and oxygen (O_2, 20.9%). These gases form the Earth's atmosphere and contribute to atmospheric pressure.

Atmospheric pressure is 101 kPa (760 mmHg) at sea level. The partial pressure of a gas is written as P, thus:

partial pressure of oxygen = PO_2,

partial pressure of carbon dioxide = PCO_2.

If the partial pressure is referred to in a specific part of the body, it is written as P with a suffix letter referring to the part of the body, e.g.

P_AO_2 = partial pressure of alveolar oxygen,

P_aCO_2 = partial pressure of arterial carbon dioxide.

The second part of Dalton's law refers to pressure exerted by saturated vapours:

The pressure exerted by a saturated vapour depends only on the temperature and the particular liquid considered.

Air is humidified on inspiration and thus contains water vapour. This will exert a pressure which will depend on body temperature. At 37 °C the pressure exerted by water vapour is 6.3 kPa. This is important, as air entering the lungs will contain a certain amount of water vapour (depending on body temperature and rate of breathing) which will exert part of the pressure of the gas contained in the alveoli.

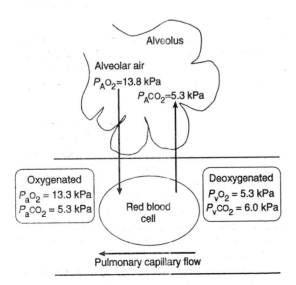

Fig. 4.2 Gas exchange in the lungs.

Boyle's law

The partial pressure of any gas is proportional to its percentage by volume in the mixture.

Example:

Air = N_2 (79%) + O_2 (20.9%) + CO_2 (0.03%).

Air at sea level has an atmospheric pressure of 101 kPa, Thus, according to Boyle's law, each gas will exert a partial pressure proportional to its percentage in air:

N_2 will exert 79% of 101 kPa = 79.8 kPa

O_2 will exert 20.9% of 101 kPa = 20.9 kPa

CO_2 will exert 0.03% of 101 kPa = 0.03 kPa

If that air is humidified, as it is on inspiration, then the pressure exerted by the water vapour in the air will depend on the temperature of the body. This is 6.3 kPa at body temperature. Thus, at a body temperature of 37 °C, the pressure of the gases on entering the alveoli will equal 101 kPa – 6.3 kPa = 94.7 kPa.

When the gas enters the lungs it mixes with carbon dioxide which has been excreted and the contents of alveolar gas are significantly different from the original inspired gas. The oxygen content of alveolar gas can be calculated using the alveolar gas equation (see box).

With perfect lung function the arterial PO_2 should theoretically equal the alveolar PO_2, However, in normal lungs the difference is usually approximately 2 kPa in youth and 3.3 kPa in old age (Oh 1990). This is known as the A–a (alveolar–arterial) oxygen gradient. The difference is due to a small amount of blood which has passed through the lungs but has not been oxygenated. An increase in the A–a oxygen gradient is evidence of an abnormality in the ventilation/perfusion ratio. The alveolar–arterial oxygen difference is calculated using the alveolar gas equation and comparing it with the measured arterial PO_2.

The following factors affect diffusion through the pulmonary capillary membrane:

1. The difference between partial pressures of the gases in the alveoli and in the pulmonary capillary.

THE ALVEOLAR GAS EQUATION

Alveolar PO_2 = [inspired PO_2 × (atmospheric pressure – water vapour pressure)] – (arterial PCO_2/respiratory quotient).

The respiratory quotient is the ratio of carbon dioxide produced to oxygen consumed, usually approximately 0.8.

---

2. The area of the respiratory membrane. Any factors that severely limit the area available for gas exchange such as emphysema or acute respiratory distress syndrome (ARDS) can have a severe effect on respiratory function.

3. The thickness of the respiratory membrane. Factors affecting this, such as cardiogenic and non-cardiogenic pulmonary oedema, will impair pulmonary function.

4. The diffusion or solubility coefficient of the gas involved. Carbon dioxide is far more soluble than oxygen and thus diffuses at a faster and more efficient rate.

The presence of nitrogen in the inspired gas has the function of acting as a gas reservoir remaining in the alveoli as it is not soluble and does not pass into the capillaries. This maintains the expansion of the alveoli, preventing collapse (atelectasis). This function is lost with very high percentages of inspired oxygen.

Ventilation/perfusion match

Another important determinant of gas exchange is the relationship between pulmonary capillary perfusion (Q) and alveolar ventilation (V). A well-ventilated alveolus should have a correspondingly well perfused capillary and the ratio of V/Q is ideally 1.

A three-compartment model of the lungs is used to illustrate ventilation/ perfusion relationships:

1. Physiological dead space—an area of wasted ventilation (i.e. V/Q > 1).

2. Perfectly matched areas of ventilation and perfusion (i.e. V/Q = 1).

3. Areas contributing to venous admixture (the mixing of non-oxygenated with oxygenated blood after passage through the lungs) where perfusion has been wasted, for example diffusion defects, right to left shunts (i.e. V/Q < 1).

There is normally a variation between the degree of perfusion and ventilation in different areas of the lungs. This is due to the effects of gravity which increases the amount of work required to force blood through the vessels further above the heart. Therefore, the lower lung lobes receive a better blood supply than the upper lobes in the erect position. The body adapts to this by preferentially ventilating the better-perfused lower lobes. This response is lost when the patient is mechanically ventilated.

A pathological cause of hypoxaemia is the presence of a right to left shunt (venous admixture). This is

SITUATIONS CAUSING RIGHT-TO-LEFT SHUNTS

- Obstructive lung disease (emphysema, bronchitis. asthma).
- Restrictive lung disease (ARDS, pneumonia, fibrotic lung disease).
- Hypoventilation for any reason (e.g. excess sedation, respiratory muscle weakness).

where poorly ventilated areas of lung continue to be perfused (e.g. atelectasis). Thus the ratio of ventilation (V) to perfusion (Q) is decreased allowing blood to pass through the lung without being oxygenated.

A right to left shunt is always increased when alveoli are:

- completely collapsed,
- totally consolidated, or
- filled with oedema fluid.

A ventilation/perfusion mismatch occurs when a poorly perfused area of lung continues to be ventilated (e.g. pulmonary embolus). Thus, the ratio of ventilation (V) to perfusion (Q) is increased as is the physiological dead space.

Two intrinsic responses to variations in ventilation and perfusion allow a certain amount of adjustment in order to maintain V/Q matching. The first involves the pulmonary capillary response to areas of low PO_2. If the alveolus is poorly ventilated the P_AO_2 will be low. This results in a correspondingly low P_aO_2 in the pulmonary capillaries supplying that area. This initiates a vasoconstrictor response—'hypoxic pulmonary vasoconstriction'—which reduces pulmonary blood flow to the affected region. The second involves a localized bronchoconstrictor response to low pulmonary capillary

SOME CAUSES OF VENTILATION/PERFUSION MISMATCH

- Pulmonary embolus.
- Partial/complete obstruction of the pulmonary artery.
- Extrinsic pressure on pulmonary vessels (pneumothorax, tumour).
- Destruction of pulmonary vessels.
- Decreased cardiac output.
- Obstruction of the pulmonary microcirculation (ARDS).

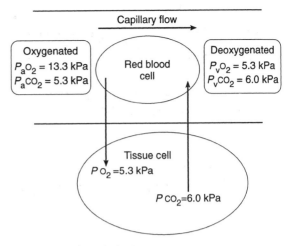

Fig. 4.3 Gas exchange in the tissues.

levels of carbon dioxide due to reduction in perfusion of the area (e.g. following a pulmonary embolus). The P_ACO_2 will remain low in the non-perfused area and the bronchioles will constrict thereby limiting ventilation of that region (Fig. 4.3).

Carriage of gases

The degree of solubility of oxygen is considerably less than that of carbon dioxide. It would be impossible to deliver the quantity of oxygen required by the body if it was simply carried as a solution. The majority is therefore carried in combination with haemoglobin. At a normal level of haemoglobin (15 g/dl), 20 ml of oxygen is carried per 100 ml of blood, whereas only 0.3 ml of oxygen is carried dissolved in the plasma. The amount of oxygen dissolved in plasma is only increased by an increase in atmospheric pressure such as that produced by a hyperbaric oxygen chamber.

The chemical structure of haemoglobin allows for a varying affinity to oxygen molecules according to the environmental PO_2 of the capillary. Thus, at a PO_2 of 13.3 kPa almost all of the oxygen-binding capacity of haemoglobin is utilized and the haemoglobin is said to be approximately 98% saturated. This is the situation found in the normal lung. Oxygen-saturated haemoglobin is termed *oxyhaemoglobin* and unsaturated haemoglobin is termed *reduced haemoglobin* on *deoxyhaemoglobin* (Fig. 4.4).

In the tissues, where oxygen is extracted, the saturation of haemoglobin is reduced to about 75% and oxygen will be released to the tissues. Three-quarters of the haemoglobin remains oxygenated providing a reservoir for conditions where oxygen demand exceeds supply (e.g. exercise and cardiogenic shock). More oxygen can be released from the haemoglobin, down to 20–30% satu-

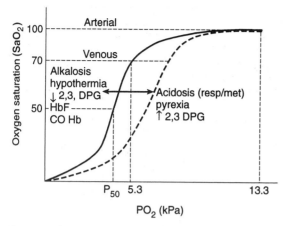

Fig. 4.4 Oxyhaemoglobin dissociation curve (Bohr). HbF = fetal haemoglobin; COHb = carbon monoxide bound to haemoglobin (carboxyhaemoglobin); P_{50} = pressure at which haemoglobin is 50% saturated; 2,3 DPG = 2,3 diphosphoglycerate.

ration in extreme circumstances, in order to maintain aerobic metabolism. Where supply fails to meet demand the tissues undergo anaerobic metabolism resulting in lactate production and a metabolic acidosis.

There are several important factors which affect oxyhaemoglobin dissociation (the detachment of oxygen from haemoglobin). In the presence of some factors the curve can shift to the right (i.e. for the same level of arterial PO_2 the haemoglobin saturation is lower therefore more oxygen is available to the tissues). However, in the presence of other factors, the curve can shift to the left (i.e. for the same level of PO_2 the haemoglobin saturation is higher therefore less oxygen is available to the tissues). In the normal range of PO_2, these shifts will have minimal effect on oxygen availability but can be highly significant in patients with a low arterial PO_2.

Shift of the dissociation curve to the right

Under conditions which shift the dissociation curve to the right, a higher level of PO_2 is required in order to maintain the same oxygen saturation of haemoglobin. Less oxygen will therefore combine with haemoglobin in the alveoli at the normal level of P_AO_2 but more oxygen will be available to the tissues where the PO_2 is low. This is the situation found in acidosis and is a compensatory mechanism to augment tissue oxygenation.

Factors causing a shift of the dissociation curve to the right include:

♦ decreased pH,

♦ increased body temperature,

♦ increased PCO_2,

♦ increased 2,3-diphosphoglycerate (2,3-DPG is a substance contained within the red blood cell formed during anaerobic glycolysis; levels are increased in response to hypoxia, anaemia, and increased pH forming a compensatory mechanism).

Shift of the dissociation curve to the left

Under conditions which shift the haemoglobin saturation curve to the left a lower level of PO_2 is required to maintain the same haemoglobin saturation. More oxygen will therefore combine with haemoglobin in the alveoli at the normal P_AO_2 but less oxygen will be available to the tissues at the normal P_aO_2.

Factors causing a shift of the dissociation curve to the left include:

♦ increased pH,

♦ decreased PCO_2,

♦ decreased temperature,

♦ decreased 2,3-diphosphoglycerate

♦ fetal haemoglobin (HbF) (this has a greater affinity for oxygen in order to enhance transfer of oxygen across the placenta),

♦ carboxyhaemoglobin (COHb) (carbon monoxide combined with haemoglobin has about 250 times the affinity of oxygen for haemoglobin. Thus, a small amount of carbon monoxide can bind large amounts of haemoglobin making it unavailable for oxygen transport).

Two further points are important in the carriage of oxygen:

1. Once haemoglobin is fully saturated, no further increase in PO_2 will increase the amount of oxygen carried by haemoglobin. The amount of oxygen carried in solution in the plasma can only be increased significantly by use of a hyperbaric oxygen chamber where atmospheric pressure can be increased.

2. The PO_2 can decrease quite considerably before any significant fall occurs in haemoglobin saturation. Thus the haemoglobin is still 90% saturated at around 8 kPa.

Oxygen delivery to the tissues is not only dependent on haemoglobin concentration and oxygen saturation (SaO_2) but also on cardiac output (see Chapter 6).

Oxygen delivery (DO_2) = cardiac output (CO) × (Hb × S_aO_2 × 1.34) + (P_aO_2 × 0.003) ml/min (1.34 ml O_2 is carried by each gram of haemoglobin).

Carbon dioxide transport

There are six different mechanisms for the movement of carbon dioxide from the tissues to the alveoli (see Table 4.4).

TABLE 4.4 Mechanisms of carbon dioxide transport

Plasma	Red blood cells	Per cent carried
1. As dissolved CO_2	4. As dissolved CO_2	~10%
2. Protein bound (the carbamino compound)	5. Carbamino-haemoglobin (combined with Hb)	1% protein bound, 20% carbaminoHb
3. As bicarbonate (HCO_3^-)	6. As bicarbonate (HCO_3^-)	~70%

Unlike oxygen, the relationship between the amount of carbon dioxide in the blood and the PCO_2 is linear over the physiological range. Thus, changes in PCO_2 will have a more direct effect on the carbon dioxide content of the blood. Carbon dioxide binding to haemoglobin is affected by the level of saturation of haemoglobin with oxygen. Deoxygenated blood enhances the loading of carbon dioxide; this is known as the Haldane effect. It is also effective in reverse, as oxygenated blood enhances the unloading of carbon dioxide.

The metabolic process in the cell to produce energy

Oxygen diffuses through the capillary membrane and tissue spaces into the tissue cells. It is combined with glucose, fatty acids, and amino acids in the mitochondria of the cell to produce energy. This process produces carbon dioxide and water as end-products as well as energy. The energy released is stored as a high-energy phosphate bond linking a third phosphate molecule to adenosine diphosphate (ADP) to form adenosine triphosphate (ATP). ATP can then be used to provide energy as required for cell functions.

Acid–base balance

A major effect of the process of CO_2 removal is the maintenance of the acid–base balance in the body. The level of acidity (pH) of the body must be maintained within certain well-defined limits in order for normal metabolic processes to continue. The mechanisms for maintaining these limits can be divided into three distinct responses to any abnormality in pH:

1. buffering (immediate);

2. respiratory response (important in first 2–3 hours);

3. renal response (over 2–3 days).

The mechanisms of the buffering and respiratory responses will be discussed here. For full details of the renal response see Chapter 9.

Carbon dioxide gas in solution may be considered to contribute to increased levels of hydrogen ions as the carbonic acid (H_2CO_3) produced is able to easily dissociate into hydrogen ions and bicarbonate ions. Thus, the removal of carbon dioxide has an important function in maintaining body pH in the normal range (see Table 4.5 for definitions).

TABLE 4.5 Definitions of terms

Term	Definition	Example/formula
Acid	A substance containing weakly held hydrogen ions which is easily split into hydrogen ions and the remaining substance	Carbonic acid $H_2CO_3 \rightarrow H^+ + HCO_3^-$
Base	A substance which can combine with hydrogen ions	Bicarbonate $HCO_3^- + H^+ \rightarrow H_2CO_3$
H^+ (hydrogen ions)	Extremely active metabolically and can have a major effect on cell function	
pH	The scale on which hydrogen ions are measured. It is a negative logarithm to the base 10 of the concentration of hydrogen ions	pH = $-\log10$ [H^+]. Normal pH range = 7.35–7.45
Acidosis	An abnormal process causing a relative increase in hydrogen ions and thus decrease in pH. It can be due to an increase in acid or a decrease in base	pH < 7.35
Alkalosis	An abnormal process causing a relative decrease in hydrogen ions and thus increase in pH. It can be due to a decrease in acid or an increase in base	pH ≥ 7.45
Buffer	A substance with the ability to bind and release hydrogen ions thus maintaining a relatively constant pH	Phosphoric acid and its salts, disodium hydrogen phosphate, and monosodium dihydrogen phosphate

The traditional view of acid-base balance is explained below, but a more recent theory suggesting that pH is a product of the strong ion difference (Sirker *et al.* 2002) may explain the body's response in a slightly different and perhaps more effective way.

Strong ions are those which dissociate entirely in solution to their ion form. In the extracellular fluid, these are most commonly Na^+ (sodium), Cl^- (chloride), and K^+ (potassium). The difference between the sum of the positive ions (cations) and the negative ions (anions) is known as the strong ion difference. Stewart's theory has shown by biochemical formulae and basic laws of biochemical physics that the factors on which the pH of the body depends are: (1) strong ion difference; (2) total weak acid in solution in the plasma (composed mostly of serum proteins, i.e. albumin and inorganic phosphate), and (3) PCO_2. Thus changes in any of these will alter the pH of the body. However, from a respiratory perspective the major determinant of acid–base balance remains the level of PCO_2.

Arterial blood gas analysis

The measurement of blood gases gives not only an indication of the respiratory status but also an important view of the metabolic environment of the body. It gauges the ability of the body to maintain homeostasis (metabolic equilibrium).

The variables measured in arterial blood gas sampling are PCO_2, PO_2, and pH. Derived variables such as bicarbonate (HCO_3) and base excess can also be used for additional interpretation of results. The normal values for these variables are given in Table 4.6.

Respiratory dysfunction can directly affect the acid–base balance in two ways:

1. by increasing the levels of CO_2 in the body and thus increasing the level of acidity (respiratory acidosis); or

2. by decreasing the levels of CO_2 in the body and thus decreasing the level of acidity (respiratory alkalosis).

An alteration in pH may not simply be the result of an alteration in PCO_2. Metabolic factors may also contribute to produce abnormalities of pH. In order to differentiate metabolic from respiratory factors, measurement of standard bicarbonate (HCO_3) and base excess must be used. When a metabolic process leads to acidosis, levels of HCO_3 and other buffer substances in the body will fall, increasing the level of hydrogen ions and thus decreasing the pH.

STANDARD MEASURES OF BICARBONATE AND BASE EXCESS

Standard bicarbonate is defined as the concentration of bicarbonate in equilibrated plasma at 37 °C and a P_aCO_2 of 5.3 kPa.

Standard base excess is defined as the milliequivalent (mEq or mmol) of strong acid necessary to titrate a blood sample at 37 °C and 5.3 kPa P_aCO_2 to a pH of 7.40.

CAUSES OF RESPIRATORY ACIDOSIS (USUALLY ASSOCIATED WITH HYPOVENTILATION)

- Obstructive lung disease
- Oversedation/other causes of depression of respiratory centre
- Neuromuscular disorders
- Hypoventilation during mechanical ventilation
- Pain, chest wall deformities, respiratory muscle fatigue, etc.

CAUSES OF RESPIRATORY ALKALOSIS (USUALLY ASSOCIATED WITH HYPERVENTILATION)

- Hypoxia
- Anxiety states
- Pulmonary embolus, fibrosis, etc.
- Pregnancy
- Hyperventilation during mechanical ventilation
- Brain injury
- High salicylate levels
- Fever
- Asthma
- Severe anaemia

TABLE 4.6 Normal values of arterial blood gases

Property	Value
pH	7.35–7.45
PO_2	4.6–6.0 kPa
PO_2	10.0–13.3 kPa
HCO_3	22–26 mmol/l
Base excess	−2 to +2
O_2 saturation	>95%

TABLE 4.7	Alterations in different types of acidosis and alkalosis		
	pH	PCO2	HCO3
Acute respiratory acidosis	pH low	PCO_2 high	HCO_3 normal
Acute respiratory alkalosis	pH high	PCO_2 low	HCO_3 normal
Acute metabolic acidosis	pH low	PCO_2 normal or low	HCO_3 low
Acute metabolic alkalosis	pH high	PCO_2 normal	HCO_3 high

There may also be mixed or combined acidosis or alkalosis due to a combination of causes.

The equation describing the relationship between bicarbonate (HCO_3) as a buffer and the partial pressure of carbon dioxide (pCO_2) is known as the Henderson–Hasselbalch equation:

$$pH = 6.1 + \log_{10} [HCO_3^-/0.03\ PCO_2].$$

It can be seen that if HCO_3 falls or PCO_2 rises then the pH will fall. When measured bicarbonate has been standardized to allow for variations in PCO_2 and temperature, any abnormality must be due to metabolic causes. Thus, standard bicarbonate is an indicator of metabolic abnormality contributing to acidosis or alkalosis.

The base excess is a reflection of the levels of bicarbonate and other bases. When bicarbonate values fall below the normal range the base excess will become negative (and can be termed 'base deficit'). Conversely, when bicarbonate levels rise there will be a positive base excess.

In interpreting the cause of any abnormality in pH the PCO_2 and the HCO_3 must be referred to, as well as the pH itself (Table 4.7).

Compensated acidosis/alkalosis

When the body responds successfully by compensating for acid–base imbalance the pH will return towards normal. This may be either by respiratory or renal compensation, depending on which system is primarily affected by the cause of the abnormality. For example, respiratory acidosis caused by hypoventilation in chronic pulmonary disease will be compensated for (over a period of time) by the kidneys producing and retaining bicarbonate.

Compensation is only complete in chronic respiratory alkalosis. In other acid–base abnormalities the pH does not usually return completely to normal (Table 4.8).

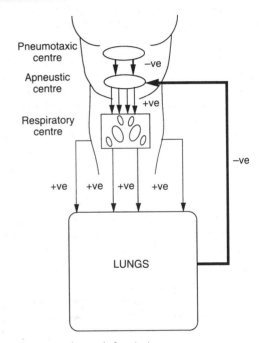

Fig. 4.5 Neuronal control of respiration.

These compensatory mechanisms have only a limited range and if the primary abnormality continues the patient may be unable to maintain a normal pH. The treatment of acid–base imbalance usually depends on determining and treating the underlying cause (see Chapter 14).

Neuronal control of respiration

The involuntary regulation of the respiratory drive is controlled from a group of respiratory neurons in the

TABLE 4.8	Alterations in compensated acidosis and alkalosis		
	PCO_2	pH	HCO_3
Compensated respiratory acidosis	PCO_2 high	pH near normal	HCO_3 high
Compensated respiratory alkalosis	PCO_2 low	pH normal	HCO_3 low
Compensated metabolic acidosis	PCO_2 low	pH near normal	HCO_3 low
Compensated metabolic alkalosis	PCO_2 high	pH near normal	HCO_3 high

medulla of the brain. These form what is usually termed the *respiratory centre* (Fig. 4.5).

The respiratory centre is moderated by the further influence of two centres situated in the pons. These are the apneustic and the pneumotaxic centres. The apneustic centre is inhibited by the pneumotaxic centre and by stimuli from receptors in the lung known as the Hering-Breuer or stretch receptors (see later).

The everyday control of respiration is further modified by a number of factors, the most important of which are stimuli from the chemoreceptors:

Central chemoreceptors

These are located bilaterally and ventrally in the medulla. Some portion of the cells making up the chemoreceptors are in direct contact with the cerebrospinal fluid (CSF). The most powerful stimulus to these receptors is an increase in hydrogen ion concentration in the CSF. This can be directly related to an increase in PCO_2 in the blood supply to the brain. The chemoreceptors act directly on the respiratory centre to increase respiratory effort.

Peripheral chemoreceptors

These are groups of oxygen-sensitive cells located at the bifurcation of the internal and external carotid arteries and on the aortic arch. They stimulate the respiratory centre to increase respiratory effort when oxygen tension falls below approximately 8 kPa/90% saturation.

Peripheral chemoreceptors are sensitive to P_aO_2 rather than O_2 content so conditions where the P_aO_2 is normal yet O_2 content is low (e.g. chronic anaemia, carbon monoxide poisoning, methaemoglobinaemia) will not stimulate an increase in respiration (Fig. 4.6).

There are a number of other factors which affect the response of the peripheral chemoreceptors:

- increase in H^+ (not due to PCO_2), for example, lactic acidosis,
- increase in temperature,
- increase in PCO_2 (minor although faster response than central chemoreceptors),
- nicotine.

Peripheral chemoreceptors can also cause:

- peripheral vasoconstriction,
- increased pulmonary vascular resistance,
- systolic arterial hypertension,
- tachycardia,
- increased left ventricular perfusion.

Other mechanisms which can influence respiration and the respiratory pattern

Hering–Breuer inflation reflex

This is generated by stretch receptors situated in the walls of the bronchi and bronchioles. When lungs overinflate the receptors are stimulated to send impulses back to the respiratory centre terminating inspiration. This appears to be a protective mechanism preventing pulmonary damage.

Deflation reflex

The rate of breathing is increased when lungs are compressed or deflated. The precise mechanism is unknown.

Irritant reflex

Receptors located subepithelially in trachea, bronchi, and bronchioles cause an increase in ventilatory rate when lungs are compressed or exposed to noxious gases. It may also cause reflex cough and bronchoconstriction.

Juxtapulmonary–capillary receptors (J-receptors)

These receptors are located in the interstitial tissues between the pulmonary capillaries and the alveoli. When they are activated they stimulate rapid, shallow breathing. They are activated by:

- pulmonary capillary congestion,
- capillary hypertension,

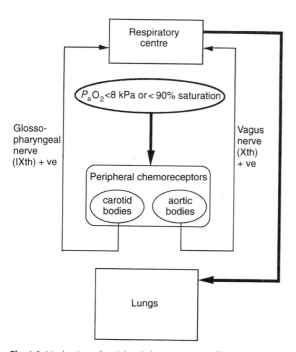

Fig. 4.6 Mechanism of peripheral chemoreceptor effect on respiration.

◆ oedema of the alveolar walls,

◆ humoral agents (e.g. 5-hydroxytryptamine (5-HT)),

◆ lung deflation.

Baroreceptors

These have a primarily cardiovascular function but when stimulated by a low blood pressure they cause an increase in ventilatory rate as well as an increase in heart rate. When stimulated by a high blood pressure they cause a decrease in ventilatory rate.

Exercise

Neural signals from the cerebral cortex to exercising muscles appear to have a collateral transmission to the respiratory centre in the medulla, producing an increased rate and depth of breathing. Movement of the limbs also transmits sensory signals up the spinal cord to the medulla. The precise mechanism of the respiratory response to the exercise stimulus has not been fully explained.

Assessment of respiratory status

In detailing the assessment of one particular system in the patient it is very easy to forget the effect that any primary dysfunction will be having on other related systems. It is thus necessary at the outset to emphasize that any respiratory problems will have an impact on cardiovascular and nutritional status, the patient's level of consciousness, and his/her emotional state. The patient's ability to perform personal needs and to maintain vital defence mechanisms will also be reduced. The nurse caring for the patient must attempt to maintain an overall view of the patient that will not neglect these other features while concentrating on the prime cause of distress. The importance of a preventative as well as a therapeutic role cannot be overemphasized.

TABLE 4.9   Useful information from history taking

1. Timespan of current problem plus any relevant past medical history, particularly the degree (if any) of chronic respiratory disability

2. Previously tried manoeuvres found to be of benefit in reducing respiratory problems and breathlessness

3. Current medications

4. Type and time of occurrence of dyspnoea (e.g. on exertion only, position-related, etc.)

5. Sputum—colour, consistency, amount

6. Pain (if any)—site, timing, modes of relief employed by patient

7. Lifestyle/social factors—smoking, drug-taking, exposure to toxic substances, etc.

8. Mood state and immediate anxieties

History

Patients admitted in acute respiratory distress are frequently unable to provide any detailed information and all efforts should be made to obtain as much as possible from alternative sources. These include:

◆ relatives and friends,

◆ GP letters,

◆ previous notes and nursing records,

◆ casualty notes and records,

◆ results of any previous investigations.

Patients in this state should not have to answer two sets of questions and so, wherever possible, the immediate nursing and medical history should be done as a collaborative process so that areas of overlap are not repeated unnecessarily. Much of the information can be obtained whilst seeing to other more urgent needs and priorities (Table 4.9).

Physical assessment

A considerable amount of information about the patient's condition can be gained from simply observing and listening.

Colour

This can range from pink and therefore relatively well oxygenated to frankly cyanosed. The patient suffering from carbon monoxide poisoning may have a characteristic 'cherry-red' colour due to the presence of carboxyhaemoglobin. The patient's buccal (mouth) mucosa as well as the peripheries should be viewed. Peripheral cyanosis is seen in conditions of poor circulation (vasoconstricted due to cold, poor cardiac output, arteriopaths, etc.) and does not indicate a low P_aO_2, but central cyanosis, seen as blue lips and buccal mucosa, is indicative of a low P_aO_2. However, a grossly anaemic patient may not exhibit this clinical sign as 5 g of reduced oxyhaemoglobin per 100 ml blood must be present before cyanosis is clinically detectable.

Patient condition

This is a general assessment of the patient's level of fatigue and potential for maintaining respiration. Useful indicators of failing respiratory function are:

1. Signs of sweating (indicates use of considerable effort to maintain function and increased sympathetic arousal).

2. Inability to speak or move limbs (indicates lack of breath and energy limitation due to poor respiratory function).

3. Restlessness and confusion as well as altered level of consciousness (may indicate cerebral hypoxia, although this can be related to other causes and should be treated with caution). The patient's ability to protect the airway should be assessed by checking the cough and gag reflex.

4. Distress.

5. Posture.

Respiratory pattern

Assess the movement of the chest wall:

1. Are both sides moving equally (pneumothorax, mechanical dysfunction, such as rib fractures and flail chest, pleural effusion, and major lobar collapse, may all cause unilateral diminished expansion)?

2. Are the normal muscles of inspiration being used (diaphragmatic splinting or paralysis, neuropathy, myopathy, Guillain–Barré syndrome, and myasthenia gravis can all affect the normal ability to use the diaphragm and intercostal muscles)?

3. Use of accessory muscles of inspiration (scalene, sternocleidomastoid, pectoralis, trapezius, and external intercostals) to assist inspiration suggest considerable extra effort required to create the increased negative pressure necessary for adequate inspiration. This can either be because inspiration is more difficult due to obstructive or restrictive disease or because the demands of the body on the lungs are greatly increased. There are other accessory muscles of expiration which include the abdominal and internal intercostal muscles. They act to increase positive pressure within the lungs to assist in expelling air when there is increased airway resistance.

4. Respiratory rate and depth should be observed and counted together to give a clear picture of respiration. A high respiratory rate with shallow breaths may indicate pain preventing normal inspiration, whereas a high rate with normal sized breaths may indicate hyperventilation.

Hypoventilation may be due to central causes including cerebrovascular accidents and head trauma. It may also be related to iatrogenic or self-administered sedatives (e.g. benzodiazepines or opiates). It is not always possible to interpret these signs correctly without looking at other data and caution should be used before attaching too great a significance to them (Table 4.10). For other respiratory patterns associated with specific neurological dysfunction see Chapter 10.

TABLE 4.10	Abnormal respiratory patterns
Name	**Characteristics**
Apnoea	Complete absence of spontaneous ventilation
Hypoventilation	Decreased alveolar ventilation with either decreased rate or depth of breaths. Results in an increased P_ACO_2 and, consequently, an increased P_aCO_2
Hyperventilation	Increased alveolar ventilation with either increased rate or increased depth of breaths. This results in a decreased P_ACO_2 and, consequently, a decreased P_aCO_2
Hyperpnoea	Increased depth of breathing, with or without increased frequency
Tachypnoea	Increased rate of ventilation
Cheyne–Stokes respiration	Periods of apnoea of between 10 and 30 s followed by a progressively increasing rate and volume of breaths which reach a peak and then decline to another period of apnoea. This pattern of respiration is associated with cerebral dysfunction
Kussmaul breathing	Increased rate and depth of breathing commonly associated with diabetic ketoacidosis. It produces a decrease in P_ACO_2 and, consequently, a low P_aCO_2
Biot's breathing	Short episodes of deep inspirations of the same volume and frequency followed by 10–30 s of apnoea. This pattern is associated with meningitis

Note: Eupnoea is the term given to normal spontaneous ventilation.

Palpation

The position of the trachea should be assessed for mediastinal shift by placing a finger either side of the trachea just above the sternal notch. Tracheal deviation is indicative of mediastinal shift caused either by large volumes of pleural air or fluid filling the pleural space and pushing the lung away from the chest wall or by lobar/lung collapse drawing the trachea towards the lung space. Tactile vocal fremitus refers to the vibrations felt when the patient speaks. Sound is usually transmitted well through solid structures and poorly through air. Thus, conditions replacing air with more solid matter in the lungs (e.g. pneumonia), may well increase the transmission of sound. If the chest is palpated with the fingertips or palm on each side and the patient is asked to speak (usually to say 'gg' several times) then a similar degree of vibration should be felt except over the heart. If there is inequality in transmission this may be due to consolidation (increased transmission) or pneumothorax/fluid (decreased transmission).

Percussion

This is not a technique frequently used by nurses and requires some practice to become skilled. The middle phalanx of the middle finger is pressed against the chest wall and struck with the tip of the other middle finger. Different sounds may be produced:

- The normal sound over the lungs is low pitched and long and described as resonant.
- Increased density (e.g. from a pleural effusion) produces stony dull (soft, short, high-pitched) sounds.
- Decreased density (such as in pneumothorax or emphysema) causes hyper-resonant (loud, lower-pitched, and longer) or tympanitic (loud, long, high-pitched, drum-like) sounds.

Auscultation

Air entry to the lung fields

This is a basic measure to ensure that there is flow of air to all areas of the lung. Causes of reduced or non-existent air entry in the self-ventilating patient vary from lobar collapse and pleural effusion to pneumothorax and hypoventilation.

Normal breath sounds

There are three *normal* types of breath sound heard over different parts of the chest:

1. *Vesicular*—low pitch, no break between inspiration and expiration, expiration is longer than inspiration, heard in the periphery of the lung.
2. *Bronchial*—high pitch, loud, pause between inspiration and expiration, expiration equals inspiration, heard over the trachea.
3. *Bronchovesicular*—combination of the above sounds, heard over major airways in most other parts of the lung.

If bronchial sounds are heard over areas of the lung other than the trachea this may be indicative of consolidation of that area or the presence of a pleural effusion just below. This is due to the transmission of the breath sounds from the main airway through the better-conducting medium of consolidated or compressed lung rather than hearing a direct flow of air. This is known as 'bronchial breathing'.

Absent or reduced/distant breath sounds may be heard over a pleural effusion or pneumothorax.

Abnormal breath sounds

1. *Crackles (fine)*—formerly called crepitations, these are high-pitched rustles related to the reopening of small airways or the presence of intra-alveolar fluid. They can be heard in pulmonary oedema and pulmonary fibrosis at the end of inspiration, and in pneumonia and bronchiectasis throughout both inspiration and expiration.

2. *Crackles (coarse)*—these are lower-pitched and usually heard over larger airways, they are indicative of sputum or fluid in these areas.

3. *Wheezes*—formerly known as rhonchi, these are heard on expiration as a result of expired air being forced through narrowed airways. These can be heard in asthma and other causes of bronchoconstriction (e.g. toxic gas inhalation or anaphylaxis). Rarely, wheeze may be heard in heart failure (cardiac asthma). Inspiratory wheeze is associated with major airway obstruction such as tumour or presence of a foreign body. This is stridor and is also heard in epiglottitis and laryngeal oedema (e.g. post-extubation). If wheezes are heard on inspiration and expiration they are often caused by excessive airway secretions.

4. *Pleural friction rubs*—rough, grating, and crackling sound heard on inspiration and expiration. It is found in areas of pleural inflammation (pleurisy) when the normally smooth surfaces of parietal and visceral pleura are roughened and rub on each other.

Pulse oximetry

It is possible to obtain reasonably accurate measures of arterial oxygen saturation using the non-invasive technique of pulse oximetry (for full details see Chapter 5). A sensor placed on the patient's skin can give an almost continuous measure of peripheral arterial oxygen saturation. The major drawback of the technique is the need for a well-perfused peripheral circulation, otherwise the sensor is unable to detect sufficiently strong signals to give an accurate read-out. The oximeter should be used with caution in cases of smoke inhalation, heavy smokers, and patients with unexplained cyanosis as types of haemoglobin, such as carboxyhaemoglobin and methaemoglobin, decrease the accuracy of the oximeter. Readings should be checked against those obtained in a co-oximeter (see Chapter 5 for further details). A saturation of >95% does not imply adequate organ perfusion. The haemoglobin may be fully saturated with oxygen but an inadequate cardiac output, or a low haemoglobin, may result in an inadequate supply of oxygen to the tissues.

NORMAL VALUES IN ARTERIAL BLOOD FOR A PATIENT BREATHING AIR

- pH : 7.35–7.45
- PO_2: 10.0–13.3 kPa
- PCO_2: 4.6–6.0 kPa
- Bicarbonate (HCO_3): 22–26 mmol/l
- Base excess: –2 to +2

The probe position should always be checked if a sharp fall in saturation occurs. Transient falls in saturation may be seen following suction and repositioning of the patient; if these falls persist arterial blood gases should be checked.

Arterial blood gases

The measurement of oxygen (PO_2) and carbon dioxide (PCO_2) tension in arterial blood can give the clearest indication of the patient's respiratory function. It should not be forgotten that the results must always be interpreted in the light of the patient's clinical condition and the inspired oxygen concentration and not purely in the abstract. It is possible for a severely tired and compromised patient to maintain a near normal PCO_2 until almost the point of collapse but clinical assessment of the patient will determine that this is at considerable cost and that intervention may be required. The functions of arterial blood gas measurement are:

1. Measurement of the oxygenation of the patient.

2. Determination of the acid-base status of the patient.

For further details refer back to the anatomy and physiology section.

Tissue hypoxia

Tissue hypoxia is an inadequate availability of oxygen for cell metabolism. This can be due to hypoxaemia (hypoxic hypoxia), anaemia (anaemic hypoxia), circulatory impairment (circulatory hypoxia), and impairment of tissue utilization (histotoxic hypoxia). Hypoxaemia will be addressed in detail in this chapter.

In *anaemic hypoxia* the oxygen tension of the arterial blood is normal but the oxygen-carrying capacity of the blood is inadequate. This can be due to either a low amount of haemoglobin in the blood or a deficiency in the ability of haemoglobin to carry oxygen such as in carbon monoxide poisoning.

In *circulatory hypoxia* the arterial blood that reaches the tissues may have a normal oxygen tension and content but the volume of blood (and therefore the amount of oxygen) delivered is insufficient to meet tissue needs. This is commonly due either to:

1. stagnant hypoxia—slow peripheral capillary flow from either a poor cardiac output, vascular insufficiency or neurochemical abnormalities, or

2. arterial-venous shunt—some tissue cells are completely bypassed by arterial blood.

Histotoxic hypoxia is impairment of the ability of the tissue cells to utilize oxygen. This occurs in cyanide poisoning.

Hypoxaemia

A low oxygen concentration (<8.0 kPa) in the blood. Tissue hypoxia does not necessarily coexist, as considerable compensation may be occurring to overcome the low level of P_aO_2, for example by an increased cardiac output, increased oxygen extraction by the tissues, or (in chronic states such as chronic obstructive airways disease or living at altitude), an increased haemoglobin.

Hypocapnia

Low carbon dioxide concentration in the blood (<4.0 kPa). Usually due to hyperventilation.

Hypercapnia

High carbon dioxide concentration in the blood (>6.0 kPa). Causes are usually hypoventilation or occasionally increased carbon dioxide production due to overfeeding with carbohydrate.

Methods of respiratory support

There is a range of levels of support from simple supplemental oxygen therapy to complete ventilatory support using mechanical ventilators (see Table 4.11).

The aims of respiratory support are:

- To correct hypoxaemia and hypercapnia.
- To assist mechanical failure (including an unprotected airway).
- To decrease associated workload: work of breathing and myocardial workload.

Priorities in caring for patients requiring respiratory support

Safety

A method of back-up ventilation for the patient must be immediately to hand. This is invariably a manual ventilation bag (e.g. rebreathe bag or Ambu bag). It is essential that it is checked as a priority safety routine by any nurse responsible for the patient.

TABLE 4.11 Methods of oxygen delivery for respiratory support

Mode of delivery	Oxygen percentage available	Associated problems	Safety priorities	Use
Nasal cannulae	2 l/min 23–28%, 3 l/min 28–30%, 4 l/min 32–36%, 5 l/min 40%, 6 l/min plus (max. 44%)	Limited % O_2 available. Inaccurate delivery of oxygen, particularly with high minute volumes. Requires patent nasal passages; if patient mouth-breathes then amount of oxygen delivered will be altered. Drying and uncomfortable for nasal passages	Regular monitoring of respiratory rate and pattern. If patient unstable use pulse oximeter to monitor O_2 saturation Positioning of cannulae inside nares. Check O_2 flow rate	Low levels of O_2 supplementation for relatively short periods only. Disposable delivery system
Semi-rigid masks (e.g. Hudson, MC, etc.)	4 l/min ~35%, 6 l/min ~50%, 8 l/min ~55%, 10 l/min ~60%, 12 l/min ~65%	Inaccurate delivery of O_2, particularly with high minute volumes. Limits patient activities such as eating and drinking. Drying for patient's mucosa and for secretions. Rebreathing may occur with high minute volumes	Regular monitoring of respiratory rate and pattern. If patient unstable use pulse oximeter to monitor O_2 saturation. Check positioning of mask and O_2 flow rate	Low to medium levels of O_2 supplementation only. Disposable delivery system
Venturi-type mask (high-flow system) (e.g. Ventimasks, Inspiron, etc.)	With use of appropriate Venturi nozzle for each %: 2 l/min 24%, 4 l/min 28%, 8 l/min 35%, 10 l/min 40%, 15 l/min 60%	Can still be drying for patient. If humidification used an extra attachment is required. Patients requiring large inspiratory flow rates may still not achieve required O_2%. Limits patient activities, such as eating and drinking	Regular monitoring of respiratory rate and pattern. If patient unstable use pulse oximeter to monitor O_2 saturation. Check positioning of mask and O_2 flow rate	Medium to high levels of O_2 supplementation. Disposable delivery system
Humified oxygen using nebulizer system (e.g. Aquapaks)	Varying rates of flow to deliver 28–60% O_2	Inaccurate delivery of O_2, particularly with high volumes and pattern. Limits patient activities	Regular monitoring of respiratory rate and pattern. If patient unstable use pulse oximeter. Check positioning of mask, O_2 flowrate, and setting of O_2 percentage on nebulizer system	Low to medium levels of O_2 supplementation. Disposable delivery system
Non-rebreathe masks with reservoir bag	90–95% depending on respiratory rate and run at 15 l/min	reservoir bag should be partially inflated at all times	Ensure reservoir bag is fully inflated before placing on patient	Emergency situations short term use only
Continuous positive airway pressure (CPAP) using high-flow generator or large-volume balloon reservoir	40–100% with tightly fitting CPAP mask. 2.5–15 cm H_2O using adjustable or exchangeable expiratory valves	Tightly fitting mask causing discomfort, pressure sores, etc. Leakage of high gas flows into eyes may cause corneal drying and abrasion. Use of nasogastric tube to decompress stomach if necessary. Air swallowing may cause gastric discomfort and increased risk of regurgitation. Eating and drinking are very difficult. Patient may experience feelings	Pulse oximetry to monitor patient O_2 saturation. Regular monitoring of respiratory rate and pattern. Provision of psychological support and comfort to assist patient tolerance	Medium to high levels of O_2 supplementation. Mask, tubing, and valve set-up disposable.

TABLE 4.11	Methods of oxygen delivery for respiratory support – *continued*			
Mode of delivery	Oxygen percentage available	Associated problems	Safety priorities	Use
		of claustrophobia due to tightly fitting mask. Increased noise associated with high flows may disturb patient. In systems without a high-flow generator, flow may be inadequate causing increased inspiratory resistance Flow generator non-disposable		
Non-invasive ventilation using standard ventilators or Bi-level assisted spontaneous breathing machines	Bi-level ventilators need entrained oxygen and only offer O_2 up to 35%. ICU ventilators can provide up to 100%	A tight-fitting mask, or helmet is required with the same problems as above	Monitoring of O_2 saturation and if there is an acute change in condition also ABGs	COPD, chest wall deformity, neuromuscular disease, failed weaning from ventilation

The appropriate sizes of oropharyngeal (Guedel) airways and facemask should also be available at the patient's bedside.

The concentration of inspired oxygen (F_iO_2) that the patient is actually receiving should be checked against that prescribed. This is done using an oxygen analyser either as part of the ventilator or as a separate piece of equipment. The method of delivery should also be considered; it should be capable of delivering the percentage required. Standard oxygen masks (e.g. Hudson masks) are incapable of delivering an accurate level of oxygen. In particular, when the patient has a high minute ventilation it is difficult to achieve an F_iO_2 above 0.4 using standard masks (see Table 4.11).

Equipment alarms are a very reliable way of identifying sudden or life-threatening changes in the patient's condition. They are, however, only as useful as the alarm limits and settings, therefore the nurse must ensure that the alarms are set appropriately.

Ventilator alarms

Alarm settings on the ventilators should be checked to ensure they are on and appropriate to the patient. For most patients:

1. Expired minute volume alarms should be set:
   - Upper at 21 above current expired minute volume.
   - Lower at 21 below current expired minute volume.

2. Airway pressure alarms should be set:

- Upper at 40 cm H_2O or as instructed by medical staff.
- Lower at 5 cm H_2O below current airway pressure reading.

3. Pulse oximeter alarms should usually be set at 90% oxygen saturation. However, this may alter according to the patient's condition.

4. Cardiac monitor alarms. These settings will reflect cardiac status but will also provide a useful warning for respiratory problems and should always be set appropriately (see Chapter 6).

Suction equipment

Suction equipment is essential both as an emergency measure and in routine use for intubated or tracheostomized patients. It should always be checked to ensure it is capable of producing the appropriate level of suction and that suction catheters are the correct size for the patient's endotracheal tube and condition of secretions (see section on suction technique later).

Problems associated with patients undergoing respiratory support

These will be divided into problems associated with supporting the patient's own compromised respiratory function and those associated with taking over the patient's respiratory function using some form of mechanical ventilation. All patients requiring a form of

DEFINITION OF RESPIRATORY FAILURE

Arterial blood gases

- PO_2 < 8.0 kPa with patient breathing air and at rest.
- ± PCO_2 > 6.5 kPa in the absence of primary metabolic acidosis.
- ± pH < 7.25 in the absence of primary metabolic acidosis.

Patient

- Respiratory rate >40 or <6–8 breaths/min.
- Deteriorating vital capacity (<15 ml/kg).

respiratory support have some degree of respiratory failure.

Respiratory failure is classically categorized into Type I and Type II:

- In Type I respiratory failure the patient is hypoxaemic but has normal levels of carbon dioxide.
- In Type II respiratory failure the patient is both hypoxaemic and hypercapnic.

Non-invasive respiratory support may be considered in the circumstances detailed in Table 4.12. Non-invasive respiratory support involves use of oxygen therapy, continuous positive airway pressure (CPAP), and non invasive ventilation (NIV) which includes intermittent positive pressure breathing (IPPB), and bilevel positive airway pressure (BiPAP).These systems deliver support through tight-fitting nasal or oral masks, full face masks, or helmets (see Table 4.11)

Hypoxaemia

Management of hypoxaemia involves oxygen therapy as per patient requirements (see Table 4.11). Chronic carbon dioxide retainers depending on a hypoxic respiratory drive should have controlled levels of F_iO_2 with continuous observation of respiratory rate and regular monitoring of P_aCO_2 levels.

Chest physiotherapy will assist in removal of secretions. Deep breathing and coughing may also help reopen areas of collapsed lung.

Positioning of the patient to optimize ventilation/perfusion matching (see section on shunting). Usually, this is upright, although if the problem is unilateral the patient should be placed on the side with the problem lung *uppermost* so that the good lung is being perfused.

Hypercapnia

Management depends on the cause: patients will require NIV or intubation and mechanical ventilation. Early management may also include respiratory stimulants such as doxapram but this is only usually a short-term option before non-invasive ventilation can be established.

National Institute for Clinical Excellence (NICE) guidelines suggest that NIV should be considered in COPD when the patient has a respiratory acidosis (pH < 7.35) and hypercapnia (National Institute for Clinical Excellence 2004)

TABLE 4.12	Indications and contraindications for use of non-invasive ventilation (NIV) (BTS Guidelines 2002)		
Indications for NIV	**Clinical condition**	**Contraindications**	**Preconditions**
Acute exacerbation of COPD	Sick but not moribund. Able to protect own airway. Haemodynamically stable. No excessive respiratory secretions	Facial injury. Vomiting. Fixed upper airway obstruction. Undrained pneumothorax	Ensure a management plan if the trial of NIV fails before commencing. Discuss/decide which environment is best for the patient
Chest wall deformity/ neuromuscular disorder	As above	As above	As above
Pulmonary oedema unresponsive to CPAP	As above but with a failed trial of CPAP	Severe hypoxaemia	ICU/HDU bed available if trial of NIV fails
Assistance to wean from mechanical ventilation	Previous failed attempts to wean from ventilation		Only in ICU

Maintenance of airway and sputum clearance

Humidification will assist clearance of thick, tenacious secretions and prevent the drying of mucosa and cilia associated with inhalation of dry oxygen (see section on humidification).

Regular assistance with deep breathing and coughing will reduce the incidence of atelectasis and help the patient to clear secretions. If necessary, suctioning via the oro- or nasal pharynx may assist in removal of sputum (see section on suction). Chest physiotherapy and postural drainage are also useful.

Fatigue related to work of breathing

Management requires the limitation of any other activity likely to produce fatigue. Provide periods specifically for complete rest without interference. Ensure that the day/night environment is preserved.

Fear and anxiety

Management involves providing comfort and reassurance by a calm and confident approach to the patient. Include the family as much as possible in care and interactions. Allow time for expression of worries and ensure that the patient is given full information expressed appropriately to ensure understanding.

Poor nutritional intake due to shortage of breath and loss of appetite

Provide frequent, small nutritious meals. Offer high-calorie hot or cold drinks in between. Encourage the family to become involved in meals and obtain details of the patient's likes and dislikes. Maintain a full record of nutritional intake and ensure that the medical staff are made aware of any continued deficit.

Impaired verbal communication due to shortage of breath and presence of mask

Provide alternative methods of communication such as an alphabet board or pen and paper. Use closed questions for specific information so that the patient can nod or shake their head to answer. Instruct the family in these methods. Anticipate the patient's information needs so that unnecessary questions can be avoided (see Chapter 3).

Drying of mouth and upper airways due to high flow of dry gases

Humidify the inspired gases (see section on humidification). Check skin turgor and the condition of the buccal mucosa. Provide mouthwashes and oral hygiene measures as necessary (see Chapter 3). Monitor fluid balance and avoid systemic dehydration unless the medical condition dictates otherwise.

INDICATIONS FOR ENDOTRACHEAL AND TRACHEOSTOMY TUBES

- To obtain or maintain a clear airway.
- To prevent aspiration of gastrointestinal contents.
- To facilitate delivery of positive pressure ventilation.
- To enable delivery of high concentrations of oxygen.
- To facilitate removal of pulmonary secretions.

SITES OF INSERTION

- Oral endotracheal tube—mouth to trachea.
- Nasal endotracheal tube—nose to trachea.
- Tracheostomy—percutaneous or surgical insertion below the cricoid and thyroid cartilages (usually between the second and third tracheal rings).
- Minitracheostomy and cricothyroidotomy—percutaneous or surgical insertion through the cricothyroid membrane.

Endotracheal intubation and tracheostomy

Positive pressure ventilation requires a closed system of delivery in the adult patient to allow effective ventilation. Thus, some form of seal in the patient's airway is essential. Non-invasive ventilation uses a tight-fitting mask to form a seal and invasive mechanical ventilation uses either an endotracheal (ET) tube or a tracheostomy tube. Endotracheal tubes are usually placed orally, although nasal placements are used in children and occasionally in adults. Tracheostomy tubes require percutaneous or surgical placement below the cricoid and thyroid cartilages (usually around the second or third ring of the trachea). The cuff also provides some protection against the aspiration of gastric secretions, food, blood, etc., although this is not complete.

The presence of a tube in the trachea is associated with a number of potential problems and complications. Some of these problems are immediately apparent but many will not become apparent until later in the patient's recovery period when decannulation highlights them.

A major factor in the development of tracheal ulceration and stenosis is the need for a cuff or balloon to seal the airway. These cuffs are now designed to be high

PROBLEMS ASSOCIATED WITH ENDOTRACHEAL TUBE PLACEMENT

- Tracheal stenosis, ulceration, necrosis
- Tracheomalacia (degeneration of the cartilaginous rings)
- Clearance of secretions
- Loss of normal humidifying and warming mechanisms
- Loss of physiological positive end expiratory pressure (PEEP) (i.e. the resistance to expiration exerted by the pharynx and upper airways which limits alveolar collapse)
- Damage to vocal cords and trauma on insertion
- Increased risk of nosocomial (hospital-acquired) pneumonia
- Maxillary sinusitis (with nasal tubes)

PROBLEMS ASSOCIATED WITH TRACHEOSTOMY TUBE PLACEMENT

- Tracheal stenosis, fibrosis, tracheomalacia
- Loss of normal humidifying and warming mechanisms
- Loss of physiological PEEP
- Increased risk of nosocomial pneumonia

in volume and low in pressure to reduce some of the complications, and are filled with air to provide the necessary seal. Capillary occlusion pressure within the tracheal wall is approximately 30 mmHg and it is important to limit the cuff pressure to less than this in order to protect the blood supply to the tracheal mucosa. The use of manometers to measure cuff pressure is essential. Cuff pressure should be checked three or four times a day and whenever an air leak is heard, in order to ensure that pressures are within this limit. Estimation by fingertip pressure on the external cuff balloon or filling until no further leak is heard is inaccurate and may lead to much higher pressure. However, when lung inflation pressures are high, cuff pressures may have to be increased over the recommended levels to prevent leaks.

Any access to the trachea bypassing the normal protective immune mechanisms will increase the likelihood of pneumonia. Endotracheal intubation is associated with a 21-fold increase in the risk of developing pneumonia (Rello and Diaz, 2003). Subglottic suctioning, either continuously or intermittently, using specially adapted ET tubes has been suggested as a way of reducing this but studies have yet to show this (Girou *et al.* 2004)

Endotracheal tubes

Oral tubes are most commonly used in adults, being easier to insert and secure.

Nasal tubes are felt to be more comfortable for the patient and avoid the hazard of being constricted by the patient's teeth. However, a smaller size is generally necessary and the angle at the nasopharynx can cause difficulty with insertion of suction catheters. Furthermore, there is a significant associated incidence of maxillary sinusitis and this should always be considered if a nasally intubated patient develops an unexplained pyrexia. They are therefore not commonly used in adults.

Types of tube used for adults

- Single use cuffed endotracheal and tracheostomy tubes made from silastic or PVC.
- Red rubber tubes should no longer be used.

There are also some special tubes:

- Double lumen ET tubes for asynchronous ventilation. One lumen opens into the trachea and the other into a bronchus (usually the left—this should be ascertained prior to insertion).
- Adjustable flange ET tubes for larger necks or problems with cuff sealing in ordinary tubes.

Note: Endotracheal tubes for children are always uncuffed as they are highly susceptible to stenotic problems related to cuff pressure, particularly in the cricoid region which is narrowed until puberty.

USUAL ADULT SIZES OF ENDOTRACHEAL TUBE

- Men: oral, 8–9 mm internal diameter (ID); nasal, 7–8 mm ID.
- Women: oral, 7–8 mm ID; nasal, 6–7 mm ID.

Tube sizes ranging from 6.0 mm to 11.0 mm ID are routinely available. The tube diameter (external) should be considerably less than the cricoid diameter to decrease the risk of damage.

Note. Tube sizes for children vary with age or body weight from 2.5 mm newborn to 8.0 mm for 12- to 15-year-olds. Various formulae are available to estimate the correct diameter for age.

Length of endotracheal tubes

Oral ET tubes should be positioned at approximately 23 cm at the incisors for men and 21 cm for women. However, this position will depend on body size and neck length and requires confirmation initially by ensuring good air entry to both lungs and, subsequently, by chest X-ray. A cause of patient agitation after recovery from intubation, paralysis, and sedation can be the tube sitting on the carina or, alternatively, the cuff herniating through the vocal cords. The end of the tube should be roughly 3–5 cm above the carina.

In the UK the tubes are generally pre-cut prior to insertion to a length 2–3 cm longer than estimated to allow secure tying of the tube. This method has been used with reasonable success in preventing endobronchial intubation.

Intubation

If at all possible this should be a calm, elective procedure made in good time according to the criteria for ventilation. Ideally, the patient should not have eaten for at least 4 h. However, it is often necessary to intubate in emergency situations so it is vital to have all equipment (see Table 4.13) readily available and kept together in one place.

Safety priorities apply whether the procedure is elective or an emergency, namely:

- Check the manual ventilation bag and suction equipment to ensure they are functioning.
- Attach the ventilator to the gas source and check it is functioning.
- Ensure emergency drugs (see Chapter 7) are to hand and that the patient has reliable intravenous access.

TABLE 4.13 Equipment for intubation over and above available safety equipment

Laryngoscopes—one curved, one straight blade (check that the light is working)

Selection of endotracheal tubes of varying internal diameter

Lubrication (e.g. KY jelly)

Magill's forceps

Introducer (Bougie)

10 ml syringe

Artery forceps

Tape to secure tube

Catheter mount

Cuff pressure manometer

Sedating and paralysing agents

A back-up manual ventilation bag and mask

Prior to intubation the procedure should be explained to the patient if there is time. In particular, the temporary loss of speech due to the presence of the tube should be emphasized to prevent anxiety.

- Prepare equipment, drugs, and ventilator.
- Pre-oxygenation via facemask for at least 5 min if the patient's condition permits.
- Cricoid pressure (pressure on the cricoid cartilage using the finger pads of the thumb, forefinger, and middle finger to compress the pharyngeal airway) preventing reflux of gastric contents in emergency intubation may be necessary.

Before administering any drugs, check that:

1. All equipment is ready and functioning (including manual ventilation bag, suction, etc.).

2. A tube has been cut ready for insertion and an intact cuff ensured.

3. A doctor has checked the settings on the ventilator. The inspired oxygen concentration should initially be set at a higher level than the anticipated requirements of the patient.

4. The patient is ideally positioned either supine with a pillow under the occiput or if the patient is orthopnoeic then remaining upright but able to be laid flat as soon as the manoeuvre begins. The position for intubation is neck slightly flexed and head extended.

Continuous observation of the patient, ECG, pulse oximetry, and blood pressure is essential. Following insertion and cuff inflation:

- Check air entry by auscultation then attach to the ventilator.
- Secure the tube—one method is shown in Fig. 4.7.
- Check cuff pressure with a manometer.
- Consider insertion of a nasogastric tube.
- Carry out a full set of respiratory observations.
- Ensure a chest X-ray has been arranged to confirm satisfactory tube position (tip sited 2–5 cm above the carina), and absence of pneumothorax.
- Arterial blood gases should be performed to confirm satisfactory P_aO_2 and P_aCO_2 levels after 10–15 min equilibration (or sooner if indicated). Ventilator settings should then be adjusted as necessary.

Specific nursing care of the intubated patient
Securing the tube

Movement of the tube can result in traumatic extubation, displacement of the tube, loss of cuff seal, and

POTENTIAL COMPLICATIONS OF INTUBATION

- Inability to intubate
- Aspiration of gastric contents
- Bleeding from trauma to the airway
- Endobronchial intubation (usually right main bronchus)
- Oesophageal intubation
- Vocal cord damage
- Perforation (rare)
- Hypotension (usually due to vasodilator effects of anaesthetic agents unmasking covert hypovolaemia; occasionally due to cardiodepressant effects of the same drugs)
- Arrhythmias (usually bradycardia due to hypoxia or vagal stimulation—atropine may be required if the patient does not respond to correction of hypoxaemia)
- Dislodged teeth

even oesophageal intubation, as well as causing considerable discomfort to the patient. Displacement of the tracheostomy tube into the pre-tracheal tissue is also possible. It is therefore vital to secure the tube and to check for any loosening of the tapes on a regular basis. Unplanned extubation has been reported in between 1 and 19% of patients and is associated with restlessness/agitation, confusion, previous accidental extubation episode, current history of smoking, medical ICU, use of physical restraint, decreased level of consciousness, and oral (versus nasotracheal) endotracheal tube (Happ 2002). The usual method of securing adult tubes uses cotton tapes which are looped around the ET tube or

through the slits in the flange of the tracheostomy tube. These are passed round the patient's head either above or below the ears and tied at one side. They should be tight enough to allow only one finger between the tape and the patient's neck (Fig. 4.7). Alternative commercially available ties use Velcro flaps on soft cotton collars but these are expensive.

Pressure from the constricting tapes or knot is a problem. Regular changing of tapes (checking the skin and lip underneath) and foam or felt covers for the tapes is of benefit. It should also be remembered that the patient's ears and the occiput may also develop pressure sores from the tapes. (*Note*: Intracranial pressure can be increased by tight tapes occluding venous return.)

Prevention of upper airway damage

Pressure within the tube cuff should be checked routinely. Ideally, cuff pressure should not exceed 30 mmHg (capillary occlusion pressure) and should be kept as low as is compatible with a good seal. High-volume, low-pressure cuffs should always be used for anything other than short-term intubation as the incidence of tracheal trauma is greatly reduced.

There is no evidence that periodic deflation of the cuff is of any benefit and it may actually cause problems if large amounts of saliva/secretions have collected above the cuff.

Secure fixation of the tube to prevent displacement (see above) is important in preventing tracheal damage. The skin and lip or nostril under the tube should be checked and cleaned whenever the tapes are changed as pressure can cause severe ulceration and necrosis.

Oral hygiene

Routine oral care may have to be increased in frequency and extra care taken, particularly with an oral tube. The lips may become excoriated and dry and should be protected with petroleum jelly or a similar barrier agent.

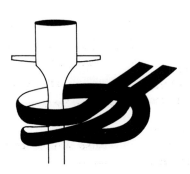

Fig. 4.7 Securing endotracheal tube (ET) tapes. Tapes should *always* be tied around the plastic of the ET tube itself, not around the connector because it is possible for the connector to dislodge.

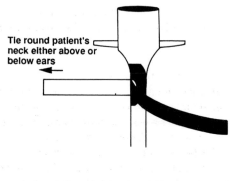

Tie round patient's neck either above or below ears

EQUIPMENT FOR EXTUBATION

- Scissors
- Syringe
- Suction—tracheal and Yankauer
- Oxygen mask and tubing (or CPAP circuit)
- Disposable towel
- Mouthwash

Extubation procedure (oral or nasal endotracheal tubes)

Preparation of the patient should include an explanation of the procedure and securing their cooperation during removal. Emergency equipment, as for intubation, should be checked. If the patient has been intubated for any length of time a pulse oximeter is useful for monitoring oxygen saturations during and after extubation. The patient should remain monitored/under close observation for the next 4–6 h to ensure that respiratory distress does not occur.

The principles of extubation are as follows:

1. Two nurses are necessary for safe extubation.

2. The patient is usually most comfortable sitting up.

3. The patient's airway and oropharynx should be as clear of secretions as possible prior to extubation.

4. One nurse will cut the tapes and deflate the cuff, the other will suction and withdraw the tube.

5. If secretions are thick or copious, suction to just below the tip of the tube should continue while the tube is withdrawn.

6. The patient will need assistance to cough up any further secretions and then should have a mouthwash or oral toilet to clear the mouth.

7. The patient will require oxygen via either an oxygen mask or CPAP depending on his/her condition.

Tracheostomy

Formation of a tracheostomy

This may be either a surgical procedure requiring a horizontal incision between the second and third tracheal rings or a percutaneous approach using a dilator system to insert the tracheostomy tube.

Tracheostomy is a procedure which carries some risk and should not be undertaken lightly. There is some evidence to suggest that the percutaneous method has a reduced incidence of complications (Freeman *et al.* 2000). A meta-analysis of studies in 236 patients showed no difference in overall operative complication rates but less peri-operative bleeding, a lower overall post-operative complication rate, and lower post-operative incidence of bleeding and stomal infection.

Following insertion, it is recommended that the tube be left in place for 5–7 days to allow formation of a tract from the skin to the trachea. It can then be changed as required. Use of tracheostomy tubes with removable inner cannulae will allow cleaning of the inner tube to avoid encrustation and blockage due to secretions. The tube should be a size that is the largest that will fit comfortably into the trachea.

Tracheostomy tubes

Types of tubes used will vary according to the length of time the patient is likely to remain tracheostomized. Commonly the first tube placed will be a PVC tube without inner cannulae or fenestration but with a cuff. This will then be changed after a period of between 5 and 7 days for a longer-term tube:

- A long-term tracheostomy tube with removable inner tubes for cleaning/regular replacement to prevent blockage and with inflatable cuff.

- A long term tracheostomy tube with fenestration (window or hole) to allow redirection of exhaled breath through the vocal cords and speech, when cuff deflation and capping of the tube are effected. This is only possible during spontaneous ventilation.

- A re-useable uncuffed silver tube (Negus), used for long-term tracheostomized self-ventilating patients.

The sizes routinely used for tracheostomy tubes range from 26 FG to 36 FG. They are usually of a standard length, although it is possible to obtain custom-made tubes for patients with problem necks which are very short or long, or to avoid damaged areas of the trachea (e.g. tracheomalacia).

PERI-OPERATIVE COMPLICATIONS OF TRACHEOSTOMY

- Haemorrhage
- Surgical emphysema
- Pneumothorax
- Air embolism
- Cricoid cartilage damage

Specific care of the patient with tracheostomy
Safety priorities

Tracheal dilators and replacement tubes of the same and a smaller size should be kept with the patient in case of accidental extubation. Routine emergency equipment including suction, manual ventilation bag, airways, catheter mount, and mask should be immediately available and checked routinely.

Care of the stoma

Following formation, a dry dressing, such as gauze or lyofoam, is used. The stoma should be cleaned routinely (~8-hourly) and the site inspected for signs of infection or bleeding. This is an aseptic procedure. Normal saline is usually sufficient, although other solutions such as chlorhexidine have been suggested. However, there is no evidence that they are more effective and therefore there is little point in their use.

If secretions from the tracheostomy are very copious, the skin should be protected with a stomahesive wafer shaped to fit and the secretions should be suctioned away as they form.

If tracheostomy tubes with removable inner cannulae are used, these should be removed and cleaned 8-hourly. The cannula can be cleaned using mouthcare sponges, small bottle brushes, or ribbon gauze soaked in antiseptic solution. If very encrusted, sodium bicarbonate may help to remove dried secretions.

Changing the tracheostomy tube

It is usual to wait 7 days or so after insertion to allow the stoma to form before changing the tube. The frequency of tube changes thereafter is usually dictated by

TABLE 4.14 Equipment for tracheostomy tube change
Emergency equipment
Tubes, one the same size, one smaller
Tracheal dilators
Lubricant jelly
Sterile gloves
Cleaning solution
10 ml syringe
Tracheostomy dressing and new tapes

unit policy but should be at least every 7 days (in a tracheostomy tube without a separate inner cannula) in order to prevent encrustation and narrowing of the inner diameter which will increase the work of breathing (Table 4.14).

Tubes can be changed by an experienced nurse, but medical back-up should always be readily available in case of problems.

Prior to assembling the equipment for the procedure, the patient should be prepared with an explanation of the need for a tube change and the steps involved.

Two nurses are necessary for safe procedure. It is an aseptic technique. After preparation of the equipment, the new tracheostomy tube should be checked to ensure even inflation of the cuff and easy withdrawal of the introducer. The patient should be well pre-oxygenated and have had mouth and trachea suctioned. The stoma should be cleaned as normal and the tapes cut. When all is prepared the cuff is deflated and the old tube removed. The new tube is inserted, the introducer withdrawn, and

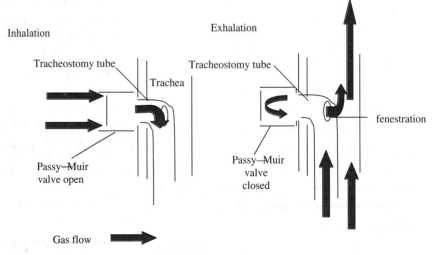

Fig. 4.8 Passy-muir valve action.

Gas flow ▶

NB: Tracheostomy cuff is always deflated

the cuff inflated. The ventilator is then reattached and air entry checked. The tube is then secured.

Use of Passy–Muir valves with tracheostomies

The Passy–Muir valve (Fig. 4.8) is a one-way valve designed to be used in both ventilated and spontaneously breathing tracheostomized patients (Bell 1996). The valve allows gas flow into the lungs from the ventilator during inspiration but closes as soon as gas flow ceases, thus redirecting exhalation out through either fenestrations or around the deflated cuff of the tracheostomy tube. Exhaled gas thus passes through the vocal cords allowing the patient to speak.

Removal (decannulation) of tracheal tubes

A patient who has had a tracheostomy tube *in situ* for some time should be fully assessed for any limiting factors associated with decannulation. Removal of the tracheostomy tube will result in a dead space increase for the patient which can translate into an increase in the work of breathing of up to 30% (Chadda *et al.* 2002). Any patients with a restrictive respiratory disease who may not cope with the increased demand will require careful assessment and a gradual approach to decannulation, perhaps by the use of smaller sized tracheostomy tubes rather than abrupt removal.

Assess the patient (Bourjeily *et al.* 2002) to ensure that there is:

1. No ongoing requirement for mechanical ventilation that cannot be met by non-invasive ventilatory support.

2. An adequate cough allowing expectoration of secretions (peak expiratory cough flows in excess of 200 l/min).

CONTRAINDICATIONS FOR THE USE OF THE PASSY–MUIR VALVE

- Unconscious and/or comatose patients
- Inflated tracheostomy tube cuff
- Foam-filled cuffed tracheostomy tube
- Severe airway obstruction
- Unmanageable, thick secretions
- Severe risk of aspiration
- Severely reduced lung elasticity
- The device is not intended for use with endotracheal tubes or other artificial airways
- Sleeping patients

Bell (1996)

---

3. No physiologically significant upper airway lesion (such as overgranulation or tracheal stenosis).

No patient should be decannulated unless they have been able to breathe for a period of at least 24 hours with the cuff deflated and the tracheal cannula itself capped off (Serra 2000). Ideally, this should be via a fenestrated tracheal tube.

Decannulation procedure

Preparation is as for changing the tube and preparation of the patient is as for extubation.

The equipment needed is similar to that for extubation but the mouthwash is unnecessary and an airtight dressing such as a stomahesive wafer or petroleum gauze and waterproof plaster should be added. No surgery is necessary as the stoma will close spontaneously over a number of days.

The principles of tracheostomy tube removal are:

1. Principles (1)–(4) for extubation apply.

2. The site should be cleaned prior to extubation.

3. The stoma should be sealed with an airtight dressing.

4. Attach an oxygen mask (or CPAP circuit).

5. A minitracheostomy may be inserted through the existing stoma after extubation if there is concern that the patient may not adequately clear secretions.

Minitracheostomy

This involves insertion of a small-diameter (4.0 mm) cuffless tube through the cricothyroid membrane. It is a reasonably safe procedure employing a guidewire and dilator (Seldinger) technique for placement. Potential complications are haemorrhage, surgical emphysema, and displacement. Its uses include:

- Suction access for sputum retention in patients who do not require intubation for any other reason (a 10 FG suction catheter can be inserted through the tube).

- Emergency insertion for life-threatening airway obstruction.

Minitracheostomy is not suitable for protection of the airway in patients without a cough or gag reflex, or in patients who require ventilatory support. However, it is possible to perform jet ventilation via a minitracheostomy in some patients.

Ventilatory support (mechanical ventilation)

The objectives of supporting ventilation are (Tobin 2001):

- To decrease the work associated with breathing.

◆ To reverse life-threatening hypoxaemia.

◆ To reverse acute progressive respiratory acidosis.

Ventilatory support includes methods of positive and negative pressure ventilation, both non-invasive and invasive, as well as high-frequency ventilation and extracorporeal support. The vast majority of ventilators used in critical care are positive pressure ventilators. These will therefore be discussed in detail, although other types of ventilators will be described briefly and referenced for further information (see Table 4.15).

Positive pressure ventilation means that ventilatory gas is driven into the airways under a positive pressure which allows inflation of the alveoli and movement of the gas from mouth to alveoli. The force required is higher than that produced in normal ventilation and the effects of this non-physiological approach are widespread. Furthermore, the gas mixture has to be propelled through tubing (i.e. the endotracheal tube) of a smaller diameter than the patient's own trachea (see endotracheal tube sizes, p. 88). This increases resistance to airflow and the pressures required to deliver the tidal volume are correspondingly higher.

There are three types of positive pressure ventilation:

1. *Pressure-cycled*. The ventilator allows inspiration to continue until a pre-set pressure is reached when it will cycle to expiration. It carries certain risks in that a sudden change in lung compliance or the existence of a large air leak may result in inadequate ventilation. Thus, the expired tidal volume and the inspiratory pressure must be closely monitored along with the patient's clinical status. This is the preferred mode of ventilation for small children where endotracheal tubes with a cuff to seal the airway are not used due to the potential for damage to the trachea.

2. *Volume-cycled*. This allows a pre-set volume of air to be delivered to the patient, and once this volume has been reached expiration then occurs. The pressure generated by the delivery of this volume will be determined by the compliance of the lung, the flow rate, and the time for inspiration. It is possible to manipulate the pressure generated by manipulating the flow rate and inspiratory time. As high airway pressures are associated with an increased incidence of lung trauma, manipulation is usually aimed at minimizing airway pressure.

3. *Time-cycled*. This can be an option on ventilators that are normally volume-cycled. The time for each breath is proportioned into inspiration, expiration, and occasionally plateau sections. This gives a ratio of time for inspiration to time for expiration (I:E ratio). This is normally set at 1:2 but can be adjusted to allow a longer period for expiration in patients, such as asthmatics, with outflow obstruction, or a longer period for inspiration in patients with non-compliant lungs, such as those with ARDS. In other words, the set tidal volume is delivered over shorter or longer proportions of the total time for each breath.

The mechanics of positive pressure ventilation

Most current ventilators are driven by the pressure of compressed air, using electronic or computerized formats for control of delivery. However, newer technologies in recent ventilators allow generation of pressure which is independent of a compressed gas source, e.g. Puritan Bennett PB 740, Respironics Esprit. Independence from a compressed gas source allows the ventilator more flexibility in terms of movement, etc. Different technologies such as pistons, electromagnetic valves, and turbines have been employed but little is known about the influence that these different technologies have on the patient.

There are similar functions or controls on most ventilators, although there may be many individually named features depending on their complexity and different styles of weaning modes (Table 4.16).

Standard ventilators (pre-1993 generation)

The older type of ventilator was developed prior to 1993 and is less able to respond to patient demand (triggering) during pressure support ventilation than the newer generation (Richard *et al.* 2002). However, for the most part they provide similar modes of ventilation and are suitable for weaning more complex intensive care patients

New generation ventilators

The more sophisticated ventilators produced after 1993 have improved triggering and pressure response and in addition some are no longer dependent on compressed air gas supply. Although they perform better in simulated patient situations, this has yet to be shown to translate into differences in weaning outcome or length of time on mechanical ventilation.

Non-invasive ventilators

These ventilators are simple positive pressure devices that provide a gas flow at two levels of pressure (inspiratory and expiratory) which can be set. They do not require an endotracheal tube, using either a nasal mask, full face mask, or helmet. The ventilator cycles between the two levels of pressure based on either sensing reversal of gas flow or timing. They deliver

TABLE 4.15 Ventilator settings

Ventilator setting	Typical range of adult patient	Typical range of ventilation capability	Function	Alarm limits	Safety checks
Inspired oxygen (F_iO_2/%O_2)	Variable according to patient need and PO_2. From 21% to 100%	F_iO_2 = 0.21–1.0. %O_2 = 21–100%	Manipulation of inspired O_2 to produce optimal patient oxygenation	Automatic alarm setting. If F_iO_2 falls/ rises from set amount then alarm is triggered	Use separate oxygen analyser in patient circuit to confirm setting. Check digital display of ventilator
Respiratory rate or (frequency/ min)	Usually 10–15 breaths/min but rate altered to manipulate MV and PCO_2/PO_2	From 0–50 breaths/min (rate above 50 usually for paediatric use)	Delivery of adequate ventilation, and can be used to manipulate PO_2 and PCO_2	Associated with expired MV alarm as resp. rate/min × V_T = V_E. MV alarms usually set manually at 2 litres above (upper alarm) and 2 litres below (lower alarm) set ventilation MV	The patient's respiratory rate/min should be manually counted hourly. If patient on IMV/spontaneous modes then ventilator display should be checked
Tidal volume (V_T/ml)	Aim is 6–8 ml/kg but may be altered outside this range to optimize PO_2 and PCO_2	0–1500 ml	Size of each breath can be altered to suit patient size and to ensure optimal alveolar ventilation without hyper-inflation	Associated with expired MV alarm as above	Check ventilator display of expired MV or tidal volume if available. If in doubt, use separate spirometer to confirm.
Minute volume (V_E or MV)	6–8 ml/kg × 10–15 breaths/min = ~2.5–12 l/min	0–75 1itres	As above	MV alarms usually set manually at 2 litres above (upper alarm) and 2 litres below (lower alarm) the set ventilator MV	Check ventilator display of expired MV. If in doubt, use separate spirometer on inspiratory and expiratory limbs
Positive end expiratory pressure (PEEP) (cmH$_2$O)	+2 to +20 cmH$_2$O. Increasing levels of PEEP carry increasing risk of barotrauma and a depressant affect on cardiac output through decreased venous return.	+2 to +20 cmH$_2$O	Maintenance of alveolar expansion during expiration giving increased time for gas exchange and thus increased PO_2. Also aids recruitment of collapsed areas of lung	None. However, increased PEEP gives increasing airway pressure so upper, lower airway pressure alarm limits should be adjusted to allow for PEEP	Observe airway pressure display on ventilator. Pressure at end of expiration should not be less than set PEEP level
Pressure support/ assist (for further details see ventilation modes, p. 97)	+ 5 to +40 cmH$_2$O. Levels set according to patient need and resulting tidal volume produced for each breath	+5 to +40 cmH$_2$O	Used to maintain patients' respiratory muscles and to wean patients by gradual reduction in the degree of assistance for each spontaneous breath. High levels can provide complete ventilatory support	Contributes to airway pressure and MV	Observe airway pressure and MV. Spontaneous breaths should show a positive pressure rise of the amount set as assist

TABLE 4.15 Ventilator settings – *continued*

Ventilator setting	Typical range of adult patient	Typical range of ventilation capability	Function	Alarm limits	Safety checks
Flow rate (V) (l/min)	Variable within limits—default is usually 60 l/min: must be adjusted to ensure required V_T is reached if inspiratory time is reduced	2–100 l/min	(1) Adjusts to achieve V_T in inspiratory time with optimal airway pressure (2) Can be used to limit peak airway pressure by manipulation in conjunction with I:E. ratio (3) Can manipulate I:E ratio in pressure control ventilation (see ventilation modes, p. 97)	None, but contributes to achieving set V_T and thus MV, so MV alarms as before	Regular checks of ABGs if flow rate is altered, as inadequate V_T will affect PO_2 and PCO_2. Observe expired MV. Particular care for COPD patients when weaning as flow must be adequate for increased inspiratory effort
Inspiratory: Expiratory ratio (I:E ratio). Ratio of time for inspiration to time for expiration in each breath	Variable from 1:1 to 1:4. Normal ratio is 1:2. Inverse ratio ventilation refers to inspiratory times which are longer than expiratory times (i.e.2:1 up to 4:1). In acute asthma it is usually 1:3/1:4	In some ventilators the range is continuous from 4:1 to 1:4. In others, ratios are limited (i.e. 1:1, 1:2, 1:3, etc.)	(1) Allows manipulation of peak airway pressure by altering inspiratory time (2) Allows time for complete expiration in severe asthmatics so avoiding risk of air trapping (incomplete expiration produces build up of air in lungs)	Contributes to airway pressure so alarm limits set at 40 cm, or as instructed (upper) and 5–10 cmH$_2$O below current AP reading for lower alarm	Observe peak airway pressure for increases. If air trapping (incomplete expiration) is suspected, inform medical staff. Check pressure and flow waveforms on ventilator graphics— if flow does not return to 0 before next breath begins then air trapping is likely
Trigger/ sensitivity alters the degree of effort required by patient to trigger a positive pressure breath from the ventilator.	Negative pressure Inspiratory effort of −0 to −10 cmH$_2$O. Reduction in base flow of between 1 and 3 l/min	Not always quantified on ventilator, may simply range from minimum to maximum sensitivity	Assists patient weaning by altering sensitivity to patient effort, thus reducing ventilator support as patient strength increases. Alters the work of breathing for the patient	None	Careful observation of patient during weaning to ensure coping with respiratory effort. ABGs to check PO_2 and PCO_2
Base flow for flow trigger system	Not applicable	Normally between 3 and 5 l/min. May vary according to ventilator breath.	Provides a constant flow through the circuit which is reduced when the patient takes a This reduction triggers full flow to support the breath	None	NB. Check base flow is on after use of nebulizer in the circuit

TABLE 4.16	Table of ventilatory modes	
Mode	Description	Clinical Use
Controlled mechanical ventilation (CMV): (a) volume-controlled, (b) pressure-controlled	(a) Pre-set tidal volume and frequency of breaths are delivered. (b)Breaths are delivered to a pre-set pressure with tidal volume varying with lung compliance	Patient requires complete mechanical ventilatory support
Assist/control (triggered)	Pre-set tidal volume breaths are delivered in response to a patient attempting a spontaneous breath. A back-up delivers a pre-set rate of breaths if the patient does not achieve the required rate	Patient is able to initiate breaths but requires ventilatory assistance to maintain oxygenation and CO_2 removal
Synchronized intermittent mandatory ventilation (SIMV)	Pre-set tidal volume breaths are delivered at a pre-set rate but spontaneous breaths can be taken in between and ventilator breaths are synchronized with the spontaneous breaths	Patient is being weaned from ventilation or for greater patient comfort/reduction of sedation requirements
Pressure support (PSV) assist	Following triggering by the patient, a breath is delivered to a pre-set pressure level, tidal volume delivered will thus depend on lung compliance	Patient is being weaned from ventilation or for greater patient comfort/reduction of sedation requirements

up to 40 cmH$_2$O pressure on inspiration and up to 20 cmH$_2$O on expiration.

The main advantage in their use is the avoidance of the need for and risks associated with, endotracheal intubation.

Physiological effects of positive pressure ventilation

The effects of positive pressure are apparent not only in the patient's respiratory status but also in a number of other systems including cardiac, renal, and vascular.

INDICATIONS FOR VENTILATORY SUPPORT

- Respiratory failure which is not corrected by other forms of respiratory support (e.g. status asthmaticus, ARDS, pneumonia, pulmonary oedema).

- Support of other failing organs, especially the heart, in order to reduce its workload.

- Support of mechanical dysfunction (e.g. Guillain-Barré, flail chest, cervical spine fractures).

- Support of ventilatory function during use of high levels of sedation and anaesthesia necessary for other problems (e.g. status epilepticus, intra-operative anaesthesia).

- Therapeutic ventilation to reduce intracranial pressure (e.g. post-head injury or extensive neuro-surgery).

Awareness of these changes is vital to any nurse caring for ventilated patients as they may have a profound effect on the patient.

Decreased cardiac output and venous return

- *Manifested by*: hypotension, tachycardia, hypovolaemia, decreased urine output, increasing metabolic acidosis.

- *Caused by*: increased intrathoracic pressure during inspiration which reduces venous return and increases right ventricular afterload. As a result, right ventricular and, consequently, left ventricular output is reduced. If PEEP is used then pressure is positive even in expiration, and may reduce venous return further according to the level of PEEP. If the patient has been greatly distressed prior to commencing mechanical ventilation there may be a sudden reduction in peripheral vascular tone related to loss of circulating catecholamines and the effects of sedation.

- *Treated by*: fluid filling, using 200 ml challenges over 10–15 min until the stroke volume (if measured) shows no further increase. Otherwise, fill until (CVP) increases by =3 mmHg after a fluid challenge and remains increased (see Chapter 6). Inotropic support may be necessary if fluid loading is not considered clinically appropriate (see Chapter 6).

Alteration of ventilatory characteristics, such as inspiratory and expiratory time, tidal volume, level of PEEP, may also be considered.

Decreased urine output

◆ *Manifested by*: oliguria.

◆ *Caused by*: reduction in cardiac output invoking release of antidiuretic hormone together with the renin–angiotensin–aldosterone response leading to salt and water retention.

◆ *Treated by*: fluid filling as above. Close monitoring of urine output.

Increased incidence of barotrauma (trauma caused by pressure) related to higher positive airway pressures

◆ *Manifested by*: high airway pressures on inspiration.

◆ *Caused by*: the higher pressures required during positive pressure ventilation to force air into airways which are resistant to airflow. Damage to the lung occurs which may be manifested clinically as pneumothorax, pneumomediastinum, etc. Resistance to flow is related to the radius of the airway to the fourth power. Lung compliance will also increase the pressures involved. This is particularly relevant in the asthmatic patient, where bronchoconstriction produces greatly increased resistance to flow and greatly increased airway pressures.

◆ *Treated by*: manipulation of inspiratory and expiratory times for each breath and by flow rates of inspiratory gas. The aim is to keep plateau airway pressures below 35 cmH$_2$O (Tobin 2001). Current practice aims at lower tidal volumes (6–8 ml/kg) (ARDS Network 2000) to reduce the pressures required.

Problems associated with mechanical ventilation (Table 4.17)

Sputum clearance and airway management

The presence of an endotracheal or tracheostomy tube means that normal humidification and warming of inspired air by the upper airway tract, in particular the nasal passages, is bypassed. The delivery of dry, cold gas, often at a high flow rate, has several deleterious effects on the trachea and bronchi:

◆ increased viscosity of mucus which may dry and encrust the airways causing inflammation and ulceration;

◆ depressed ciliary function;

◆ microatelectasis from obstruction of small airways by thickened mucus.

The overall effect of this is to grossly impair movement or clearance of secretions. This may result in obstruc-

tion of major segments of lung or blockage of the tube itself.

Two other factors contribute to the problem:

◆ The decreased ability of the intubated patient to cough. This is due either to the presence of the tube itself or to suppression of the cough reflex by sedation or analgesia.

◆ The loss of the natural periodic sigh. This is a periodic breath of increased tidal volume which occurs at regular intervals in the spontaneously ventilating patient. It expands the base of the lungs and alveoli that may not be fully expanded during normal breathing.

If the patient is dehydrated, the moisture content of the mucus will be reduced and extra humidification will be required. The accumulation of secretions will cause airway blockage leading to atelectasis and collapse of areas of lung with an associated shunt due to limited availability for gas exchange. The degree to which this will cause problems is related to the underlying disease process. Thus, patients with pneumonia who are producing large amounts of purulent secretions or those with cystic fibrosis or bronchiectasis will require greatly increased intervention.

Methods of managing sputum clearance

Humidification   Ideally, the chosen method of humidification should:

◆ allow inspired gas to be delivered to the trachea at 32–36 °C with a water content of 33–43 g/m^3;

◆ be a simple and easy to use device;

◆ be adaptable for a variety of methods of oxygen therapy and ventilation;

◆ avoid any increase in airway resistance or compliance;

◆ avoid any added risk of infection.

There are a number of types of humidification available:

SPUTUM CLEARANCE REQUIRES:
1. Adequate humidification.
2. Suctioning and bronchial hygiene.
3. Chest physiotherapy.
4. Systemic hydration.
Note: The underlying disease process will affect the intensity of each intervention.

TABLE 4.17 Problems associated with mechanical ventilation

Problem	Details/action	
High airway pressure	Manifested by:	Airway pressure alarm sounds, persistent rise in peak airway pressure, evidence of patient distress, haemodynamic instability
	Causes	
	(a) Life-threatening (i.e. investigate and rule out/treat at once)	ET (or ventilator tubing) obstruction, pneumothorax, severe bronchospasm
	(b) Other	Build-up of secretions in airway. Patient breathing out of synchronization with ventilator ('fighting'). Patient coughing. Increased peak airway pressure resulting from a tidal volume set too high for patient, or inspiratory time set too short, or addition of PEEP. Displacement of the ET tube either downwards, causing coughing from irritation of the carina or usually slipping down the right main bronchus and meeting smaller airways with increased resistance, or upwards, causing cuff herniation through the larynx, resulting in patient discomfort and agitation
	Intervention	1. If patient is severely compromised remove from ventilator and manually ventilate using rebreathe bag and 100% oxygen. Assess lung compliance (the degree of resistance to inspiration) and symmetry of inflation while bagging. Call for senior and medical help
		2. Perform suction to clear any secretions and to determine whether tube is patent. If secretions are very thick, review humidification and instill 2–3 ml normal saline down ET tube prior to suctioning. Repeat as necessary
		3. If the cause is complete obstruction of the ET tube, emergency reintubation will be necessary. If there is no one immediately available to reintubate it is possible to ventilate the patient following extubation using a Guedel airway and tight-fitting facemask with manual ventilation. It is important to have the patient's neck resting on one pillow and to lift the jaw forwards to maintain a patent airway. If trained and proficient in its use, a laryngeal mask airway is an alternative to either reintubation or facemask bagging
		4. Auscultate lungs for signs of wheezing, reduction in air entry, and altered breath sounds
		5. If the cause is a pneumothorax and there is cardiovascular compromise immediate insertion of a chest drain or large needle will be necessary (by medical staff) to allow relief of tension (for details see chest drains, p. 113)
		6. If the patient is stable, attempt to ascertain the cause of increased airway pressure
		7. Reassure and attempt to alleviate any cause of distress if the patient is restless and distressed by ventilation ('fighting'). This is suggested by tachypnoea, breathing out of synchronization with the ventilator, and continually coughing or gagging
		8. Check blood gases if restlessness and distress continues and/or peripheral oxygen saturation remains low. Increase F_iO_2 and consult with medical staff
		9. If the patient is restless and unable to settle on the ventilator but otherwise cardiovascularly stable with appropriate blood gases, review sedation and inform senior or medical staff if an increase ± muscle relaxant is indicated
		10. Review ventilator settings and discuss with senior or medical staff if settings seem inappropriate or addition of PEEP appears to have caused a problem.

TABLE 4.17 Problems associated with mechanical ventilation – *continued*

Problem		Details/action
Low airway pressure	Manifested by:	Sounds of air leak, decreased expired minute volume (MV), low airway pressure reading
	Causes:	
	(a) Life-threatening	Disconnection or major leak from the ventilator, burst cuff on endotracheal/ tracheostomy tube
	(b) Other	Leak in the ventilator circuits, loss of seal on cuff, bronchopleural fistula (with massive air leak through chest drain), ventilator dysfunction
	Intervention	1. Check the patient is attached to the ventilator
		2. Check connections on ventilator tubing for leaks, tears, or cracks
		3. Check cuff pressure to ensure a seal is present. Use cuff pressure manometer to check the cuff pressure is less than 30 mmHg. If the leak continues inflate cuff further if necessary
		4. Check inspired tidal volume to ensure the ventilator is delivering its set amount
		5. Check ventilator function
		6. Check levels set for pressure alarm limits are appropriate
		7. If low airway pressure continues and the tidal volume is not being delivered the ET tube or the ventilator may need changing. Manually ventilate the patient and inform senior nursing or medical staff
Low minute volume	Manifested by:	Low MV alarm sounding, MV read-out shows less than set MV, audible cuff leak, patient may appear distressed and haemodynamically compromised, oxygen saturation may drop and the patient may appear cyanosed
	Causes:	
	(a) Life-threatening	Disconnection from the ventilator, inappropriate ventilator settings (i.e. flow rate may be too low to allow set volume in time allocated by set respiratory rate), hole in ventilator tubing
	(b) Other	Leak caused by tubing connections working loose, loss of seal on cuff, presence of bronchopleural fistula with chest drain *in situ*
	Intervention	1. Unless the cause of low MV is immediately apparent, manually ventilate patient
		2. Check ventilator tubing from machine to patient, testing connections, and looking for holes
		3. Review ventilator settings to ensure MV is capable of being delivered and that ventilator is not malfunctioning
		4. Auscultate the trachea to detect any leak around the cuff. Refill cuff as before
		5. Monitor air leak through chest drain if present. If increased inform medical staff. Ventilation may have to be increased or altered to allow for leak
High minute volume	Manifested by:	Sounding of high MV alarms, patient making respiratory effort
	Causes:	
	(a) Life-threatening	Possible ventilator malfunction
	(b) Other	Patient making respiratory effort which is excessive, inappropriate ventilator settings
	Intervention	1. Check causes of patient's tachypnoea such as pain, hypoxia, hypercapnia
		2. Review ventilator settings with senior and/or medical staff

1. Heat/moisture exchangers (HMEs). These are filters which are hygroscopic on the patient side and hydrophobic on the gas source side (Fig. 4.9). The hygroscopic material picks up moisture and heat from the patient's exhaled breath which is then transferred to the inhaled gas as the patient inspires.

- *Advantages*: decreased infection risk (most HMEs are bacteriostatic); light and disposable.

TABLE 4.17 Problems associated with mechanical ventilation – *continued*

Problem		Details/action
Hypoxaemia	Manifested by:	Peripheral O_2 saturation <90%, arterial blood gases show fall in PO_2 to below 8–10 kPa, patient is restless (unless heavily sedated ± paralysed), tachycardic, possibly hypotensive, and cyanosed
	Causes:	
	(a) Life-threatening	Pneumothorax, pulmonary embolus, sputum plug, or other body obstructing major airway, severe haemodynamic compromise, severe bronchospasm, severe pulmonary oedema, ventilator malfunction
	(b) Other	Build-up of thick secretions, increase in severity of disease, atelectasis, bronchospasm, repositioning of patient causing increase in shunt, leak in ventilator tubing, patient fighting ventilator, pulmonary oedema
	Intervention	1. If hypoxaemia is severe and/or causing haemodynamic compromise ventilate patient on 100% oxygen. Call for help
		2. Check ventilator is delivering set ventilation and that alarm limits are appropriate
		3. Check arterial blood gases and ensure that pulse oximeter is picking up a good signal
		4. Auscultate chest for air entry and abnormal breath sounds, depending on findings, suction and/ or chest physiotherapy may be necessary. Observe symmetry of lung movement and consider pneumothorax
		5. Ascertain cause of hypoxaemia—reposition patient if recently placed on side, in consultation with medical staff consider need for chest X-ray, review haemodynamic causes such as decreased cardiac output. Review need for further sedation
		6. In consultation with medical staff, ventilator settings such as F_iO_2, tidal volume, I:E ratio, etc., may be altered
Hypercapnia	Manifested by:	PCO_2 > 6.0 kPa, patient appears restless and agitated with tachypnoea if on weaning modes or possibly showing signs of respiratory effort if on controlled ventilation. *Note:* Habitual CO_2 retainers (chronic COPD, etc.) may tolerate or even require much higher levels of CO_2 to maintain normal pH values as renal compensation will have adjusted for levels of bicarbonate. In patients with severe pulmonary disease, such as ARDS where there is risk of further lung damage with the high airway pressures necessary to reduce PCO_2, it may be preferable to tolerate high levels of CO_2 providing acidosis is adequately compensated ('permissive hypercapnia')
	Causes:	
	Life-threatening	No urgently life-threatening causes but long-term uncorrected hypercapnia may cause severe metabolic problems
	Other	Inadequate MV either from patient if in weaning modes or ventilator settings. Compensation for metabolic alkalosis, carbohydrate overload, or increased CO_2 related to increased metabolic rate (see Chapter 12), air trapping (intrinsic or auto-PEEP)
	Intervention	1. Ensure the patient is receiving the set MV or if weaning, that the patient is achieving the MV required
		2. Check air entry and perform suction to discount any sputum plugging or obstruction
		3. Review ventilator settings with medical staff and alter MV if necessary. A decrease in ventilation may be necessary if the patient is air-trapping

♦ *Disadvantages*: the level of humidification available is fixed and may be insufficient for high gas flow rates or very thick secretions; the presence of the HME may increase resistance to air flow in the circuit.

2. Nebulizers. These devices deliver aerosolized water particles. The water particles are produced by: (a) a jet of gas passed through a film of fluid or creating a suction and fine spray from a reservoir;

TABLE 4.17 Problems associated with mechanical ventilation – *continued*		
Problem		**Details/action**
Auto-PEEP (intrinsic PEEP, air-trapping)	Manifested by:	Failure of alveolar pressure to return to zero at the end of exhalation (Pepe and Marini 1982)
	Causes:	Increased resistance to airflow and increased work of breathing. Incomplete/impeded exhalation either as a result of high MV (>10 1/min) or in respiratory or cardiac disease, particularly chronic airway limitation (Ruggles 1995)
	Interventions:	1. Ensure low-compressible volume ventilator tubing is used
		2. Review ventilator settings with medical staff and decrease MV by decreasing respiratory rate or alter inspiratory flow rate to decrease inspiratory time and increase expiratory time
		3. Reduce metabolic workload to reduce respiratory demand

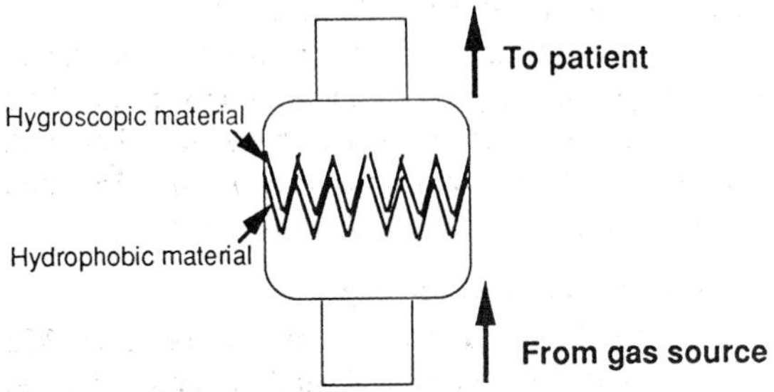

Fig. 4.9 Heat/moisture exchanger.

(b) a spinning disc which creates droplets using centrifugal force; (c) ultrasonic frequency vibrating transducers. The droplets produced are deposited in the upper airway, bronchi, and alveoli depending on their size. Particles smaller than 1 μm reach the alveoli, those of 5 μm are deposited in the bronchi, and those of 7–10 μm are deposited in the upper airway (Oh 1990, p.172).

♦ *Advantages*: (a) The amount of humidification can be increased and decreased according to patient need. (b) The quantity of water delivered is not limited by temperature and with ultrasonic nebulizers supersaturation is possible. (c) Delivery of topical medication is possible.

♦ *Disadvantages*: (a) Risk of infection is higher from bacterial contamination of the water (sterile water should always be used). (b) Gross overhydration is possible, particularly in ultrasonic nebulizers where supersaturation may occur. (c) There may be increased airway resistance due to the presence of the nebulizer in the circuit.

3. Hot water bath humidifiers. Gas is driven over or through a heated water bath. Humidity can only be achieved at temperatures between 45 and 60 °C. As

the humidified gas passes through the tubing to the patient it cools and condenses producing a gas at about 37 °C which is fully saturated.

♦ *Advantages*: Effective and efficient humidification.

♦ *Disadvantages*: (a) Infection is a hazard. Water temperatures of 45 °C provide an effective growth medium for contaminating bacteria such as *Pseudomonas pyocyneus*. Temperatures must be maintained near the 60 °C level to limit the growth of contaminants. The water bath and tubing must be changed every 24 hours. (b) Efficiency is not constant and may be altered by gas flow, water temperature, and surface area of the vaporizing surface. (c) There is a risk of scalding the airway. Thermostatic control and temperature sensors situated at the patient end of the circuit are vital.

4. Cold water humidifiers. Gas from an oxygen flowmeter passes via a Venturi system allowing alteration of oxygen concentration through a water reservoir. Most types are disposable and provide oxygen concentrations from 28% to 60%, although these are not reliable at high minute volumes. The oxygen is only partially humidified, depending on gas flow rates, but is not completely saturated.

5. Instillation of normal saline. Boluses of normal saline (3–5 ml) instilled into the trachea may be used as an adjunct to other forms of humidification. They are thought to be helpful in conjunction with suction and chest physiotherapy for clearing secretions by thinning them (Bostick and Wendelgass 1987). However, the evidence for this is equivocal and an association with decreased P_aO_2 has been suggested (Ackerman 1993). There may also be lower airway contamination with upper airway organisms (Hegler and Traver 1994). Further research is required, but

this method currently remains a useful adjunct to suction and physiotherapy.

Suctioning and bronchial hygiene Removal of secretions using a suction catheter placed in the trachea is essential for maintaining airway patency. It may be performed intermittently when evidence of secretions in the large airways is heard as crackles or wheezes, or routinely in conjunction with chest physiotherapy.

An important precaution in suctioning borderline hypoxaemic patients is the use of pre-oxygenation using 100% oxygen and possibly hyperinflation (Stone *et al.* 1989, Mancinelli-Van Atta and Beck 1992). The use of closed suction systems is also thought to reduce the degree of desaturation associated with suctioning (Harshbarger *et al.* 1992)

The deleterious effects of suctioning include:

- decreased S_vO_2 (mixed venous oxygen saturation) due to falls in cardiac output and arterial oxygen saturation (Clark *et al.* 1990),

- decreased P_aO_2,

- cardiac arrhythmias associated with vagal stimulation and hypoxia,

- microatelectasis,

- haemodynamic instability,

- increased intracranial pressure,

- laryngospasm (in the non-intubated patient),

- bronchoconstriction,

- tissue damage, haemorrhage.

The evidence for tissue damage is from research done between 40 and 20 years ago and it is likely that improvements in catheter construction and limitations of negative pressure levels have reduced the risk of mucosal trauma. However, Donald *et al.* (2000) found that suction was consistently applied at higher (mean = 359 mmHg) than the recommended limits of 200 mmHg by 64 nurses and physiotherapists even when they were shown continuous manometer readings of pressures attained.

Some of the desaturation problems can be reduced by the use of hyperoxygenation (usually 100%) for 1–2 min prior to suctioning or more controversially the use of controlled hyperinflation (1.5 times tidal volume; Stone *et al.* 1989) via a manual resuscitation bag, rebreathe bag, or the ventilator.

Closed suction systems have gradually become the accepted norm for many critical care areas. Their advantages for the patients are:

- decreased levels of contamination by organisms leading to VAP (Combes *et al.* 2000);

- reduced episodes of desaturation during suction (Harshbarger *et al.* 1992);

- possible reduced incidence of bacterial keratitis (eye infection) through splash contamination from withdrawal of suction catheters (Parkin *et al.* 1997);

- no requirement to break the ventilator circuit in order to suction which may result in loss of PEEP.

The closed suction system consists of a suction catheter positioned within a T-shaped catheter mount and protected by a flexible plastic sleeve. An instillation port is available for saline to either inject into the endotracheal lumen or to be used to wash through the suction catheter and system (see Fig. 4.10).

The manufacturers recommend changing the closed suction system every 24–48 hours to prevent build up of bacterial colonization, but a study by Kollef *et al.* (1997) showed no increase in incidence of VAP when suction systems were changed as necessary.

Safety principles for suctioning

1. Suction levels should be set below 26.6 kPa (200 mmHg, or 260 cmH$_2$O) and preferably around 13.3–16 kPa (100–170 mmHg or 130–160 cmH$_2$O) to minimize trauma associated with suction.

2. If used, hyperinflation should commence 3–5 breaths prior to suctioning and for 1–2 breaths after the last suction catheter is passed. This is to reopen any alveoli which may have been collapsed by the negative suction pressure and reduce any atelectasis. The technique should be aseptic:

   - hand-washing (or use of alcohol gel) prior to the procedure
   - wear clean gloves.

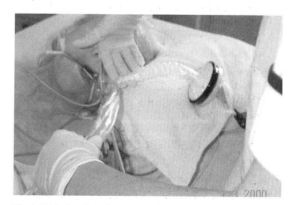

Fig. 4.10 A closed suction system.

3. For an *open suction system*:
   - catheters should be sterile and inserted only once prior to discarding (see later for exceptions);
   - a clean or sterile disposable second glove should be worn on the dominant hand (suction catheter handling hand) with each catheter.

4. For a *closed suction system* the catheter and sleeve should be examined regularly to ensure that the catheter is patent and the sleeve is intact.

5. When suction is complete:
   - The suction catheter should always be washed through with normal saline.
   - The suction catheter should always be withdrawn so that the black marker line is visible in the sleeve. If the catheter remains in the endotracheal tube or catheter mount itself, it will occlude the lumen and increase airway resistance.

6. The correct size of suction catheter is important. It should not exceed one-half of the internal diameter of the endotracheal tube.

7. The catheter should be inserted to just above the carina if trauma to the trachea is to be minimized. In some patients, it may be necessary to insert the catheter further; it will usually pass into the right main bronchus due to the anatomy of the bronchi.

8. Suction should be applied only as the catheter is withdrawn.

9. The whole procedure of insertion and withdrawal should not take longer than 30 s (suction itself should be less than 15 s), otherwise the patient may experience hypoxaemia and distress.

10. Observation of ECG and SpO_2 should be continuous during the procedure.

11. Catheters used should have an end of catheter lumen and more than one side lumen to minimize trauma. A single side lumen is more likely to cause tracheal trauma.

The experience is most unpleasant for the patient and has been described as feeling like choking or loss of breath (Bergbom-Engberg and Haljamäe 1989). It should therefore be performed as briefly and effectively as possible to maximize efficacy and minimize trauma.

Chest physiotherapy The use of a number of techniques, such as vibration, postural drainage, percussion, and hyperinflation can all improve clearance of secretions. These techniques should be taught by an experienced physiotherapist and practised under guidance.

1. *Vibration*: The chest wall is shaken using two hands at a frequency of about 200 per minute throughout patient exhalation. It is designed to loosen and move secretions into the major airways where they can be coughed up or suctioned out.

2. *Postural drainage*: Movement of secretions using gravity by altering the patient's position so that different areas of the lung are drained. (*Note*. Remember there is increased perfusion to the dependent lung so that the shunt/venous admixture may increase if the dependent lung has very poor air entry.)

3. *Percussion*: This technique is infrequently used in critically ill patients because of the incidence of arrhythmias and other problems of haemodynamic instability. It is performed in association with postural drainage. Loosening and movement of secretions may be helped by beating cupped hands (gently at first) over the patient's chest from the least dependent to the most dependent area.

4. *Hyperinflation*: Delivery of a breath to the patient which is approximately 1.5 times the tidal volume of the patient. A rebreathing or manual hyperinflation bag is commonly used to hyperinflate the lungs, although most ventilators now have a hyperinflation facility and are thought to be as effective (Berney and Denehy 2002). The purpose of hyperinflation is to re-expand collapsed alveoli (atelectasis), mobilize and remove excess bronchial secretions, and improve oxygenation by introducing larger volume breaths. Care must be taken to limit the airway pressures generated by these larger breaths. A study of hyperinflation in 100 stable ventilated patients found that static compliance, P_aO_2:F_iO_2 ratio and A–a gradient were all significantly improved for some time after hyperinflation (Patman *et al.* 2000).

The safest method using the manual hyperinflation bag is to position a manometer (pressure gauge) within the manual hyperinflation bag circuit and to limit pressure generated to less than 40 cmH$_2$O. The standard manual hyperinflation bag has a volume of about 2 litres as it is necessary to provide a reservoir of gas plus a flow rate of 15 l/min or more. The potential volume possible in each breath is therefore considerably larger than necessary to provide 1.5 times the normal tidal volume. Thus, the full volume of the bag should not be used as a guide for the size of the breath to be delivered. During the procedure the patient's chest should be observed to ensure inflation with the bag produces a rise followed by a fall during deflation.

Patient needs All of the above techniques involve discomfort and distress for the patient. It should be a nursing priority that the patient is given full explanation prior to any intervention and as much information as possible to explain the necessity of carrying out these procedures. The patient's cooperation should always be sought as this will lessen the negative nature of these unpleasant procedures.

Communication difficulties associated with endotracheal intubation

These problems affect the patient themselves, the family, and the staff who care for them.

The first priority is to explain the cause to the patient and reassure them that their inability to talk is a temporary situation which will revert when the tube is removed. Alternative methods of communication must be sought and established so that patient, family, and carers become familiar and practiced with the methods that work best.

The presence of an endotracheal or tracheostomy tube tends to reduce communication to closed questions requiring only a positive or negative answer. This is obviously extremely limiting and should only be a temporary measure until the patient can adopt an alternative method (see Chapter 3 for more details).

It is vital that the amount of information/communication offered by staff and family to the patient is not limited and encompasses more rather than less than would normally be communicated.

Methods of non-verbal communication

◆ The patient's family will need encouragement and help to continue talking to their relative as though they are able to reply fully, particularly with regard to expressing their thoughts and feelings to them.

◆ The speech and language therapy department are invaluable in providing assistance and technical aid and should be contacted early for the long-term patient. They are also able to assist with any swallowing or upper airway problems associated with the complications of tracheostomy and endotracheal tubes.

◆ The family need involvement in determining topics of interest to the patient. Provision of newspapers, radio, tapes, television, etc., will all assist the patient to remain in touch.

Psychological problems associated with intubation and ventilation

Most patients on ventilatory support or requiring intensive care have greatly increased levels of anxiety and stress. This is discussed in detail in Chapter 3. This is naturally compounded by their inability to express this. It is very important that the nurse recognizes symptoms of anxiety and stress and responds to them.

Nutritional problems associated with intubation and ventilation

This will be discussed in detail in Chapter 11 on gastrointestinal problems. Obviously, a standard oral diet is impossible for the intubated patient, although patients with tracheostomies may manage very well if the cuff can be deflated and they have regained normal swallow capability. Alternative forms of nutritional support, including enteral and parenteral feeding, must be utilized. The effects of malnutrition on the critically ill patient are severe and efforts should be made to establish appropriate levels of intake as soon as possible.

In the patient who is weaning from ventilation, particular problems can be encountered:

1. Overfeeding of carbohydrate will cause the body to lay down fat stores. This process produces considerably more CO_2 than that produced by the breakdown of food for energy. The patient must therefore increase his/her minute volume in order to remove the excess CO_2. This will increase the workload the patient must perform and may prove too much for weakened respiratory muscles. In these circumstances provision of half of the non-protein calories as fat should be substituted.

2. Depletion of important minerals and trace elements, such as zinc, magnesium, and phosphate, will also have a deleterious effect on respiratory muscle function. Repletion of muscle mass is not possible without these minerals thus respiratory muscle degeneration will not improve if supply is inadequate.

> ## FACTORS CONTRIBUTING TO PSYCHOLOGICAL PROBLEMS
>
> ◆ Discomfort
> ◆ Fear
> ◆ Loss of control
> ◆ Disorientation
> ◆ Disease pathology

3. Patients exhibiting the septic response (i.e. fever, high levels of urinary nitrogen excretion, high metabolic rate; see Chapter 12), seem unable to utilize nutrition to regenerate depleted muscle mass and weaning should only be attempted slowly.

4. Malnourished patients have an increased risk of developing pneumonia and other complications due to the associated dysfunction of the immune system and the possible limitation of surfactant production seen with fatty acid deficiency.

5. Malnutrition is associated with a reduced diaphragmatic mass, reduced maximal voluntary ventilation, and reduced respiratory muscle strength. All of these will seriously detract from the patient's ability to wean from the ventilator. Patients who do not require ventilatory support may also have problems maintaining adequate nutritional intake when they have oxygen masks *in situ* and experience dyspnoea when attempting to eat.

Strategies for assisting the breathless patient to eat include:

♦ nasal cannulae to continue oxygen delivery during meals;

♦ nutritional supplements such as high-calorie (fat and carbohydrate) drinks;

♦ small, frequent, nutritious, and tempting(!) meals;

♦ upright and comfortable positioning to eat;

♦ thoughtful timing of meals (i.e. not just after physiotherapy!).

Increased infection risk associated with intubation and ventilation

The presence of a 'foreign body' in the airway increases the likelihood of infection in a number of ways:

1. The tube bypasses normal physical and physiological mechanisms of resistance such as cilia and the mucous membrane of the upper airways.

2. Trauma associated with the presence of the tube and suctioning provides a portal for bacterial colonization. In addition the cuff of the tube is not a perfect seal and secretions from upper airways and gastric regurgitation may trickle into the lungs.

3. Interventions such as suctioning require scrupulous attention to aseptic principles in order to avoid direct delivery of any bacterial contamination to the bronchi and respiratory lobules.

4. Critically ill patients are usually already greatly at risk from infection due to the high level of instrumentation (cannulae etc. penetrating the body for access and monitoring). They also frequently have a compromised immune response due to the underlying pathology.

Alternative modes of ventilation and respiratory support

Improving ventilation

There is no doubt that the maintenance of at least some spontaneous breathing effort by the patient will improve the likelihood of eventual discontinuation of mechanical ventilation and wherever possible this should be continued in whichever mode of ventilation best supports this. The posterior sections of the diaphragm move more actively with spontaneous breathing and this ensures better ventilation of dependent lung regions in the supine position (Putensen *et al.* 2002). Other advantages include retention of diaphragmatic muscle bulk and less need for high sedation levels.

Inverse ratio ventilation

This technique consists of reversing the normal inspiratory–expiratory ratio and controlling the inspiratory gas flow by limiting the airway pressure, slowing or decelerating the rate of inspiratory flow, or adding an additional end inspiratory pause.

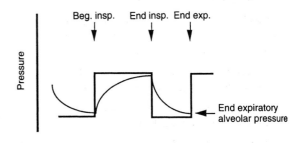

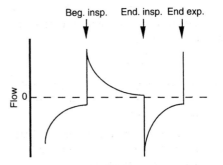

Fig. 4.11 Pressure and flow in pressure-controlled inverse ratio ventilation (= airway pressure; = alveolar pressure) (after Marcy and Marini 1991).

Two methods are generally used to administer inverse ratio ventilation:

1. The ventilator is time-cycled with a pre-set inspiratory pressure limit and a long inspiratory phase. This is pressure-controlled inverse ratio ventilation (PC-IRV) (Fig. 4.11).

2. The ventilator is volume-cycled with an end inspiratory pause and a slow or decelerating inspiratory flow rate. This is volume-controlled inverse ratio ventilation (VC-IRV).

Both methods ensure that inspiration occurs when there is still expiratory flow and therefore some degree of auto-PEEP is maintained at the end of the expiratory phase.

Advantages of VC-IRV include:

- availability of this mode on all adult ventilators,

- the delivery of a guaranteed tidal volume,

- precise manipulation of the inspiratory flow pattern,

- decreased peak inspiratory flow rates with similar or lower shear force (Marcy and Marini 1991).

Disadvantages of VC-IRV include:

- changes in peak alveolar pressures may occur and may exceed the optimal level if peak inflation pressures are not carefully monitored.

Advantages of PC-IRV include:

- possibly better gas distribution than constant flow VC-IRV due to the decelerating flow pattern.

Disadvantages of PC-IR V include:

- variation in tidal volume delivered with alterations to respiratory system compliance and resistance,

- opposing pressure exerted by any level of auto-PEEP may reduce the volume delivered,

- compared with VC-IRV greater shear forces may be generated by the fast flow associated with the beginning of inspiration; this may contribute to tissue injury (Marcy and Marini 1991).

Limitations of inverse ratio ventilation

1. The breathing pattern imposed (I:E ratio of greater than 1:1) is difficult for a patient to tolerate unless well sedated and/or paralysed.

2. Air trapping can occur in alveoli with high expiratory resistance leading to hyperinflation and possibly an increased incidence of barotrauma.

3. In PC-IRV, the longer inspiratory time allows equilibration between alveolar and airway pressure causing an increase in peak alveolar pressure compared with volume controlled ventilation where peak airway pressure always exceeds alveolar pressure.

4. Rises in mean airway pressure and auto-PEEP may affect cardiac output and venous return as well as increasing right ventricular afterload.

Other measures for supporting respiration

In the situation of severe ARDS or other acute lung pathology, where conventional ventilation is unable to support adequate PO_2 levels and ensure CO_2 excretion (even allowing for some permissive hypercapnia) there are further options.

Supporting adequate oxygenation
Nitric oxide gas inhalation

Nitric oxide (see Chapter 12) is a pulmonary vasodilator, which when inhaled crosses the alveolar membrane and acts locally on the pulmonary vasculature, dilating vessels and increasing blood flow. This has the effect of improving ventilation/perfusion (V/Q) matching and therefore gas exchange as the blood flow is only increased in the ventilated areas. As soon as it enters the blood, nitric oxide is bound to haemoglobin and has no further systemic (i.e. hypotensive) effect.

Nitric oxide gas is added to the gas delivery of the ventilator or in the inspiratory limb, volumes are measured in parts per million (ppm) by a monitor. Optimal delivery levels are identified by titrating the nitric oxide against either PO_2 or SpO_2. Levels should be re-titrated at least once a shift. Withdrawal of nitric oxide should be slow as there may be rebound pulmonary hypertension and hypoxaemia.

Although significant increases in oxygenation are seen in up to 60% of patients with inhaled nitric oxide this is not associated with an improvement in overall mortality (Dellinger *et al.* 1998)

Safety aspects:

- Nitric oxide will combine with oxygen to produce a small amount of the toxic substance nitrogen dioxide and levels of this must be closely monitored in exhaled gases. Levels of nitrogen dioxide >0.005 ppm are rarely seen, and only levels above 5 ppm are considered dangerous.

- Nitrogen dioxide can further combine with water to produce nitric acid, so catheter mounts and ventilator circuits should be used with HME filters and prevented from developing high levels of condensation or water pooling.

◆ Some patients may also develop significant (>5% total haemoglobin) methaemoglobinaemia (formed when NO combines with haemoglobin) after several days on nitric oxide and this should be monitored.

Prone positioning

The severely injured lung is likely to have a range of dysfunctional areas from irreversible damage and alveolar collapse to potentially reversible areas of infiltration and consolidation. This lack of homogeneity means that potentially functional areas of ventilation and perfusion are likely to be poorly matched. This problem may be compounded by the supine position that most patients are nursed in, which tends to favour ventilation of the anterior portions of the lung. Placing patients in the prone position improves oxygenation in a proportion (termed 'responders'), and although the mechanism is still not established, this is now used as an adjunct to maintain levels of oxygen in hypoxaemic patients requiring high F_iO_2.

However, a multicentre randomized controlled study in 304 ARDS patients, half of whom underwent prone positioning, has shown no difference in survival, although levels of oxygenation were improved (Gattinoni et al. 2001).

Not all patients can be turned prone and the risk–benefit of any manoeuvre must be evaluated.

Safe prone positioning will require at least four personnel and preferably five, with one person responsible purely for turning the patient's head and taking care of the endotracheal tube.

Some units use special beds which will allow alteration of the support pressures to reduce support under the abdomen and increase support at the head, chest, and pelvis. This allows the abdomen to be expanded during inspiration. If a special bed is not used, pillows should be placed under the pelvis and chest and a specific head support or two pillows used.

Positioning of the arms is important, and a variety of positions have been recommended. The 'swimmers' position has one arm above the head and one by the patient's side, alternatively both arms can be placed above the head. Some units use special boards to allow the arms to be extended to the side.

The whole bed should be tilted up at the head end in a reverse Trendelenberg position.

Further details about the technique can be found in Balas (2000).

Reducing hypercapnia
Tracheal gas (oxygen) insufflation

Insufflating a continuous flow of oxygen via a narrow catheter close to the carina via an endotracheal tube is

---

RELATIVE CONTRAINDICATIONS TO PRONE POSITIONING

◆ Spinal instability

◆ Increased intracranial pressure

◆ Abdominal compartment syndrome

◆ Shock

◆ Multiple trauma

◆ Massive resuscitation or haemodynamic instability

◆ Pregnancy

◆ Abdominal surgery

◆ Extreme obesity

Balas (2000)

---

occasionally used to reduce hypercapnia. The mechanism for action is believed to be washout of CO_2 in the anatomical deadspace during end expiration.

Gas flows should be limited to less than 6 l/min otherwise increased airway pressures and tidal volumes may be damaging. The gas flow must be warmed and humidified if possible as it is passing directly into the trachea.

High-frequency ventilation

High-frequency ventilation (HFV) incorporates techniques using ventilation frequencies of greater than 60–2000 breaths/min and tidal volumes of between 1 and 5 ml/kg. Two types currently used are high-frequency oscillation and high-frequency jet ventilation.

Delivery requires a specialized ventilator, as conventional ventilators provide an insufficient tidal volume at high frequencies due to compression of gas within the ventilator itself.

PROBLEMS ASSOCIATED WITH THE PRONE POSITION

◆ Facial and conjunctival oedema

◆ Pressure ulcers on knees, shoulders, iliac crests, and face

◆ Limited access to endotracheal and nasogastric tubes

◆ No immediate access for resuscitation in the event of cardiac arrest

High-frequency oscillation

A rapidly oscillating gas flow is created by a device that acts like a woofer on a loudspeaker, producing a high-frequency rapid change in direction of gas flow. Most of the experience with this has been in the paediatric population, but recent work has been carried out in adults with severe ARDS suggesting it may be beneficial.

The oscillator is set using DELTA P which is the measure of the pressure swing between inspiration and expiration, the frequency (in hertz) and the mean airway pressure.

Further details are available in Brice and Davis (2004).

High-frequency jet ventilation (HFJV)

High-pressure air and oxygen are blended and supplied to a non-compliant injection (jet) system. The normal pressure of this gas (known as the driving pressure) is around 2.5 atmospheres (atm). This can be adjusted to alter the rate of flow from the maximum (2.5 atm) down to zero. Added (warmed and humidified) gas is entrained from an additional circuit via a T-piece attached to the endotracheal tube. The entrainment circuit should provide at least 30 l/min of flow. Highly efficient humidification (usually via a hot-plate vaporizer humidifier) is necessary due to the high flows of otherwise dry gas.

The usual frequency set is between 100 and 200 breaths/min delivering tidal volumes of 2–5 ml/kg.

In an entrainment system, the tidal volume delivered by the ventilator increases with driving pressure and decreases with respiratory frequency. It remains the same with alterations in I:E ratio. The system requires either a special jet endotracheal tube or a cannula via an adapter fixed to a standard endotracheal tube.

This mode of ventilation has advantages for specific groups of patients but as yet there is no evidence that there is any improvement in survival or length of stay in patients who are ventilated with HFJV. It requires considerable skill to maintain a patient successfully on HFJV and as such this mode of ventilation is used only in a minority of ICUs for problem patients with specific disorders.

Extracorporeal respiratory support

Extracorporeal membrane oxygenation (ECMO) was first reported by Hill *et al.* (1972). The technique consists of an extracorporeal circuit incorporating a membrane with high surface area, a gas flow of variable percentage oxygen/air, and a blood pump. ECMO is defined as an extracorporeal system requiring 50% of cardiac output to pass via a venoarterial circuit. Exposure of venous blood to the membrane allows some oxygenation and removal of carbon dioxide across the

---

INDICATIONS FOR THE USE OF HIGH-FREQUENCY JET VENTILATION

- Bronchopleural fistula where air leak flow causes failure of conventional ventilation.
- Severe acute respiratory failure with high airway pressures and reduced respiratory compliance.
- Emergency situations during which tracheal intubation is impossible.
- During anaesthesia in order to minimize movement of lung fields, to allow clear access to respiratory tract surgery, and to limit stone movement during lithotripsy.

---

membrane using concentration gradients. It is theoretically possible to provide adequate oxygenation and removal of CO_2, but in practice it is usual to supplement oxygenation with mechanical ventilation of 8–12 breaths/min and F_iO_2 of <0.5.

Its use has been proven in children and neonates but is currently limited to a few centres in adults.

Extracorporeal carbon dioxide removal (ECCO$_2$R) aims only to remove CO_2 by the extracorporeal circuit at flow rates of only 20–30% of cardiac output. Oxygenation is provided by apnoeic oxygenation (a continuous flow of oxygen with a respiratory rate of zero) or tracheal insufflation of oxygen (100% oxygen is delivered into the trachea via a cannula inserted to just above the carina). Some oxygen can be delivered across the extracorporeal membrane as above depending on the patient's need. Carbon dioxide can be removed through a low blood flow–high gas flow circuit as it has a much higher solubility coefficient than oxygen. The main goal of this support is to avoid elevated peak airway pressures and F_iO_2 and to abolish specific hyperventilation. Atelectasis is avoided by the use of low-frequency positive pressure ventilation (LFPPV) at a rate of 3–4 breaths/min with a limited peak airway pressure (35–45 cmH$_2$O) and a constant level of PEEP (20–30 cmH$_2$O). The theory behind the use of ECCO$_2$R is that it will lessen further lung injury and allow time for the diseased lungs to heal.

Cannulation is usually venovenous using large (34 FG) catheters in femoral-femoral or femoral–jugular positions

Complications:

- Bleeding is the most frequent complication due to the need for systemic anticoagulation to preserve the extracorporeal circuits. Heparin is infused to maintain activated clotting times (ACT) of 180–200 s.

However, the development of heparin-bonded circuits has reduced the risk of bleeding considerably.

- Infection risk is high due to the highly invasive nature of the system and scrupulous aseptic precautions are necessary, particularly if extracorporeal support continues for several days.

Weaning from mechanical ventilation

The majority of patients who are mechanically ventilated have little difficulty weaning once the disease process has been resolved. However, a small but significant group of patients prove difficult to reduce support and may never wean completely. This group includes patients with chronic airflow limitation, neuropathies such as critical illness polyneuropathy, or respiratory paralysis such as myasthenia gravis, poor left ventricular function, complications following postabdominal, and cardiac surgery (see Chapter 8), and prolonged ventilation (Fig. 4.12).

Short-term weaning

- The decision to wean is made following assessment of the patient's physiological and physical status.

- The precipitating illness/factor should be resolved and the patient's haemodynamic and respiratory status should be stable. The patient should be able to make respiratory efforts and have an intact cough reflex.

- Weaning criteria may be of use (see Table 4.18) but the clinical state of the patient is as important.

- Use of the rapid shallow breathing index (RSBI) is recommended (Ely 2001). This is a test of the patient's ability to generate sufficiently deep breaths without becoming too tachypnoeic. The patient is placed on CPAP via the ventilator (i.e. no pressure support or intermittent ventilatory breaths). After 1 min the respiratory rate is divided by the average tidal volume of breaths for that minute (see box).

- If the f/V_T is >105 then the patient is likely to wean and should be given a spontaneous breathing trial either via a T-piece or through a responsive, sensitive trigger ventilator for between 30 and 120 min.

- The patient is considered to have failed the spontaneous breathing trial when any of the following criteria are met:
respiratory rate >35 for >5 min
oxygen saturation <90% for >5 min
heart rate increased or decreased by >20% for >5 min
systolic BP >180 or <90 mmHg continuously for at least 1 min
agitation, anxiety, and diaphoresis occur and are present for >5 min.

- Weaning should start during the day.

- The patient should have a full explanation with the opportunity to ask any questions.

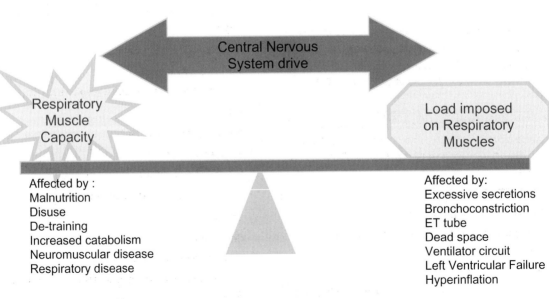

Fig. 4.12 The balance required for weaning.

TABLE 4.18	Causes of ventilator dependence
Cause	**Description**
Neurological control	Central drive (respiratory centre or brain stem damage etc.). Peripheral nerves (disease/damage). Cervical spinal cord damage
Respiratory system	Mechanical loads: respiratory system mechanics, e.g. reduced compliance, imposed loading
	Ventilatory muscle properties: inherent strength/endurance; metabolic state/nutrients/oxygen delivery and extraction
	Gas exchange properties: vascular properties and ventilation/perfusion matching
Cardiovascular system	Cardiac tolerance of ventilatory muscle work; peripheral oxygen demands
Psychological issues	

- The patient should be suctioned and made comfortable in a sitting position to allow expansion of lung bases.

- A T-piece with accurate oxygen delivery from a humidified source should be used.

- Close observation and monitoring of ECG and pulse oximetry should continue throughout the weaning period.

- Quarter-hourly respiratory rate, and tidal volume should be recorded with arterial blood gases after 20 min.

- If all is well after 30 min the patient can be extubated.

- If the patient has not weaned after 30 min, CPAP with 5 cmH$_2$O PEEP should be attached to the T-piece (to compensate for the loss of laryngeal PEEP).

SCREENING THE PATIENT USING THE RSBI

The patient breathes at a respiratory rate of 20 producing an expired minute volume of 8 litre over 1 min:

respiratory rate (f) = 20,

minute volume (V_E) = 8 litre

average tidal volume (V_T) = V_E/f = 8/20 = 400 ml (or 0.4 litre)

RSBI = f/V_T = 20/0.4 = 50.

Yang and Tobin (1991)

- If sputum clearance is a problem the patient may manage with a minitracheostomy.

Methods of long-term weaning

Current evidence suggests that the strategy (or protocol) employed for weaning will influence the duration of mechanical ventilation (Ely *et al.* 1996) but there does not seem to be a clearly superior mode of weaning with either pressure support ventilation (PSV) or spontaneous breathing trials (SBT) producing similar results (Brochard *et al.* 1994, Esteban *et al.* 1995). However, in both these studies, the most *inferior* weaning mode was intermittent mandatory ventilation (IMV) which resulted in a weaning period almost three times longer than PSV or SBT.

Recommendations based on these and many other studies showed that the use of a daily weaning screen for readiness to wean followed by a spontaneous breathing trial of between 30 to 120 min resulted in over 88% of patients being extubated. Of these, 94% remained extubated for more than 3 days (Ely 2001). When patients fail on more than three occasions, the likely cause for weaning failure should be investigated:

1. If possible, the factors listed in Table 4.18 should be resolved or optimized prior to attempting weaning.

2. The first six steps of short-term weaning also apply to long-term weaning.

3. In the ventilation modes of weaning, safety is maintained by the usual ventilator alarms for apnoea, etc.

FACTORS LIKELY TO PREVENT WEANING

- Sepsis

- Increased CO$_2$ production

- Electrolyte/fluid imbalance

- Decreased magnesium and phosphate levels

- Pain

- Haemodynamic instability

- Metabolic alkalosis

- Extreme malnutrition

- Untreated/unresolved respiratory problems

- Sedation

- Heart failure

- High intra-abdominal pressures

- Neurological factors such as reduced conscious level

However, continuous monitoring of ECG and S_aO_2 with regular arterial blood gases is important to monitor the patient.

4. If CPAP is instigated, close observation and monitoring of the patient is essential for signs of distress. ECG and pulse oximetry must be continuous. Respiratory rate, tidal, and minute volumes must be recorded quarter-hourly until the patient is evidently stable and coping with the weaning mode.

5. A full record of weaning attempts and achievement should be kept and referred to so that a logical, consistent, and structured approach can be continued.

6. The level of support provided by the chosen weaning method is gradually reduced until the patient is able to breathe without support (other than that required to overcome ventilator resistance) for more than 24 hours.

7. The patient is extubated and may be placed on mask CPAP or oxygen via mask. Observation at this point should be as per point (4).

Long-term weaning is frequently a trial and error situation with limited progress frequently followed by a set-back. No one weaning method has been shown to produce consistently superior results and each individual patient is different.

The patient's psychological state has a marked effect on his/her ability to wean and a positive attitude should be fostered and maintained.

In this group of patients, the multidisciplinary approach is by far the most likely method to succeed, with contributions from physiotherapy, speech and language, dietitian, and occupational therapy professionals forming the major part of successful support.

In prolonged ventilatory dependence, there is increasing evidence that specialist centres are more likely to succeed in weaning patients and once a patient has been ventilated for more than 3 months, the possibility of transferring patients to these centres should be considered.

Specific respiratory problems

Pneumothorax and bronchopleural fistula

A pneumothorax is the presence of air between the visceral and parietal pleura. It occurs when trauma or a spontaneous rupture results in a hole between the alveolar or bronchial wall and the pleura, allowing air to escape into the pleural space. The loss of an area of lung for gas exchange can severely compromise patients whose lung function is already limited.

Tension pneumothorax

A tension pneumothorax can develop when the rupture in the alveolar wall acts as a one-way valve. Thus, air escapes into the pleural space on inspiration but cannot return into the lung on expiration. A build-up of air within the pleural space occurs which rapidly increases in pressure until the lung on the affected side is collapsed. Displacement of the mediastinal structures towards the unaffected lung then occurs. The clinical effects of this are life-threatening and immediate.

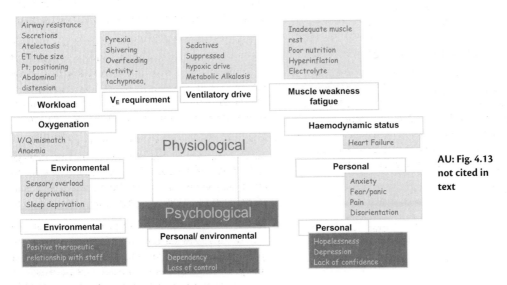

AU: Fig. 4.13 not cited in text

Fig. 4.13 Contributory factors to weaning failure.

Clinical effects of tension pneumothorax:

- Tachycardia and rise in blood pressure followed by a fall in blood pressure as the cardiac output decreases. This is due to the rise in intrathoracic pressure which impedes venous return and compresses the heart.

- Cyanosis, respiratory distress, and agitation. If the patient is being monitored by pulse oximetry the O_2 saturation will be seen to fall rapidly.

- If ventilated, airway pressures will increase dramatically, and expired minute volume may fall.

- If not treated, cardiovascular collapse and cardiac arrest will occur.

On examination, the patient will have unilateral chest movement. Air entry and breath sounds will be greatly decreased on the affected side. There will be a displaced apex beat and hyper-resonance on percussion. The trachea may be shifted from the midline towards the unaffected side.

Bronchopleural fistula

A fistula connecting lung and pleural space will produce the same effect as a pneumothorax. It is, however, less likely to close spontaneously and may require surgical intervention.

Interventions

1. *Tension pneumothorax* is an emergency situation and help must be sought immediately. Relief of the tension by percutaneous insertion of a large gauge needle or a 12/14 g IV cannula in the second intercostal space in the mid-clavicular line is performed as an emergency measure. Patients on positive pressure ventilation cannot suck in air through the needle or cannula unless they are making spontaneous breathing efforts. A chest drain is then inserted and attached to underwater seal drainage (see below).

2. *Pneumothorax.* If the pneumothorax is not 1ife-threatening the diagnosis and position will be confirmed by CXR and a drain can then be inserted (by medical staff) in an appropriate position under aseptic conditions. It is possible for other fluids, including effusions, to occupy the pleural space. Treatment is by needle aspiration or insertion of a chest drain or pigtail catheter.

Insertion and care of underwater seal chest drains

Chest drains are inserted into the pleural space to allow one-way drainage of:

- air,

- blood,

- pleural effusions,

- parenteral feed and other infusions,

- chyle (digested fat drained by the lymphatic system),

- empyema (pus in the pleural cavity).

Chest drains are large (18–32 FG) tubes inserted percutaneously through an intercostal space in the chest wall into the pleural space. The size of the chest drain will depend on what is to be drained, the largest sizes being required for the drainage of blood. The technique requires an aseptic procedure to cut down into the chest wall and insert the drain. The recommended site of insertion is in the mid or posterior axillary line. The second intercostal space of the anterior chest wall in the mid-clavicular line can be used for an anterior pneumothorax

Insertion

1. The patient should be informed of the procedure and explanation given.

2. If awake, the patient is usually placed in a comfortable upright or semi-upright reclining position for insertion of the drain either leaning over pillows placed on a bed-table in front of him/her or lying on the opposite side.

3. The underwater seal system bottle is primed with an amount of sterile water sufficient to cover the drainage tube. This prevents back-flow of air or fluid into the pleural space. The initial water level should be clearly marked to allow measurement of any subsequent drainage.

4. As with any insertion procedure the site is cleaned and covered with sterile towels. The area is infiltrated with local anaesthetic and a skin incision is made.

5. The chest drain is then inserted without the trocar in place to reduce the risk of significant trauma. A blunt dissection technique is used to form a track through the intercostal muscles and the parietal pleura is opened. The drain is then placed through the track into the pleural space and connected to the drainage system.

6. The drain is positioned in the uppermost chest for pneumothorax and in the dependent area for drainage of fluid. When the chest drain is correctly positioned air or fluid will drain out and there will be movement of the fluid level in the drainage tube with respiration.

7. The chest drain is sutured in place. To prevent any leak of air following removal of the drain a suture (purse string) may be sewn round the site of entry at this point although this is not always necessary. A dressing of either petroleum gauze, gauze soaked in

collodion, or plain gauze may be applied followed by an outer airtight strapping. This will prevent air leaks and anchor the drain firmly.

8. A CXR should be taken to check the position of the drain and lung re-inflation.

Problems associated with insertion and drainage

1. Puncture of the lung is possible if the drain is inserted in the wrong position and the trochar is used; for this reason, insertion is by blunt dissection.

2. Any blockage of the drainage system may result in a tension pneumothorax or a build-up in pressure within the pleural space. For this reason chest drains should never be clamped and drainage of a haemopneumothorax may require milking or stripping (applying pressure to the drainage tubing with a roller) to prevent obstruction from a clot.

3. Milking or stripping should not be carried out routinely as the negative pressures generated can be dangerously high (–100 to –400 cmH$_2$O; Duncan and Erickson 1982), resulting in further trauma to the lung tissue. Stripping should only be considered if there is reason to suspect obstruction of drainage by a clot (as in haemothorax and haemopneumothorax). Irrigation of the drain with saline may be prescribed in these cases.

4. Leaks may occur either at insertion site, connection between drain and tubing, or connection between tubing and bottle. They must be secured to prevent redevelopment of the pneumothorax.

5. Continuous bubbling of air which continues in spite of checking for leaks may indicate a bronchopleural fistula.

6. Suction (usually at –5 kPa) can be added should the lung fail to re-inflate despite a well-placed drain.

7. If drainage is greater than 1000 ml or continues at more than 200 ml for 4 hours there may be trauma to a major blood vessel. A doctor should be informed and the patient may need referral to a thoracic surgeon.

Principles of care
Securing the drain

1. Suture at time of insertion.

2. Use adhesive tape to secure at the insertion site and further down the chest wall.

3. Adhesive tape can also be placed round connections between the drain and tubing, although this may cause problems if it becomes lax and allows connections to part but remains stuck to the tubing.

Avoiding/managing leaks and obstructions

1. Check drain, tubing, and drain bottle for signs of leak. Continuous bubbling not related to respiration and leakage of fluid round connections are signs of leakage. Make all connections secure and if there is still a leak examine the site itself to ensure the drain has not slipped out. Inform medical staff.

2. Check drainage for signs of obstruction. Loss of fluid swing with respiration in the drain tubing, especially if accompanied by signs of distress and lack of drainage, may be signs of obstruction. These signs may also occur as the pneumothorax or haemothorax resolves, so patient condition/situation should be evaluated. Inform medical staff.

3. Do not clamp drain or tubing if the patient is ventilated. The risk of tension pneumothorax is high. Clamping for more than a few seconds is not recommended for any patient apart from post-pneumonectomy.

4. Obstruction of the drain by blood clot may need stripping or milking and possible irrigation. This should be considered with caution as the high pressures produced can cause further trauma and discomfort.

5. The drainage bottle should always be positioned below the level of the patient's chest to avoid backflow of water into the lung.

Prevention of infection

1. The dressing should be checked daily and changed if obviously wet or soiled, using routine aseptic technique.

2. Hands should be washed and gloves worn for handling the drain or redressing the site.

Removal of chest drains

1. Re-expansion of the lung should be checked on X-ray following previous discontinuation of any suction. There should be no air leak or drainage.

2. There is no need to clamp drains prior to removal but suction should be discontinued just prior to removal.

3. Full explanation is given and if possible patient co-operation is obtained. Analgesia should be given in good time prior to removal to allow it to have full effect.

4. An aseptic technique is essential.

5. If a purse string suture is used, two people are needed to remove the drain. The securing suture is removed and the ends of the purse string are freed and tied loosely.

6. The drain is removed on end inspiration to prevent indrawing of air on removal of the drain. The purse strings are pulled tight and secured.

7. An airtight dressing, such as gauze soaked in flexible collodion or petroleum gauze, under waterproof strapping is applied.

Acute respiratory distress syndrome (ARDS)

ARDS is a form of respiratory failure resulting from a variety of direct and indirect pulmonary injuries producing similar pathophysiological changes. It is the pulmonary manifestation of multi-organ dysfunction (see Chapter 12), and reflects similar changes in other organs. The lung may be affected to a greater or lesser degree. A full description of pathophysiology and management of the patient with ARDS can be found in Chapter 12.

ARDS is defined by the following clinical findings:

- Diffuse acute pulmonary infiltrates seen on CXR associated with decreased pulmonary compliance.

- Increased alveolar–arterial oxygen difference (despite supplemental oxygen).

- Pulmonary artery wedge pressure <18 mmHg. (i.e. non-cardiogenic factors)

- A precipitating factor (see box).

The details of pathology, management, and support for ARDS are given in Chapter 12.

Acute asthma

Asthma is an acute, reversible airway restriction caused by bronchospasm in response to a range of stimuli. These include allergens, infections, and exercise. Bronchospasm invokes smooth muscle constriction, mucosal oedema, and excessive mucus production.

DISORDERS ASSOCIATED WITH ARDS

- Infection: septicaemia, pneumonia (due to various agents)
- Trauma
- Aspiration: gastric acid, hydrocarbons, near-drowning
- Inhalation: smoke, corrosive gases
- Haematological: massive blood transfusion, post-cardiopulmonary bypass
- Metabolic: pancreatitis, acute liver failure
- Drug overdose: heroin, barbiturates
- Miscellaneous: eclampsia, amniotic fluid embolism, etc.

Management
Reduction of bronchospasm and inflammation

1. Use of bronchodilators (β_2-agonists, e.g. salbutamol). Usually inhaled but may be given IV.

2. Steroids, such as hydrocortisone or prednisolone, are used to reduce hypersensitivity, although this takes a number of hours to begin working. Beclomethasone may also be inhaled.

3. Aminophylline given IV to relax bronchial smooth muscle.

4. Anticholinergics, such as ipratropium bromide, may be inhaled to relax smooth muscle.

5. In severe cases, adrenaline can be used either subcutaneously, by nebulizer, or inserted down the endotracheal tube.

6. Antibiotics for infective causes of exacerbations

Support of respiratory function

- Oxygen therapy: high concentrations are given as necessary.

- Humidification and fluid hydration to avoid mucus plugging.

- Physiotherapy and bronchoscopy, if necessary.

- CPAP.

- Ventilation if:
  P_aCO_2 is rising,
  patient is obtunded,
  patient is fatigued,
  P_aO_2 is falling,
  patient does not respond to treatment.

- Sedatives should not be given unless the patient is about to be ventilated as they can reduce the respiratory drive causing hypoventilation and precipitating respiratory failure.

- Antibiotics are only given if there are obvious signs of infection (fever, increased white cell count).

Avoidance of iatrogenic complications

1. Air trapping (intrinsic PEEP, auto-PEEP). This is evidenced by rising end expiratory pressure (see Table 4.15) and can be suggested by auscultation of expiratory wheeze continuing right up to commencement of the next breath and by increased chest girth. A long expiratory time should be used either a prolonged I:E ratio (1:3) or a slow respiratory rate, with close observation of respiratory status. Occasionally, disconnection from the ventilator and

manual chest decompression is required. Use of flow and volume graphic waveforms on the ventilator will allow identification of air trapping as the flow will not return to zero before the next breath.

2. Barotrauma. Positive pressures applied to bronchoconstricted lungs with low compliance carry a high risk of barotrauma and peak airway pressures should be kept below 35 cmH$_2$O. This can be achieved with: small tidal volumes (e.g. 6–8 ml/kg), low respiratory rate (e.g. 6–10 breaths/min), long expiratory times (1:1 or longer), acceptance of hypercapnia, providing pH is >7.2, low inspiratory flow rates, and adequate sedation/relaxants to prevent 'fighting' (Armstrong et al. 1991)

3. Avoidance of drugs potentially likely to stimulate histamine release (e.g. 'natural' opiates or derivatives thereof).

4. Sputum plugging and lobar collapse. Rigorous chest physiotherapy and frequent bronchial hygiene with high levels of humidification will be effective in most cases. The patient's own level of hydration is also important. In severe cases, use of halothane or other inhalational anaesthetics has been successful and intravenous ketamine has also been tried as a bronchodilator. High-dose magnesium sulphate has also been used to relax smooth muscle.

Chronic obstructive pulmonary disease (COPD)

COPD is a product of chronic bronchitis, bronchiectasis, emphysema, and asthma. Most patients have a mixture of chronic bronchitis and emphysema. Acute exacerbations usually occur as a result of infection but may also be related to atmospheric pollution or surgery (use of inhalational anaesthetics). Inappropriate use of sedatives or high-concentration oxygen therapy can precipitate acute decompensation.

Management

This is similar to asthma although it may be unresponsive to steroids. In most cases, infection is the precipitating cause of the exacerbation and antibiotics should be given if there is purulent sputum (Stoller 2002).

Support of respiratory function

1. Oxygen therapy. Caution is required with oxygen therapy as many patients with COPD have become dependent on hypoxic stimulation of respiratory drive due to chronic retention of high levels of carbon dioxide resulting in loss of their hypercapnic drive. Where this is the case, higher concentrations (those greater then 28%) should be delivered via an accurate delivery system (see Table 4.11), such as a Ventimask and arterial blood gases should be monitored on a regular basis for evidence of increasing CO$_2$ retention. The level of P_aO_2 aimed for should be relative to the usual range; this may be considerably lower than that of the normal person. However, the patient should not be allowed to become excessively hypoxaemic and the question of whether or not to ventilate mechanically must be discussed, ideally at an early stage (see later). Judicious use of non-invasive ventilation, such as BiPAP, has been shown to be highly effective in these patients (Keenan et al. 2003) or the early use of CPAP may also be of some benefit.

2. Physiotherapy.

3. Respiratory stimulants, such as doxapram or nikethamide, are now only recommended if NIV is not available and can be used if the P_aCO_2 continues to rise with deteriorating consciousness (National Institute for Clinical Excellence 2004).

4. Mechanical ventilation. The decision to intubate and ventilate patients with COPD should be carefully considered, preferably at some time well in advance of an immediate need for ventilation. Weaning from ventilation is difficult and the quality of life and survival can be very poor afterwards. If there is a reversible precipitating factor, such as recent surgery or a treatable infection, then ventilation may provide support until recovery has taken place. However, if respiratory failure is the result of a continuing deterioration in the disease itself then ventilation simply prolongs life without prospect of improvement. Weaning may be impossible and quality of life deteriorates further. There is a need for advance discussion by all members of the team with the patient and his/her relatives to decide whether ventilation is appropriate. The responsibility for initiating this should rest with the physician rather than the intensive care team. Ventilation should aim to maintain the patient's normal P_aCO_2 and to reduce an elevated P_aCO_2 slowly to prevent an acute alkalosis. Weaning is a prolonged pro-cess due to the patient's poor respiratory reserve and nutritional state. It benefits from the use of pressure support and gradual increase in patient effort (see ventilation modes, Table 4.16).

5. Nutrition. Patients with COPD are usually chronically malnourished due to impairment of appetite, dysp-

noea during meals, and chronic ill health. It is important to start early nutritional support. During weaning, these patients are least likely to be able to cope with any excess CO_2 production related to carbohydrate overload (see Chapter 11). Care should be taken to ensure that equal amounts of fat and carbohydrate contribute to calorie intake.

Pulmonary embolus (PE)

Pulmonary embolus is the occlusion of a pulmonary artery by a thrombus. The embolus is most commonly thrown off from a deep vein thrombosis of the pelvic or leg veins. The severity of effect is directly related to the size of the embolus and thus the size of the vessel which has been blocked.

Symptoms

These are tachypnoea, tachycardia, dyspnoea, and chest pain.

Diagnosis is made on clinical presentation (including a raised CVP), CXR (reduced blood flow 'oligaemia' to an area of lung, evidence of pulmonary infarction—classically a wedge-shaped shadow), ECG (right axis deviation, S1, Q3, T3 configuration, right ventricular strain pattern, partial right bundle branch block—see Chapter 6), hypoxaemia, and exclusion of other likely causes. If the patient is stable, a spiral CT scan with contrast pulmonary angiography and V/Q scans may be performed, otherwise emergency surgery should be considered.

Management
- Anticoagulation using heparin.
- Thrombolytic therapy.
- Respiratory support (oxygen, CPAP, mechanical ventilation).
- Pulmonary embolectomy.
- Prevention of any further deep vein thrombosis using elastic support stockings, exercises, and mobilization.
- If cardiovascular embarrassment is evident, the patient must be fluid loaded to ensure optimal right ventricular filling.

For further management see Chapter 6.

Pneumonia

Pneumonia is an inflammatory process caused by bacterial, viral, fungal, protozoan, rickettsial, or, rarely, chemical (e.g. gastric aspiration) causes. It is characterized by purulent respiratory secretions, pyrexia, and commonly CXR opacity associated with the area of the infection. Treatment depends on the aetiology and infecting agent but all patients require similar support and management. Hospital-associated pneumonia is defined as pneumonia occurring either after the first 48 hours of hospital admission or in intubated patients. Aspiration is the main route for pneumonia in intubated patients as the endotracheal tube holds the vocal cords open facilitating aspiration (Rello and Diaz 2003)

Management
- Antibiotic therapy.
- Oxygen therapy, CPAP, and mechanical ventilation may all be necessary to maintain PO_2.
- Chest physiotherapy and bronchial hygiene to clear secretions.
- Postural drainage and position changes.
- Adequate nutrition to prevent complications associated with malnutrition (see Chapter 11).
- Prevention of further infection.

Test yourself
Questions

1. What are the key components of respiratory assessment in a mechanically ventilated patient?
2. What are the main priorities of care to prevent problems associated with an endotracheal tube?
3. What are the main problems identified by the intubated patient?
4. What are the advantages of a closed suction system?
5. Which groups of patients will find weaning more difficult?

Answers

1. *The patient*: skin colour, sweating, distress, restlessness; respiratory rate, use of accessory muscles, pattern and effort; auscultation of air entry, equal R and L, added breath sounds etc.; monitoring—O_2 saturations, tachycardia (bradycardia), blood pressure; arterial blood gases.
The ventilator: airway pressure; tidal and minute volumes; inspired oxygen; graphic waveforms for pressure and flow.

Secretions: colour; consistency; volume.

2. Humidification and warming of inhaled gases; assistance to clear secretions; prevention of infection due to bypassing of normal protective mechanisms.

3. Inability to communicate verbally; discomfort from the tube, and the tapes securing it; feelings of suffocation associated with suction.

4. Decreased risk of infection and ?decreased risk of corneal contamination; suction-associated desaturation may be decreased; haemodynamic compromise may be decreased.

5. COPD patients; patients with limited cardiac reserve; patients with long-standing ventilation; patients with neuromuscular disorders.

References and bibliography

Ackerman, M.H. (1993). The effect of saline lavage prior to suctioning. *American Journal of Critical Care* **2**, 326–30.

Armstrong, R.F., Bullen, C., Cohen, S.L., *et al.* (1991). *Critical Care algorithms*, p. 26. Oxford University Press, Oxford.

Balas, M.C. (2000). Prone positioning of patients with acute respiratory distress syndrome: applying research to practice. *Critical Care Nurse* **20**, 24–36.

Baun, M.M., Flones, M.J. (1984). Cumulative effects of three sequential endotracheal suctioning episodes in the dog model. *Heart and Lung* **13**, 148–54.

Bell, S.D. (1996). Use of Passy-Muir tracheostomy speaking valve in mechanically ventilated neurological patients. *Critical Care Nurse* **16**, 63–8.

Benito, S. (1991). Pulmonary compliance. In: *Mechanical Ventilation* (ed. F. Lemaire), pp. 86–98. Springer, Berlin.

Bergbom-Engberg, I., Haljamäe, H. (1989). Assessment of patients' experience of discomforts during respirator therapy. *Critical Care Medicine* **17**, 1068.

Berney S., Denehy, L., (2002). A comparison of the effects of manual and ventilator hyperinflation on static compliance and sputum production in intubated and ventilated intensive care patients. *Physiotherapy Research International* **7**, 100–8.

Bethune, D. (1989) Humidification in ventilated patients. *Intensive and Critical Care Digest* **8**(2), 37–8.

Bostick, J., Wendelgass, S.T. (1987). Normal saline instillation as part of the suctioning procedure: effects on PaO_2 and the amount of secretions. *Heart and Lung* **16**, 532–40.

Bourjeily, G., Habr, F., Supinski, G. (2002). Review of tracheostomy usage: complications and decannulation procedures. Part II. *Clinical Pulmonary Medicine* **9**, 273–8.

Brathwaite, C., Borg, U., (1990). Ventilatory support. Use of pressure modes in critically ill patients. *Critical Care Report* **1**, 300–7.

Brice, J, Davis, D. (2004). High Frequency Ventilation in the Adult. *Clinical Pulmonary Medicine* **11**, 101–6.

British Thoracic Society (2002). Non-invasive ventilation in acute respiratory failure. *Thorax* **57** (3), 192–211.

Brochard, L, Rauss, A., Benito, S. *et al.* (1994). Comparison of three methods of gradual withdrawal from ventilatory support during weaning from mechanical ventilation. *American Journal of Respiratory and Critical Care Medicine* **150**, 896–903.

Chadda, K., Louis, B., Benaissa, L, *et al.* (2002). Physiological effects of decannulation in tracheostomized patients. *Intensive Care Medicine* **28**, 1761–7.

Clark, A.P., Winslow, E.H., Tyler, D.O., *et al.* (1990). Effects of endotracheal suctioning on mixed venous oxygen saturation and heart rate in critically ill adults. *Heart and Lung* **19**, 552–70.

Combes, P., Fauvage, B., Oleyer, C. (2000). Nosocomial pneumonia in mechanically ventilated patients, a prospective randomized evaluation of the Stericath closed suctioning system. *Intensive Care Medicine* **26**, 878–82.

Dellinger, R.P., Zimmerman, J.L., Taylor, R.W., *et al.* (1998). Effects of inhaled nitric oxide in patients with acute respiratory distress syndrome: results of a randomized phase II trial. *Critical Care Medicine* **26**, 15–23.

Des Jardins, T.R. (1988). *Cardiopulmonary Anatomy and Physiology: Essentials for Respiratory Care.* Delmar Publishers, New York.

Donald, K.J., Robertson, V.J., Tsebelis, K. (2000) Setting safe and effective suction pressure: the effect of using a manometer in the suction circuit. *Intensive Care Medicine* **26**, 15–19.

Duncan, C., Erickson, R (1982). Pressures associated with chest tube stripping. *Heart and Lung* **11**, 166–71.

Ely, E.W. (2001). Weaning from mechanical ventilation (part 1): evidence supports the use of protocols. In: *Yearbook of Intensive Care and Emergency Medicine 2001* (ed. J.-L. Vincent, pp. 481–95). Springer, Berlin.

Ely, E.W., Baker, A.M., Dunagan, D.P *et al.* (1996). Effect on the duration of mechanical ventilation of identifying patients capable of breathing spontaneously. *New England Journal of Medicine* **335**, 1864–9.

Esteban, A., Frutos, F., Tobin, M.J. *et al.* (1995). A comparison of four methods of weaning patients from mechanical ventilation. *New England Journal of Medicine* **332**, 345–50.

Freeman, B.D., Isabella, K., Lin, N., *et al.* (2000). A meta-analysis of prospective trials comparing percutaneous and surgical tracheostomy in critically ill patients. *Chest* **118**, 1412–18.

Gattinoni, L., Tognoni, G., Pesenti, A., *et al.* (2001). Effect of prone positioning on the survival of patients with acute respiratory failure. *New England Journal of Medicine* **345**, 568–73.

Gellinger, R.P.,Zimmerman, J.L., Taylor, R.W., *et al.*(1998). Effects of inhaled nitric oxide in patients with acute respiratory distress syndrome: results of a randomized phase II trial. *Critical Care Medicine* **26**, 15–23.

Gift, A.G., Bolgiano, C.S., Cunningham, J. (1991). Sensations during chest tube removal. *Heart and Lung* **20**, 131–7.

Girou, E., Buu-Hoi, A., Stephan, F., *et al.* (2004). Airway colonisation in long-term mechanically ventilated patients. Effect of semi-recumbent position and continuous subglottic suctioning. *Intensive Care Medicine* **30**, 225–33.

Griggs, W.M., Myburgh, J.A., Worthley, L.I.G. (1991). A prospective comparison of a percutaneous tracheostomy technique with standard surgical tracheostomy. *Intensive Care Medicine* **17**, 261–3.

Guyton, A. (1985). *Anatomy and Physiology*. Holt Saunders, Philadelphia.

Happ, M.B (2002). Treatment interference in critically ill patients: an update on unplanned extubation. *Clinical Pulmonary Medicine* **9**, 81–6.

Harshbarger, S.A., Hoffman, L.A., Zullo, T.G., *et al.* (1992). Effects of a closed tracheal suction system on ventilatory and cardiovascular parameters. *American Journal of Critical Care* **1**, 57–61.

Hegler, D.A., Traver, G.A. (1994). Endotracheal saline and suction catheters: sources of lower airway contamination. *American Journal of Critical Care* **3**, 444–7.

Hill, J.D., O'Brien, T.G., Muray, J.T. (1972). Prolonged extracorporeal oxygenation for acute post-traumatic respiratory failure (shock-lung syndrome). *New England Journal of Medicine* **286**, 629–34.

Hubmayr, R., Abel, M., Rehder, K. (1990). Physiologic approach to mechanical ventilation. *Critical Care Medicine* **18**, 103–13.

Keenan, S., Sinuff, T., Cook, D., *et al.* (2003). Which patients with acute exacerbation of chronic obstructive pulmonary disease benefit from noninvasive positive-pressure ventilation?: A systematic review of the literature. *Annals of Internal Medicine* **138**, 861–70.

Knebel, A.R. (1992). When weaning from mechanical ventilation fails. *American Journal of Critical Care* **1**(3), 19–29.

Kollef, M., Shapiro, S.D, Silver, P., *et al.* (1997). A randomized controlled trial of protocol-directed versus physician-directed weaning from mechanical ventilation. *Critical Care Medicine* **25**, 567–74.

Lemaire, F. (ed.) (1991). *Mechanical Ventilation*. Springer, Berlin.

Mancinelli-Van Atta, J., Beck, S.L. (1992). Preventing hypoxemia and hemodynamic compromise related to endotracheal suctioning. *American Journal of Critical Care* **3**, 62–79.

Marcy, T.W., Marini, J.J. (1991). Inverse ratio ventilation in ARDS: rationale and implementation. *Chest* **100**, 494–504.

National Institute for Clinical Excellence (2004). *Chronic Obstructive Pulmonary Disease*, Guideline 12. NICE, London (www.nice.org.uk/CG012NICEguideline).

Parkin, B., Turner, A., Moore, E., *et al.* (1997). Bacterial keratitis in the critically ill. *British Journal of Ophthalmology* **81**, 1060–3.

Patman, S., Jenkins, S., Stiller, K. (2000). Manual hyperinflation—effects on respiratory parameters. *Physiotherapy Research International* **5**, 157–71.

Pepe, P., Marini, J. (1982). Occult positive end expiratory pressure in mechanically ventilated patients with airflow obstruction. *American Review of Respiratory Disease* **126**, 166–71.

Pierce, J.D., Piazza, D., Naftel, D.C. (1991). Effects of two chest clearance protocols on drainage in patients after myocardial revascularization surgery. *Heart and Lung* **20**, 125–30.

Putensen, C., Hering R., Wrigge, H. (2002) Controlled versus assisted ventilation. *Current Opinion in Critical Care* **8**, 51–7.

Rello, J., Diaz, E. (2003). Pneumonia in the intensive care unit. *Critical Care Medicine* **31**, 2544–51.

Richard, J.C., Carlucci, A., Breton, L., *et al.* (2002). Bench testing of pressure support ventilation with three different generations of ventilators. *Intensive Care Medicine* **28**, 1049–57.

Ruggles, L. (1995). Auto-PEEP: measurement issues and nursing interventions *Critical Care Nurse* **15**(2), 30–8.

Serra, A. (2000). Tracheostomy care. *Nursing Standard* **14**, 45–55.

Sirker, A.A, Rhodes, A., Grounds, R.M., *et al.* (2002). Acid–base physiology: the 'traditional' and the 'modern' approaches. *Anaesthesia* **57**, 348–56.

Stoller, J.K. (2002). Acute exacerbations of chronic obstructive pulmonary disease. *New England Journal of Medicine* **346**, 988–94.

Stone, K.S., Vorst, E.C., Lanham, B., *et al.* (1989). Effects of lung hyperinflation on mean arterial pressure and postsuctioning hypoxemia. *Heart and Lung* **18**, 377–85.

Tobin, M.J. (1991). Weaning assessment. In: *Ventilatory Failure, Update in Intensive Care and Emergency Medicine 15* (ed. J.J. Marini, C. Roussos). Springer, Berlin.

Tobin, M.J. (2001). Medical progress: advances in mechanical ventilation. *New England Journal of Medicine* **344**, 1986–96.

Villar, J., Slutsky, A.S. (1991). Alternative modalities for ventilatory support. In: *Update in Intensive Care and Emergency Medicine 14* (ed. J.L. Vincent), pp. 345–56. Springer, Berlin.

Yang, K.L., Tobin, M.J. (1991). A prospective study of indexes predicting the outcome of trials of weaning from mechanical ventilation. *New England Journal of Medicine* **324**, 1445–50.

Monitoring the critically ill patient

Introduction

Monitoring of physiological variables is essential in the care of the critically ill patient. The aims of monitoring are:

- to detect changes in the patient's clinical condition,
- to assess the response to treatment strategies,
- to act as a diagnostic tool.

Monitoring may be continuous or intermittent. Although individual readings can be significant for both types of monitoring, it is important to analyse trends from serial data, and to assimilate and interpret information from all forms of patient monitoring including clinical observation.

In order to act correctly on information provided by the various monitoring devices, the nurse must have a thorough understanding of the relevant physiology, practical expertise in the procedures, and an awareness of the reliability of the equipment or technique involved.

Reliability and safety of monitoring devices

- All monitoring devices are manufactured to specific standards and recommendations are given for the conditions of their use. It is important that these are adhered to in order to ensure the accuracy of information obtained.

- Most monitoring devices are powered by mains electricity and/or rechargeable battery units. The immediate area surrounding the patient therefore often contains a large number of electrical items. Cables must be treated with care to avoid undue stretching or tension and vital plugs, such as to the ventilator, should be easily identifiable. Extreme care must be taken not to allow spillage of fluid on to plugs and sockets (particularly if using extension leads). Position equipment so that leads do not drape across the patient and ensure there is easy access around the bed area.

• Some items of monitoring equipment are very heavy and care must be taken when attaching them to items, such as drip stands, in order to avoid breakage or injury to the patient or staff.

• When large amounts of monitoring equipment surround the bed area they must be positioned such that the nurse can see their visual displays at all times.

• If alarm systems are incorporated within the monitoring devices these must used and the alarm limits set according to the patient's condition. Alarm settings should be checked at the beginning of every shift and reviewed if the patient's condition changes.

Types of monitoring

Methods of monitoring may be non-invasive or invasive. Details of specific neurological, metabolic, and respiratory monitoring devices are discussed in the relevant chapters. The following techniques will be discussed in this chapter:

• *Non-invasive*: observation; monitoring fluid balance; investigations; the ECG and arrhythmias; the 12-lead ECG; pulse oximetry; end tidal carbon dioxide monitoring; blood pressure; gastrointestinal tonometry; Doppler techniques; bispectral index.

• *Invasive*: pressure monitoring; arterial cannulation; central venous pressure; pulmonary artery catheterization; cardiac output determination—the Fick method, oesophageal Doppler, lithium dilution cardiac output, pulse contour cardiac output, thermodilution methods.

Non-invasive monitoring

Simple monitoring of the patient can be achieved without the use of equipment. The nurse can obtain a great deal of clinical information by merely watching, touch-

TABLE 5.1   Non-invasive monitoring: observation

Observation	Appearance	Possible cause
Skin		
Touch	Dry	Fluid depletion
	Cool, clammy	Hypoperfusion states, excess vasoconstriction
	Hot, flushed	Pyrexia vasodilatation
	Tense, pitting	Oedema
Colour	Pale	Anaemia
	Cherry pink	Carbon monoxide poisoning
	Cyanosed (peripheral or central)	Hypoxaemia (central cyanosis). Poor perfusion (peripheral cyanosis)
	Jaundiced	Biliary obstruction, haemolysis, liver dysfunction
Other	Petechiae, bruising, bleeding from puncture/cannulae sites	Clotting disorders
	Decreased limb perfusion (white, cold, mottled, loss of pulse)	Arterial occlusion, rhabdomyolysis, compartment syndrome
	Limb warm, painful, swollen	Venous occlusion
	Blisters, rashes	Allergic reactions (drugs, dressings)
Neurological		
Conscious level	Reduced	Neurological deterioration. Drug therapy. Uraemia. Metabolic causes. Hypoperfusion states
Behaviour	Restlessness, agitation, aggressiveness, confusion	Hypoxaemia. Sepsis. Neurological deterioration. Metabolic causes. Pain, discomfort. Need to open bowels. Full bladder or stomach. Haemorrhage. Reaction to the environment and illness. Drug therapy
Expression	Grimacing, worried	Pain, discomfort, fear, anxiety

ing, and listening to the patient. The patient's posture, facial expressions, behaviour, and conscious level can all reveal important information (see Table 5.1). For respiratory observations see Chapter 4.

Monitoring fluid balance

All critically ill patients should have their fluid intake and output measured, at minimum, on an hourly basis. This includes wound and nasogastric drainage, urine output, and all drug and fluid infusions (preferably administered via volumetric pumps or syringe drivers to aid accuracy). Fluid balance must be reviewed and assessed regularly in combination with haemodynamic and respiratory data.

Investigations

Regular haematological, microbiological, and biochemical investigations enable the early identification of physiological deterioration or improvement and must be evaluated in conjunction with data from other monitoring devices.

Routine blood tests will include arterial blood gas analysis, full blood count, clotting studies, glucose, urea, creatinine, and electrolytes, liver function tests, and urinary electrolytes and creatinine. Many other investigations, such as amylase and endocrine function tests, may also be performed depending on the patient's presumptive diagnosis.

Most units will routinely send specimens of sputum, urine, blood, wound discharge, etc., for microbiological culture if infection is suspected. Many other specific investigations, such as computed tomography (CT), ultrasound, echocardiography, and X-rays, also play an important part in the monitoring and identification of disease processes and are used according to the patient's clinical condition.

The electrocardiogram (ECG)

All critically ill patients will require continuous ECG monitoring. The aims of cardiac monitoring are:

1. The early detection of changes in heart rate and rhythm.

2. To assess the effectiveness of treatment strategies.

There are many types of cardiac monitors but the essential components of ECG monitoring are the same.

Basic principles of ECG monitoring

◆ Electrodes are placed on the chest wall to detect the electrical activity initiated by the heart. Electrical activity that is moving towards an electrode will produce an upward (positive) deflection on the recording and activity that is moving away from the electrode will produce a downward (negative) deflection. The baseline (isoelectric line) is where the positive and negative deflections begin and end.

◆ The electrodes are connected by a patient cable to an oscilloscope that displays a continuous waveform reflecting each phase of the heart's electrical activity.

◆ The impulses produced by the cardiac activity would be too small to be seen on an oscilloscope naturally and are therefore amplified by the monitor so that their height is increased about a thousand fold.

◆ The waveform on the monitor can be adjusted so that the optimal size, brightness and position of the ECG are seen. A choice of leads is possible but lead II is usually selected. This is because the direction of electrical current as it passes through the ventricles is directed towards lead II, resulting in a large, positive waveform that can be easily interpreted.

Placement of ECG electrodes

The electrodes are small, disposable, adhesive pads. These are pre-gelled (to facilitate conduction) and are attached to the chest wall by simply peeling off the backing paper and pressing firmly to the skin. The skin must be clean and dry and it may be necessary to shave chest hair to facilitate contact. It is imperative to have good contact between the skin and electrode or the ECG waveform will be distorted and artefacts will appear.

Usually, three electrodes are used (see Fig. 5.1), but some equipment may require four or five electrodes to allow multiple views of the heart.

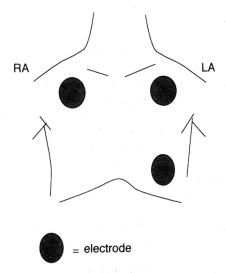

Fig. 5.1 Placement of ECG electrodes.

The electrodes can remain *in situ* for several days, as the gel does not usually dry out. However, skin irritation can occur due to the adhesive used on the electrode or the conducting jelly. The electrode positions should be rotated regularly to avoid soreness, and the skin checked for sensitivity.

Thin wires snap or clamp on to the electrodes and are connected to designated leads on the patient cable. These are usually designated RA (right arm), LA (left arm), and RL (right leg or earth) and should be connected to the corresponding electrode. The patient cable is then connected to the cable socket of the monitor.

Adjusting the monitor

The displayed waveform must be clear and distinct. Fine adjustments to the brightness and size of the waveform can be made on the monitor. The amplitude of the R wave is of particular importance as the monitor calculates the heart rate by recognizing and counting this wave. If the height of the wave cannot be increased sufficiently to record an accurate heart rate the position of the electrodes, or the lead displayed, may need to be changed to obtain a greater electrical potential.

High- and low-rate alarm limits should be set according to the patient's clinical condition. Frequent false alarms undermine the rationale for alarm setting and may cause the patient undue anxiety.

Most rate meters count the number of ventricular beats (R waves) per minute and display this as the heart rate. In fact, most meters will count all large, upward deflections as they are unable to distinguish ventricular beats from muscle potentials caused by contraction of skeletal muscle. This means that movement by the patient or muscle tremors may cause falsely elevated heart rate readings.

Falsely high rates can also be seen if the R and T wave of the ECG waveform (p. 125) are the same size and the monitor is recognizing both as the R wave. To rectify this the amplitude of the waveform should be increased until the R wave is higher than the T wave, or the electrode positions or ECG lead displayed should be changed.

Falsely low heart rates will occur if the R wave is of insufficient size to be detected by the monitor (the amplitude should be increased until this is recognized), or if there is a disturbance in the transmission of the signal from the skin to the monitor. This may be due to a defective electrode, separation of the electrode from the skin, or disconnection of one of the patient leads.

Electrical interference can occur from other electrical devices at the bedside. This will appear as a series of fine, rapid spikes (artefact) which distort the baseline of the ECG. This may be due to incorrect earthing and the device responsible should be identified and checked. Artefact may also be caused by shivering of the patient (particularly if the electrodes are positioned over skeletal muscle) or loose connections at the patient's cable.

A wandering baseline can occur when the isoelectric line regularly moves up and down rather than in a straight line. This is invariably due to movement of the chest wall during respiration. The only solution is to alter the electrode position and place the electrodes to the lowest ribs and apex of the chest (Table 5.2).

Arrhythmias and conduction disturbances

Disorders of cardiac rhythm are one of the commonest problems experienced by critically ill patients. Monitoring of the ECG allows prompt recognition of these disorders and immediate intervention where necessary. It is worth remembering, however, that all ECG rhythms should be examined in the context of the patient's clin-

TABLE 5.2 Summary of problems associated with EGG monitoring		
Problem	**Cause**	**Action**
Falsely high rate	Patient movement, fitting, tremors	Ensure electrodes are not placed over skeletal muscle
	T wave same height as R wave	Increase amplitude, change position of electrodes
Falsely low rate	Lead disconnection	Check leads
	Separation of electrode from skin	Check/replace electrodes
	Insufficient height of R wave	Increase amplitude, change position of electrodes
Artefact	Shivering, tremors	Ensure patient is warm
	Electrical equipment	Check other electrical equipment in use at bedside (e.g. electric razors, fans)
	Poor connection of leads or electrodes	Check all connections are firm, change electrodes
Wandering baseline	Respiration causing chest wall movement	Adjust patient position. Reposition electrodes to lowest ribs to minimize effect

ical condition and intervention decided on according to this, rather than the rhythm itself.

ECG definitions

There are a number of definitions that provide a background for understanding the ECG:

- *Sinus rhythm*: a rhythm originating in the sinoatrial (SA) node of >60 and <100 beats per minute (bpm).

- *Sinus tachycardia*: a rhythm originating from the SA node of >100 bpm.

- *Sinus bradycardia*: a rhythm originating in the SA node of <60 bpm.

The above rhythms usually reflect either a normal heart or a normal physiological response to an external factor.

- *Tachycardia*: heart rate >100 bpm.

- *Bradycardia*: heart rate <60 bpm.

- *Isoelectric line*: the baseline of the ECG tracing (i.e. no electrical activity is occurring).

- *Positive deflection*: upward movement of the ECG tracing from the baseline.

- *Negative deflection*: downward movement of the ECG tracing from the baseline.

- The *P wave* corresponds to atrial depolarization and is seen in normal sinus rhythm (see later). P waves are best seen in leads II, III, VI, and V2. (No P waves are seen in atrial fibrillation while a peaked wave is classically seen with chronic pulmonary hypertension and an M-shaped wave with mitral valve disease.)

- The *PR interval* should be in the range 0.12–0.2 s. A longer interval (>0.2 s) is seen with first degree heart block while a shorter interval (<0.12 s) is seen with rapid atrioventricular (AV) conduction (e.g. Wolff–Parkinson–White (WPW) syndrome).

- The *QRS complex* (Fig. 5.2) corresponds to ventricular depolarization and the width should be less than 0.12 s. A greater width is seen with delayed conduction through the ventricular conducting system (e.g. bundle branch block). The QRS height is useful in assessing left or right ventricular hypertrophy (see later). A pathological Q wave is seen in myocardial infarction and should be at least 25% of the height of the following R wave and exceed 0.04 s in width (see myocardial infarction).

- The *Q–T interval* varies with heart rate and is approximately 0.35–0.43 s long when the heart rate is 60 bpm. It is prolonged in hypocalcaemia and shortened by hypercalcaemia.

- The *ST segment* is elevated (in convex shape) from the baseline (isoelectric line) in myocardial infarction and depressed during myocardial ischaemia (see later). Concave ST segment elevation is seen in pericarditis.

- The *T wave* corresponds to ventricular repolarization and should normally be 'positive' (i.e. pointing upwards) in leads I, II, V4, V5, and V6. An inverted T wave may be seen in myocardial ischaemia and infarction, and in types of bundle branch block (see later). It is peaked during hyperkalaemia and flattened by hypokalaemia.

Timing of the ECG

The paper used to record the ECG trace is made up of small and large squares. Each small square measures 1 mm and each large square measures 5 mm. The paper is then run at a standard speed of 25 mm/s. Thus, each small square takes 0.04 s to pass the recording pen and each large square takes 0.2 s. This allows the timing and rate of the ECG trace to be calculated.

Systematic analysis of the ECG rhythm strip

When first attempting to identify arrhythmias it is helpful to use a step-by-step sequence to ensure all aspects of the rhythm are analysed and to avoid missing important information. Ideally, a recorded strip (traditionally of lead II, but any monitoring lead can be used) should be taken and used to analyse the rhythm systematically.

One suggested sequence is:

1. Determine the rate.

2. Determine the regularity of the rhythm.

3. Identify the P wave and its shape.

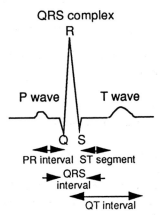

Fig. 5.2 The QRS complex.

4. Identify the QRS complex.

5. Determine the relationship between P waves and QRS complexes (i.e. is there one P wave to every QRS?).

6. Calculate the P–R interval.

7. Examine the shape and width of the QRS complex.

Classification of arrhythmias

Arrhythmias can be classified as disorders of impulse formation or impulse conduction:

1. Disorders of impulse formation. This may be due to dysfunction of the pacemaker rate of the sinoatrial node allowing escape rhythms from other pacemakers. In conjunction, excessively rapid impulse generation may produce atrial, junctional, and ventricular tachycardias via re-entry pathways (see Table 5.3). These are discussed below.

2. Disorders of impulse conduction. This refers to situations where conduction is either slowed, blocked, or uses an alternative pathway (see Table 5.4).

TABLE 5.3 Disorders of impulse formation

Site	Disorder
Ventricular	Ventricular ectopic beats
	Ventricular tachycardia
	Torsades de pointes
	Ventricular fibrillation
Junctional	AV nodal (junctional) premature beats
	AV nodal (junctional) tachycardia
Supraventricular	Sinus arrhythmia
	Sinus bradycardia
	Atrial ectopic beats
	Sinus tachycardia
	Atrial flutter
	Atrial fibrillation (AF)
	Sick sinus syndrome

TABLE 5.4 Disorders of impulse conduction

Slowed or blocked conduction	First degree atrioventricular block
	Second degree atrioventricular block
	Third degree atrioventricular block
	Bundle branch block
Alternative pathways	Wolff–Parkinson–White (WPW) syndrome
	Lown–Ganong–Levine syndrome

Precipitating causes of arrhythmias

As well as the focal arrhythmias associated with cardiac disease itself, alterations of underlying physiology may also precipitate arrhythmias. The patient's condition should always be reviewed for precipitating treatable causes. These include:

1. Myocardial ischaemia due to poor coronary perfusion related to low cardiac output states, hypoxaemia or sepsis.

2. Autonomic control may be affected by central neurological damage.

3. Alterations in electrolyte and acid–base balance (e.g. hypo- and hyperkalaemia, -calcaemia, -magnesaemia, -phosphataemia, metabolic and respiratory acidosis).

4. Endocrine influence, particularly thyroid.

5. Effects of drugs.

Disorders of impulse formation

1. Sinus arrhythmia (Fig. 5.3):
   Spacing between normal P and QRS complexes varies regularly, usually with respiration in young patients due to increased venous return on inspiration.
   Aetiology: It is physiological in most young patients but is occasionally associated with inferior myocardial infarction.
   Treatment: None.

2. Sinus tachycardia (Fig. 5.4):
   The P and QRS complexes are normal but the rate is increased to greater than 100 bpm.
   Aetiology: It is physiological in exercise and emotional slates. It is pathologically associated with underlying fever, fluid volume deficit, heart failure, anaemia, thyrotoxicosis, stimulants, such as amphetamines, and drugs such as atropine and epinephrine.
   Treatment: This is directed at finding and treating the underlying cause.

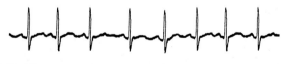

Fig. 5.3

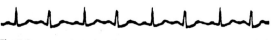

Fig. 5.4

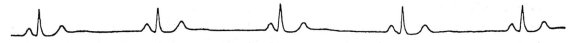

Fig. 5.5

3. Sinus bradycardia (Fig. 5.5):
   Normal P and QRS complexes but the rate is less than 60 bpm.
   Aetiology: It is physiological in athletes and fit people. It is pathologically associated with myocardial infarction, sick sinus syndrome, myxoedema, obstructive jaundice, raised intracranial pressure, glaucoma, and drugs such as beta-blockers, digoxin, verapamil, and cholinergic drugs.
   Treatment: Usually only necessary if the blood pressure is compromised or where cardiac failure means the patient will be unable to compensate for the slow rate with increased myocardial contraction. Atropine 0.3 mg, followed by supplemental doses as necessary, may be used to block vagal tone and increase the rate. Occasionally, in sick sinus syndrome transvenous pacing may be necessary.

4. Atrial ectopic (premature) beats (Fig. 5.6):
   A stimulus for a beat occurs earlier than expected, arising not in the sinoatrial node but in another part of the atrium. The distance between the previous beat and the ectopic beat is much shorter than normal and it may be followed by a longer than normal interval before the next beat occurs ('compensatory pause').
   Aetiology: These beats are often present in the normal heart but may be induced by stimulants such as caffeine, nicotine, and stress. They may occur pathologically as a result of infections, ischaemia, electrolyte imbalance, underlying heart disease, and drug toxicity such as excess theophylline and digoxin.

Treatment: Only indicated in the healthy person if the ectopic beats are symptomatic or precipitate atrial tachycardia. Avoidance of recognized provoking factors is usually sufficient. Digoxin or beta-blockers may be used if symptomatic.

5. Supraventricular tachycardia (SVT) (Fig. 5.7):
   A rapid, regular rhythm, with a rate of between 140 and 250 bpm, usually of sudden onset. P waves may be present but abnormal or obscured by the rapid rate QRS complex. There may be difficulty in distinguishing SVT with aberrant ventricular conduction from a ventricular tachycardia. Carotid sinus massage (see below) or IV adenosine (initially 3 mg followed by 12 mg if no effect in 1–2 min) can slow the rate sufficiently to allow diagnosis of the tachycardia.
   Aetiology: SVT can occur in patients with healthy hearts but may also occur in heart disease and WPW syndrome. It is distinguished from sinus tachycardia by its sudden onset or cessation.
   Treatment: Supraventricular tachycardia is usually successfully treated with IV amiodarone (300 mg over 15 min followed by an infusion of 10–20 mg/kg/24 h). Alternatives include beta-blockers or verapamil (5–10 mg bolus). Verapamil should be given with great care to patients in heart failure and those receiving beta-blockers as severe hypotension and bradycardia may result. Other options include cardioversion and overdrive pacing.

6. Atrial flutter (Fig. 5.8):
   Atrial flutter is an ectopic atrial rhythm, which produces characteristic 'sawtooth' or 'picket fence' P waves. The atrial rate is usually between 250 and

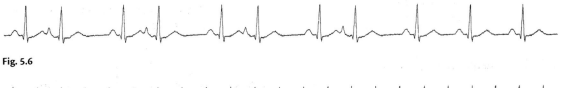

Fig. 5.6

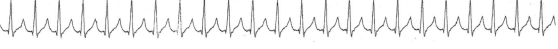

Fig. 5.7

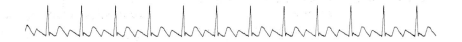

Fig. 5.8

300 bpm. The ventricular rate is variable depending on the degree of AV nodal block. If one QRS occurs to every two P waves then the ventricular rate is 125–150 bpm. If one QRS occurs to every three P waves then the ventricular rate is 75–100 bpm. The QRS is normal unless there is aberrant conduction.

Aetiology: Usually, there is underlying heart disease, such as ischaemic or rheumatic heart disease.

Treatment: If there is haemodynamic compromise or a very fast ventricular rate then synchronized DC cardioversion should be considered. If the rate is acceptable, and the patient stable, then IV amiodarone (dose as above), verapamil (dose as above), or digoxin can be given. The loading dose of digoxin is 0.5–1.5 mg IV, given as periodic infusions of 0.5 mg, followed by 0.25 mg daily until the ventricular rate is slowed to 60–100 bpm. The dose may then have to be reduced further.

7. Atrial fibrillation (Fig. 5.9):
   An irregular QRS pattern with no discernible P waves. The QRS width is usually normal. The atria are fibrillating at a rate of about 400–600 bpm. The QRS rate is usually greater than 100 bpm.

   Aetiology: Chronic atrial fibrillation can occur as a result of heart disease and paroxysmal atrial fibrillation occurs as a result of a variety of acute disorders as well as WPW syndrome. Digoxin toxicity may cause atrial fibrillation and should be suspected if the ventricular rate is slow, or there is evidence of AV block, with associated ventricular ectopics.

   Treatment: In chronic atrial fibrillation, the aim is to control the ventricular rate with digoxin. In paroxysmal atrial fibrillation, the aim is to restore sinus rhythm following treatment of the primary cause. If there is haemodynamic compromise, cardioversion may be required but if the AF is chronic the patient should be adequately anticoagulated first to reduce the risk of emboli. Amiodarone IV (dose as above) can be used to restore sinus rhythm. Digoxin IV (dose as above) will slow the rate but will not convert the rhythm to sinus rhythm.

8. AV junctional (nodal) premature beats (ectopics) (Fig. 5.10):
   A premature stimulus occurs arising from the atrioventricular node. This is conducted simultaneously through the ventricle and retrogradely through the atria. The QRS is usually normal.

   Aetiology: AV junctional ectopics may occur in the normal person but are most commonly associated with heart disease. They can be a sign of digoxin toxicity.

   Treatment: Management is similar to atrial ectopics.

9. Junctional (nodal) tachycardia (Fig. 5.11):
   A rapid regular rhythm originating in the atrioventricular node. There are no upright P waves but inverted P waves may be visible. QRS waves are normal unless there is aberrant conduction. Rate is up to 140 bpm. Differentiation between atrial and junctional tachycardia may be difficult at fast rates.

   Aetiology: Paroxysmal junctional tachycardia is classified and treated as SVT. A non-paroxysmal or accelerated junctional rhythm may be caused by digoxin toxicity, myocardial infarction, rheumatic fever, and myocarditis.

   Treatment: As for SVT if paroxysmal. Discontinuing digoxin treats accelerated junctional rhythm caused by digitalis toxicity. Correction of any underlying physiological disturbance may be sufficient to terminate the arrhythmia.

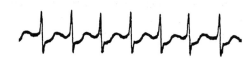

Fig. 5.11

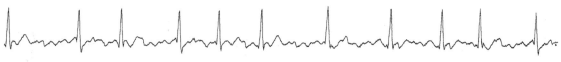

Fig. 5.9

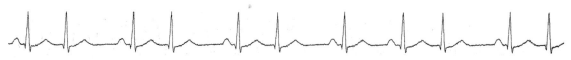

Fig. 5.10

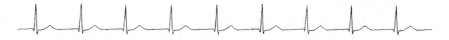

Fig. 5.12

10. Junctional (nodal rhythm) (Fig. 5.12):

Failure of the SA node to generate impulses will result in the AV node taking over as pacemaker. There are no discernible P waves. The QRS is normal unless there is aberrant conduction. The intrinsic rate is slower (40–70 bpm) and the rhythm is regular.

Aetiology: Junctional rhythm can occur in the normal person. It is usually associated with myocardial infarction or increased vagal tone. Occasionally seen in digoxin toxicity.

Treatment: Discontinue digoxin if toxicity is suspected. Treatment is usually only necessary if there are symptoms or haemodynamic compromise. Atropine 0.3 mg IV can be given if excessive vagal tone is suspected.

11. Sick sinus syndrome (Fig. 5.13):

A variety of disruptions to rhythm occur including SA node bradycardia, SA node arrest, wandering pacemaker (the origin of the impulse occurs in different parts of the atria), and atrial ectopic beats. These may be accompanied by episodes of rapid atrial arrhythmias, such as atrial fibrillation, atrial flutter and SVT.

Aetiology: Intrinsic disease of the sinoatrial node and conducting system produces symptoms of palpitations and episode of fainting (Stokes–Adams attacks). These may be idiopathic in the elderly but can be associated with infarction affecting the atria, rheumatic heart disease, and pericarditis.

Treatment: Permanent pacing is often required with pharmacological control of tachyarrhythmias if necessary (e.g. with beta-blockers).

12. Ventricular premature contractions (ectopics) (Fig. 5.14):

A stimulus arises earlier than expected from the Purkinje fibre network in the ventricles. There is no P wave present prior to the beat, although an inverted P wave from retrograde conduction may be seen after the beat. The QRS is widened and bizarre in shape with a notch and increased amplitude. A compensatory pause may follow the beat. Bigeminy occurs when each normal beat is accompanied by an ectopic beat. Trigeminy occurs when every second normal beat is followed by an ectopic beat. Multifocal ectopic beats appear as different shaped QRS complexes and arise from different areas within the ventricle.

Aetiology: A common arrhythmia that can occur in any age at any time. They are common in myocardial disease or as a result of increased myocardial irritability (e.g. hypoxia, hypokalaemia, and digoxin toxicity). Ectopic beats are associated with heart disease in the over 40s, if they are frequent, occur in runs, and are multifocal.

Treatment: Occasional ventricular premature contractions require no treatment. If they are multifocal, occur in runs, are frequent (>5/min) or occur very close to the apex of the T wave of the previous beat then they may require treatment if the patient is symptomatic. Correction of underlying disorders, such as hypokalaemia, digoxin toxicity, and hypoxia is essential.

13. Ventricular tachycardia (Fig. 5.15):

A ventricular ectopic focus stimulates a series of rapid and regular beats. There are no P waves pres-

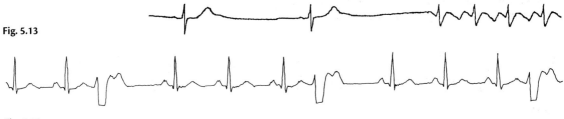

Fig. 5.13

Fig. 5.14

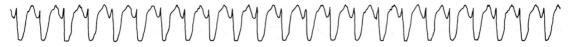

Fig. 5.15

ent and the QRS complex is bizarrely shaped and widened. The rate is between 100 and 220 bpm.

Aetiology: Occurs commonly following myocardial infarction or as a result of digoxin toxicity. The stimulus arises in the Purkinje fibres and it is thought to continue as a re-entry mechanism (see later). The fast rate and the loss of coordinated atrial contraction into the ventricles produces a severe drop in cardiac output which may require cardiopulmonary resuscitation (CPR).

Treatment: Defibrillation is the treatment of choice if there is haemodynamic deterioration. If the patient is stable, amiodarone IV (dose as above) should be given. Potassium and magnesium levels should be checked, and other underlying physiological disorders corrected.

14. Torsades de pointes (Fig. 5.16):
    This is a specific variety of ventricular tachycardia. Torsades de pointes means 'twisting of the points'. The QRS complex is ventricular in origin and broadened but the axis changes from positive to negative and back again. It appears to be a transitional rhythm between ventricular tachycardia and fibrillation. It is associated with a prolonged Q–T interval.

    Aetiology: Development of torsades de pointes is more likely with a prolonged Q–T interval (>0.44 s). Precipitating conditions include hypokalaemia, hypocalcaemia, and hypomagnesaemia; or antiarrhythmic agents, such as disopyramide, which will increase the Q–T interval. Prolonged Q–T with torsades has also been reported with tricyclic antidepressants and phenothiazines (e.g. haloperidol) as well as insecticide poisoning.

    Treatment: It is important that the rhythm is recognized and treated accordingly as conventional treatment for ventricular tachycardia will cause the condition to worsen. Correction of any underlying electrolyte imbalance and discontinuation of any pharmacological cause is the first step. IV magnesium is now considered the treatment of choice.

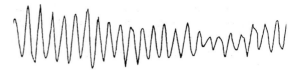

Fig. 5.16

15. Ventricular fibrillation (Fig. 5.17):
    Rapid, chaotic and ineffectual contractions of the ventricle. It is always accompanied by complete loss of cardiac output and unless CPR is carried out immediately the patient will die.

    Aetiology: Associated with ischaemic heart disease, hypoxia, metabolic disturbances, following electrocution, and as a result of drug toxicity (e.g. digoxin, tricyclic antidepressant overdose).

    Treatment: Immediate defibrillation is the only treatment of ventricular fibrillation (see Chapter 7). Following successful defibrillation the patient may be treated with an antiarrhythmic such as lignocaine or amiodarone (dose as above).

Disorders of impulse conduction

16. First degree heart block (Fig. 5.18):
    Delay in impulse conduction occurs at the AV node. The PR interval is greater than 0.20 s.

    Aetiology: First degree block can occur in normal or diseased hearts. It may be a precursor to second or third degree block.

    Treatment: First degree block does not require treatment and is only significant if it precedes second or third degree block.

17. Second degree heart block.
    There are two types of second degree heart block: Mobitz type I (Wenkebach) and Mobitz type II.
    In Mobitz type I (Wenkebach) (Fig. 5.19) a delay at the AV node gradually increases through a series of beats until conduction of the impulse does not occur. The whole process is then repeated. The QRS complex is normal.

Fig. 5.17

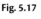

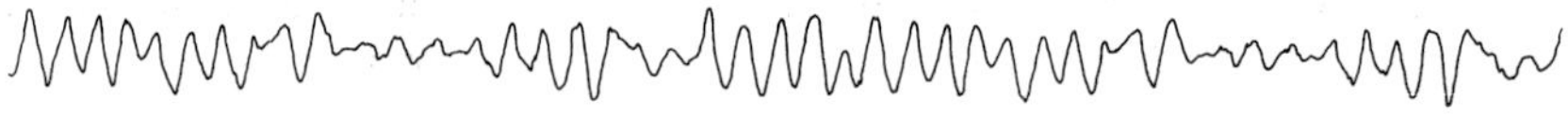

Fig. 5.18

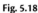

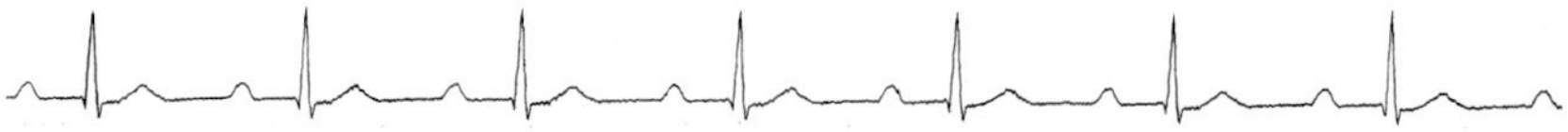

Fig. 5.19 Mobitz type I.

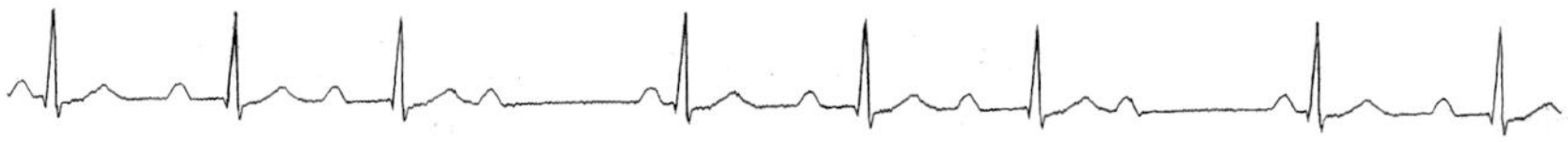

Aetiology: Mobitz type I is usually associated with acute reversible conditions and is relatively benign.

Treatment: Treatment is only necessary if there is haemodynamic compromise associated with the block.

In Mobitz type II (Fig. 5.20), a varying ratio of QRS to P waves are conducted through the AV node (e.g. two P:one QRS or three P:one QRS, etc.). The PR interval in conducted beats remains constant.

Aetiology: Mobitz type II block indicates more severe impairment of AV conduction and is associated with myocardial infarction. It may precede complete heart block.

Treatment: Monitoring is essential but treatment depends on the cardiac output. If this is compromised or the ventricular rate is very slow then treatment is indicated. Atropine IV may be used. Alternatively, transvenous pacing may be required.

18. Third degree (complete) heart block (Fig. 5.21):
There is a complete block of conduction between atria and ventricles at the AV node. The atrial rate continues at a normal or slightly faster rate but the QRS rate will be slower. There is no relationship between the P and the QRS complexes. If the QRS originates in the AV node then the rate will be between 50 and 60 bpm and the QRS will be normal. If the QRS originates in the ventricles then the rate will be between 30 and 40 bpm and the QRS will be widened and enlarged.

Aetiology: The commonest causes are acute myocardial infarction and idiopathic degeneration of the conducting system with age. It can occur following cardiac surgery, particularly on the mitral or aortic valves.

Treatment: In anterior myocardial infarction treatment is urgent and occurrence of complete heart block is associated with more extensive infarction. In other patients, treatment will depend on symptoms and haemodynamic compromise. The definitive treatment is transvenous pacing, although external cardiac pacing (see Chapter 7) can be used for short periods to maintain cardiac output. If this is not available IV atropine can be tried.

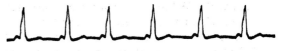

Fig. 5.22

19. Wolff–Parkinson–White syndrome (Fig. 5.22):
This syndrome consists of episodes of paroxysmal tachyarrhythmia characterized by a shortened PR interval and a widened QRS complex. In the non-tachyarrhythmic state the QRS complex has a notch known as the delta wave which is indicative of early ventricular stimulation via the accessory conduction pathway which bypasses the AV node. The PR interval is shortened due to rapid conduction through the accessory pathway which unlike the AV node does not slow conduction.

Aetiology: There is a faulty embryonic development of the AV ring of fibrous tissue whereby strands of myocardial tissue act as a bridge of conducting tissue across the non-conducting AV ring. This conduction pathway is known as the bundle of Kent. The accessory pathway is capable of supporting arrhythmia's, most commonly atrial fibrillation (AF) and paroxysmal supraventricular tachycardias (PVST).

Treatment: If haemodynamically unstable in AF or PSVT, cardioversion is carried out. Amiodarone IV is the treatment of choice. Digoxin should be avoided as it lengthens AV nodal block and may increase conduction via the aberrant pathway.

Mechanisms of tachyarrhythmias

Re-entry tachycardias: re-entry is thought to occur in the following circumstances:

- There is more than one available route for conduction of an impulse.

- Circumstances such as ischaemia, high potassium levels, and blockage of the Purkinje system produce an area of depressed conduction such that stimuli can be conducted in only one direction in one of the available routes.

- Conduction is slow so that the normally functioning route is repolarized and available for a second depolarization.

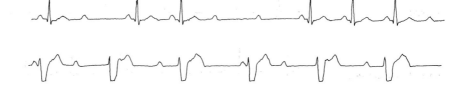

Fig. 5.20 Mobitz type II.

Fig. 5.21

TABLE 5.5 Arrhythmias caused by metabolic changes

Metabolic change	Disorder
Hyperkalaemia	Tall ('tented') T waves
	± Wide QRS complexes
	± Absent P waves
Hypokalaemia	Flattened T waves
	U waves (wave seen after T wave)
Hypercalcaemia	Short Q–T interval
Hypocalcaemia	Prolonged Q–T interval
Hypothermia	J wave (small wave appearing immediately after QRS complex)·
	Bradycardia
Digoxin effect	ST depression
	Inverted T wave ('reverse tick'); not a sign of toxicity
	Any arrhythmia may occur with toxicity

A stimulus is therefore conducted down the normal conduction route but blocked through the depressed area in that direction. The impulse is then slowly propagated retrogradely through the depressed area in the opposite direction and then restimulates the normal route, which has by now repolarized. Re-entry tachycardias can occur in any area of the conduction systems and are probably the cause of various supraventricular and ventricular tachycardias.

Monitoring the Q–T interval

The normal value for the Q–T interval depends on the heart rate. As it increases, the Q–T interval shortens and as it decreases the Q–T interval lengthens. The formula for correcting the Q–T interval for heart rate (QTc) is:

$$QTc = QT/\sqrt{R-R}$$

where QT is the interval measured from beginning of QRS to end of T wave and $\sqrt{R-R}$ is the square root of time between two successive R waves.

The QTc is prolonged if it exceeds 0.44 s. A prolonged QTc interval is associated with hypokalaemia, hypocalcaemia, hypomagnesaemia, and tricyclic drugs. It can lead to torsades de pointes.

The 12-lead ECG

This is performed in order to:

● make a clinical diagnosis and

● monitor cardiac changes.

The frequency of recording a 12-lead ECG will depend on the patient's clinical condition and diagnosis. In the absence of cardiac problems this may be on a daily or alternate day basis, but those who have undergone cardiac surgery or have cardiac dysfunction (e.g. myocardial infarction, unstable angina) may require more frequent recordings.

The 12-lead ECG records the flow of current in several planes so that a more comprehensive view of the heart's electrical activity can be obtained. This is achieved by placing one electrode on each limb and six electrodes on the chest wall. The electrode placed on the right leg acts as an earth and is not an electrical lead.

The electrodes should be placed over positions of least muscle mass to avoid interference from skeletal muscle (i.e. the inside of the wrist and the inner aspect of the ankle). Ideally, the electrodes should be in the same position for each serial ECG.

The standard leads (limb leads)

Three major planes of electrical activity can be viewed using the limb leads, which record the differences in electrical forces between each of the limb electrodes. The three limb leads are termed I, II, and III (see Table 5.6).

These views form a hypothetical triangle with the heart at the centre. Electrical current flows between a negative and a positive pole. When current flows towards a positive pole the ECG shows an upward (positive) deflection. When current flows away from a positive pole the ECG shows a downward (negative) deflection. The positions of the positive and negative electrodes in leads I, II, and III are shown in Fig. 5.1.

The complete 12-lead EGG consists of:

● three limb leads: I, II, and III,

● three augmented (modified) limb leads termed: aVL (augmented view left); aVR (augmented view right); and aVF (augmented view foot or left leg)

● six chest leads: V1, V2, V3, V4, V5, and V6.

TABLE 5.6 The 12-lead ECG

Lead	Electrode 1 (negative)	Electrode 2 (positive)
I	RA	LA
II	RA	LL
III	LA	LL
VR	RA	LA and LL
VL	LA	RA and LL
VF	LL	RA and LA

RA, right arm; LA, left arm; LL, left leg.

Electrodes recording the limb and augmented limb leads
These show the direction of viewing the heart (from electrode 1 to electrode 2); thus each lead will have characteristic upward and downward deflections.

The chest leads

The positions of the chest leads are:

◆ V1: fourth intercostal space to the right of the sternum,

◆ V2: fourth intercostal space to the left of the sternum,

◆ V3: midway between V2 and V4,

◆ V4: fifth intercostal space mid-clavicular line,

◆ V5: anterior axillary line at same level as V4,

◆ V6: mid-axillary line at same level as V4.

All 12 leads will show different electrocardiographic patterns due to the different positions of the electrodes. The direction of deflection depends on the view of the heart in that particular electrical lead. Some waves may change polarity (a normally negative deflection becomes a positive one) due to disease. Figure 5.23 shows a 12-lead EGG taken from a patient with a normal heart.

The EGG should he analysed for rate, rhythm, axis, P wave, PR interval, QRS complex, QT interval, ST segment, and T wave to enable diagnosis of:

◆ abnormal rhythms and conduction,

◆ changes secondary to ischaemic heart disease,

◆ changes secondary to pericardial disease,

◆ changes secondary to metabolic and other diseases,

◆ ventricular hypertrophy.

Axis

This is the sum of the ventricular electrical forces during depolarization. Figure 5.24 shows the orientation of the limb leads. The normal axis of the heart lies between −30° and +90° (i.e. towards the left as the left ventricular mass is greater than the right). If the axis lies outside −30° this is termed left axis deviation, and if greater than +90°, right axis deviation. The axis is determined by determining the vector of the forces between lead I (0°) and lead aVF (+90°) (see Fig. 5.25).

Analysis of 12-lead EGG

A variety of disease processes can be assessed from 12-lead EGG analysis.

Changes secondary to ischaemic heart disease The area of the heart affected by injury, ischaemia, or infarction can be determined by observing which leads show abnormal changes as shown in Table 5.7:

◆ Changes in the anteroseptal area are indicated by leads V1–V4.

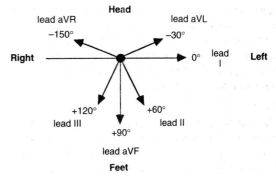

Fig. 5.24 Orientation of the limb leads.

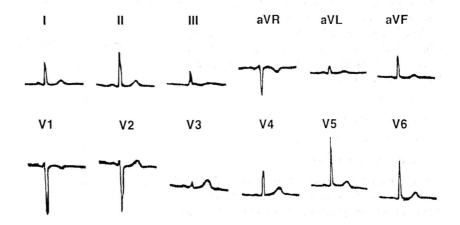

Fig. 5.23 Waveforms of the 12-lead EGG in a patient with normal heart function.

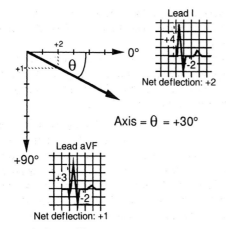

Fig. 5.25 Calculation of the axis.

TABLE 5.7	Changes secondary to ischaemic heart disease

Change in ECG	Cause
ST segment depression	Myocardial injury/ ischaemia
ST segment elevation (convex)	Myocardial injury/ischaemia. If prolonged may be suggestive of an aneurysm
Pathological Q wave	Myocardial infarction
T wave inversion	Myocardial injury/ischaemia/ infarction

* Changes in the anterolateral area are indicated by leads I, aVL, V5,and V6.

* Changes in the inferior area are indicated by leads II, III, and aVF.

* Changes in the posterior area are indicated by a mirror-image (i.e. upside-down changes) seen in leads Vl and V2.

Changes secondary to pericardial disease   Concave ST segment elevation and tachycardia may be seen in acute pericarditis while low voltages (and, occasionally, alternating QRS complexes) may be seen with a large pericardial effusion.

Changes due to ventricular and atrial hypertrophy   Large QRS complexes are suggestive of hypertrophy. This finding may be normal in adults under 35 years old. Left ventricular hypertrophy is present when the sum of the R wave in V5 or V6 plus the S wave in Vl exceeds 35 mm. In right ventricular hypertrophy a 'dominant' R wave is seen in lead Vl (i.e. a large R wave relative to the S wave), but a normal-width QRS complex.

A 'strain pattern' is seen when ST depression and T wave inversion coexist in the appropriate leads and is suggestive of ischaemia in the hypertrophied ventricle.

Changes due to other diseases   ECG changes of pulmonary embolism are those of acute right heart strain and include:

* sinus tachycardia,

* right axis deviation,

* 'S1–Q3–T3'—deep S wave in lead I, pathological Q wave and inverted T wave in lead III,

* right ventricular strain,

* partial right bundle branch block (i.e. M-shaped QRS complex but width <0.12 s),

* peaked P waves,

* atrial fibrillation.

Pulse oximetry

Pulse oximetry is used to continuously monitor the oxygen saturation of arterial blood (S_aO_2). It provides immediate detection of hypoxaemic episodes without the discomfort and hazards of repeated arterial puncture.

A probe is attached to the patient. Various types of probe are available but they must be placed over a pulsating arteriolar bed (e.g. the finger or earlobe). The probe is connected to a monitor which will give a con-

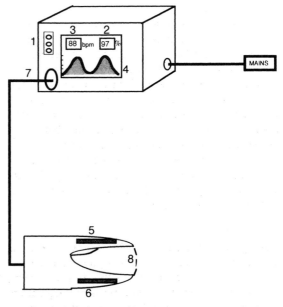

Fig. 5.26 The pulse oximeter: 1, on/off, alarm settings; 2, S_aO_2 display; 3, heart rate display; 4, pulse waveform; 5, light-emitting diodes; 6, photodetector; 7, patient cable display; 8, patient's digit.

tinuous digital display of the oxygen saturation. Some monitors will also show the heart rate and a pulsatile waveform (see Fig. 5.26).

Pulse oximetry works by measuring the variations in light absorption across the vascular bed. The calculation of oxygen saturation is based on the principles of Beer's law.

Beer's law states that the concentration of an unknown solute dissolved in a solvent can be determined by light absorption (Lynne *et al.* 1990). The intensity of light transmitted through a substance depends on the amount of incident light, the concentration of the substance (in this case haemoglobin), and the distance that the light travels.

The probe

The probe consists of two light-emitting diodes, which emit light at two specific wavelengths: 660 nm (red) and 940 (infrared). At these wavelengths the absorption characteristics of reduced haemoglobin and oxyhaemoglobin are quite different (Lynne *et al.* 1990). The light passes through the tissue and is sensed by a photodetector at the base of the probe (see Fig. 5.26). During its passage, the majority of light is absorbed by skin, bone, connective tissue, pigmentation, and venous vessels and this amount is constant with time (the baseline measurement). The only relevant fluctuations in absorption are caused by the increase in blood flow during systole. The peaks and troughs of the pulsatile and baseline absorption for each wavelength are detected by the photodetector, and the ratios of each are compared. There is no mathematical correlation between these ratios and the oxygen saturation which is calculated by a microprocessor using a calibration curve obtained from experimental data.

Dedicated probes are used for each site. The digit (finger or toe) is the most common position, but alternative sites are the earlobes, the nasal bridge, above the eyebrow in the adult, or the arch of the foot in the neonate. Low-perfusion probes are available.

There may be potential problems of pressure on the skin from the probe, for this reason the probe site should be changed at least every 8 hours in the adult and 4-hourly in the neonate.

Accuracy of the pulse oximeter

The oxygen saturation displayed by the pulse oximeter does not give an indication of the oxygen content of the blood as this is determined by the oxygen-carrying capacity of the blood (i.e. how much haemoglobin is present to carry oxygen). Therefore, if the patient is anaemic the oxygen saturation may read 100%, since all the available haemoglobin is fully saturated, but in fact the oxygen content of the blood may be markedly low. In severe anaemia (<5 g/dl) a 'low perfusion' alarm may be displayed.

Although the pulse oximeter is generally accurate if the oxygen saturation is in the range 70–100%, there are specific conditions that will make the readings inaccurate. These are described below:

1. *The presence of dysfunctional haemoglobins*. The light source in the probe uses only two wavelengths of light and can therefore only determine the concentrations of two substances (reduced (deoxy-) haemoglobin and oxyhaemoglobin). The oxygen saturation calculated by the pulse oximeter is termed the 'functional' saturation of haemoglobin. In order to take into account the concentration of other types of haemoglobins, additional wavelengths must be used. A co-oximeter (spectrophotometric haemoximeter) is a more accurate method of measuring oxygen saturation as it uses four or more wavelengths of light and is therefore able to identify the concentration of additional haemoglobins, such as methaemoglobin and carboxyhaemoglobin. The oxygen saturation calculated in this way is termed the 'fractional' oxygen saturation of haemoglobin (Hb) (Lynne *et al.* 1990). For the pulse oximeter:

$$\text{'Functional' saturation} = \frac{\text{oxyHb}}{\text{oxyHb} + \text{deoxyHb}}$$

For the co-oximeter:

$$\text{'Fractional' saturation} = \frac{\text{oxyHb}}{\text{oxyHb} + \text{deoxyHb} + \text{dysfunctional Hb}}$$

Thus, in the following situations, oxygen saturation measured by pulse oximetry may be inaccurate:

- Smoke inhalation. This raises carboxyhaemoglobin levels. The pulse oximeter interprets carboxyhaemoglobin as oxyhaemoglobin because the absorption coefficients of both are very similar. Therefore, in the presence of carboxyhaemoglobin the pulse oximeter will give false high readings compared with measurements by a co-oximeter (Barker and Tremper 1987).

- The administration of drugs that cause methaemoglobinaemia. These include lidocaine (lignocaine), nitrates, and metoclopramide. Normal cellular mechanisms usually prevent the accumulation of methaemoglobin (formed when the iron in haemoglobin is oxidized from the ferrous state to the ferric state), but significant levels may be induced by these drugs (Smith and Olson 1989).

• The administration of certain dyes and pigments. These include methylthioninium chloride (methylene blue), indigo carmine, and indocyanine green. Methylene blue absorbs light at a similar frequency to reduced haemoglobin and the pulse oximeter may give false low readings of oxygen saturation (Sidi *et al.* 1987). There are contradictory data on the effect on pulse oximetry readings in patients with hyperbilirubinaemia (Lynne *et al.* 1990); and if there is any uncertainty, the readings should be checked on a co-oximeter.

2. *Low perfusion.* If there is poor perfusion to the vascular bed over which the probe is placed it will be difficult for the photodetector to distinguish the pulsatile and baseline absorption. Often the monitor will flash a 'low perfusion' alarm but false low readings may be displayed. The probe should be moved to a different site or a low-perfusion probe used. Low readings must be checked by arterial puncture and co-oximeter calculation. Poor perfusion may be due to hypovolaemic states, hypotension, septicaemia, or peripheral vascular disease. The digits and earlobe sites are most commonly affected in these conditions.

3. *Other conditions to avoid.*

   • Avoid application of the probe distal to blood pressure cuffs, venous, or arterial catheters and intravenous lines, as any increased venous or arterial pulsations can affect the readings.

   • Nail varnish must be removed from fingers and toes.

   • Do not use restrictive tape at the probe site.

   • Light interference should be minimized from surgical lamps, direct sunlight, infrared warming lamps, and phototherapy lamps. These may cause light to be sensed by the photodetector without first passing through the tissue. If necessary, the probe may be covered with an opaque material.

Specific nursing interventions

• High and low alarm limits should be set according to the patient's clinical condition.

• The probe site should be rotated regularly and the area checked for pressure or irritation.

• The probe must be securely attached.

• Pulse oximetry should be used as a continuous guide to arterial oxygen saturation and not for its absolute values. Abnormal readings should be checked by arterial blood gas analysis or co-oximetry.

End tidal carbon dioxide monitoring (ETCO$_2$)

Peak end tidal carbon dioxide concentrations can be measured at the end of expiration and be continually displayed as a waveform or digital reading. This can be used as a guide to arterial CO$_2$ tension ($P_a CO_2$).

Measurement is achieved by placing a sensor between the patient's endotracheal tube and the ventilator tubing. A transducer detects the amount of infrared radiation that is absorbed by the expired gas and the ETCO$_2$ is derived from the level of radiation absorbed by carbon dioxide.

Alveolar CO$_2$ levels, in the presence of normal ventilation/perfusion relationships, can accurately reflect the adequacy of alveolar ventilation and a good correlation is seen between arterial and alveolar CO$_2$ levels. It is less accurate when ventilation/perfusion mismatch occurs, or if there is significant air trapping (e.g. in asthma).

This technique is particularly useful as a guide to CO$_2$ elimination in patients who do not have arterial access for blood gas analysis. It can also be used to verify the correct placement of an endotracheal tube in the trachea at intubation, and a spontaneous cardiac output during CPR.

Blood pressure (BP)

The technique for recording blood pressure using a sphygmomanometer and cuff will not be discussed, as this should be more than familiar. However, several points may need emphasis:

1. *Cuff size.* To ensure accurate blood pressure recording the correct size of cuff is important. If the cuff is too narrow or applied too loosely the BP will be falsely high, and if it is too wide it will under-read. The bladder width should ideally be 40–50% of the upper arm circumference. The bladder length should encircle 80% of the arm. The cuff should also be at the level of the heart to maintain a true zero level.

2. *Comparing blood pressure recorded by different techniques.* There are occasions when a BP recorded by one technique may need to be verified using a different technique. It must be remembered that each are methodologically different and measure different phenomena. Direct intra-arterial measurements record pressure impulses and indirect measurements record volume displacement (oscillometry) or flow detection (Doppler). Values obtained by auscultation may be lower than those obtained by direct measurement, since blood flow begins before sound is heard and the sound may also be absorbed by the surrounding tissues. Even with accurate techniques,

direct intra-arterial pressure can be expected to be 5–20 mmHg greater than by indirect measurement. Potential inaccuracies occur in all techniques and this makes direct comparison difficult, even when the BP is recorded simultaneously. Such inaccuracies in indirect measurements include wrong cuff size and placement, personal variations, lack of stethoscope sensitivity, poor technique, and instrument errors.

Oscillometry

A more reliable method for measuring BP non-invasively is by oscillometry. An automated machine uses a cuff to compress the limb and measures BP by sensing the arterial pulsations (oscillations) as a function of cuff pressure. The sensor on the cuff is placed in the correct position (an arrow on the cuff indicates its placement over an artery) and the cuff is automatically inflated. As the cuff deflates the arterial pressure becomes equal to the cuff occluding pressure and blood begins to flow through the artery. The oscillations in the artery wall are small but as the cuff continues to deflate flow is increased and the amplitude of the oscillations reaches a maximum. As the cuff completely deflates the oscillations in the arterial wall lessen. This is due to the reducing resistance to flow as the cuff occluding pressure is less than the diastolic pressure. The rapid increases and decreases in oscillations correspond to the systolic and diastolic pressures and the mean pressure is the lowest cuff pressure with the greatest oscillations.

Oscillometry may be less useful when used on severely hypotensive patients as the oscillation amplitude may be too small to be accurate.

Gastrointestinal tonometry

Gut tonometry is used to calculate the intramucosal pH (pH$_i$) of either the stomach or (less commonly) the sigmoid colon. This has been shown to reflect oxygen delivery to the mucosa and a low level is said to be indicative of splanchnic ischaemia.

There is evidence that the blood supply to the gut is the first to be affected when oxygen delivery is reduced for whatever reason (e.g. myocardial dysfunction, haemorrhage, and hypoxaemia). If this can be detected then effective treatment strategies can be instituted early in the hope of preventing subsequent organ failure.

The technique

The gastric tonometer is a modified nasogastric tube which, by the addition of an extra lumen, allows gastric aspiration, enteral feeding, and pH$_i$ measurement. At the tip of the tube is a silicone balloon that is permeable to carbon dioxide.

To make a measurement the tubing and balloon are primed with 0.9% sodium chloride to remove any air. The balloon is then filled with 2.5 ml of sodium chloride and left *in situ* for at least 20 min to allow equilibration to occur. The solution is then aspirated (the first millilitre is discarded as this has been in the tubing), and the remaining 1.5 ml is passed through a blood gas analyser to determine the PCO_2. Neither device does this sampling automatically. An arterial blood gas is drawn at the same time for measurement of bicarbonate. The saline CO_2 and the arterial bicarbonate (assumed to be the same as the bicarbonate level in the gastric mucosa) are placed in a modified Henderson–Hasselbach equation to enable calculation of pH$_i$:

$$pH_i = 6.1 + \log_{10} \frac{[HCO_3]}{PCO_2 \times K \times 0.03}$$

where 6.1 is the pK for the HCO$_3$/CO$_2$ system in plasma (i.e. the pH value where concentrations of bicarbonate and carbonic acid are equal), [HCO$_3$] is the actual arterial bicarbonate concentration, PCO_2 is the CO$_2$ tension in tonometer saline, K is the equilibration period correction factor and 0.03 is the solubility of CO_2 in plasma at 37 °C.

The theory

The principle underlying this technique is that in low oxygen delivery states, anaerobic respiration will occur and CO_2 will be produced. The PCO_2 of the saline in the balloon reflects the PCO_2 level in the gastric mucosa, which, in turn, reflects the CO_2 tension in the capillaries supplying the mucosa. Therefore, if the pH$_i$ falls, indicating an acidotic state with a surplus of CO_2, it may be assumed that blood supply to the gastric mucosa is inadequate for tissue oxygen requirements.

There are two consequences of this, which may have clinical significance. First, the patient may initially compensate for a low-perfusion state and there may be no other detectable signs of reduced tissue oxygen delivery. Secondly, the gut can be rendered 'leaky' if allowed to become ischaemic, resulting in translocation of bacteria and endotoxins into the surrounding structures. However, this translocation has not yet been conclusively demonstrated in humans (see Chapter 11).

A number of drawbacks are evident; for example, if gastric acid is present in the lumen of the stomach this may react with alkaline bile refluxing back through the pylorus and produce CO_2. This would invalidate the tonometer measurement of PCO_2 as a measure of gut mucosal CO_2. An H$_2$ antagonist (e.g. ranitidine) or a proton pump inhibitor (e.g. omeprazole) must then be administered to block gastric acid production. The effect of enteral nutrition in the stomach remains unknown. There are also a number of assumptions inherent in the technique, e.g. arterial bicarbonate is used as a substitute for gut mucosal bicarbonate and any metabolic acidosis present in the blood will automatically produce a low pH_i. This prompts some investigations to assess the size of the arterial CO_2 tonometer gap rather than the pH_i. A low pH_i or increased gap is associated with a worse outcome, though few studies have demonstrated survival benefit through its use.

Doppler techniques

Doppler ultrasound can be used to measure blood flow in a variety of vessels. An ultrasonic transducer transmits a single frequency of ultrasound at the blood vessel. The same or another transducer (depending on the type of ultrasound used) picks up the ultrasound waves reflected back off the moving blood corpuscles. These waves have shifted in frequency according to the velocity of the moving blood. These Doppler frequency shifts can be converted into audible signals or, after computer analysis, displayed on a monitor as velocity–time waveforms. The velocity–time integral i.e. the waveform area, represents the distance a column of blood travels with each pump ('stroke') of the heart. The product of this 'stroke distance' and the cross-sectional area of the vessel is the volume passing through the vessel with each heart beat. For total stroke volume (SV), blood flow velocity measurement (by Doppler) and cross-sectional area (measured by echocardiography or estimated via a nomogram) of the ascending aorta is performed.

A Doppler probe can be placed in the suprasternal notch and aimed at the ascending aorta. A drawback of this approach is the inability to hold the probe in place, thereby preventing continuous measurement. An approach via the oesophagus can also be used to measure blood flow continuously in the descending thoracic aorta (see later). An estimate of cardiac output to some 85–90% accuracy can be provided using a nomogram incorporating the patient's age, height, and weight. This approach makes a number of assumptions about flow going to the head and neck and the aortic cross-sectional area but has proven to be a reliable, non-invasive alternative to pulmonary artery catheterization (see later).

Doppler probes can also be used by the nurse at the bedside to check for the presence of pulsatile flow in ischaemic limbs, particularly following distal vascular surgery. In these cases, they are used to check primarily that there is blood flow (a pulse that can be heard) rather than to calculate flow volume and can be extremely useful in detecting a pulse that is difficult to palpate.

Bispectral Index™ (BIS)™

The BIS monitor uses a processed electroencephalogram (EEG) parameter to provide a non-invasive, direct means of measuring the effects of anaesthetic agents on the brain. The monitor uses a sensor on the forehead to capture the EEG signals, which are translated into a single number ranging from 100 (for wide awake) to zero (indicating the absence of brain electrical activity).

It was primarily developed to enable anaesthetists to easily observe a patient's level of consciousness and make the necessary adjustments to ensure the patient remains unconscious during, and wakes up rapidly after, surgery. However, it has several important potential uses and limitations in the critical care area.

The monitor can easily be attached to ventilated patients who have been given muscle relaxants and sedation can be titrated to the BIS score. This may lead to a reduction in the cumulative dose of sedative drugs that these patients receive.

It can also be useful in patients admitted with status epilepticus where subclinical seizures can be detected and therapy titrated against the BIS value. In brain injured patients, particularly those with hypoxic or ischaemic injury, the BIS value correlated well with neurological outcome. However, as the score was derived from healthy patients undergoing anaesthesia, the effects of sepsis, encephalopathy, and other factors affecting critically ill patients have yet to be established. Usual levels during general anaesthesia are approximately 30–40.

Invasive monitoring

Invasive methods of monitoring are now commonplace on the ICU but the potential value of such techniques must be carefully considered prior to insertion. They can be potentially hazardous for the patient due to complications that can arise either from their insertion or by remaining *in situ*. However, they can also provide invaluable information for the monitoring of disease processes and manipulation of treatment strategies.

The nurse must be fully aware of the operating techniques and the potential hazards and complications of the equipment used in order to minimize risk to the patient.

Each device will have its associated complications, but the very fact that it is an invasive procedure means infection is a potential problem. Local policies and practices should be followed for dressing changes and changes of cannulae and tubing (including transducers). Routine infection control measures should be instituted. These should include:

♦ effective hand-washing,

♦ the use of a strict aseptic technique when inserting or re-dressing cannulae,

♦ clear semi-permeable dressings over cannula sites to allow regular inspection,

♦ minimal disturbance of the dressing; re-dress as necessary rather than routinely,

♦ minimal use of three-way taps to limit potential entry for infection,

♦ labelling of lines and transducers with the date and time that they were last changed.

Most invasive lines will be sutured in position and these should be well secured to prevent accidental removal by the patient. Some devices, such as pulmonary artery catheters (with associated cardiac output leads), are quite heavy and the weight will need to be supported by securing these to the pillow or bedding.

Pressure monitoring

Most patient monitors have the facility to display pressures continuously from invasive monitoring. These can include systemic arterial, pulmonary artery, and central venous pressures.

Transducers are needed in the monitoring circuit to measure and transmit the pressure recorded within the heart or blood vessel to the monitor. Transducers come in varying shapes and forms depending on the manufacturer and the type of monitor used. These can be obtained already assembled with all the patient tubing attached and are very easy to prepare (see Fig. 5.27). Some older equipment may still require each part of the transducer to be connected separately with individual sterile domes and separate tubing and taps.

In general, transducers are small, fluid-filled devices. Tubing from the patient cannula is connected to one side of the transducer and from the other side a giving set is connected to a bag of 0.9% saline solution. This solution must be kept under continuous pressure (usually 300 mmHg for arterial lines but less for venous lines) to prevent a back-flow of blood from the patient into the circuit. Adjacent to the transducer is a flushing device which ensures the continuous delivery of fluid (3 ml/hour) through the patient's cannula and allows the tubing to be manually flushed at any time (such as after taking blood samples). The flushing device keeps the cannula patent.

Pressure is transmitted from the cannula through the fluid-filled pressure tubing to the transducer. From here it is relayed via an electrical cable to the monitor where it is usually displayed as both a waveform trace and as a digital readout providing systolic, diastolic, and mean pressure measurements.

There are several points to remember to ensure accurate pressure readings:

♦ The transducer must always be level with the zero reference point. This is usually the right atrium (mid-axilla). If the patient is moved, the transducer must be realigned.

♦ The transducer must be calibrated to atmospheric pressure ('zeroed') before use, intermittently while in use (e.g. at the beginning of each shift), and whenever the patient tubing or transducer is changed or disconnected. This procedure will vary according to the type of monitor being used but basically entails turning the three-way tap in the circuit 'off' to the patient, thus exposing the transducer to atmospheric pressure (air), and pressing a zero button on the monitor. When the monitor shows a zero reading the three-way tap can be turned back 'on' to the patient and placed at the zero reference point. The transducer will now read an arterial or venous pressure calibrated to atmospheric pressure.

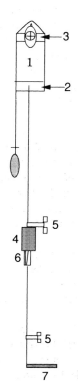

Fig. 5.27 Transduced pressure monitoring system: 1, infusion fluid; 2, pressure bag; 3, pressure gauge; 4, transducer; 5, three-way tap; 6, flush device; 7, patient cannula.

◆ Only dedicated manometer tubing should be used throughout the system. This is rigid tubing with a low compliance and small diameter. Soft, flexible tubing should not be used, as the pressure changes will not be accurately conducted.

◆ Excessively long tubing or air bubbles in the tubing or transducer may cause a 'dampened' trace with consequent inaccurate readings. The presence of three-way taps in the circuit will also 'dampen' the trace.

Arterial cannulation

Intra-arterial cannulation can be utilized for optimizing patient management and for rapid reassessment. It allows continuous monitoring of blood pressure and frequent blood sampling without patient disturbance and repeated vessel puncture.

The radial, femoral or dorsalis pedis arteries are the most commonly used. The radial artery is preferred as the hand usually has a good collateral circulation, the artery is near to the skin surface, and the cannula site is easily observed. However, in patients with Raynaud's disease or an inadequate ulnar circulation, hand ischaemia and skin necrosis can occur. The Allen test (occlusion of radial and ulnar arteries to blanch the hand, followed by release of the pressure on the radial artery to check the quality of the collateral circulation provided by the ulnar artery) has been shown to give unreliable results. If in doubt, Doppler ultrasound of the arteries may give an idea of patency.

The femoral artery is often cannulated in severely hypotensive patients because the femoral pulse is often the most easily palpable and its superficial location makes it easy to access. However, if blood flow to the limb is compromised the patient is exposed to a potentially large area of ischaemia. Regular assessment of pedal pulses and skin temperature should be carried out. Since the groin cannot be continually exposed and therefore observed, unseen haemorrhage at this site can have dire consequences. It is imperative that lower alarm limits are set on the monitor and a clear waveform is visible so that any accidental disconnection is discovered immediately. This is not the preferred cannulation site for diabetic patients (who may have poor wound healing and microcirculation problems) or patients with occlusive vascular disease.

The dorsalis pedis artery can also be used but the vessel is small and often difficult to cannulate. It also makes mobilization difficult for the patient, and it can be difficult to obtain a good waveform. It should be avoided if possible in patients with peripheral vascular disease or diabetes. Thrombosis can occur and the toes should be observed for ischaemia. Due to the greater distance from the heart and the smaller vessel lumen, the blood pressure recorded from the dorsalis pedis (and the radial artery also) will be higher than that in the femoral artery, and may not necessarily reflect the perfusion pressure in other regions.

The brachial artery should not be used except for short-term placement when no other cannulation sites are available/accessible. As it is an end artery, vessel damage/thrombosis at this point may result in loss of the blood supply to the forearm. Haematoma formation at the cannula site can result in median nerve compression. Nerve damage and reduced joint mobility can occur as well as the universal potential complication of embolization. This site is also uncomfortable for the patient as mobility is reduced.

In summary, whichever artery is chosen:

◆ there should be a good collateral blood supply to the limb,

◆ it must be easily observable with access for nursing care,

◆ it should not be located in an area prone to contamination or where a wound exists,

◆ it should not be sited in limbs that have vascular prostheses.

Complications of intra-arterial cannulation

Specific complications have been mentioned above. In addition to thrombus formation, embolization, infection, and exsanguination due to disconnection, the following are also recognized complications:

◆ accidental intra-arterial injection of drugs

◆ air embolus (from air within the flush system)

◆ arteriovenous fistula

◆ pain

◆ aneurysm

◆ local haematomas

◆ necrosis of skin and digits.

Removal of the cannula

When the catheter is removed digital pressure must be applied for as long as necessary to achieve haemostasis. Assess the peripheral circulation, as thrombosis can occur after removal.

The arterial waveform

This reflects the pressure generated in the arterial tree following contraction of the left ventricle after elec-

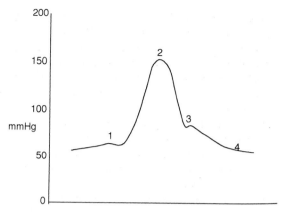

Fig. 5.28 The arterial waveform: 1, anacrotic notch; 2, peak systolic pressure; 3, dicrotic notch; 4, diastolic pressure.

trical activation. Hence, when the arterial waveform is evaluated in conjunction with the ECG the electrical activity will occur before the mechanical activity. It should be stressed that the arterial pressure does not equate to cardiac output. For example, a high blood pressure may be produced by the vasoconstriction response to hypovolaemia while a low blood pressure may be associated with a high-flow, vasodilated state, as seen in sepsis (see Fig. 5.28):

1. *The anacrotic notch.* This is only seen in central aortic pressure monitoring or in some pathological conditions. During the second phase of ventricular systole there is a pre-systolic rise in pressure which occurs before the opening of the aortic valve. This is the anacrotic notch.

2. *The peak systolic pressure.* This is the maximum left ventricular systolic pressure. The sharp upward rise in pressure is generated by the outflow of blood from the ventricle into the arterial system.

3. *The dicrotic notch.* The dicrotic notch reflects the closure of the aortic valve caused by a rise in pressure in the aorta. When the pressure in the aorta is greater than in the left ventricle the blood attempts to flow backwards causing the valve to close. On the waveform trace the dicrotic notch marks the end of systole and the onset of diastole. The dicrotic notch wave is markedly elevated in patients with decreased cardiac output and increased peripheral vascular resistance.

4. *The diastolic pressure.* The diastolic pressure is related to the degree of vasoconstriction in the arterial system and the diastolic time during the cardiac cycle. During diastole there must be sufficient time for blood to drain into the smaller arteriolar branches. If

there is a short diastole, as in a fast heart rate, there is insufficient time for this drainage to occur and, consequently, the diastolic pressure may be higher.

Pulse pressure (PP)

The pulse pressure is the difference between the systolic and diastolic pressure. Factors which may affect this include changes in stroke volume (affects systolic pressure) or changes in vascular compliance (affects diastolic pressure).

Mean arterial pressure (MAP)

Most monitors have the ability to calculate the MAP from the arterial waveform. This value is the average pressure in the arterial system during one complete cycle of systole and diastole. Since at normal heart rates systole usually requires one-third of the cardiac cycle time and diastole two-thirds this is reflected in the equation for calculating MAP:

$$MAP = DBP + \frac{SBP - DBP}{3}$$

or

$$MAP = \frac{SBP + (DBP \times 2)}{3}$$

where SBP is systolic pressure and DBP is diastolic pressure.

Observation of the arterial waveform can also provide information in some clinical conditions:

1. *Atrial fibrillation.* The characteristic ECG rate and rhythm irregularity is reflected on the pressure monitor by variable amplitudes of the arterial waveform. This equates to the variable stroke volumes produced as a consequence of altered diastolic filling times during atrial fibrillation. A 12-lead ECG is needed to make a firm diagnosis of atrial fibrillation as multiple supraventricular ectopic beats can mimic the irregular rhythm.

2. *Pulsus alternans.* There is a regular alternating of peak systolic pressure amplitude with the patient in sinus rhythm and is classically seen in patients with left ventricular failure.

3. *Aortic stenosis.* This may produce a narrow pulse pressure since the systolic pressure is lower and the slowed ventricular ejection through the stenotic valve causes a delayed systolic peak. The dicrotic notch is not well defined because the valve leaflets close abnormally at the onset of diastole.

4. *Aortic regurgitation.* This causes a wide pulse pressure and (usually) a higher peak systolic pressure due to

the left ventricle receiving more blood as it back-flows through the incompetent valve during diastole.

Normal respiration can also cause changes in amplitude of systolic pressure due to changes in intrathoracic pressure. During inspiration in the spontaneously breathing person, intrathoracic pressure is lower (i.e. more negative) thereby causing a pooling of blood in the pulmonary vasculature. This causes less blood to reach the left side of the heart and peak systolic pressure may be 3–10 mmHg lower. At expiration, the blood that had pooled in the pulmonary bed is shunted to the left side of the heart increasing the left ventricular filling volume and causing a higher peak systolic pressure. The opposite is seen with mechanical positive pressure ventilation.

'Pulsus paradoxus' is a term used when the difference in peak systolic pressure is greater than 10 mmHg between inspiration and expiration. This is an accentuation of the normal pattern and an exaggerated swing in systolic pressure over the respiratory cycle in seen on the monitor. Causes of this include pericardial disease (e.g. pericardial tamponade) which impedes ventricular filling, exaggerated inspiration by the patient, or pathological causes that result in gross changes in intrathoracic pressure during respiration (e.g. asthma). Probably the commonest cause of an exaggerated 'respiratory swing' in the critically ill patient is hypovolae-mia, particularly when the patient has concurrently high airway pressures.

Specific nursing care

Safety   Accidental disconnection can result in considerable blood loss unless detected immediately. For this reason the cannula site should always be visible (unless the femoral artery is used). Alarm limits (particularly the lower limit) must be set on the monitor if the cannula is transduced; this will allow disconnection to be recognized immediately. If the femoral artery is used this is essential as the site will not be continuously visible.

All connections within the circuit should be Luer locked and firmly connected. A loose connection can cause loss of pressure within the circuit, back-flow of blood from the patient, and blood loss at the connection site.

Inadvertent administration of drugs can have dire consequences and arterial lines must be labelled clearly to avoid confusion with venous lines.

Limb perfusion   Perfusion distal to the cannula site must be observed regularly. Occlusion of the artery by a thrombus or adjacent haematoma can severely reduce blood flow to the area supplied by that vessel. *If the limb becomes cold, white, or painful senior medical staff must be informed immediately.* The cannula should be removed and circulation must be assessed manually by capillary refill or the use of Doppler to identify pulsatile flow. If

TABLE 5.8 Summary of problems associated with arterial cannulae		
Problem	**Cause**	**Action**
'Damped' trace leading to underestimated BP (blunt pressure peak, loss of dicrotic notch)	Loss of pressure or no fluid in the infusion pressure bag	Inflate pressure bag to 300 mmHg. Check there is sufficient flushing solution
	Thrombus/fibrin formation at tip of catheter	Withdraw blood and then flush catheter
	Air in tubing or transducer	Disconnect tubing from catheter and flush through to expel air before reconnecting. If necessary, change transducer
	Too many three-way taps in the circuit	Remove excess taps
	Long length of tubing between catheter and transducer	Shorten tubing
	Poor position of limb, tip of catheter against vessel wall, kinked tubing	Manipulate catheter and/or limb to achieve a better trace
No arterial waveform (straight line)	Taps turned off to patient or transducer	Check taps are on to patient and transducer
	Disconnection of catheter	Check catheter site—reconnect immediately
	Disconnection of transducer cable to monitor	Check connections—reconnect
	Poor catheter position (tip against vessel wall)	Manipulate position of cannula or limb, flush catheter
	Asystole	Institute CPR
Backflow of blood from catheter towards transducer	Loose tap connection within the circuit	Check all connections are secure
	Flush bag pressure too low (below patient's BP)	Inflate bag to 300 mmHg pressure

collateral circulation is good, the limb may be saved but there is a danger, particularly if the brachial artery has been used, that circulation may not be restored.

Arterial spasm can also result in blanching and pain in the limb. This can be caused by very cold and frequent administrations of flush solution or the accidental injection of a drug into the cannula. The cannula should be removed. The other limb can be warmed to encourage reflex vasodilatation but the affected limb should not be warmed directly as this increases the metabolic rate. In the absence of a restored circulation, it may hasten and worsen the ischaemia. In the case of accidental drug administration into the arterial line the cannula should be flushed vigorously using the flushing device. An additional treatment option for persisting arterial spasm is to inject papaverine intra-arterially (see also Table 5.8).

Intra-arterial blood gas electrode

A very thin probe containing specialized electrodes can be placed through the cannula into the artery and will continuously measure the arterial PO_2, PCO_2, and pH, which are displayed on a monitor. Studies have shown a good correlation between the values derived from arterial samples and the intra-arterial electrodes. The oxygen measurement in particular is prone to drift and thus the sensor requires recalibration at intervals of 12–24-hours. The probe may also 'dampen' the arterial waveform trace by partially occluding the cannula. It does, however, provide a continuous guide to arterial blood gases allowing direct assessment of the effect of interventions and the early recognition of problems. Potentially spurious results must be confirmed by arterial sampling.

Central venous pressure (CVP) and right atrial pressure

In order to monitor the CVP, a catheter is usually inserted into the internal jugular or subclavian veins, though long lines inserted via the femoral or brachial veins can also be used. The tip of the catheter does not need to lie inside the right atrium but can be within one of the larger veins leading to the heart, though it should be within the thoracic cavity. The CVP at this point equals right atrial pressure which, in turn, equals right ventricular end diastolic (filling) pressure. The pressure within the right atrium does not necessarily reflect either intravascular volume status or left heart pressures. It therefore has limitations in the acute stages of critical illness. However, the resultant access to a large vein enables the infusion of hypertonic solutions, solutions that are irritant to peripheral veins and drugs that require a rapid effect.

Single, double, triple, and quadruple lumen catheters are available. Multiple-lumen catheters are particularly useful as they allow dedicated lumens for inotropes, separate infusions of fluids that should not be mixed with others (such as total parenteral nutrition, sodium bicarbonate), and the bolus administration of drugs without the inadvertent flushing of other drug infusions.

The catheter is inserted under sterile conditions, usually by the Seldinger technique. An introducer (a large-bore needle or cannula) is inserted into the vessel, a flexible wire is fed into the vein via the introducer, and the introducer is then withdrawn completely. The catheter is then inserted over the wire to a satisfactory depth (usually 15–20 cm for jugular or subclavian lines) and the wire is then removed.

The catheter position is usually confirmed by X-ray before drugs or infusion fluids are administered. The tip position should be ascertained and any complications such as pneumothorax excluded. Recent guidelines encourage the use of ultrasound guidance. This is particularly applicable with anatomically difficult patients (e.g. short, fat neck) or other previous failed attempts. There must also be an easy withdrawal of blood from all lumens of the catheter.

When the correct position is confirmed, a transducer system or giving set can be attached and drugs or infusions administered as necessary.

Potential complications associated with the insertion of a CVP catheter

1. *Arrhythmias.* These may occur during insertion, especially when the introducer guidewire makes contact with the tricuspid valve or the catheter is inserted too far. If this occurs, the wire or catheter should be withdrawn several centimetres. Rarely, drugs or cardioversion may be necessary.

2. *Pneumo/haemothorax.* This can result from accidental puncture of the pleura during the procedure. The patient's haemodynamic and respiratory status must be monitored closely during and after insertion. The post-insertion chest X-ray should be carefully examined. Not only may the patient be compromised if a pneumothorax is present, but if fluids and drugs are infused into the pleural space a potentially disastrous situation can result. The consequent pleural effusion may cause respiratory deterioration and the drugs and infusion fluids given would be ineffective, as they have not entered the systemic circulation. The catheter must be removed immediately and pleural aspiration/drainage may be required while supportive respiratory care is given.

3. *Haematoma caused by trauma to the vein and/or surrounding tissue.* Observe the site for bleeding, bruising, and

swelling. An artery may be accidentally punctured by the introducer while attempting insertion. If this is known to have occurred, particular attention must be focused on the site to identify bleeding or swelling. Prolonged direct pressure may be necessary to stop bleeding although this cannot be achieved if the subclavian artery has been punctured. Occasionally, thoracotomy is necessary to control excess bleeding.

4. *Catheter in incorrect position.* Occasionally, the catheter may follow a path away from the heart towards the head or down the arm. This will not give an accurate reading of the CVP and rapid fluid infusions may cause discomfort. The catheter should be repositioned.

5. *Air embolus.* This may occur if the catheter is not properly connected to the appropriate tubing, or if one of the portals or three-way taps is left 'open to air' and the patient is making spontaneous breathing efforts (negative intrathoracic pressure sucking the air in). The catheter and tubing should be primed with fluid prior to insertion.

Measuring the CVP

The CVP may be measured using a transducer system (see Fig. 5.27), or manually using a manometer (this method is uncommon within the ICU, as it is far less accurate). Manual measurement allows only intermittent recordings to be made and requires a fluid-filled manometer tube to be connected to the catheter. The manometer is aligned so that the point on the scale of the manometer that is level with the right atrium of the patient is regarded as zero. The manometer is filled with fluid from a bag of 0.9% sodium chloride or 5% glucose to a level well above the expected CVP. The manometer tap is then turned so that fluid runs down the manometer into the patient. It will come to rest at a level, which is the CVP, and the reading can be made from an adjoining scale. The fluid in the manometer should gently rise and fall with respiration.

A transduced catheter will give a continuous display of the CVP on a monitor. The waveform on the monitor should show small undulations reflecting the changes in pressure within the right atrium during the cardiac cycle (see Fig. 5.29). Excessive undulations are seen with tricuspid regurgitation or if the tip is within the right ventricle.

The normal range for CVP measurements is 3–10 mmHg. It must be remembered that any increase in intrathoracic pressure such as positive pressure ventilation or positive end expiratory pressure will increase the CVP measured relative to atmospheric pressure. The juxtacardiac pressure (i.e. CVP minus intrathoracic pressure) may be considerably lower. Hypovolaemia can thus be camouflaged by a seemingly normal or high CVP, especially in the presence of concurrently high intrathoracic pressures.

The right atrial pressure waveform has three characteristic positive deflections corresponding to the electrical events of the ECG:

1. The *A wave*. This reflects right atrial contraction and follows the P wave on the ECG. The descent after this represents atrial relaxation. An elevated A wave may be associated with right ventricular failure or tricuspid stenosis.

2. The *C wave*. This represents tricuspid valve closure and follows the QRS on the EGG tracing. The distance A–C should be the same as the P–R interval.

3. The *V wave*. This represents the pressure generated to the right atrium by the contracting right ventricle despite the tricuspid valve being shut. It corresponds to the latter half of the T wave on the ECG. An elevated V wave is associated with tricuspid regurgitation.

TABLE 5.9	Conditions affecting the CVP
Increased values	Right ventricular failure
	Pericardial tamponade
	Fluid overload
	Pulmonary hypertension
	Tricuspid regurgitation
	Pulmonary stenosis
	Peripheral vasoconstriction (e.g. cold, excess norepinephrine)
	Superior vena caval obstruction
Decreased values	Hypovolaemia
	Peripheral vasodilatation (including sepsis, drugs, regional analgesia, sympathetic dysfunction)

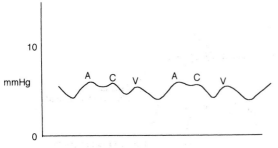

Fig. 5.29 The right atrial pressure waveform (A, C, and V waves).

Table 5.9 summarizes conditions that affect the CVP.

Removal of the CVP catheter

In order to reduce the risk of an air embolism the patient should lie flat or, if their condition allows, with the head tipped down, when the catheter is withdrawn. After removal a sterile, occlusive dressing should be placed over the site.

Pulmonary artery catheterization

In many critically ill patients, particularly those with pulmonary disease or isolated right heart or left heart dysfunction, the measurement of right atrial pressure gives no indication of the function of the left side of the heart. If the determinants of cardiac function (see below) can be known and manipulated, better targeted treatment strategies can be instituted. This can be achieved using a pulmonary artery catheter.

The pulmonary artery catheter

The pulmonary artery (PA) catheter is inserted to measure (or derive) a range of intracardiac and pulmonary artery pressures, vascular resistance, and cardiac output.

The standard pulmonary artery catheter consists of three or four lumens, is 110 cm long, and is marked in 10 cm increments to aid placement (see Fig. 5.30). Various modifications exist including:

- extra lumens for drug/fluid administration,
- thermistor and computer connector for cardiac output measurement,
- continuous mixed venous oxygen saturation,
- a pacing wire or external electrodes for temporary pacing,

- measurement of right ventricular volume and ejection fractions.

1. *The proximal lumen*. This lumen opens 30 cm from the tip of the catheter. Therefore, when the tip of the catheter is in the pulmonary artery the opening of the proximal lumen should lie within the right atrium. It is used to inject fluid into for thermodilution cardiac output measurements, or to monitor right atrial pressure, but it can also be used for drug/fluid infusions.

2. *The distal lumen*. This runs the entire length of the catheter opening at the tip, which lies in the pulmonary artery. It is connected to a transducer, which continually monitors the pulmonary artery pressure and permits the recording of pulmonary artery wedge pressure. During insertion of the catheter it is used to monitor all intracardiac pressures as it passes through the heart. Blood samples can be withdrawn from this lumen to obtain blood. Blood withdrawn from PA or RV outflow tract is known as 'mixed venous' blood (i.e. where blood from the inferior vena cava (IVC) and superior vena cava (SVC) are well mixed).

3. *The thermistor connection*. This is connected to the monitor cable to enable core and injectate fluid temperatures to be detected.

4. *The thermistor*. This lies 4 cm from the tip of the catheter and senses blood temperature. Two insulated wires run the length of a lumen to end at the thermistor connection.

5. *Balloon inflation lumen*. This lumen is used to inflate and deflate the balloon when recording the pul-

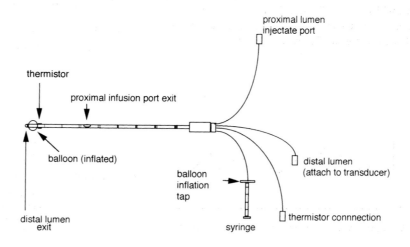

Fig. 5.30 The standard pulmonary artery catheter.

monary artery wedge pressure. A 1.5 ml capacity syringe is attached at this point and a tap allows the lumen to be turned off to the syringe when not in use. All catheters for adults will accommodate the full 1.5 ml of air in the balloon and this should be inflated only while the wedge pressures are being taken. Overinflation by injection of extra volumes may result in balloon rupture.

Insertion of the catheter

The most common insertion sites for the pulmonary artery catheter are the internal jugular and subclavian veins. The external jugular, antecubital, and femoral veins can be also be used but it is considerably more difficult to 'float' the catheter into a correct position from these sites. The subclavian vein approach may result in kinking in the catheter for anatomical reasons and this can cause a dampened waveform.

Before insertion, all lumens of the catheter are flushed with a standard saline solution, and the integrity of the balloon is checked by inflating it with 1.5 ml of air. The balloon should be seen to inflate evenly and symmetrically. A sterile sleeve adapter is placed over the catheter before insertion and this allows later manipulation while keeping the enclosed catheter portion sterile.

The catheter is inserted under strict aseptic conditions. Using the Seldinger technique a larger size introducer cannula is first inserted into the vessel and the pulmonary artery catheter is then passed through a

self-sealing valve at the top of the introducer into the vessel itself.

The distal lumen of the catheter is connected to the transducer and, by observing the monitor during placement, the location of the catheter tip can be determined by the changes in waveform and pressure.

The catheter is advanced, with the balloon deflated, until it is beyond the end of the introducer cannula; it can then be inflated. If the internal jugular or subclavian veins are used, the catheter tip should enter the right atrium at 15–20 cm (femoral vein distance is 30 cm and right antecubital fossa 40 cm). The characteristic right atrial (RA) waveform will be seen at this point (see Fig. 5.31).

The catheter is advanced until a right ventricular (RV) waveform is displayed on the monitor and ventricular systolic and diastolic pressures are noted. This should be achieved within 10–15 cm of entering the right atrium. Failing this, the balloon should be deflated, the catheter withdrawn, and the procedure repeated until the right ventricular waveform is seen. If the right ventricle is not entered, the catheter may advance down the vena cava or into the coronary sinus (which may give the impression of a 'wedged' trace (see later) which is achieved well before the expected 50 cm insertion distance).

The catheter is further advanced, through the pulmonary valve, into the pulmonary artery where a change in waveform occurs (a rise in diastolic pressure). This point will be approximately 40–45 cm from the insertion site if the internal jugular vein is used.

The catheter is then advanced a further 5–10 cm until it is in a 'wedge' or occluded position. If the catheter is not wedged at this length there may have been some coiling in the right ventricle. The balloon should not be left inflated for more than 15 s and a distinct pulmonary artery waveform should always be seen on the monitor.

Waveform characteristics

1. *Right ventricular pressure.* The waveform shows tall upright peaks corresponding to ventricular systole. The baseline corresponds to ventricular diastolic pressure. This is similar to RA pressure due to the low resistance across the tricuspid valve. As the catheter is passed through the ventricle particular attention must be paid to the ECG monitor as ventricular arrhythmias can occur (due to irritation of the ventricular wall by the catheter tip or its passage through the tricuspid valve). If ventricular ectopics occur, one can continue with the procedure, but if ventricular tachycardia occurs the catheter should

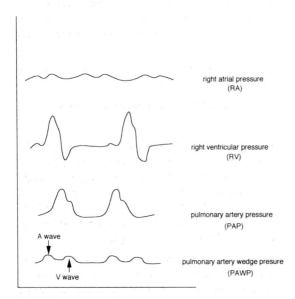

Fig. 5.31 Pressure waveform characteristics during insertion of the pulmonary artery catheter.

right atrial pressure (RA)

right ventricular pressure (RV)

pulmonary artery pressure (PAP)

pulmonary artery wedge presure (PAWP)

A wave

V wave

be withdrawn from the ventricle. This normally self-corrects, though lidocaine (lignocaine) may be necessary if this recurs on reinsertion.

2. *Pulmonary artery pressure.* Rapid ejection of blood from the right ventricle into the PA represents the pulmonary artery systolic pressure (PASP). Since the pulmonary valve is open at this point, PASP is equal to RV systolic pressure. At the end of systole the PA pressure falls and the pulmonary valve closes, creating a dicrotic notch on the waveform. The PADP is usually 5–10 mmHg higher than the right ventricular diastolic pressure (RVDP).

3. *Pulmonary artery wedge pressure (PAWP).* When the balloon is inflated in a branch of the pulmonary artery, this occludes flow completely. Thus all influences on pressure measured at the catheter tip resulting from flow from the right side of the heart are removed. The pressure at the tip of the catheter therefore reflects only the pressure ahead of it. Assuming an open circuit through the pulmonary vasculature and into the left heart, the left ventricular end diastolic pressure equals the left atrial pressure, the pulmonary venous pressure and the pulmonary capillary pressure. The pulmonary artery wedge (or occlusion) pressure is thus a good reflection of the left venticular end diastolic pressure (LVEDP) except in certain circumstances (see later). The PAWP waveform is characteristic of the pressure changes within the left atrium. Small A and V waves can be distinguished which represent left atrial and left ventricular systole. The pressure in the left atrium is usually slightly higher than in the right atrium and slightly less (1–3 mmHg) than the PADP. The PAWP is measured at the end of the A wave (i.e. at the end of ventricular diastole, and at the end of expiration). At this point, the intrathoracic pressure is closest to barometric pressure against which the pressure transducer is zeroed.

Measuring the PAWP

♦ Whilst watching the monitor, *slowly* inflate the balloon until the characteristic flattened waveform is seen. The balloon is now occluding blood flow in the vessel and is said to be 'wedged' (Fig. 5.32).

♦ Stop inflating as soon as this waveform is seen.

♦ Freeze the monitor screen if the monitor has this facility (if not, read the wedge pressure from the monitor display; if the patient is mechanically ventilated, the lowest value should be taken as this corresponds to the PAWP at the end of expiration).

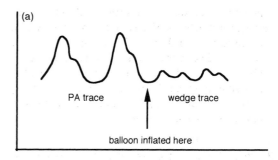

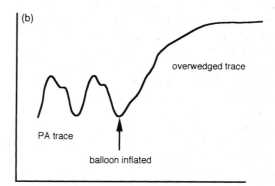

Fig. 5.32 The pulmonary artery wedge trace: (a) waveform showing a wedge trace; (b) waveform showing an overwedged trace caused by overinflation of the balloon.

♦ Deflate the balloon rapidly. The balloon should not be left inflated for more than 15 s.

♦ If a screen freeze facility is available, ascertain the wedge pressure by moving the cursor control on the monitor to the correct position on the waveform (see Fig. 5.32).

♦ Unfreeze the screen to restore the continuous pulmonary artery waveform.

♦ Ensure that a pulmonary artery waveform is present.

Special points:

♦ Do not use more than 1.5 ml of air to inflate the balloon or there is a risk of rupture of the balloon or vessel. If less than 1.2 ml of air is required to obtain the wedged waveform the catheter tip is too far advanced. As this also carries an increased risk of pulmonary artery rupture the balloon should be deflated and the catheter withdrawn slightly.

♦ The catheter is 'overwedged' if the trace rises sharply while the balloon is being inflated. This is due to the high pressure within the over-inflated balloon being transmitted to the transducer (see Fig. 5.32). If this occurs when the balloon is inflated with less than

1.2 ml of air the catheter tip is situated in a small vessel; the balloon should be *immediately* deflated and the catheter withdrawn to a more proximal position.

- Inflation time must be kept to a minimum and the balloon should not remain inflated for more than 15 s (approximately two to three cycles of respiration).
- Never flush the catheter when the balloon is inflated.
- Never inject fluid into the inflation port.

The correct wedge pressure can be easily achieved in a patient who is mechanically ventilated, but it is more difficult to gain accurate readings in patients who are breathing spontaneously (with or without ventilatory assistance), particularly if deep breaths are being taken as this may result in large 'respiratory swings' on the monitor.

During spontaneous respiration the PA and PAWP both fall during inspiration (i.e. as the intrathoracic pressure becomes more negative) and rise with expiration. All pressures are recorded at the end of expiration (i.e. closest to atmospheric pressure), therefore this is just before the pressures start to fall on the waveform trace. The opposite occurs in ventilated patients because positive pressure ventilation causes the intrathoracic pressure to increase with inspiration causing an increase in PA and PAWP. As the patient exhales, the pressures fall. Thus, in a ventilated patient, readings

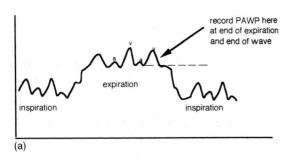

(a)

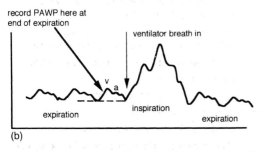

(b)

Fig. 5.33 Where to measure the PAWP: (a) in a patient breathing spontaneously; (b) in a mechanically ventilated patient.

are made just before the trace on the waveform begins to rise (see Fig. 5.33).

There are certain conditions where PAWP does not accurately reflect LVEDP—PAWP is greater than LVEDP in:

- greatly raised intrathoracic pressure,
- pulmonary venous obstruction,
- mitral stenosis,
- left atrial myxoma.

Catheter position in the pulmonary artery

The catheter tip should be located in a main branch of the pulmonary artery. Changes in the position of the catheter tip can cause potential risks to the patient. The catheter may migrate into a more distal branch of the pulmonary artery when the balloon is deflated, causing it to be partially or completely wedged. This can be identified by the characteristic wedged tracing on the waveform. The catheter must not remain in this position due to the potential risk of pulmonary artery occlusion or rupture and must be repositioned (usually by withdrawing the catheter by 1–2 cm).

Occasionally, the tip of the catheter may slip back into the right ventricle giving a ventricular waveform tracing. The tip may cause irritability to the ventricle and predispose to ventricular arrhythmias (ventricular fibrillation, tachycardia, or ectopics). If this occurs, the balloon should be inflated and refloated into the pulmonary artery.

The position of the catheter tip in the lung is important for accurate PAWP recordings. The lungs have three physiological ('West') zones of blood flow depending on the interaction of alveolar, pulmonary, arterial, and venous pressures (West 1990). In order to reflect left atrial pressure the catheter tip should lie in zone III where flow is continuous (see Fig. 5.34). If it is placed in zones I or II, alveolar pressures are reflected and may give a spuriously high reading of LVEDP. These zones are not fixed anatomically and will change gravitationally with body position. Hypovolaemia and positive end expiratory pressure (PEEP) will increase the proportions of zones I and II. Thus, the zone within which the catheter tip is located may change with body position, hypovolaemia, or PEEP. Paradoxically, therefore, the wedge pressure may rise with hypovolaemia. The correct position can be identified on a lateral chest X-ray where the tip of the catheter should be below the level of the left atrium. An alternative means of confirming a satisfactory zone III position is to increase the level of PEEP temporarily (e.g. by 5 cmH$_2$O) and see that the

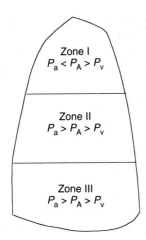

Fig. 5.34 Lung zones as described by West (1990). The tip of the pulmonary artery catheter should lie in zone III to provide accurate recordings of PAWP. P_A, pulmonary alveolar pressure; P_a, pulmonary artery pressure; P_v, pulmonary venous pressure.

wedge pressure does not increase by at least half the increase in PEEP (e.g. 2–3 mmHg).

- *Zone I.* The alveolar pressure is greater than the pulmonary arterial and venous pressure, therefore there is no blood flow from the pulmonary capillary beds.

- *Zone II.* The alveolar pressure is higher than the pulmonary venous pressure but the arterial pressure is high enough to allow some blood flow. PAWP recordings will be less accurate than if the tip is in zone III. PEEP may increase the alveolar pressure, causing zone II to be similar to zone I.

- *Zone III.* The pulmonary venous pressure is higher than the alveolar pressure and all pulmonary capillaries are open.

Specific complications of pulmonary artery catheterization (Table 5.10)

- Pulmonary artery rupture, or perforation due to the catheter tip, or overinflation of the balloon. This is particularly important in patients with pulmonary hypertension and the elderly as they have less distensible arteries.

- Rupture of the right atrium.

- Air embolism due to rupture of the balloon.

- Ventricular arrhythmias. These can occur on insertion or removal of the catheter, or if the tip migrates back into the right ventricle.

- Pulmonary artery infarction. This results from loss of blood supply to a branch of the pulmonary artery

TABLE 5.10 Summary of problems associated with pulmonary artery catheterization		
Problem	**Potential cause**	**Action**
Unable to obtain wedge when balloon is inflated	Catheter tip not in correct position	Inform medical staff. Catheter needs to be advanced
	Balloon rupture	Remove catheter
	Pulmonary hypertension	May not obtain wedge, use other readings (e.g. PADP)
Overwedged trace when balloon inflated	Incorrect position of catheter: tip is advanced too far and lies in a smaller vessel	Inform medical staff. Catheter needs to be pulled back into larger vessel
Blood in syringe when air removed from balloon	Rupture of balloon	Inform medical staff. Turn off stopcock to syringe. Catheter must be removed
Spontaneous wedge (wedge trace seen when balloon not inflated)	Catheter has migrated into a small vessel	Inform medical staff. Catheter must be withdrawn urgently until PA waveform is seen otherwise there is a risk of pulmonary infarction
RV waveform instead of PA trace	Catheter has slipped back into the right ventricle	Inform medical staff. Potential for ventricular arrhythmias. Catheter must be repositioned in the PA
'Damped' pressure trace	Loose connections	Inform medical staff. Check connections are secure
	Catheter tip against vessel wall	Reposition catheter
	Low pressure in pressure bag	Check pressure bag inflated to 300 mmHg
	Excessive length of tubing from transducer	Remove any excess tubing
	Air bubbles or blood in transducer	Check transducer: change if necessary
	Fibrin deposition at tip	Flush catheter or replace (use a 2 ml syringe to aspirate or for a high-pressure flush)

due to the catheter spontaneously wedging if the catheter migrates forwards, or if the balloon remains inflated for long periods.

♦ Valvular damage. This can occur if the balloon is inflated while the catheter is withdrawn.

♦ Right-sided valvular vegetations. The proportion leading to clinically significant endocarditis or valve dysfunction is open to question.

♦ Insertion problems such as arterial puncture, pneumothorax, etc.

♦ Knotting of the catheter during insertion.

Removal of the pulmonary artery catheter

The PA catheter alone can be removed leaving the introducer *in situ*; therefore ascertain if only the catheter or both are to be removed. Infusions via the PA catheter should be transferred to the side arm of the introducer or other infusion sites and any cardiac output equipment should be disconnected.

Emergency equipment for defibrillation should be at hand as there is a potential risk of ventricular arrhythmias as the catheter passes through the ventricle.

The procedure is carried out aseptically:

♦ Assemble equipment.

♦ Explain procedure to patient.

♦ Lay patient in supine position to reduce the risk of air embolism.

♦ Ensure the balloon is deflated and a PA waveform is shown on the monitor.

♦ Unclip the sleeve adapter from the introducer sheath.

♦ Remove the dressing and cut sutures.

♦ Remove during expiration in the spontaneously breathing patient or time removal with the inspiratory cycle of the ventilator: this reduces the risk of air embolism.

♦ Whilst observing the ECG monitor, gently withdraw the catheter. As the catheter tip passes from PA to RA the characteristic change in waveforms will be seen. Particular observation of the ECG is necessary as the tip passes through the RV. If ventricular arrhythmias occur, continue withdrawing the catheter as these will often terminate once the catheter is removed.

If there is any difficulty in withdrawing the catheter, discontinue the procedure immediately. On no account use force as this resistance may be due to knotting or kinking of the catheter, or it may be caught on a valve or other structure. Seek medical help. If the catheter is in the RV and unable to be withdrawn, and ventricular arrhythmias are occurring, consider inflating the balloon and advancing the catheter forward to try and stop the arrhythmias.

♦ When the PA catheter has been completely removed a haemostatic valve closes over the entrance in the introducer. This should prevent entry of air and exit of blood but can occasionally be damaged by the passage of the catheter. A sterile occlusive cap should therefore be placed over the exit site.

♦ If the introducer is also to be removed, it is easier to remove the PA catheter first and then remove the introducer. Ensure haemostasis by manual pressure and cover with an occlusive dressing.

Cardiac output determination

There are a variety of methods for measuring cardiac output.

The Fick method

The measurement of cardiac output is based upon the principle of Adolph Fick. The Fick principle states that the amount of substance that is taken up by an organ is equal to the organ's blood flow rate and its arterial–mixed venous difference. Commonly in clinical practice, the Fick method uses the lungs as the organ and oxygen as the substrate. Cardiac output (CO) can be calculated as follows:

$$CO = \frac{\text{oxygen consumption (ml/min)}}{\text{A} - \text{V oxygen difference}}.$$

It is a cumbersome method, and unsuitable for use in critically ill patients as the method demands a steady physiological state. The error in CO measurement by the Fick method is estimated to be approximately 10%.

Oesophageal Doppler

Oesophageal Doppler monitoring is a relatively non-invasive technique for continuously measuring a variety of haemodynamic parameters. Compared with pulmonary artery catheterization it is simple to insert, cost-effective and safe.

The technique involves passing an ultrasonic flow probe down the oesophagus, attaching it to a monitor and obtaining a waveform display that accurately reflects blood flow in the descending thoracic aorta. By analysis of various characteristics of the waveform the haemodynamic parameters can be displayed.

The Doppler machine The machine consists of a probe containing transducers mounted at its tip and a monitor that gives a visual display of the blood flow velocity profiles. The probe continuously emits ultrasound waves at a frequency optimal for the depth of penetration and sensitivity required for measuring blood flow in the descending thoracic aorta (4 MHz).

Waveform characteristics   A stylised normal blood velocity profile as displayed on the monitor is shown in Fig. 5.35.

The *x*-axis denotes time and the *y*-axis shows the blood flow velocity. The basic signal resembles a row of triangles sitting on the time line. The triangle itself represents the blood flow profile as a bolus of blood is pumped through the aorta. The base of the triangle represents the duration of systolic blood flow and is known as the flow time.

Blood moving away from the transducer is plotted above the time axis while blood flowing towards the transducer is plotted below the time axis.

Regurgitant flow in the descending aorta, as seen in moderate to severe aortic regurgitation, produces a reverse flow signal throughout all of diastole.

- *The cycle time*. This is the time from the beginning of one systole to the beginning of the next. It is expressed in seconds and is analogous to the R–R interval on the ECG. The flow time (systole) and the filling time (diastole) are affected by heart rate. The flow time can be corrected to a heart rate of 60 bpm by the following equation:

$$\text{Corrected flow time} = \frac{\text{flow time}}{\sqrt{\text{cycle time}}}$$

The normal corrected flow time is 330–350 ms.

- *Stroke distance*. This is the area within the triangle and is defined as the distance a column of blood travels down the descending aorta with each left ventricular

stroke. The stroke volume of blood passing down the descending thoracic aorta is the stroke distance multiplied by the cross sectional area of the aorta at the observation point.

- *Peak velocity*. The peak of the waveform represents the maximum velocity at which blood is moving during systole

- *Mean acceleration*. This is the peak velocity divided by the time to reach peak velocity from the beginning of systole.

Potential errors in the estimation of cardiac output using oesophageal Doppler   Potential errors may arise because the machine makes certain assumptions when calculating cardiac output. These are:

- The probe is facing the descending aorta at an angle of 45°.

- The stroke volume is computed using a nomogram. Although this has been formulated by measurements from many patients, it remains an average value.

- The proportion (approximately 70%) of blood passing through the observation point in the descending aorta (approximately 30% goes to coronary circulation, carotid, and upper limbs) is not significantly changed by alterations in cardiac output or blood pressure.

Contraindications for use   The oesophageal Doppler will not be accurate in the following circumstances:

- during aortic vascular surgery when the aorta is cross-clamped,

- when an intra-aortic balloon is *in situ* (causes local turbulence),

- with aortic coarctation.

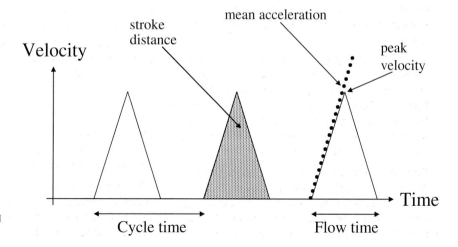

Fig. 5.35 Normal blood velocity profile of oesophageal Doppler.

Electrocautery during surgery interferes with the Doppler signal; however, this is not a contraindication to its use.

Cautions/contraindications to its use include:

◆ Patients who have oesophageal pathology (e.g. oesophageal varices).

◆ Patients who have undergone recent surgery to the mouth, oesophagus, or stomach.

◆ Patients who have severe bleeding disorders.

Probe placement   At a depth of approximately 35–40 cm from the teeth in the normal sized adult, the descending aorta lies parallel and very close to the oesophagus in the region of the T5–T6 vertebrae. The appropriate depth will change in very tall or short people; this should be considered when the probe is inserted otherwise it may be inadvertently focused on other vessels (e.g. pulmonary artery or coeliac axis) which may look similar to the aortic waveform.

At the correct depth, the probe detects blood flow from three structures—the heart, the azygos vein, or the descending thoracic aorta—depending on the orientation of the probe tip. The signals from each are distinct and can be easily recognized with experience.

Once *in situ* the probe may be rotated or moved slightly up or down until a clear aortic waveform appears on the monitor. The 'ideal' waveform should have a black central portion and a sharp outline in red, orange, yellow, and white. The colours correspond to the proportion of blood cells moving at a given speed at that point in time. White indicates the speed at which most of the blood cells are moving. Red shows the velocity at which few cells are moving and black indicates no movement at all.

Insertion of the probe

◆ Position the patient appropriately.

◆ Explain the procedure and ensure the patient is adequately sedated.

◆ Lubricate the probe tip with lubricating jelly.

◆ Gently insert the probe orally into the oesophagus.

Never force the probe. If firm resistance is encountered stop the procedure and seek medical advice. Occasionally, the probe needs to be inserted under direct vision using a laryngoscope, as there may be difficulty in bypassing the region adjacent to the endotracheal tube.

◆ Continue gently inserting the probe until the patient's teeth are midway between the external depth markers (indicating 35–40 cm from the tip).

◆ Connect the probe to the monitor.

◆ Confirm the position by achieving a correct waveform display.

◆ The probe can be secured with paper tape to the endotracheal tube or catheter mount to prevent movement.

The probes are disposable and there is no recommended time limit for how long they may be left *in situ*. Care should be taken to avoid pressure effects of the probe on the lips and mouth.

Interpretation of the waveform   Certain pathological conditions show characteristic changes in the waveform shape and can therefore give immediate information concerning haemodynamic status (Fig. 5.36). Studies have shown a close relationship between myocardial contractility and the peak velocity of the waveform, and an inverse relationship between increased systemic vacular resistance (SVR) and the corrected flow time (Singer *et al.* 1989).

1. *The corrected flow time (FTc).* The normal range is 330–350 ms. A value below this suggests vasoconstriction and a high SVR. This is usually due to hypovolaemia but can also be due to cold, excessive vasopressor drugs, or obstruction (e.g. due to tamponade). A value higher than normal suggests vaso-

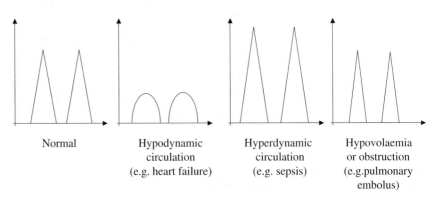

| Normal | Hypodynamic circulation (e.g. heart failure) | Hyperdynamic circulation (e.g. sepsis) | Hypovolaemia or obstruction (e.g.pulmonary embolus) |

Fig. 5.36 Stylized normal and pathological waveforms.

dilatation. During hypovolaemia, unless extreme, the peak velocity is usually maintained within age-related values and produces a narrow, peaked waveform. However, in the presence of left ventricular dysfunction, the peak velocity is normally reduced producing a short, rounded waveform.

2. *The peak velocity (PV).* The normal range seen within the descending thoracic aorta decreases with age. Normal values are:

at 20 years old: 90–120 cm/s
at 50 years old: 60–90 cm/s
at 70 years old: 50–80 cm/s.

Values that fall below this range suggest a hypodynamic circulation such as cardiogenic shock, while values above suggest a hyperdynamic circulation such as that seen in sepsis or pregnancy.

3. *Clinical profiles*:

 ◆ Septicaemia. A patient with septicaemia (usually a hyperdynamic circulation) would show an increase in peak velocity and an increase in corrected flow time (provided the patient is fluid resuscitated).

 ◆ Cardiac failure. A patient in cardiac failure (a hypodynamic circulation) would show a flattened waveform with a decrease in peak velocity and a fall in corrected flow time because of compensatory vasoconstriction.

 ◆ Hypovolaemia. A patient with hypovolaemia or flow obstruction (e.g. due to pulmonary embolus) would show a normal or slightly low peak velocity, and a short corrected flow time.

Clinical utility of waveform analysis   Alterations in preload, afterload, and inotropic status produce consistent changes in the corrected flow time and peak velocity (Fig. 5.37). Preload changes predominantly affect FTc, inotropic changes affect PV, while changes in afterload affect both FTc and PV.

Oesophageal Doppler can also be used for non-invasive optimization of left ventricular filling as immediate changes can be seen in the size of the waveform. Preload can be increased by fluid challenge or decreased by diuretics or nitrates. Afterload can also be decreased by administering short-acting nitrates.

Inotropes, vasodilators, vasopressors, fluid, and ventilator settings can be thus titrated to optimize cardiac output. Inotropes and vasopressors, which produce an excessive narrow waveform, can be corrected by adequate administration of fluid or co-administration of a vasodilator.

Dye dilution methods

This method involves the injection of a dye or chemical into the blood (usually through a central venous catheter) and measuring the subsequent dilution after a designated time. The dilution of the dye will indicate the amount of fluid that it was added to. The traditional dye is indocyanine green and its subsequent dilution can be measured by a densitometer downstream of where it was injected. Serial measurements are taken over a period of time and a dye dilution curve is produced. From this, the cardiac output can be calculated.

Lithium dilution cardiac output (LiDCO™)   This method uses the dye dilution method but involves the

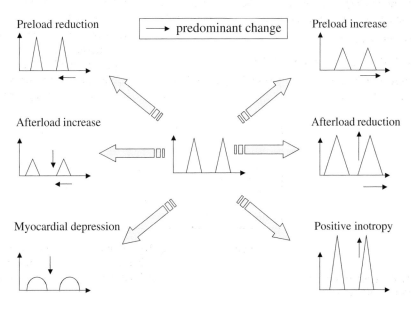

Preload reduction

predominant change

Preload increase

Afterload increase

Afterload reduction

Myocardial depression

Positive inotropy

Fig. 5.37 Waveform responses to clinical interventions.

use of an indicator solution of lithium chloride (LiCl) instead of indocyanine green. The technique requires only an arterial line and a central venous catheter and therefore is less invasive than pulmonary artery catheterization, and without many of its associated complications.

The lithium chloride is injected as a bolus via the central venous catheter and an arterial plasma concentration curve is measured by means of a sensor. The sensor is disposable and consists of a polycarbonate flow-through cell housing a lithium-selective electrode. When making a measurement, blood is sampled through this cell with a peristaltic pump, which limits the flow to 4 ml/min. The voltage across the lithium-selective membrane is related by the Nernst equation to plasma lithium concentration. A correction is applied for plasma sodium concentration because of the relatively low selectivity of the membrane for Li^+ over Na^+. The voltage is measured using an isolated amplifier and, then digitized on-line and analysed and stored.

The cardiac output is calculated as follows:

$$\text{Cardiac output} = \frac{\text{LiCl dose} \times 60}{\text{area} \times (1 - \text{PCV})}\ \text{l/min}$$

where LiCl dose is in mmol, area is the integral of the primary curve, and PCV is packed cell volume.

The dose of lithium used is 1/300th of the therapeutic dose and should not cause any adverse effects. It is, however, recommended that measurements are limited to 10 a day and it should not be used in patients on lithium therapy. The device also cannot be used in patients who are being given non-depolarizing neuromuscular blocking agents as these adversely affect the sensor.

Pulse contour cardiac output (PiCCO™, PulseCO™)

These provide an alternative to continuous monitoring and are less invasive, requiring only existing arterial and peripheral/central venous access.

The PulseCO™ system must be calibrated regularly (at least 12 hourly), for example with a lithium indicator dilution procedure (the LiDCO™ system), and will give a continuous display of cardiac output, systemic vascular resistance, stroke volume, and oxygen delivery. Once calibrated, the PulseCo™ utilizes only arterial line information to provide these parameters.

The PiCCO™ involves the insertion of a very thin catheter into the femoral artery and uses transpulmonary thermodilution and arterial pulse contour for measurement of stroke volume, continuous cardiac output, systemic vascular resistance, intrathoracic blood volume and extravascular lung water. Few data

are available to show the accuracy of the pulse contour technique in rapidly changing haemodynamic situations.

Cardiac output measurement using these techniques may also be inaccurate in the presence of aortic valve disease, arrhythmias, and a dampened arterial waveform.

Thermodilution methods

Pulmonary artery catheter   This method involves the injection of an exact amount of cold fluid into the right atrium via a PA catheter. Its dilution by the blood is calculated by serial changes in pulmonary artery temperature.

Measured amounts (5 or 10 ml) of preferably ice-cold 5% glucose (although glucose at room temperature can also be used) are injected into the proximal lumen of the PA catheter. Greater accuracy is achieved when using 5 ml volumes if it is ice-cold. The injection must be rapid (within 4 s), and enters the blood in the right atrium. As the solution mixes with the blood the blood is cooled temporarily. A thermistor at the tip of the PA catheter senses the blood temperature and a time–temperature curve can be plotted. A cardiac output computer is required to compute the output and takes into consideration the injectate volume, blood and injectate temperature, and the specific heat and gravity of the blood and injectate. As the fluid is injected a curve will be displayed on the cardiac output monitor. This represents the change from a cooler to warmer temperature and the area under the graph is inversely proportional to the cardiac output.

A closed injectate set is available whereby syringes of injectate can be drawn without disconnecting the circuit. Alternatively, pre-filled syringes can be prepared and used at room or iced temperature.

A computer constant must be fed into the monitor before cardiac output measurements are made. This constant depends on the make and model of catheter, the volume of injectate fluid used, and the temperature of the injectate.

Once selected, the temperature of the injectate must be within a defined range for each set of measurements that are taken. The computer constants are found accompanying the catheter.

For problems encountered when determining cardiac output see Table 5.11.

Thermodilution continuous cardiac output   Continuous cardiac monitoring can be obtained at the bedside by using a modified pulmonary artery catheter and a cardiac output computer. The catheter has a special

TABLE 5.11 Summary of problems associated with measuring cardiac output (CO)

Problem	Potential cause	Action
Difficulty injecting solution through proximal lumen	Proximal lumen ·occluded/kinked	Inform medical staff.·Unkink/replace catheter
	Catheter tip against wall of vessel	Reposition catheter
Blood temperature not displayed	Faulty thermistor. Fibrin growth on thermistor	Replace catheter
Injectate temperature not displayed	Faulty injectate temperature probe	Replace probe
Wide discrepancies in serial CO recordings	Inaccurate amounts of injectate drawn up	Ensure exact injectate volume is drawn up
	Poor technique (uneven injection)	Inject evenly and within 4 s
	Arrhythmias (atrial fibrillation, ventricular ectopics)	Observe ECG, avoid injection during arrhythmias
	Valvular disease (tricuspid insufficiency) causing turbulent flow	Use alternative method for obtaining CO
	Patient movement during recordings	Limit patient movement during measurements
	Malfunction of CO computer	Replace computer
Inappropriately high values for CO	Incorrect injectate volume (usually too low or leaking connection)	Check correct volume to be used (5 or 10 ml)
	Injectate temperature too low	Check temperature of injectate
	Incorrect computer constant	Check computer constant
	Poor injection technique	Inject evenly within 4 s
Inappropriately low values for CO	Incorrect injectate volume (usually too much)	Ensure correct injectate volume
	Injectate temperature too high	Check temperature of injectate. Do not hold barrel of syringe when injecting
	Start button pressed after beginning of injection	Press start button at the same time or just before beginning the injection
	Incorrect computer constant	Check computer constant
	Delivery of injectate longer than 4 s	Ensure injection is within 4 s
	Concomitant infusions at high flow rates (>150 m/h) through distal lumen	If possible, turn off concomitant infusions during measurements

10 cm long thermal filament, which lies between the RA and RV when correctly positioned. The energy signal is emitted from this filament.

The intermittent method of measuring cardiac output uses an injectate that is cooler than blood, but for continuous measurement the catheter emits pulses of energy in a repetitive on–off sequence. The algorithm in the computer identifies when the change in pulmonary artery temperature matches the input signal. Cross-correlation of the input and output signal produces a thermodilution wash-out curve. The modified Stewart–Hamilton equation is applied to determine the cardiac output value. This process occurs every 30–60 s and the values are averaged to produce a continuously displayed parameter. However, on average, data are collected over 2–7 min and are not, therefore, strictly 'con-tinual' as rapid changes are detected as artefact by the software.

Pulse contour analysis   The PiCCO and LiDCO techniques described earlier rely on discrete injection of dye/lithium/cold fluid. To provide a continuous measure the devices incorporate pulse contour analysis. Pulse contour methods analyse the region of the arterial pressure waveform between the start of ventricular ejection and the dicrotic notch in order to determine stroke volume. All devices using pulse contour analysis require a direct measurement of cardiac output in order to calibrate the pulse contour algorithm.

The pulmonary artery catheter controversy

The main disadvantages of using pulmonary artery catheters are the time taken and the complications associated with their insertion and use. In addition, despite the huge amount of information that can be obtained from them, no outcome improvement has been demonstrated through their use. Consequently, there has been considerable debate as to whether it is justifiable to continue using pulmonary artery catheters (Robin 1987, Dalen and Bone 1996).

The controversy was fired anew by a study by Connors *et al.* (1996) which suggested that patients receiving a pulmonary artery catheter on day 1 of their ICU admission were 39% more likely to die compared with patients matched for disease and illness severity who did not receive a catheter.

It was not clear from the study whether the excess mortality was due to a selection bias, to complications directly attributable to the catheters, or to an adverse response to treatment initiated on the basis of measurements made using the catheters. A similar study (Murdoch *et al.* 2000) of 4132 intensive care patients, 44% of whom had pulmonary artery catheters, showed no beneficial effect of pulmonary artery catheters, but concluded that they did not cause an increase in mortality.

The study by Connors *et al.* has been heavily criticised (Singer 1998) but has served as a catalyst for debate and acknowledgement that there is a lack of conclusive data showing benefit or harm.

Whilst invasive measurement of cardiac output is coming under increasing scrutiny the merits of non-invasive technology, such as oesophageal Doppler and pulse contour analysis techniques, become more apparent. However, these too have not been yet shown to influence outcome in the critical care setting.

Test yourself

Questions

1. What is 'Pulsus paradoxus' and what are the causes of it?

2. Which specific conditions make pulse oximetry unreliable?

3. What is the definition of first degree heart block?

4. What is the dicrotic notch, as seen in the arterial waveform?

5. What are the normal values of systemic vascular resistance, pulmonary vascular resistance, stroke volume, and cardiac output?

6. What is the difference between Mobitz type 1 and Mobitz type 2 heart block?

Answers

1. 'Pulsus paradoxus' is a term used when the difference in peak systolic pressure is greater than 10 mmHg between inspiration and expiration. This is an accentuation of the normal pattern and an exaggerated swing in systolic pressure over the respiratory cycle is seen on the monitor.

   Causes of this include pericardial disease (e.g. pericardial tamponade) which impedes ventricular filling, exaggerated inspiration by the patient, or pathological causes that result in gross changes in intrathoracic pressure during respiration (e.g. asthma). Probably the commonest cause of an exaggerated 'respiratory swing' in the critically ill patient is hypovolaemia, particularly when the patient has concurrently high airway pressures.

2. Pulse oximetry is unreliable in the presence of dysfunctional haemoglobins. These can be found in:

   ◆ Smoke inhalation when carboxyhaemoglobin levels are raised. The pulse oximeter interprets carboxyhaemoglobin as oxyhaemoglobin because the absorption coefficients of both are very similar.

   ◆ The administration of drugs that cause methaemoglobinaemia such as lidocaine (lignocaine), nitrates, and metoclopramide.

   ◆ The administration of certain dyes and pigments such as methylthioninium chloride (methylene blue) and indocyanine green, because they absorb light at a similar frequency to reduced haemoglobin and may give false low readings of oxygen saturation.

   Other causes include:

   ◆ poor perfusion to the vascular bed where the probe is placed

   ◆ nail varnish

   ◆ restrictive tape or blood pressure cuffs distal to the probe

   ◆ light interference from sunlight and lamps.

3. First degree heart block is caused by a delay in conduction at the AV node and is characterized by a prolonged P–R interval of greater than 0.20 s.

4. The dicrotic notch reflects the closure of the aortic valve caused by a rise in pressure in the aorta. When the pressure in the aorta is greater than in the left ventricle the blood attempts to flow backwards causing the valve to close. On the waveform trace the

dicrotic notch marks the end of systole and the onset of diastole.

5. Normal values are (1 dyn = 10^{-5} N):
SVR: 800–1200 dyn s/cm^5
PVR: <250 dyn s/cm^5
SV: 60–100 ml
CO: 4–8 litre/min.

6. In Mobitz type 1 a delay at the AV node gradually increases through a series of beats until conduction of the impulse does not occur. The whole process is then repeated. The QRS complex is normal. In Mobitz type 2, a varying ratio of QRS to P waves are conducted through the AV node (e.g. two P:one QRS). The P–R interval in conducted beats remains constant.

References and bibliography

Abbott Laboratories (1994). *Continuous, Non-invasive Cardiac Monitoring Training Manual*. Abbott Laboratories, Abbott Park, IL.

Barker, S., Tremper, K. (1987). The effects of carbon monoxide inhalation on pulse oximetry and transcutaneous PO_2. *Anaesthesiology* **66**, 677–9.

Bone, R., Balk, R. (1988). Noninvasive respiratory care unit: a cost effective solution for the future. *Chest* **93**, 390–4.

Brunel, W., Cohen, N.H. (1988). Evaluation of the accuracy of pulse oximetry in critically ill patients. *Critical Care Medicine* **16**, 432.

Castor, G., Klocke, R.K., Stoll, M. *et al.* (1994). Simultaneous measurement of cardiac output by thermodilution, thoracic electrical bioimpedance and Doppler ultrasound. *British Journal of Anaesthesia* **72**, 133–8.

Connors, A.F. Jr, Speroff, T., Dawson, N.V. *et al.* (1996). The effectiveness of right heart catheterization in the initial care of critically ill patients. SUPPORT Investigators. *Journal of the American Medical Association* **276**, 889–97.

Dalen, J.E., Bone, R.C. (1996). Is it time to pull the pulmonary artery catheter? (editorial). *Journal of the American Medical Association* **276**, 916–18.

Deltex Medical (1999). *CardioQ Operating Handbook* (English version), part number 9051–5201, revision 1.01. Deltex Medical, Chichester.

Drew, B.J. (1993). Bedside electrocardiogram monitoring. *AACN Clinical Issues in Critical Care Nursing* **4**, 26–33.

Edwards, D. (1988). Principles of oxygen transport. *Care of the Critically Ill* **4**, 13–16.

Fiddian-Green, R.G. (1992). Tonometry; theory and applications. *Intensive Care World* **92**, 60–5.

Hathaway, R. (1978). The Swan–Ganz catheter: a review. *Nurses Clinics of North America* **13**, 380–407.

Gardner, P. (1993). Pulmonary artery pressure monitoring. *AACN Clinical Issues in Critical Care Nursing* **41**, 98–118.

Gorney, D.A. (1993). Arterial blood pressure measurement technique. *AACN Clinical Issues in Critical Care Nursing* **4**, 66–79.

Hanowell, L. (1987). Ambient light affects pulse oximeters. *Anaesthesiology* **67**, 864–5.

Hartmann, M., Montgomery, A., Jonisson, K. *et al.* (1991). Tissue oxygenation in haemorrhagic shock measured as transcutaneous oxygen tension and gastrointestinal intramucosal pH in pigs. *Critical Core Medicine* **19**, 205–10.

Headley, J.M. (1989). *Invasive Haemodynamic Monitoring: Physiological Principles and Clinical Applications*. Baxter Healthcare Corporation, Edwards Critical-Care Division, Irvine, CA.

Kadota, L.T. (1985). Theory and application of thermodilution cardiac output measurement: a review. *Heart and Lung* **14**, 605–14.

Kaye, W. (1983). Invasive monitoring technique: arterial cannulation, bedside pulmonary artery catheterization, and arterial puncture. *Heart and Lung* **12**, 395–424.

Kidd, J.F. (1988). Pulse oximeters: basic theory and operation. *Care of the Critically Ill* **4**, 10–13.

Low, J.M. (1990). Haemodynamic monitoring. In: *Intensive Care Manual*, 3rd edn (ed. T.E. Oh.), pp. 578–91. Butterworth, London.

Lynne, M., Scnapp, M.D., Neal, H., *et al.* (1990). Pulse oximetry: uses and abuses. *Chest* **98**, 1244–50.

Mackenzie, S.J. (1992). Haemodynamic monitoring in intensive care. In: *Intensive Care in Britain* (ed. M. Rennie). Greycoat, London.

Murdoch, S.D., Cohen, A.T., Bellamy, M.C. (2000). Pulmonary artery catheterization and mortality in critically ill patients. *British Journal of Anaesthesia* **85**, 611–15.

Neff, T. (1988). Routine oximetry: a fifth vital sign? *Chest* **94**, 227.

Oh, T.E. (ed.) (1990). *Intensive Care Manual*, 3rd edn. Butterworth, London.

Peruzzi, W.T., Gould, R., Brodsky, L. (2003). Minimally invasive haemodynamic monitoring. In: *Yearbook of Intensive Care and Emergency Medicine* (ed. J.L. Vincent), pp. 521–9. Springer, Berlin.

Pittman, J.A.L., Gupta, K.J. (2003). Cardiac output monitoring: will new technologies replace the pulmonary artery catheter? In: *Yearbook of Intensive Care and Emergency Medicine* (ed. J.L. Vincent), pp. 481–3. Springer, Berlin.

Pulmonary Artery Catheter Consensus Conference: consensus statement (1997). *Critical Care Medicine* **25**, 910–25.

Ramsey, M. (1991). Blood pressure monitoring: automated oscilloscope devices. *Journal of Clinical Monitoring* **7**, 56–67.

Rithalia, S.V.S., Edwards, D. (1992). Intra-arterial oxygen electrode. *British Journal of Intensive Care* **2**, 29–33.

Robin, E.D. (1987). Death by pulmonary artery flow-directed catheter. Time for a moratorium? (editorial). *Chest* **92,** 727–31.

Sidi, A., Paulus, D., Rush, W. *et al.* (1987). Methylene blue and indocyanine green artificially lower pulse oximetry readings of oxygen saturation: studies in dogs. *Journal of Clinical Monitoring* **3**, 249–56.

Singer, M. (1998). Cardiac output in 1998. *Heart* **79**(5), 425–8.

Singer, M. Clarke, J., Bennett, E.D. (1989). Continuous haemodynamic monitoring by oesophageal Doppler. *Critical Care Medicine* **17**, 447–52.

Smith, R., Olson, M. (1989). Drug induced methaemoglobinaemia on pulse oximetry and mixed venous oximetry. *Anaesthesiology* **70**, 112–17.

Spralka, J.M., Strickland, D. Gomez-Marin, O., *et al.* (1991). The effect of cuff size on blood pressure measurements in adults. *Epidemiology* **2**, 214–17.

Urban, N. (1991). Haemodynamic clinical profiles. *AACN Clinical Issues in Critical Care Nursing* **1**, 123–4.

Veyckemans, F., Baele, P., Guillaume, J.E. *et al.* (1989). Hyperbilirubinaemia does not interfere with haemoglobin saturation measured by pulse oximetry. *Anaesthesiology* **70**, 118–22.

West, I. B. (1990). R*espiratory Physiology—the Essentials*, 4th edn, pp. 41-3. Williams and Wilkins, Baltimore, MD.

White, K.M. (1993). Using continuous SvO_2 to assess oxygen supply/ demand balance in the critically ill patient. *AACN Clinical Issues in Critical Care Nursing* **4**, 134–45.

Woods, S.L., Osguthorpe, S. (1993). Cardiac output determination. *AACN Clinical Issues in Critical Care Nursing* **4**, 81–94.

APPENDIX Abbreviations used in text

Abbreviation	Term	Definition	Normal value
CVP	Central venous pressure	Pressure recorded within a vein near to the heart	3–10 mmHg
RA or RAP	Right atrial pressure	Pressure within the right atrium	3–8 mmHg
MRAP	Mean right atrial pressure	Mean pressure of right atrium	4–6 mmHg
RVSP	Right ventricular systolic pressure	Systolic pressure in right ventricle	15–25 mmHg
RVDP	Right ventricular diastolic pressure	Diastolic pressure in right ventricle	3–8 mmHg
PASP	Pulmonary artery systolic pressure	Systolic pressure in pulmonary artery	15–25 mmHg
PADP	Pulmonary artery diastolic pressure	Diastolic pressure in pulmonary artery	8–12 mmHg
PAWP or PAOP or PCWP	Pulmonary artery wedge pressure (also known as PA occlusion pressure or pulmonary capillary wedge pressure)	Closely reflects ventricular filling pressure (or left ventricular end diastolic pressure)	6–12 mmHg
LA or LAP	Left atrial pressure	Pressure in left atrium	6–12 mmHg
MAP	Mean arterial pressure	MAP = [SBP + (DBP × 2)]/3	70–105 mmHg
SV	Stroke volume	Volume of blood ejected from the left ventricle per beat: SV= CO/HR	60–100 ml
CO	Cardiac output	Volume of blood expelled by left ventricle per minute	4–8 1/min
CI	Cardiac index	Cardiac output related to body size: CI = CO/BSA	2.4–4.0 1/min
EF	Ejection fraction	Stroke volume expressed as a percentage of EDV	60–70%
EDV or LVEDV	End diastolic volume	Amount of blood left in left ventricle at end of diastole	120–150 ml
ESV	End systolic volume	Amount of blood left in left ventricle at end of systole	50–70 ml
SVR	Systemic vascular resistance	Measures resistance to the left ventricle: SVR = [(MAP – RAP) × 80]/CO	800–1200 dyn s/cm^5
PVR	Pulmonary vascular resistance	Measures resistance to the right ventricle: PVR = [(MPAP – PCWP) × 80]/CO	<250 dyn s/cm^5
FTc	Corrected flow time	Time from beginning of one systole to the next: FTc = flow time/v(cycle time)	330–360 ms
PV	Peak velocity	Maximum velocity at which blood moves at systole	90–120 cm/s (at 20 yr), 60–90 cm/s (at 50 yr), 50–80 cm/s (at 70 yr)

BSA, body surface area; MPAP, mean pulmonary artery pressure.
1 dyn = 10^{-5} N.

Cardiovascular problems

Anatomy and physiology

The principal functions of the cardiovascular system are as follows (Fig. 6.1):

1. Carriage of oxygen to the tissues from the lungs.
2. Carriage of carbon dioxide from the tissues to the lungs.

Anatomy and physiology

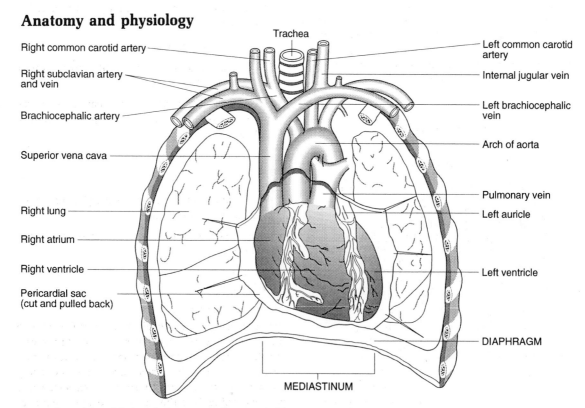

Right common carotid artery

Right subclavian artery and vein

Brachiocephalic artery

Superior vena cava

Right lung

Right atrium

Right ventricle

Pericardial sac (cut and pulled back)

Trachea

Left common carotid artery

Internal jugular vein

Left brachiocephalic vein

Arch of aorta

Pulmonary vein

Left auricle

Left ventricle

DIAPHRAGM

MEDIASTINUM

Fig. 6.1 General view of the heart in the anatomically correct position.

3. Carriage of nutrients from the digestive tract to the tissues.

4. Carriage of metabolic waste from the tissues to the kidneys.

5. Carriage of hormones from endocrine glands and other sources to site of action.

6. Transport and radiation of excess heat.

The cardiovascular system includes:

1. The pulmonary circulation consisting of the pulmonary artery, pulmonary capillaries, and pulmonary veins. This is supplied by the right ventricle.

2. The systemic circulation consisting of the aorta, arteries, capillaries, and veins of the rest of the body. This is supplied by the left ventricle.

Flow of blood through the heart

Venous blood returns to the right atrium via the inferior and superior venae cavae. The atria act as a top-up system which forces extra blood into the respective ventricles immediately prior to ventricular contraction (Fig. 6.2).

The pressure created by commencement of ventricular contraction closes the valves between the atria and ventricle. Continuing ventricular contraction then forces blood out from the right ventricle into the pulmonary artery and from the left ventricle into the aorta. Due to the disparity of pressures between pulmonary and systemic circulations, the left ventricle is considerably thicker and more muscular than the right. It also has a globular shape as opposed to the half-moon shape of the right ventricle.

Pressure changes during a cardiac cycle

Ventricular pressure changes

In the left ventricle:

♦ Peak pressure of ~120 mmHg during systole (this pressure rises with age).

♦ During diastole, the pressure falls to a thoracic cavity pressure of ~0 mmHg.

♦ Left ventricular pressure changes are therefore 120/0 mmHg.

In the right ventricle:

♦ Maximum pressure of ~25 mmHg. The same volume of blood is ejected as the left ventricle but at a lower pressure.

♦ During diastole the pressure falls to the thoracic cavity pressure of ~0 mmHg,

♦ Right ventricular pressure changes are therefore 25/0 mmHg.

Aortic pressure changes

♦ The peak pressure is the same as left ventricular pressure, namely ~120 mmHg.

♦ During diastole, aortic pressure is maintained by the elastic recoil of arterial walls and pressure falls to ~80 mmHg.

♦ Aortic pressure changes are therefore ~120/80 mmHg.

Pulmonary artery pressure changes

♦ Maximum pressure is the same as right ventricular pressure, namely ~25 mmHg.

♦ During diastole, pulmonary artery pressure falls to ~8 mmHg.

♦ Pulmonary artery pressure changes are therefore 25/8 mmHg.

Atrial pressure changes

Pressure changes are much more complex due to bulging of the tricuspid and mitral valves during ventricular systole, and downward movement of the atrioventricular ring following opening of the pulmonary and aortic valves. Upward return of the atrioventricular ring and filling from the venae cavae and pulmonary veins cause an increase in atrial pressures until the

Anatomy and physiology

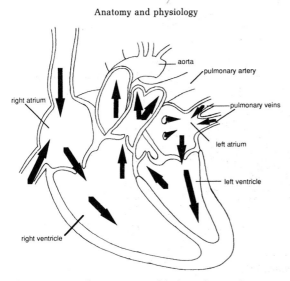

Fig. 6.2 Diagram of a cross-section of the heart showing direction of flow.

mitral and tricuspid valves open again and atrial contraction occurs.

Excitation, contraction, and conduction

Features of cardiac muscle

Syncytium

Cardiac muscle is similar to skeletal muscle apart from the lattice-like interconnection of fibres between muscle cells. This is known as a syncytium and forms a complex network that allows almost simultaneous spread of excitation and contraction. The atria form one syncytium, and this is divided from the ventricular syncytium by fibrous tissue. This division is important to allow separate atrial and ventricular contraction.

Automatic rhythmicity

Some areas of muscle fibre have the ability to depolarize rhythmically without external stimulation. This occurs because the membrane of the muscle fibre is permeable to sodium allowing a continual leak of sodium ions into the cell. This increases the electrical charge until it hits a 'threshold' level triggering an action potential. After the action potential occurs the membrane is temporarily less permeable to sodium ions but more permeable to potassium ions. Potassium thus leaks out, creating a negative charge across the membrane.

The speed of rhythmic depolarization is determined by the length of time it takes to increase the membrane potential to the 'threshold' level once more. Sinoatrial node fibres have the fastest inherent rhythmicity and thus act as the pacemaker.

> ### MEMBRANE POTENTIAL
>
> All cells have an electrical potential across the cell membrane, which is negative inside the cell in resting conditions. The potential is due to the differences between ion composition in intracellular and extracellular fluids. This is maintained by the Na^+/K^+ pump, which transports sodium ions to the outside of the cell while transporting potassium ions inside. The membrane is very permeable to potassium ions but much less permeable to sodium ions. Potassium ions tend to leak out, leaving large negatively charged ions inside the cell that produce the relative negative charge.

TABLE 6.1   Duration in seconds of contraction and repolarization

Event	Duration (s) at rate of 75 bpm	Duration (s) at rate of 200 bpm
Cardiac cycle	0.80	0.30
Systole	0.27	0.16
Action potential	0.25	0.15
Absolute refractory period	0.20	0.13
Relative refractory period	0.05	0.02
Diastole	0.53	0.14

Prolonged muscle contraction

The action potential includes a plateau phase that lasts for about 0.3 s before returning to baseline due to the slow repolarization of cardiac muscle.

Increased speed of contraction and repolarization with increased cardiac rate

This is partly due to a shortened period of systolic ejection, but mostly to a shortened diastolic period. Thus, in prolonged tachycardia, time for muscle rest and coronary blood flow is greatly reduced. The absolute refractory period is protected to prevent tetanic or chaotic excitation (Table 6.1).

Depolarization

A stimulus alters the permeability of the polarized cell membrane by inactivating the Na^+/K^+ pump and allowing sodium ions to diffuse rapidly into the cell via 'fast sodium channels' in the cell membrane. This results in a reversal of the electrical charge. When polarity reduces from the resting potential of –80 mV to –35 mV, the calcium channels of the cell membrane are opened. There is an immediate influx of calcium ions that, combined with the continuing sodium ion influx, increases the polarity across the membrane to +30 mV. When this threshold point is reached the cells on either side are stimulated and membrane permeability altered, thus depolarization becomes self-propagating. This is known as an action potential and calcium release is triggered to allow muscular contraction (see below). If the critical level of depolarization is not reached, then depolarization will remain local to the cell and calcium release will not be activated.

Repolarization

The first phase of repolarization is closure of the 'fast' sodium channels. Potassium begins to move out of the cell and there is an influx of calcium and sodium ions into the cell via slow channels. This is the plateau phase of repolarization (phase 2), which is represented on the electrocardiogram (ECG) as the ST segment. During phase 3, the slow channels close and the influx of calcium and sodium ions is halted. There is increased permeability to potassium ions and further movement of potassium ions out of the cell until the negative polarity of the cell's resting state is restored. This appears as the T wave on the ECG. Finally, phase 4 of repolarization reactivates the Na$^+$/K$^+$ pump, allowing the ratio of sodium to potassium ions inside the cell to be regained.

The refractory period

Cardiac muscle cells will not respond to further stimulation between phases 0 and 3 of the action potential. This is known as the refractory period. The *absolute* refractory period covers phases 0 to 2 of depolarization and repolarization. No stimulus will be able to elicit a response during this period. On the ECG, this is denoted by the period from the beginning of the QRS complex to just after the beginning of the T wave. The *relative* refractory period covers phase 3 of repolarization when membrane potential is more negative than –50 mV. A relatively strong stimulus will cause a response but conduction is slower than when fibres are fully repolarized. This period is represented by the majority of the T wave. The occurrence of an ectopic stimulus during the relative refractory period can initiate life-threatening dysrhythmias. This is known as an 'R on T' ectopic.

Mechanical response to depolarization

In response to an action potential, calcium ions are released from the sarcoplasmic reticulum that sur-

rounds the sarcomere within the cell (Fig. 6.3). Calcium influx can also occur into the cell through opening of calcium channels in the cell membrane.

Free calcium ions activate contraction ('systole') by combining with the protein troponin that is situated on the actin filaments. Calcium-bound troponin acquires a slightly different position on the filament, thereby uncovering binding sites on the actin, which can then interact and form cross-bridges with the myosin filaments. Release of energy from ATP allows the two filaments to move past each other, shortening the distance between two Z bands. This shortening is the basis of myocardial contraction. Calcium is taken up again by the sarcoplasmic reticulum and contraction ceases as the binding sites are once again covered. The sarcomere lengthens and relaxation occurs.

Conduction (Fig. 6.4)

In order for virtually simultaneous contraction to take place throughout the individual chambers of the heart, there must be a very fast conduction pathway. Electrical stimulation can be conducted from cell to cell but this is too slow to provide optimal contraction.

All specialized cells within the conduction pathway possess automaticity but the discharge rate varies. The fastest discharge rate (60—100 bpm at rest), and thus the normal pacemaker of the heart, is the sinoatrial (SA) node.

Movement of the action potential through the atria is via a number of tracts. This means that the action potential from different atrial areas will arrive at the atrioventricular (AV) node at different times. The AV

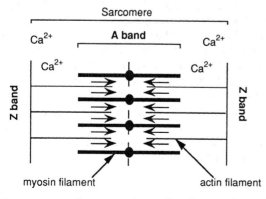

Fig. 6.3 Diagram of a sarcomere (arrows show direction of contraction).

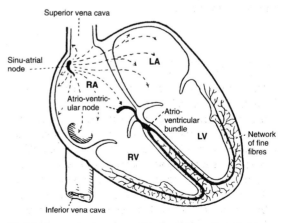

Fig. 6.4 The conduction system of the heart. (From Ross, J.S., Wilson, K.J.W. (1973). *Foundations of Anatomy and Physiology*, 3rd edn, p. 144, Fig. 120, Churchill Livingstone, Edinburgh, with permission.)

AUTOMATIC DISCHARGE RATE OF CARDIAC TISSUES

- Sinoatrial (SA) node: 60–100 bpm.
- Atrioventricular (AV) node: 40–60 bpm.
- Ventricular tissue: 20–40 bpm.

node is normally the only electrical pathway between atria and ventricles and thus the action potential is delayed here to allow all action potentials to be conducted to the ventricles at the same time. The normal AV nodal delay is approximately 0.1 s. The AV node is continuous with the bundle of His and excitation spreads rapidly down this bundle, then into right and left bundle branches, the Purkinje fibres, and the rest of the ventricles.

Depolarization starts on the left of the ventricular septum and passes to the right across the mid-portion. It then moves down to the apex and out to the ventricular walls. The electrical events of the cardiac cycle are seen on the ECG. This records fluctuations in electrical potential from the heart. These fluctuations (currents) are conducted by body fluids containing large quantities of electrolytes which conduct current and are measured on the body surface (Fig. 6.5). The principles of recording the ECG are detailed in Chapter 5.

External regulation of the heart rate

The heart rate is influenced by two major external controls:

- the autonomic nervous system,
- circulating catecholamines.

Autonomic influence

Both the SA and the AV nodes are innervated by parasympathetic and sympathetic fibres. Some myocardial fibres are also innervated by sympathetic nerve fibres. Parasympathetic stimulation via the vagus nerve causes release of acetylcholine near the nodal cells, causing:

- decreased heart rate by delayed depolarization,
- decreased force of contraction,
- delayed conduction of impulses through the AV node.

Sympathetic stimulation releases noradrenaline near the nodal cells. This stimulates specific receptor sites (β_1-adrenergic receptors), causing:

- faster heart rate, mediated by an increase in the rate of nodal depolarization,
- increased strength of cardiac contraction,
- increased rapidity of cardiac impulse conduction.

Influence of catecholamines

The release of adrenaline and noradrenaline into the bloodstream by the adrenal medulla will also have a direct effect on the heart in the same way as sympathetic nervous stimulation.

Heart rate and blood pressure

Two reflexes adjust heart rate to blood pressure (BP) via the cardioregulatory centre in the medulla.

The aortic reflex

Aaortic and carotid sinus baroreceptors respond to alterations in systemic blood pressure and sensory impulses sent to the cardioregulatory centre produce the responses shown in Table 6.2.

The Bainbridge effect

Receptors in the venae cavae stimulated by an alteration in venous return send sensory impulses to the cardioregulatory centre (Table 6.3).

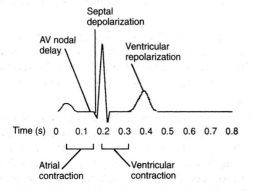

Fig. 6.5 Electrical and mechanical events during the cardiac cycle.

TABLE 6.2	The aortic reflex	
Alteration in BP	**Cardioregulatory centre response**	**Physiological response**
Raised BP	Increase in vagal stimulation or a decrease in sympathetic stimulation	Lower heart rate causing a decrease in cardiac output and BP
Lowered BP	Increase in sympathetic stimulation or a decrease in vagal stimulation	Increased heart rate and force of contraction causing a rise in cardiac output and BP

TABLE 6.3	The Bainbridge effect	
Alteration in venous return	Cardioregulatory response	Physiological response
Increased venous return	Increase in sympathetic stimulation and a decrease in parasympathetic stimulation	Increased heart rate
Decreased venous return	Increase in parasympathetic stimulation and decrease in sympathetic stimulation	Decreased heart rate

Haemodynamics

Under certain physiological conditions the normal heart should be able to meet the metabolic demands placed upon it. However, a diseased heart or alterations in the peripheral circulation may mean that attempts to maintain adequate cardiac performance is impaired.

Determinants of cardiac performance can be divided into the following components:

- cardiac output
- preload
- heart rate
- afterload
- stroke volume
- contractility.

When assessing the patient's haemodynamic status the interrelationships of all these factors must be taken into account.

Cardiac output

The cardiac output (CO) is the amount of blood ejected from the left ventricle in 1 min. It is determined by the stroke volume and heart rate, therefore manipulation of either can alter CO:

CO = heart rate × stroke volume.

The usual range of CO is 4–7 l/min. The CO can be adjusted to body size by dividing it by body surface area (BSA). This is termed the cardiac index (CI):

$$CI \ (l/min/m^2) = \frac{CO \ (l/min)}{BSA \ (m^2)}$$

The normal value for CI is 2.5–4.0 l/min/m². Body surface area is determined using a nomogram derived from height and weight. Cardiac output normally decreases by about 1% per annum after the age of 35 years.

Heart rate

Elevated heart rates can compromise cardiac output by:

- increasing the amount of oxygen consumed by the myocardium,
- reducing the diastolic time, resulting in less time for perfusion of the coronary arteries,
- shortening the ventricular filling phase of the cardiac cycle, causing a decreased blood volume to be pumped on the next contraction.

Decreased heart rates may also be detrimental. Although a longer filling time may initially increase cardiac output, if the heart is diseased the myocardium may be so depressed that that the muscle cannot contract long enough to eject this volume, resulting in a decrease in CO. A healthy heart should be able to tolerate a range of heart rates from 30 to 170 bpm for relatively prolonged periods; however, if cardiac function is compromised this range may be considerably narrower.

Other factors affecting the heart rate include temperature, psychological state, thyroid function, adrenal function, and arrhythmias.

Stroke volume

Stroke volume (SV) is the amount of blood ejected by the left ventricle during one contraction. It is the difference between the end diastolic volume (EDV: the amount of blood left in the ventricle at the end of diastole) and the end systolic volume (ESV: blood volume left in the ventricle at the end of systole).

The volume of blood ejected by each ventricular contraction (stroke volume) is dependent on:

- myocardial muscle contractility,
- preload (the volume of blood filling the ventricle),
- afterload (the resistance to blood flow from the ventricle),
- heart rate (tachycardia reduces the time for diastolic filling).

The normal range of stroke volume is 60–100 ml.

The stroke volume can be expressed as a percentage of the end diastolic volume and is then called the ejection fraction (EF) (see Chapter 8 for further details).

Preload

This refers to the degree of stretch of the muscle fibres at the end of diastole. The greater the volume of blood in the ventricle, the more the degree of muscle fibre stretch. This is a self-regulatory system allowing force of contraction to equal the volume of blood required to be ejected. Starling's law of the heart states that

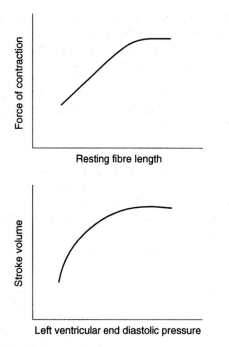

Fig. 6.6 Starling's law.

the force of myocardial contraction is determined by the length of the muscle cell fibres (Fig. 6.6).

The volume of blood in the ventricle at diastole is dictated by venous return (the volume of blood returning to the heart) and the ability of the ventricle to contract. There is an optimal range of stretch beyond which force of contraction is reduced rather than increased.

TABLE 6.4 Factors influencing ventricular preload	
Decreased preload	Volume loss—haemorrhage, vomiting, polyuria
	Vasodilatation—pyrexia, drugs (e.g. nitrates), septicaemia, neurogenic shock, anaphylactic shock
	Tachycardia (potentially insufficient diastolic filling time)
	Impeded venous return (e.g. high intrathoracic pressure, pericardial tamponade, pulmonary embolus)
Increased preload	Volume gain—renal failure, excess blood products, excess IV fluids
	Vasoconstriction—hypothermia, drugs (e.g. epinephrine, dopamine >5 mg/kg/min, norepinephrine), heart failure, pain, anxiety
	Bradycardia

The hypothesized cause of the end point of myocardial stretch is that beyond a certain distance there are too few actin–myosin binding sites overlapping to provide adequate contraction.

The factors affecting ventricular preload are shown in Table 6.4. Specific causes of a decreased left ventricular preload include pulmonary embolus and mitral stenosis. Since preload is difficult to measure at the bedside, the pressures required to fill the ventricles are used as indirect guides to ventricular end diastolic volume; that is, the right ventricular end diastolic (filling) pressure (= central venous pressure) for the right ventricle and the left ventricular end diastolic (filling) pressure (= pulmonary artery wedge pressure) for the left ventricle.

Afterload

Afterload is the resistance to the outflow of blood that must be overcome by the ventricles during systole. The most important factor determining afterload is the vascular resistance. The pulmonary vascular resistance dictates right ventricular afterload and the systemic vascular resistance dictates left ventricular afterload.

The bedside measurement of 'afterload' is the systemic vascular resistance (SVR) for the left ventricle and the pulmonary vascular resistance (PVR) for the right ventricle. Resistance is derived from the cardiac output (CO) and mean arterial pressure (MAP):

$$SVR = \frac{(MAP - RAP) \times 80 \text{ dyn s/cm}^5}{CO}$$

and

$$PVR = \frac{(MPAP - PAWP) \times 80 \text{ dyn s/cm}^5}{CO}$$

where MPAP is mean pulmonary artery pressure, PAWP is pulmonary artery wedge pressure, and RAP is right atrial pressure. 80 is a conversion factor to present the units of resistance as dyn s/cm^5 (1 dyn = 10^{-5} N). The normal range of SVR is 800–1200 dyn s/cm^5 and of PVR is 50–200 dyn s/cm^5.

Afterload has an inverse effect on ventricular function. As the resistance to ejection increases so does the workload of the ventricle. A dysfunctional ventricle, in particular, may not be able to maintain or increase the stroke volume (the amount of blood ejected from the ventricle in one beat) against a high resistance, thus the cardiac output frequently falls in the face of increasing peripheral vasoconstriction.

The opposite is seen with vasodilatation: the heart has less resistance to pump against and cardiac output usually increases as a consequence. This explains why increases in blood pressure often results in decreased flow (i.e. cardiac output). A satisfactory blood pressure that allows an adequate perfusion pressure of the vital organs must be achieved without compromising blood flow (and thus organ perfusion).

Factors affecting afterload are shown in Table 6.5. Specific causes of increased right ventricular afterload include pulmonary valve disease, pulmonary embolus, and pulmonary hypertension. Specific causes of increased left ventricular afterload include aortic valve stenosis and systemic hypertension.

Contractility

Contractility refers to the ability to shorten the myocardial muscle fibres without actually altering their length or preload. The force of contraction of myocardial muscle cells alters in response to neural stimuli

TABLE 6.5 Factors affecting afterload

Increased afterload	Vasoconstricting drugs (e.g. norepinephrine)
	Anxiety
	Hypovolaemia
	Hypothermia
	Cardiogenic shock
	Atherosclerosis
Decreased afterload	Vasodilatating drugs (e.g. nitrates, hydralazine, sodium nitroprusside)
	Anaphylactic shock
	Septicaemia
	Hyperthermia
	Neurogenic shock

TABLE 6.6 Factors affecting contractility

Increased contractility	Positive inotropic drugs
	Endogenous catecholamines
	Aerobic metabolism
	Hypervolaemia
	Hyperthyroidism
Decreased contractility	Negative inotropic drugs
	Functional loss of myocardium
	Anaerobic metabolism (intracellular acidosis)
	Hypocalcaemia
	Hypomagnesaemia
	Hypovolaemia
	Hypoxia

and levels of circulating catecholamines. Noradrenaline is liberated at sympathetic neuromuscular junctions and binds to β_1-adrenergic myocardial membrane receptors. The mechanism is mediated by cyclic AMP and protein kinase A, producing an increase in intracellular levels of calcium and ATP thereby facilitating excitation–contraction coupling. Factors affecting contractility are shown in Table 6.6.

Blood flow

The heart generates the pressure which forces blood into the circulation. However, the actual rate of blood flow will depend on the difference between the pressure produced by the heart and the pressure at the end of the vessel:

Rate of blood flow ∝ pressure difference (i.e. difference between MAP and CVP).

(MAP is mean arterial pressure and CVP central venous pressure). Thus, if the pressure in the arterioles is high due to vasoconstriction, there will be a lower blood flow for the same pressure induced by ventricular contraction. Other factors affecting flow include the diameter of the vessel, the viscosity of the blood, and the vessel length. These form the resistance to blood flow.

Poiseuille's law states that the ability of blood to flow through any given vessel is:

♦ proportional to the pressure difference between the two ends of the vessel, and to the fourth power of the vessel diameter,

♦ inversely proportional to the vessel length and blood viscosity.

That is:

$$\text{Blood flow} = \frac{\text{pressure} \times (\text{diameter})^4}{\text{length} \times \text{viscosity}}$$

Regulation of blood flow

The main regulators of blood flow in the different tissues are the arterioles. These vessels produce the greatest decrease in diameter and thus the highest resistance to flow. Their tiny size, and the fact that resistance is inversely proportional to the fourth power of their diameter, means that any alteration in diameter will result in a major change in blood flow. This alteration in diameter is mediated by the strong muscular wall, which can alter diameter by three- to five-fold.

The smooth muscle within the vessel wall responds to two regulatory stimuli:

- the local requirements of tissues when nutrient supply falls below need or exceeds demand, i.e. autoregulatioin

- autonomic signals, particularly sympathetic stimulation.

Autoregulation of blood flow

In most tissues the most powerful stimulus for autoregulation is the need for oxygen. The exceptions are the kidney, as the concentration of electrolytes and metabolic waste play a major role in renal blood flow regulation, and the brain where the carbon dioxide concentration will also control cerebral blood flow. The alteration of flow to match oxygen requirements allows automatic and immediate response to increases in cell activity. If tissue PO_2 falls then arteriolar dilatation occurs producing increased blood flow; conversely, if tissue PO_2 rises then arteriolar constriction occurs and blood flow is reduced. The system allows oxygen delivery to be adjusted according to cellular activity and blood flow to be redirected to areas of need.

Autonomic control of blood flow

Arteries, veins, and, in particular, arterioles are supplied by sympathetic nerves which moderate the state of vasoconstriction by transmitting a continuous stream of impulses. This maintains vasomotor tone. Vasoconstriction is produced by increased sympathetic impulses and vasodilatation by reduced sympathetic impulses. Autonomic control allows distribution of blood flow to major regions of the body.

Factors altering autonomic control of blood flow are:

- body temperature
- exercise
- changes in blood volume.

Blood pressure

Arterial pressure is the product of cardiac output and vascular resistance. Thus, either a change in cardiac output or a change in vascular resistance will alter blood pressure.

Normal regulation of blood pressure

The mechanisms involved are:

1. Neural control of vasoconstriction and contractility.

2. Capillary fluid shift mechanism altering blood volume.

3. Renal excretory and hormonal mechanisms which alter blood volume and vasoconstriction.

HEART RATE AND CONTRACTILITY

- Increased sympathetic stimulation = increased heart rate + increased force of contraction.

- Decreased sympathetic stimulation = decreased heart rate + decreased force of contraction.

- Increased parasympathetic stimulation = decreased heart rate + decreased force of contraction.

VASOMOTOR TONE

- Increased sympathetic activity = vasoconstriction. The decrease in arteriolar diameter and the venous reservoir will initially venous return and blood pressure.

- Decreased sympathetic activity = vasodilatation. The increase in arteriolar diameter and the venous reservoir will decrease venous return and blood pressure.

Neural control

The vasomotor centre in the brainstem controls vasomotor tone and heart rate via the sympathetic and parasympathetic nervous systems. Vasomotor tone is primarily controlled by sympathetic nervous outflow. Heart rate and contractility are controlled by the balance of sympathetic and parasympathetic stimulation and inhibition. The vagus nerve is the primary parasympathetic pathway; stimulation will reduce heart rate and decrease contractility. Sympathetic stimulation increases heart rate and the force of contractility.

The *baroreceptor system* consists of receptors that are sensitive to the degree of stretch exerted by pressure in the arteries. These receptors are situated in the aortic arch and carotid sinuses. They transmit impulses that increase in rate as the blood pressure rises. These impulses inhibit sympathetic outflow from the vasomotor centre so heart rate and contractility as well as vasomotor tone are reduced. If the blood pressure falls, the baroreceptors are stimulated less, thus impulses decrease. The vasomotor centre loses its inhibition and increases sympathetic signals to the heart and vessels.

Capillary fluid shift mechanism

This is a longer-term mechanism for regulation of blood pressure which is particularly important when blood volume tends to become either too low or too high. Increased circulating blood volume will raise systemic pressure and hydrostatic pressure within the capillaries. This will increase the shift of fluid across capillary membranes into the interstitial space.

A decrease in circulating blood volume will lower capillary hydrostatic pressure and allow the oncotic pressure exerted by plasma proteins to pull fluid by osmosis from the interstitial space into the capillaries. This response takes between 10 min and several hours to readjust the arterial pressure back towards normal.

Renal excretory and hormonal mechanisms

The kidneys play an important role in the long-term control of blood pressure and circulatory volume. Formation of urine by the kidneys is regulated by pressure in the renal arteries. A fall in blood pressure will produce a fall in renal artery blood flow, which will decrease or stop the formation of urine. Alternatively, a rise in blood pressure will produce an increased urine output.

A secondary hormonal mechanism—the renin–angiotensin system (described fully in Chapter 9)—will respond to falls in blood pressure that reduce renal perfusion. Angiotensin II, a hormone produced by this mechanism, is a potent vasoconstrictor that increases blood pressure. It also stimulates the adrenal cortex to secrete aldosterone which acts on the distal tubules and collecting ducts of the kidney to increase reabsorption of sodium and water. This results in an increase in circulating volume, which will increase blood pressure.

The vasomotor centre can be stimulated by higher cerebral centres. The limbic system and hypothalamus are thought to mediate emotionally induced alterations in blood pressure such as vasovagal collapse brought on by bad news. The midbrain is thought to mediate the initial hypertension associated with severe pain and the later fall in blood pressure following prolonged severe pain.

An elevated intracranial pressure can produce reflex increases in arterial blood pressure due to medullary hypercapnia and hypoxia. The increase in arterial pressure increases medullary perfusion thus potentially reducing the hypercapnia and hypoxia by increasing minute ventilation.

Diagnostic and investigative procedures

Electrocardiography is discussed in detail in Chapter 5. Other relevant procedures are detailed here.

Echocardiography

Ultrasound waves emitted in pulses by a probe directed at the heart are reflected back to the probe off the different surfaces and interfaces within the heart. A composite picture of these 'echoes' is built up and rebuilt multiple times per second producing a structural representation of the heart in motion, either in one dimension ('M mode' echo) or two (2D echo). As these can be viewed in real-time, movement of the atrial and ventricular walls and opening and closing of the valve leaflets through the cardiac cycle can be imaged.

More sophisticated echocardiography machines have a Doppler ultrasound facility incorporated to measure the degree and direction of blood flow within the heart. This is particularly useful for assessing and quantifying valvular regurgitation and stenosis and septal defects non-invasively. The cardiac output can also be measured by Doppler echocardiography, using the Doppler ultrasound to measure blood flow velocity through either mitral or aortic valves, and the echocardiographic image to measure the valvular cross-sectional area.

The probe can be placed on the skin surface ('transthoracic') in various locations such as the parasternal, apical (over the apex of the heart), or epigastric regions. The patient can either be resting supine or rolled onto his/her left-hand side. These changes in posture and probe site help to facilitate the view of a particular region of the heart. Signal acquisition is improved by smearing a conducting gel over the probe tip.

As ultrasound travels poorly through air, patients with hyperinflated lungs (e.g. emphysema) or after sternal opening (e.g. post-cardiac surgery) may be difficult to image. Likewise, patients with a thick chest wall may prove awkward to image. Use of trans-oesophageal echocardiography overcomes these problems as high-quality signals are obtained from behind the heart with minimal artefact. This technique can be performed in conscious, sedated patients but is also being used successfully in mechanically ventilated patients in the operating theatre and ICU environments. However, these probes are very expensive and require considerable expertise to use.

Uses of echocardiography

1. *Pericardial disease.* A pericardial effusion or haemopericardium can be imaged and drained. Constrictive pericarditis can also be diagnosed, e.g. as seen in tuberculosis.

2. *Myocardial disease:*

   ◆ *Wall motion abnormalities.* Lack of movement (akinesia) of a region of ventricle during systole indicates infarction or ischaemia, though the latter is often temporary. Reduced (hypokinetic) or abnormal (dyskinetic) movement of a ventricular segment may also be seen with ischaemia. Paradoxical movement of a region (i.e. in the wrong direction during systole) indicates a ventricular aneurysm.

♦ *Wall thickness.* Hypertrophy can be diagnosed.

3. *Chamber size.* The size of the four heart chambers can be estimated and dilatation or underfilling diagnosed. This can be used for therapeutic assessment of drugs and other therapies such as PEEP. The left and right ventricular ejection fraction, i.e. (end diastolic volume – end systolic volume)/(end diastolic volume), can also be calculated as a guide to contractility.

4. *Valvular defects.* Valvular stenosis and regurgitation can be diagnosed by characteristic movement of the valves and by the appearance of abnormal flow jets using colour-flow Doppler. The latter technique can also be used to quantify the pressure gradient across stenotic or regurgitant valves.

5. *Septal and congenital defects.* Atrial and ventricular septal defects, either congenital or acquired (e.g. post-infarction) can be readily imaged. The colour-flow facility, and/or injection of microbubbles or radiocontrast, enables the operator to determine whether a left-to-right or a right-to-left shunt exists, and its significance.

6. *Cardiac output estimation.*

7. *Thrombi, vegetations, pulmonary emboli, and neoplasms.* Although a negative result does not exclude the presence of either intramural thrombi or valvular vegetations, echocardiography is a very useful diagnostic technique, especially for larger lesions. The trans-oesophageal approach is superior in view of the better picture quality obtained. Atrial myxomas can also be readily imaged by this technique. A large pulmonary embolus cannot be directly imaged but its presence is suggested by marked right ventricular strain and left ventricular under-filling.

8. *Aortic aneurysm.* The trans-oesophageal approach is well suited for imaging the aortic root, arch, and descending thoracic aorta for the presence of an aneurysm.

Other diagnostic techniques

Electrocardiography and echocardiography can be performed at the bedside of a critically ill patient whereas other imaging techniques require transfer of the patient to an appropriate facility. As a consequence, other techniques are performed infrequently and used only occasionally in the critically ill patient for diagnostic purposes.

Nuclear scans

Radionuclide ventriculography involves the injection of ^{99}Tc-labelled blood (or albumin). A gamma camera is placed over the heart and counts the amount of radioactivity emitted by the technetium in the heart chambers at different points in the cardiac cycle. This is achieved by connection ('gating') to an electrocardiogram and is known colloquially as a 'MUGA' scan (multiple gated analysis). The difference in counts at the end of diastole and systole can be used to determine the ejection fraction of both left and right ventricles. Regional wall motion abnormalities can also be detected.

Regional myocardial perfusion can be assessed by injection of ^{201}Tl, which is taken up into the muscle. Non-perfused areas of muscle produce a defect on the subsequent scan. This can be permanent after an infarction, or transient in the case of ischaemia, which can be produced by exercise, or infusion of dipyridamole or dobutamine.

Technetium pyrophosphate is also not taken up by normal myocardium and can be used as a diagnostic tool for myocardial infarction when either the ECG or cardiac enzyme results are inconclusive, not available, or non-interpretable.

Angiography

Cardiac catheterization involves insertion of a catheter through either a vein into the right heart (see pulmonary artery catheterization in Chapter 5) or via an artery (usually brachial or femoral) into the left heart under fluoroscopy (X-ray imaging). The latter is usually performed in a specialized laboratory and enables a number of investigations and procedures:

1. Visualization of the coronary arteries by placement of the catheter into the individual coronary artery orifices followed by injection of a radiopaque dye, the path of which is recorded on to cinefilm. The patency of the vessels (including previous bypass grafts) and the degree of collateral flow can be determined.

2. Assessment of the degree of stenosis or regurgitation of a damaged valve with quantification of the pressure gradient across the valve.

3. Angioplasty ± stent insertion, or valvuloplasty (i.e. dilatation of an artery or a stenosed valve) can be performed by inflation of a balloon sited near the tip of the catheter. More recent techniques include recannulation of a stenosed artery by laser.

4. Diagnosis of a dissecting aortic aneurysm.

5. Diagnosis and assessment of intracardiac pressures, ejection fraction, congenital heart disease, shunts, etc., as well as the ability to perform an endomyocardial biopsy (e.g. cardiomyopathy, histological evidence of rejection of transplanted heart).

6. Sampling of blood for measure of oxygen saturation within the different heart chambers (used in diagnosis and quantification of intracardiac shunts).

As with any invasive procedure, cardiac catheterization does carry a recognized morbidity and mortality, including the potential to arrhythmias, thromboembolism, vessel dissection, and infection.

Pacing

Pacing refers to the technique of stimulating a myocardial contraction using a small current electrical energy delivered to the heart. Pacing may be either *temporary* or *permanent*:

◆ temporary pacing utilizes a pulse generator external to the body;

◆ permanent pacing utilizes an implanted pulse generator.

There are two types of pacing electrode:

1. *Unipolar* has only one conducting wire and electrode. Electrical current returns to the pacemaker via body fluids. These are used with permanent pacing systems.

2. *Bipolar* has two conducting wires and two electrodes. The impulse passes down one wire to (usually) the distal electrode. The circuit is then completed via the second electrode and wire back to the pacemaker.

Pacing routes

Transvenous endocardial

The wire passes down a vein (usually the subclavian) to the endocardial surface of the septal region of the right ventricle. It is a bipolar electrode wire to which an inflatable balloon may be incorporated to aid flotation of the catheter during 'blind' placement. Placement of pacing wires without balloons is usually carried out under X-ray imaging (fluoroscopy). The wire is advanced through the right atrium into the right ventricle where it is positioned against the ventricular septal wall. Positioning is confirmed using ECG monitoring. Right atrial stimulation produces large P waves and right ventricular stimulation produces large, widened QRS complexes occurring at the rate set on the pacing box. A pacing spike (a deflection of the ECG

trace) is seen prior to each stimulated complex. The voltage threshold should then be checked for good electrode placement suggested by a threshold of less than 0.5 V (see later).

Epicardial

Electrodes are sutured on the pericardial surface of the heart during cardiac surgery (see Chapter 8). One or two epicardial electrodes may be used. If only one is used, a skin surface electrode is used to complete the circuit.

External (transcutaneous)

Large surface area, adhesive skin electrodes are placed on the patient's chest and back. Three ECG electrodes are connected from the external pacer to the usual positions on the patient's chest. Current is passed between the skin electrodes inducing a paced heartbeat (see Chapter 7). This is the method of choice in an emergency as it is rapidly placed and effective, requiring little operator skill.

Trans-oesophageal

A difficult and unreliable method of pacing in an emergency, using an electrode placed in the patient's oesophagus.

Modes of pacing

Most temporary pacemakers are only capable of single-chamber demand or fixed-rate pacing. More advanced models have the ability to synchronize pacing in dual chambers.

Fixed rate

The heart is stimulated at a fixed rate per minute and will not alter in response to any intrinsic activity. This is rarely used unless there is no evidence of any underlying rhythm as arrhythmias may result if the pacing beat occurs close to the patient's intrinsic beat.

Demand

An impulse is initiated if a pre-set interval elapses without an intrinsic stimulation of the ventricle. The interval is determined by the rate at which the pacemaker is set. For example, a setting of 60 bpm on the pacemaker will only initiate pacing if the patient's own rate falls below 60 bpm.

Synchronous

Electrodes placed in both the right atria and ventricle will allow synchronization of the stimulus in both cardiac chambers. For example, a sensing electrode in the atria will sense an atrial contraction and stimulate a ventricular beat via a pacing electrode sited in the ven-

THE INTERSOCIETY COMMISSION FOR HEART DISEASE (ICHD) PACEMAKER CODE

Chamber(s) paced (I):

0 = none

A = atrium

V = ventricle

D = dual (atria and ventricle)

Chamber(s) sensed (II):

0 = none

A = atrium

V = ventricle

D = dual (atria and ventricle)

Mode of responses (III):

0 = none

T = triggered

I = inhibited

D = dual (triggered and inhibited)

Note: Other categories for programmable and anti-tachycardia functions are available but are not relevant for temporary pacing in the ICU.

TABLE 6.7 Types of pacing

Type of pacing	Indications
Ventricular demand (VVI)	Emergency situations: life-threatening bradycardias
AV sequential (DVI)	Impaired AV conduction with atrial bradycardia
Atrial synchronous ventricular inhibited (VDD)	Normal sinus rhythm with impaired AV conduction
AV universal (DDD)	Different functions according to underlying problem

Overdrive pacing for terminating tachycardias

Pacing at rates of 10–15 beats above the spontaneous rate may suppress ventricular or atrial arrhythmias. Arrhythmias suitable for overdrive pacing are paroxysmal supraventricular tachycardias, atrial flutter, and ventricular tachycardia. However, it is not effective in slowing sinus tachycardia or atrial fibrillation.

Care of the patient with a pacemaker

Electrical safety

The pacing wire provides a direct efficient conduction route for electrical current into the heart. This is a particular problem with older forms of temporary pacing generator. Therefore, contact with any poorly insulated source of electrical current could prove dangerous to the patient. Any connections between pacemaker and pacing wire should be securely fixed and if necessary protected with gauze or tape.

Monitoring

In the acute setting, the patient with temporary pacing should be monitored in the ECG lead which gives the clearest picture. The paced rhythm can be clearly seen as a 'spike' either negatively or positively on the ECG. Any failure in pacing will cause an absence of the spike or a spike without a following QRS complex. Note that battery failure can be a cause of loss of pacing. Pacing box batteries should always be checked prior to use and if failure is suspected.

Failure to capture

Absence of a QRS complex following a spike is known as 'failure to capture' and can be due to an increase in threshold (see below) or displacement of the pacing electrode. An increase in delivered current may overcome an increase in threshold, or the pacing wire may have to be re-sited or replaced.

tricle. This allows atrial contraction to fulfil its role of optimally filling the ventricle.

AV sequential

Stimulation of both atria and ventricles can be accomplished when necessary with a set interval between atrial and ventricular stimulation. This allows optimization of atrial filling for ventricular contraction.

Fixed-rate pacing would be designated V00 or A00 under the ICHD code because the atria or the ventricle is the chamber paced but there is no sensing in either chamber and therefore no response to sensing.

Ventricular demand pacing would be designated VVI because the ventricle is the paced chamber, the ventricle is the sensed chamber and the pacemaker is inhibited by the sensed beat.

Atrial synchronized pacing would be designated VAT because the ventricle is the paced chamber, the atria is the sensed chamber and the ventricular pacemaker is triggered by the sensed atrial beat (P wave) (see Table 6.7 for types of pacing).

Pacing threshold

This is the minimum level of current required to consistently pace the heart. This is measured when the pacemaker is first attached and should be <1.0 mA (milliampere). It should then be checked daily or if there is a change in monitored rhythm. Ideally, the pacemaker current should be set at 2–3 mA above the threshold to allow for minor variations and the usual increase in threshold level that occurs over a period of days after pacing is initiated. The threshold increase is thought to be due to fibrosis at the electrode tip.

Patient assessment

Assessment of the ICU patient with a cardiac disorder is achieved by using information derived from a variety of sources. These include:

- history
- physical assessment
- ECG
- non-invasive and invasive monitoring
- serum biochemical and haematological tests
- chest X-ray
- other diagnostic tests (e.g. echocardiogram, angiography; see earlier).

History

Details should include: type of pain, length of history, precipitating factors, relieving factors, social history (smoking, alcohol, drugs, etc.), and any relevant family history.

Physical assessment

Full details of physical assessment are given in Chapters 4 and 5. Table 6.8 gives observations that are particularly important in the patient with a cardiac disorder.

The assessment of pain can be an important diagnostic tool and may help differentiate pain of cardiac origin from that of respiratory, oesophageal, or musculoskeletal disorders.

Characteristic descriptions of chest pain

Stable angina

Typically constricting, retrosternal pain, radiating to the arms (predominantly the left), neck, or jaw. It often occurs in response to stimuli that increase the oxygen demand of the heart (e.g. physical exertion or emotion) and is relieved by resting.

Unstable angina

As in stable angina but the periods of pain are prolonged, may occur at rest, and have no precipitating factors.

Myocardial infarction

Typically severe, crushing, retrosternal pain which may extend to the arms, neck, jaw, or back and often lasts >30 min. It is often accompanied by nausea, vomiting, and sweating. The onset of pain is not always associated with exertion and is not relieved by rest. Some patients, however, may have little or no pain, especially the elderly and diabetics.

Pericarditis

The pain is usually sharp and retrosternal and may be more apparent on inspiration. It is often worse when lying flat but is relieved when sitting up and leaning forward.

Pleuritic pain

This is usually a sharp, localized pain, worse on inspiration and coughing.

Pulmonary embolism

The pain is usually pleuritic in nature and may be associated with haemoptysis and breathlessness.

Oesophageal pain

Oesophageal pain is usually associated with, or eased by, food, and typically worse when lying flat. It may also be relieved by nitrates. Oesophageal rupture is usually preceded by vomiting.

TABLE 6.8 Physical assessment in the patient with a cardiac disorder

	Observation	Note particularly if:
Skin	Colour, touch	Pale, cyanosed, mottled, cold, clammy, hot, presence of ankle oedema
Respiration	Rate, depth	Tachypnoeic, dyspnoeic, using accessory muscles, orthopnoeic (breathless lying flat)
Pulse	Feel, rate	Thready, full volume, bounding tachycardia, irregular
Pain	Site, duration, severity	Associated with movement, respiration, at rest, position, eating
Other		Oliguria, nausea, vomiting, presence of cough possibly due to pulmonary oedema. Anxious, restless

Aortic dissection

The patient experiences a 'tearing' pain (as opposed to the crushing pain of myocardial infarction). This pain is typically felt in the back.

Musculoskeletal pain

Pain due to spinal or muscular disorders can usually be identified by the effect of movement and position. Unlike the other conditions, the chest wall is tender to touch at the specific location.

ECG: 12-lead and continuous monitoring

When making a diagnosis the 12-lead ECG must be viewed in conjunction with the patient's history, physical examination, and the results of blood tests. If the ECG shows unequivocal changes then it can be extremely valuable, particularly in confirming a diagnosis of myocardial infarction.

Non-invasive and invasive monitoring

Full details of non-invasive and invasive monitoring are given in Chapter 5. The extent of monitoring will depend on the patient's condition. Increasingly complex regimens (e.g. for the treatment of cardiogenic shock) will require an increased complexity of monitoring.

Treatment strategies should be guided by data gained from invasive monitoring and used in conjunction with the assessment of physical signs (e.g. cool peripheries, pallor, confusion), biochemical tests, chest X-ray, and urine output.

Serum biochemical and haematological tests

Routine blood tests will include:

♦ cardiac enzymes,

♦ urea and electrolytes,

♦ haemoglobin,

♦ glucose,

♦ clotting studies (usually only if anticoagulant therapy has been administered),

♦ cholesterol and triglyceride levels.

Other biochemical and haematological tests:

♦ arterial blood gas analysis will be indicated if acidosis or hypoxaemia are suspected,

♦ other specific tests that may be indicated (e.g. digoxin levels).

Chest X-ray

Usually taken on admission and thereafter according to the patient's condition. It provides valuable information on heart size, the presence of pulmonary oedema, and aortic dissection.

Priorities of care

The main function of the cardiovascular system is to maintain tissue perfusion in order to deliver an adequate supply of oxygen and nutrients, and to remove carbon dioxide and other waste substances. The priority in caring for any critically ill patient is to support the ability of the cardiovascular system to carry out its functions:

♦ support and maintenance of tissue perfusion and oxygenation

♦ prevention or early detection of arrhythmias.

Adequate monitoring is essential to allow assessment of cardiac function. This should include a minimum of ECG monitoring and arterial blood pressure monitoring (preferably continuous). Central venous pressure, pulmonary artery pressure, and mixed venous oxygen saturation monitoring may also be indicated. Urine output will provide a guide to renal perfusion.

Emergency equipment should be available (see Chapter 3) and familiarity with the use of defibrillators and external pacing systems is imperative (see Chapter 7).

Oxygenation and oxygen transport

Any patient with a compromised cardiovascular system may have impaired tissue perfusion and will require increased levels of tissue oxygenation. This will attempt to redress the oxygen deficit induced when oxygen transport is limited by cardiovascular function or impaired tissue perfusion. Ensuring that tissues are well supplied with oxygen should be a target for treatment in the critically ill in order to prevent tissue hypoxia and subsequent organ dysfunction and failure.

Oxygen delivery

This is the amount of oxygen delivered to the tissues by the blood and depends on the blood flow and the amount of oxygen carried in the blood. Blood flow to the tissues is measured by the cardiac output while the amount of oxygen carried in the blood is determined by the haemoglobin concentration and oxygen saturation Therefore, if cardiac output, arterial oxygen saturation and haemoglobin level are known, the delivery of blood to the tissues can be calculated:

Oxygen delivery $(DO_2) = CO \times (1.34 \times Hb \times S_aO_2) \times 10$

where CO is cardiac output (l/min), 1.34 ml of O_2 carried by 1 g Hb, Hb is the haemoglobin content of the blood (g/100 ml), S_aO_2 is the % saturation of arterial Hb, and the factor 10 is used to convert ml of O_2 per 100 ml blood to ml/l. Normal DO_2 for the resting adult is approximately 1000 ml/min.

When oxygen has been extracted from the blood by the tissues there remains an oxygen reserve in the venous blood. If the demand for oxygen by the tissues increases, the venous oxygen reserve may decrease if the oxygen supply does not improve to meet the increased demand.

Oxygen consumption

This is the amount of oxygen used by the tissues over one minute (VO_2). It can be calculated by measuring the arteriovenous oxygen difference (i.e. the difference in oxygen content between arterial and venous blood). Blood taken from the pulmonary artery is considered true mixed venous blood and the percentage oxygen saturation of this blood is termed the mixed venous oxygen saturation (S_vO_2). Venous blood is aspirated from the pulmonary artery and a sample is taken from an arterial line. The oxygen saturation of both are measured in a co-oximeter. This can then be used to calculate the oxygen extraction ratio (O_2ER), which is the amount of oxygen extracted by the peripheral tissues divided by the amount of oxygen delivered:

$$O_2ER = \frac{\text{arterial} - \text{venous } O_2 \text{ saturation}}{\text{arterial } O_2 \text{ saturation}}$$

The normal value in an adult is about 25%.

Factors increasing the O_2 extraction ratio are:

- decreased cardiac output,
- increased oxygen consumption (not compensated by improved oxygen delivery,
- anaemia,
- decreased arterial oxygenation.

The venous oxygen reserve is the oxygen content in the venous blood over 1 min:

Venous oxygen reserve $= CO \times (1.34 \times Hb \times S_vO_2) \times 10$

Oxygen consumption = oxygen delivery – venous oxygen reserve.

The normal range in an adult is 225—275 ml/min.

DO_2 and VO_2 can be adjusted for the patient's size by dividing by the body surface area to produce the oxygen delivery index (DO_2I) and the oxygen consumption index (VO_2I). The normal range for the oxygen consumption index is 125–165 ml O_2/m^2.

Methods of increasing oxygen delivery

Physiological responses

When the body's requirement for oxygen increases (e.g. during exercise), this need stimulates mechanisms in the respiratory and circulatory systems that will effectively increase oxygen delivery to the tissues.

In the *respiratory system* respiratory effort is increased to augment oxygen intake and CO_2 elimination. In the *circulatory system*:

- venous return is increased (and thus preload),
- heart rate is increased (due to adrenergic stimulation),

TABLE 6.9	Interventions to improve oxygen delivery		
System	**Manipulation**	**Rationale**	**Intervention**
Cardiovascular	Optimize preload. Reduce afterload (if possible). Increase contractility Increase heart rate (if bradycardic)	Blood flow to the tissues will be increased	Serial fluid challenges until no further increase in SV (Starling curve). Reduce afterload (e.g. with nitrates) to normalize SVR. Inotropes to increase cardiac output (e.g. dobutamine, dopexamine, epinephrine)
Blood	Maintain Hb level within normal limits	The oxygen carrying capacity of the blood will be maximized	Transfuse to keep Hb above a certain threshold e.g. 8 g/dl
Respiratory	Maintain arterial oxygen saturation >95%. Respiratory support if patient is fatigued or hypoxaemic	The blood reaching the tissues will be adequately oxygenated. The work of breathing may in itself increase oxygen demand	Increase inspired oxygen to maintain S_aO_2. Hyperoxygenate prior to suction procedures if necessary

♦ contractility is increased (due to adrenergic stimulation).

All of these mechanisms serve to increase cardiac output.

Clinical interventions

Critically ill patients are often unable to increase oxygen delivery sufficiently by their own physiological mechanisms. If delivery does not match consumption, specific cardiovascular and respiratory interventions (see Table 6.9) can be instituted. The technique of measuring oxygen transport is given in Chapter 5.

When oxygen transport is limited by cardiac output (e.g. cardiogenic shock), oxygen consumption by the tissues is maintained by increased oxygen extraction from the blood. The normal S_vO_2 is 70–75% but if increased oxygen extraction occurs, it may drop well below 50%. An $S_vO_2 < 40\%$ is associated with a serious disturbance in the oxygen supply–demand relationship.

General principles of care

Hypotension

There is no level of blood pressure that can define hypotension as this depends on the clinical condition of the patient and their pre-morbid state (e.g. history of chronic hypertension). However, a patient is usually considered to be hypotensive when the MAP falls below 60 mmHg or is associated with clinical symptoms of organ hypoperfusion and a MAP 40 mmHg or more below usual values. It is important to note that impaired organ perfusion can still be present despite a normal or elevated blood pressure.

The aims of treatment of hypotension should to:

♦ establish and treat the cause,

♦ maintain tissue oxygenation where appropriate by increasing cardiac output, haemoglobin, and/or arterial oxygen saturation,

♦ maintain tissue perfusion pressures by increasing the systemic blood pressure.

Ensure that the blood pressure recording is correct. If a cuff is being used, confirm it is the right size and correctly applied to the arm. Repeat the measurement. If an arterial line is being transduced, check for damping of the trace (e.g. air bubbles in the circuit), kinking (e.g. wrist movements), the position of the transducer relative to the left atrium, and that it is zeroed correctly. If doubt exists regarding transducer accuracy, confirm a low reading by a cuff measurement.

CAUSES OF HYPOTENSION:

♦ Hypovolaemia.

♦ Cardiogenic causes: cardiac failure; tachy/brady arrhythmias; valvular stenosis/incompetence.

♦ Obstructive causes: cardiac tamponade; pulmonary embolism; tension pneumothorax.

♦ Sepsis/inflammation.

♦ Anaphylactic reactions.

MANIFESTATIONS OF ORGAN HYPOPERFUSION:

♦ Kidneys: oliguria.

♦ Skin: pallor, cool peripheries.

♦ Brain: confusion, drowsiness, agitation, syncope.

♦ Metabolic acidosis.

♦ Compensatory tachycardia.

Treatment strategies and choice of drugs may vary amongst different intensive care units and will be influenced by the methods of monitoring that are available. However, the underlying principles of managing hypotension will be the same.

Blood pressure should be restored by one or more of the following:

♦ Ensuring circulating volume is adequate before positive inotropic drugs are used.

♦ Administering inotropic drugs to attain adequate cardiac output and organ perfusion.

♦ Administering vasopressor drugs, rather than inotropes, in the hypotensive patient with a high cardiac

HYPOVOLAEMIA CAN BE CAUSED BY:

♦ Haemorrhage (e.g. trauma, dissecting/ruptured aortic aneurysm, bleeding ulcers).

♦ Fluid loss (e.g. vomiting, diarrhoea, burns).

♦ Pooling of fluid in extravascular spaces (e.g. increased capillary permeability secondary to an insult, ileus following bowel surgery.

♦ Inadequate fluid input.

♦ Relative vasodilatation and loss of peripheral vascular tone.

output and low systemic vascular resistance (e.g. sepsis, anaphylaxis).

♦ Specific treatment where appropriate (e.g. drainage of a tension pneumothorax).

Hypovolaemia as a cause of hypotension
Management of hypovolaemia

The underlying cause must be identified and treated. The usual cardiovascular pointers in the hypovolaemic patient are tachycardia, hypotension, oliguria, decreased cardiac output, and a high SVR. However, the young, fit patient can compensate by increased vasoconstriction and can often maintain a normal blood pressure until the hypovolaemia is well advanced. It is therefore important not to rely solely on blood pressure as an indicator of shock.

Immediate treatment is by rapid administration of fluid guided by monitored haemodynamic variables. If there is no stroke volume measuring technique *in situ*, intravascular fluid status can be guided by CVP measurements. Fluid challenges should be repeated until the CVP rises by ≥3 mmHg 5–10 min after the challenge has been completed. If the CVP rises ≥3 mmHg and MAP remains <60 mmHg in the presence of oliguria then cardiac output monitoring may provide additional valuable information. No response in stroke volume to a fluid challenge—in the absence of continued bleeding—suggests that vasoactive drugs such as inotropes will be necessary. Heart rate, blood pressure, urine output, and level of consciousness/orientation can also provide a guide to improvement in organ perfusion.

The fluid used to restore intravascular volume is partly related to custom; however, blood will be needed if the Hb level drops too low and clotting products such as fresh frozen plasma will be needed for severe coagulopathy. No overall difference has been found between crystalloid and colloid, or between different types of colloid. Millilitre for millilitre, colloid has a quicker and longer-lasting effect than crystalloid but high volumes may induce a coagulopathy. If hypovolaemia is due to major haemorrhage, fluid should be given until cross-matched blood is available. Group-specific or O rhesus-negative blood should be used if haemorrhage is particularly severe. Fluids should be administered rapidly, under pressure if necessary, and continued until organ perfusion and blood pressure are maintained at adequate values.

If hypovolaemic hypotension is due to excessive fluid loss from vomiting, large nasogastric aspirates, diarrhoea, or pooling of extravascular fluid, colloid or crystalloid can be given rapidly as a series of fluid challenges. Blood pressure, urine output ± stroke volume ± CVP ± PAWP should be checked after each challenge. If the CVP, PAWP, and BP remain unchanged and the stroke volume (if measured) continues to rise, fluid challenges should be given repeatedly until adequate pressures and organ perfusion are achieved. Adequate organ perfusion is sometimes achieved at surprisingly low blood pressures. Following resuscitation, the hourly fluid requirements of the patient should be reviewed and a crystalloid solution, such as 0.9% sodium chloride, may need to be given or increased to replace fluid losses.

Cardiogenic causes of hypotension

These include arrhythmias (e.g. tachyarrhythmias, heart block), myocardial pump failure, intracardiac shunts, and valvular dysfunction. If hypotension is secondary to a tachy- or bradyarrhythmia, the arrhythmia must be treated to restore the circulation.

Cardiogenic shock results from failure of the heart to maintain adequate organ perfusion (see later for full details). Such patients will require intensive monitoring and complex treatment strategies. The initial treatment for cardiogenic hypotension is with inotropes to restore an adequate perfusion pressure. However, fluid challenges should also be considered as hypovolaemia often coexists.

Treatment of the severely hypotensive patient should not be withheld while a pulmonary artery catheter or other monitoring is being inserted. Empiric 'best guess' therapy may be needed in the interim. Dobutamine and epinephrine are inotropic drugs commonly given and dosages are titrated according to response. If systemic vascular resistance is high, a vasodilator (e.g. glyceryl trinitrate) may be infused and titrated according to changes in pressure, flow, organ perfusion, and symptomatic response. Reducing afterload is an important means of improving cardiac efficiency since peripheral resistance and hence left ventricular work is decreased. Cardiac over-distension should also be treated by decreasing venous return. Care must be taken to ensure that the intravascular volume is maintained while vasodilators are given, otherwise further hypotension may result.

Obstructive causes of hypotension

These include cardiac tamponade, pneumothorax, and pulmonary embolus. The cause must be identified and treated to restore blood pressure and organ perfusion (see also Chapters 4 and 13).

'Inflammatory' causes of hypotension

Infection, or other insults, such as burns, pancreatitis, and trauma, will stimulate a generalized inflammatory response resulting in loss of peripheral vascular tone and increased capillary leak. The resultant vasodilatation, relative hypovolaemia, loss of vascular tone ('hyporeactivity'), and, possibly, myocardial depression from circulating toxins and mediators may cause hypotension. More details on causes and management of inflammatory hypotension are given in Chapter 12.

The management of sepsis syndrome is aimed at identification of the source of infection, prescribing appropriate antibiotic therapy, and maintaining organ perfusion and tissue oxygenation. Monitoring of vital signs will usually show low central venous, pulmonary artery wedge, and systemic arterial pressures, a low SVR, tachycardia, pyrexia, and a high cardiac output. These represent a hyperdynamic circulation and are frequently, but not always, seen in such patients. The skin may feel hot to the touch and the patient may have a bounding pulse.

A minority of such patients may present with hypotension but are apyrexial with a low cardiac output. This may be due to pre-existing poor cardiac function or to inflammatory mediator-induced myocardial depression.

Fluid resuscitation is usually the first treatment. However, for severe hypotension, empiric therapy with epinephrine or norepinephrine may also be needed while adequate monitoring is being inserted, to rapidly restore a satisfactory perfusion pressure.

Fluid restoration has the aim of optimizing stroke volume. Large volumes may be required and infusion should continue until no further improvement in stroke volume is seen. Due to capillary leak, intravascular volume expansion may still be required, even if there is evidence of oedema. If respiratory function is severely compromised with coexisting ARDS it may be necessary to institute vasopressors at an earlier stage and to restrict the amount of fluid given.

If the patient remains hypotensive after fluid resuscitation, vasopressors will be required; high dosages are often necessary. Norepinephine (or high-dose dopamine) is the drug of choice as it is an effective vasoconstrictor. If myocardial dysfunction is present and afterload is raised, then epinephrine, dobutamine, or milrinone may be of benefit as they increase myocardial contractility. Care should be exercised with dobutamine, milrinone, and other phosphodiesterase inhibitors as they may cause excessive vasodilatation. The new agent levosimendan may also be beneficial as it acts by calcium sensitization, thereby increasing cardiac contractility without increasing cardiac work.

Anaphylaxis as a cause of hypotension

The acute reaction to an allergenic substance can cause severe hypotension or even cardiovascular collapse. Severe anaphylactic reactions may require full cardiorespiratory resuscitation. Allergenic substances (e.g. food, blood, drugs, insect stings) can result in degranulation of mast cells. These release histamine and other mediator substances that cause vasodilatation, smooth muscle constriction, and increased capillary permeability. Hypotension is caused by vasodilatation and loss of fluid from the capillaries resulting in a relative hypovolaemia.

Hypotension and tachycardia may be severe. There may be dyspnoea and cyanosis due to bronchospasm or laryngeal obstruction, skin flushing, urticarial rash, soft tissue swelling, nausea, vomiting, and diarrhoea.

Immediate treatment for anaphylactic hypotension is to provide respiratory support if required, epinephrine, and fluid infusion (often colloid). Epinephrine (0.5–1 mg) is given intramuscularly but may be given intravenously in situations where severe shock may impede absorption from muscle. Epinephrine should not be given subcutaneously for this reason. An intravenous infusion may also be necessary. Hydrocortisone 200 mg and chlorphenamine 10 mg are also given intravenously. Colloid should be given rapidly to correct hypovolaemia, ideally guided by stroke volume or CVP measurements. In their absence, treatment should be titrated against blood pressure, heart rate, urine output, and physical assessment.

The causative agent of the reaction should be identified in order to avoid re-exposure. If an anaphylactic reaction occurs during a transfusion of blood or blood products, the bag of fluid should be retained and sent back to the haematology department for analysis. A sample of the patient's blood should also be taken for subsequent analysis (see Chapter 14 for further details).

Summary of changes in haemodynamic parameters

Table 6.10 shows common changes seen in many patients, but they are by no means universal to all (Table 6.15 lists the drugs used for treating hypotension).

TABLE 6.10 Hypotension: haemodynamic parameters			
Cause of hypotension	CO	PAWP	SVR
Hypovolaemia	↓	↓	↑
Cardiogenic	↓	↑ or → ←	↑
Inflammatory	↑	↓	↓
Obstructive	↓	↑ or → ←	↑
Anaphylactic	↑	↓	↓↑

↑, increased; ↓, decreased; → ←, unchanged.

Hypertension

Hypertension can be defined as a sustained, raised BP above that which would be considered normal for the patient's age. The 'normal' BP is difficult to quantify because it is a statistical range of values based on the mean of the population, therefore the level of BP at which treatment should be started is not clear-cut. Before diagnosing a patient as chronically hypertensive, the BP must be recorded correctly, and be consistently elevated. Chronic antihypertensive therapy is generally begun if the resting diastolic blood pressure is consistently above 90–95 mmHg. However, acute treatment may be started at lower pressures for specific conditions such as dissecting aortic aneurysm to minimize the risk of further deterioration.

If the cause of the hypertension cannot be identified it is termed 'primary' (or 'essential') hypertension. If there is an identifiable cause it is termed secondary hypertension. Primary hypertension exists in 90–95% of patients with hypertension and is diagnosed by elimination of the identifiable causes of secondary hypertension. Hypertension may be a natural response to pain and stress and this will require the appropriate treatment (e.g. analgesia, anxiolysis).

Blood pressure is regulated by multiple endocrine, neuronal, humoral, renal, and other factors that moderate vasomotor and vasoconstrictor responses (see earlier). However, the mechanisms involved in causing primary hypertension remain complex and are not fully understood.

Vascular tone is important in maintaining blood pressure. If arterioles become narrowed due to an increase in vascular tone, there is an increase in peripheral vascular resistance. This increase in peripheral resistance causes hypertension. In the early stages this can be effectively reversed by vasodilator drugs. However, over time, the tunica media (the smooth muscle layer of the arterioles) becomes permanently hypertrophied due to the chronically raised pressure (medial hypertrophy). The effect of this is to narrow the lumen of the vessel, reducing blood flow to the tissue it supplies, and possibly resulting in ischaemic damage. Any of the body tissues can be affected but since a large proportion of cardiac output flows to brain, heart, and kidneys, these organs are particularly vulnerable in hypertension. Unfortunately, in chronic hypertension, patients are often asymptomatic until there is irreversible damage.

Management of an acute hypertensive crisis

If symptomatic (headaches, confusion, drowsiness, fits, agitation), the aim of treatment is to reduce BP urgently, yet smoothly, and not aiming for an excessive fall. A mean BP of approximately 120 mmHg may be an appropriate initial target, though the rate of fall depends on the underlying condition. It can be achieved over 2–3 hours for hypertensive encephalopathy, 6–12 hours for subarachnoid haemorrhage, and over days to weeks for strokes. Sudden drops in blood pressure should be avoided. If the cause of the hypertension is a raised ICP,

---

CAUSES OF SECONDARY HYPERTENSION

- Endocrine: phaeochromocytoma, Conn's syndrome (primary hyperaldosteronism), Cushing's syndrome, acromegaly

- Renal: chronic glomerulonephritis, chronic pyelonephritis, renal artery stenosis, polycystic disease, polyarteritis nodosa

- Pregnancy-induced

- Intracranial haemorrhage

- Coarctation of the aorta

- Drug-related (e.g. withdrawal of antihypertensive drugs, clonidine, monoamine oxidase inhibitors (MAOIs) antidepressants with tyramine-containing foods, e.g. cheese)

MANIFESTATIONS OF HYPERTENSION

- Neurological: headache, dizziness, transient ischaemic attacks, focal disturbances, confusion, fits, coma (hypertensive encephalopathy), strokes

- Cardiovascular: palpitations, left ventricular failure (causing pulmonary oedema), angina, myocardial infarction, retinopathy

- Renal: renal failure, proteinuria

- Other: retinopathy

DISORDERS THAT MAY CAUSE AN ACUTE HYPERTENSIVE CRISIS INCLUDE:

- Malignant hypertension

- Phaeochromocytoma

- Pre-eclampsia/eclampsia

- Any cause of raised intracranial pressure (ICP)

- Drug-related (withdrawal of clonidine, reaction of MAOIs with foods containing pressor amines)

the BP is usually allowed to remain high to maintain an adequate cerebral perfusion pressure.

Intravenous drug therapy is often required, and continuous BP monitoring is essential. The choice of hypotensive drug will depend on the cause of the hypertension and its urgency of treatment. Adequate pain relief should be confirmed. The most commonly used in the ICU are sodium nitroprusside, which produces a rapid effect and can be finely controlled, glyceryl trinitrate, labetalol, and hydralazine, which can all be given by infusion. The drug dosage should always be titrated against response. Nifedipine can be used, although sublingual administration has a variable absorption rate and a variable, often abrupt, hypotensive effect.

Hypertensive encephalopathy

This can be caused by uncontrolled hypertension from any cause. In addition to organ damage, it is characterized by neurological signs resulting from reduced cerebral blood flow. There may be areas of cerebral infarction, haemorrhage, or transient ischaemia. Symptoms are initially severe headaches and nausea but can progress to deteriorating level of consciousness, seizures, and coma. If the hypertension is treated early, changes may be reversible but mortality is high.

Malignant hypertension

Malignant hypertension is a distinct pathological condition where there is progressive severe hypertension (diastolic pressure may exceed 140 mmHg). Patients can develop severe organ damage such as renal failure, heart failure, retinal haemorrhages, papilloedema, and hypertensive encephalopathy. If untreated, mortality is 90% within 1 year of onset. Treatment is strict bed-rest and antihypertensive drugs (e.g. nitroprusside or labetalol) to reduce the blood pressure slowly but not excessively to a diastolic of 110–120 mmHg. Overaggressive reduction may result in poor perfusion and a stroke.

Acute coronary syndromes

These are syndromes usually associated with chest pain that are due to myocardial infarction or ischaemia.

Myocardial infarction

Myocardial infarction (MI) arises when a region of the myocardium becomes irreversibly necrosed. It is usually due to thromboembolic occlusion of the coronary artery supplying that area of heart muscle, although MI can occasionally follow direct trauma or electrocution. It is the commonest single cause of death (approximately 25–30% of all deaths, higher in males). Approximately 40% die before arrival in hospital and a further 5–10% will die while in hospital. Recent advances in care, notably the use of thrombolysis, have significantly improved outcomes. Numerous large-scale international multicentre trials are being continually undertaken to improve prognosis and function still further.

Risk factors for MI are well recognized, particularly smoking, hyperlipidaemia, and hypertension. Other factors include obesity, age, diabetes, family history, and geographical and environmental factors (Scotland, Northern Ireland, and Finland have a particularly high incidence, whereas Mediterranean countries have a low incidence). The incidence of MI has dropped considerably in the United States over the last two decades as a direct result of health education and primary prevention programmes.

Assessment

Physical assessment:

◆ *Pain.* Classically, the patient presents with crushing central chest pain, with or without radiation of pain down the left arm, neck, or jaw. Unless relieved by medication, the pain usually lasts more than 30 min and is not eased by posture or food. 'Silent' infarcts, that is, without chest pain are not infrequent, especially in elderly or diabetic populations, and the pain may occasionally be atypical (e.g. short-lived or epigastric in location).

◆ *Skin.* The patient may be sweating, pale, grey or cyanosed, and peripherally constricted.

◆ *Respiratory.* The patient may be tachypnoeic or dyspnoeic and there may be evidence of pulmonary oedema (see Chapter 4).

◆ *Other physical signs.* Nausea and vomiting may occur.

Psychological assessment:

◆ *Anxiety.* The patient usually appears distressed and anxious and may require considerable comfort and reassurance.

◆ *Confusion.* The patient may appear confused due to hypoxaemia or poor cerebral perfusion.

Physiological assessment:

◆ *Blood pressure.* May be normal, elevated, or depressed.

◆ *ECG monitoring.* May show tachycardia, and arrhythmias may occur.

◆ *Urine output.* May be oliguric due to poor renal perfusion.

◆ *Blood glucose.* May be raised due to sympathetic activity (see later).

Investigations

12-lead ECG

Depending on the time from onset of symptoms, a 12-lead ECG will initially show convex ST elevation and T wave inversion (implying injury and ischaemia) in the leads adjacent to the infarcted area. Leads opposite the area will show inverse changes (e.g. V1, V2 in posterior MI). Pathological Q waves will then develop, although this can vary from minutes to days. Approximately 20% of patients with subsequently proved infarction will present without ST elevation or clearly identifiable Q waves. Occasionally, no Q waves (non-Q wave infarction) or other electrocardiographic evidence will develop despite conclusive proof from other sources (e.g. rise in cardiac enzymes). Coexisting left bundle branch block may also obscure ECG signs of an acute MI. Serial ECGs and cardiac enzyme estimations should be taken over three days to confirm the occurrence of an acute MI and to show its evolution.

Cardiac enzymes

The myocardium releases enzymes into the blood as a consequence of cardiac injury and measurement of these can assist in the diagnosis of myocardial infarction. These enzymes peak at different times following the insult, but elevations are not synonymous with cardiac injury and a diagnosis of myocardial infarction must be made in conjunction with ECG changes and clinical findings.

The measurement of either cardiac troponin T or I is now considered the gold standard for the diagnosis of cardiac injury. Three further enzymes, creatine kinase (CK), aspartate transaminase (AST), and lactic dehydrogenase (LDH) are also measured; however, these are of variable specificity to cardiac muscle as they are also released from other damaged body tissues. Greater specificity can be obtained by measurement of the creatine kinase isoenzyme (CK-MB), which is only released from cardiac tissue and may clarify whether a cardiac event has occurred in the preceding 48 hours.

1. *Troponins*. Troponins are structural protein components of striated muscle. There are three types: troponin C, T, and I. Troponins T and I are found solely in cardiac muscle and are released following cardiac damage. They will not rise unless myocardial injury has occurred. Troponin I rises after 3–6 hours and peaks at about 20 hours. At 12 hours the sensitivity is generally good enough to exclude a myocardial infarct. Both troponins remain elevated for a much longer time than either CK, AST, or LDH. Troponin I is detectable in the blood for up to 5 days, and troponin T for 7–10 days following myocardial

infarction. This allows a myocardial infarction to be diagnosed, or excluded, in a patient who presents late with a history of chest pain.

Although elevations of troponins T and I are absolutely indicative of cardiac damage, this can also occur as a result of myocarditis, severe cardiac failure, cardiac trauma from surgery or road traffic accidents, sepsis, coronary artery spasm from cocaine, and pulmonary embolism. Both troponins T and I may also be elevated in patients with chronic renal failure and indicate a higher long-term risk of death. In this case, the levels are sustained rather than rising and falling as in myocardial infarction.

2. *Creatine kinase*. This is released up to 3 days post-infarction. Levels peak at 30–60 hours. Skeletal muscle is also rich in CK and false positive results may arise in patients who have had intramuscular injections, recent vigorous exercise, trauma, surgery, or rhabdomyolysis.

3. *Aspartate transaminase*. Released 1–3 days post-infarction. Levels peak at 24–48 hours. Diseases of the liver, brain, kidney, and lung may all give false positives.

4. *Lactate dehydrogenase*. Released 2–10 days post-infarction. Peak levels occur at 3 days. Red cells also contain LDH and any cause of haemolysis may produce false positive results.

Traditionally, cardiac enzymes are measured on admission and over the next 2 days (Fig. 6.7). An early rise in creatine kinase to diagnostic levels (more than twice the normal level) in the absence of other causes such as trauma is highly suggestive of MI. This rise may take up to 4–8 hours and, if early doubt persists, a repeat CK level should be performed within hours of the first measurement. The levels of cardiac enzymes

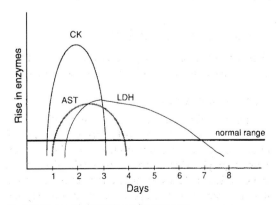

Fig. 6.7 Temporal change in cardiac enzymes.

CAUSES OF CENTRAL CHEST PAIN

- Angina
- Gastritis and peptic ulceration
- Pericarditis
- Pancreatitis
- Myocarditis
- Pneumonia
- Oesophagitis
- Pulmonary embolism
- Pleurisy
- Acute aortic dissection
- Chest wall—intercostalsmyalgia, costochondritis, pre-rash shingles

peak earlier, and are often higher, following successful thrombolytic therapy due to the 'washout' of enzymes from the infarcted area as reperfusion occurs.

A particular concern in making a correct diagnosis is with acute aortic dissection. In this situation, administration of thrombolysis is contraindicated as catastrophic bleeding may occur. A good history, in particular noting the duration, character and radiation of the pain, precipitating, temporal and relieving factors, and associated symptoms, in conjunction with a careful examination and appropriate investigations, may enable MI to be distinguished from other causes of chest pain. Sometimes, however, definitive diagnosis still proves difficult and the patient may receive treatment purely on a strong presumptive basis. Glyceryl trinitrate (GTN) may also relieve the pain of oesophageal spasm and therefore should not be considered diagnostic.

Priorities of care

Intervention should occur promptly while undertaking a rapid assessment of the patient, obtaining a brief but pertinent history, and performing appropriate assessment and investigations. The patient's cardiorespiratory status must be adequately evaluated and resuscitative measures commenced as appropriate. If diagnostic doubt exists more time may be spent before instituting certain steps (e.g. administration of thrombolysis):

- High-concentration, high-flow oxygen should be administered.
- Two to four puffs of GTN spray or one sublingual GTN tablet.
- An aspirin tablet (150 mg) should be chewed.

- Continuous ECG and pulse oximetry monitoring, regular BP recording.
- Wide-bore peripheral venous access.
- Intravenous opiate (e.g. diamorphine 2.5—5 mg) and anti-emetic if in pain or distress. The opiate dose should be repeated as necessary.
- Appropriate investigations (including 12-lead ECG, cardiac enzymes, potassium, glucose, lipids, and chest-X-ray).
- Thrombolytic agent (unless contraindicated) plus heparin (see later).
- A beta-blocker should be commenced (unless contra-indicated).
- Consider early angioplasty, particular in younger patients with anterior MI.
- Management of complications (cardiac arrest, pulmonary oedema, cardiogenic shock, life-threatening or haemodynamically compromising arrhythmias).
- Relief of patient anxiety and distress using skilled, competent care, and providing information appropriate to the situation is essential.
- Assist patient into a comfortable position and reduce effort and stress.

Principles of care

The patient should then be admitted to a high-dependency area, such as a coronary care unit (CCU), although admission to an intensive care unit may be warranted if complications are present. Thrombolysis should ideally not be delayed until the patient is transferred to a CCU. Indeed, some centres give pre-hospital thrombolysis while others admit patients directly to a chest pain unit to prevent unnecessary delays in diagnosis and treatment.

The patient without complications should be on strict bedrest with continuous ECG and regular BP monitoring for the first 24 hours. Both patient and family should be reassured and provided with information about rehabilitation and suggestions for lifestyle alteration. Blood glucose estimations should be performed regularly as an MI often results in glucose intolerance and hyperglycaemia. This will often settle over the following week, although may occasionally need either short- or long-term insulin or oral hypoglycaemic treatment. Euglycaemic control is important for improving outcome. Pyrexia is common for the first 2–3 days.

On day 2 the patient may be allowed to mobilize slowly. Discharge to a general ward often takes place after 1–2 days. Most hospitals have their own mobilization regimens with the patient being discharged at approximately 7 days, by which time he/she will have climbed a staircase and performed a treadmill test. After hospital discharge the patient will be advised to undertake a slowly increasing exercise regimen and will be followed up in cardiac rehabilitation classes and the out-patient clinic. Return to work is generally delayed for 2–6 months depending on the type of activity involved. Further investigations, such as angiography, may be indicated, particularly in a young person or if complications develop or the treadmill test is positive. Surgery or angioplasty may then be recommended if appropriate.

Therapies
Thrombolysis

As coronary thromboembolism is the predominant cause of myocardial infarction, administration of a thrombolytic agent to dissolve the clot will hopefully recanalize the occluded coronary artery and reperfuse the affected region of myocardium. If the area has fully infarcted then little can be achieved by thrombolysis. However, early administration may reverse, or at least minimize, the amount of permanently necrosed muscle. Large multicentre trials have conclusively shown mortality benefit. Ideally, the thrombolytic agent should be given as soon as possible, preferably within 4–6 hours of the onset of symptoms. However, treatment has been shown to be effective for up to 24 hours.

Two choices are available—either naturally occurring thrombolytics such as streptokinase (or occasionally urokinase), or agents produced by recombinant therapy, e.g. tissue plasminogen activator (rTPA). Although the latter agents are specific for newly formed clot and are less likely to cause allergic or anaphylactic reactions, they are considerably more expensive and have a much shorter half-life, necessitating the use of intravenous heparin for a few days to prevent reocclusion of the vessel.

Some centres consider rTPA or equivalents as first-line therapy in young patients (<45 years), in large anterior MI presenting early (<4 hours), and in cardiogenic shock. However, rTPA should not be used more than 6 hours after the onset of symptoms (except when streptokinase has been previously given), in patients over 75 years old (greater risk of cerebrovascular accidents), and in the absence of diagnostic ECG changes.

Little difference has been seen in terms of clinical benefit between the different fibrinolytic agents, although the GUSTO study (Global Utilization of Streptokinase and tPA for Occluded coronary arteries) suggested that an increased risk of stroke exists with rTPA (3–4/1000), especially in older and/or hypertensive patients. This may offset any mortality reduction advantage, thus the risk:benefit ratio should always be considered on an individual patient basis.

Contraindications to thrombolysis are shown in Table 6.11 and may either be absolute or relative. Thrombolysis may be given even when relative contraindications exist when the mortality risk from the MI (e.g. with associated hypotension) outweighs the risk of bleeding.

Arterial and/or central venous cannulation should not be delayed following commencement of thrombolysis if clinically indicated. Cannulation should be performed by an experienced operator, avoiding the subclavian route.

If considerable haemorrhage does occur from either attempted cannula insertion or other causes (e.g. peptic ulcer), this can often be reversed by stopping the infusion, giving fresh frozen plasma, and either (1) aprotinin 500 000 units over 10 min, then 200 000 units

---

CONTRAINDICATIONS TO THE USE OF STREPTOKINASE

- Previous reaction
- Previously treated with streptokinase within the previous 5 days to 54 months
- Recent streptococcal infection (<1 month)
- Imminent surgical or invasive procedure anticipated

TABLE 6.11	Contraindications to thrombolysis
Absolute contraindications	Active gastrointestinal bleeding
	Aortic dissection
	Neurosurgery/head injury/cerebrovascular accidents within 2 months
	Intracranial neoplasm/aneurysm
	Proliferative diabetic retinopathy
	Serious trauma, major surgery within 10 days
	Systolic BP >200 mmHg
Relative contraindications	Traumatic or prolonged CPR
	Recent obstetric delivery
	Prior organ biopsy
	Bleeding diathesis
	Recent puncture of major vessel

DRUG DOSES OF THROMBOLYTIC AGENTS

- Streptokinase: 1.5 million units in 100 ml 0.9% saline IV over 1 hour.

- rTPA: 100mg IV over 90 min (15 mg bolus, 50 mg/ 30 min, 35 mg/60 min).

over 4 hours; or (2) tranexamic acid 10 mg/kg repeated after 6–8 hours.

Revascularization arrhythmias are common following thrombolysis. Of these, over 90% are benign and do not require treatment. If these occur during infusion, temporary cessation may be all that is necessary. Allergic or anaphylactic reactions to streptokinase (e.g. hypotension and rash) are relatively rare and should be treated by stopping the infusion and giving hydrocortisone 200 mg IV, chlorpheniramine 10mg IV, and ranitidine 50 mg IV. The circulation should be supported if necessary with the aim of restarting thrombolytic therapy; rTPA may be given instead.

Aspirin/heparin

Unless there is a known contraindication, the patient should be given aspirin 150–325 mg once daily as soon as possible after MI, This should preferably be first given by the GP, ambulance personnel, or doctor who first sees the patient in the casualty department. Aspirin is given for its antiplatelet aggregation effect (see Table 6.12). Unless the patient has received a short-acting thrombolytic, such as rTPa, there is no added benefit to aspirin by giving heparin.

TABLE 6.12 Summary of benefits of therapy

Agent	Benefit at 1 month	Groups that particularly benefit
Aspirin	20–30 lives/1000	All suspected MI or unstable angina. Continue after hospital discharge.
Thrombolytic therapy	30+ lives/1000	All suspected MI with ST elevation or bundle branch block within 24 hours of onset (ideally within 4–6 hours).
ACE inhibitors	5 lives/1000 (10 lives/1000 high-risk groups)	Anterior or previous MI, or if developing heart failure. Start early, continue long-term
Heparin, magnesium, oral nitrates	Minimal	

Beta-blockers

The early large multicentre studies that pre-dated thrombolytic therapy concentrated on the effects of beta-blockers. Although benefit was shown, particularly when an early IV dose was given, and they proved generally safe, a major effect on outcome is not seen with mortality being reduced by only 1% (i.e. an extra one hospital survivor per 100 hospital admissions). There is also evidence for reduced morbidity and long-term myocardial damage. Most hospitals have developed their own post-infarction treatment protocol, which usually includes beta-blocker therapy.

Other agents

1. Angiotensin-converting enzyme (ACE) inhibitors have been shown to improve outcome in patients with chronic heart failure and a number of large-scale trials have been undertaken to assess their efficacy post-myocardial infarction. Apart from reducing cardiac work by their afterload-lowering properties, they also appear to reduce wall stress within the heart thereby limiting infarct expansion and excessive ventricular dilatation The ISIS-4 study of 58 000 patients from 1000 hospitals in 30 countries showed a small but significant improvement in survival with captopril, while the AIRE study using ramipril confirmed long-term efficacy.

2. Despite early reports suggesting benefit from intravenous magnesium, both meta-analysis and the ISIS-4 study demonstrated no effect.

3. Although small-scale trials and meta-analyses suggested that oral nitrate therapy may be of use, the ISIS-4 study failed to reveal an overall improvement in survival.

4. Lipid lowering agents will not have any effect on short-term survival, although long-term benefits have been clearly demonstrated.

Complications of MI

Complications of MI include:

- arrhythmias

- heart failure/cardiogenic shock

- hypertension

- post-infarction angina

- pericarditis

- rupture of papillary muscle, ventricular septal defect, LV aneurysm formation

- cardiac rupture.

Hypertension may occur for a variety of reasons after myocardial infarction. Pain and anxiety are two causes, although excessive vasoconstriction, perhaps due to inappropriate use of diuretics, may also contribute. If treatment is necessary, this should aim to bring about a gradual rather than precipitate reduction. Hypotension post-infarction may also be due to hypovolaemia secondary to inappropriate diuretic usage or be drug-related (e.g. beta-blockade, ACE inhibition). It should not be automatically assumed that the cause is pump failure.

Post-infarction angina has to be treated aggressively (see later) and is one of the indications for angiography with a view to either angioplasty or bypass surgery. This pain can usually be distinguished from pericarditis, which may either occur within a few days of the infarct or after a period of 2–6 weeks. This latter situation, known as Dressler's syndrome, is thought to be related to the formation of autoantibodies against the myocardium. Other causes and management of pericarditis are described later.

Papillary muscle rupture results in disruption of the mitral valve. It usually presents with acute pulmonary oedema. Echocardiography will reveal severe mitral regurgitation and the damaged valve. The patient should be treated as for severe heart failure and also referred for urgent cardiac surgery.

A ventricular septal defect may occur after septal infarction. It usually presents several days after the MI as acute heart failure. Colour-flow Doppler echocardiography will reveal the abnormal flow jet across the defect while sampling of blood from right atrium and right ventricle will reveal a 'step-up' in oxygen saturation due to the left-to-right shunt. Again, the patient should be treated for heart failure and also considered for urgent cardiac surgery.

Ventricular aneurysm formation usually develops over weeks to months after the infarction. Clues are persistent elevation of ST segments on electrocardiography and a bulge in the cardiac contour on chest X-ray. Echocardiography or angiography will reveal the abnormal and often paradoxical movement of the aneurysmal area during the cardiac cycle and, possibly, an associated mural thrombus. Complications that may develop include arrhythmias, heart failure, and systemic embolization. Cardiac rupture is recognized, although is invariably a terminal event. Treatment depends on the size of the aneurysm and the degree of compromise or complications caused. It may either be conservative or surgical (aneurysmectomy).

Angina pectoris

The usual cause is critical narrowing of one or more coronary arteries leading to a myocardial oxygen debt and ischaemia during periods of increased demand such as exercise. Angina at rest or on minimal exertion indicates severe stenosis of the artery and is a recognized major risk factor for infarction. Approximately 20% of patients with unstable angina will die within 1 year if left untreated. Prinzmetal angina is chest pain occurring at rest and is due to coronary artery spasm. Rarer causes of angina include aortic stenosis or hypertrophic obstructive cardiomyopathy, where both aortic and coronary blood flow may be severely compromised, and severe anaemia where the oxygen-carrying capacity of the blood is significantly reduced. Significant arrhythmias may also compromise cardiac output leading to the development of angina.

Assessment

Physical assessment includes evaluation of the following features:

- *Pain.* Ischaemia of the myocardium results in a build-up of lactic acid and the development of pain, which is classically crushing and retrosternal. This pain may radiate down the left arm or both arms, or up to the neck or jaw. Occasionally, chest pain may be absent. The pain generally lasts less than 30 min and is usually exertion-related but may also be precipitated by cold weather, anxiety, or during a meal. The pain is not eased by posture or food but is usually relieved by either rest and/or sublingual glyceryl trinitrate. Development of anginal pain at rest, or of increasing severity on minimal exertion is termed 'unstable angina'.

- *Skin.* The patient may be sweaty and appear pale, grey, or cyanosed. There may be peripheral vasoconstriction and the patient will feel clammy.

- *Respiratory.* The patient may become dyspnoeic or tachypnoeic.

- *Other symptoms.* The patient may complain of nausea or actually vomit.

Investigations

A 12-lead ECG may reveal ST segment elevation and T wave flattening or depression. It may be normal outside an attack, but should be repeated if possible during pain to confirm electrocardiographic changes of myocardial ischaemia. Cardiac enzyme estimation over several days will show no serial rise. Further tests include stress testing (usually treadmill, cycle, dipyridamole, or dobutamine), electrocardiography, and thallium radionuclide scanning. An angiogram may be necessary, especially if the diagnosis is uncertain,

Priorities of care

- Administration of high-flow, high-concentration oxygen.
- Pain relief by administering sublingual GTN tablet or spray, repeated as necessary. Diamorphine may be necessary in severe pain.
- Aspirin ± clopidogrel (another antiplatelet agent)
- Heparinization.
- Nitrates.
- Beta-blockade (unless contraindicated)

Principles of care

1. *Rest*. If the pain does nor resolve quickly, occurs with much greater frequency than normal, is brought on by minimal exertion, or occurs at rest, this is termed 'unstable' (or crescendo') angina and warrants hospital admission, bedrest, aggressive medical treatment, and investigation with a view to a coronary revascularization procedure (angioplasty or bypass surgery).

3. *Relief of anxiety*. The patient will require reassurance in the form of competent and skilled nursing care, appropriate, information, and empathetic listening.

3. *Drug therapy*. Unless a certain drug type is specifically contraindicated, medical treatment of unstable angina consists of intravenous nitrates, beta-blockade, full heparinization, and aspirin ± clopidogrel. The mnemonic MONA (morphine, oxygen, nitrates, aspirin) is a useful way of remembering this. Thrombolysis is of no benefit. If the symptoms do not resolve quickly with this aggressive pharmacological therapy, an infusion of a IIb/IIIa inhibitor (such as Rheopro) should be commenced and angiography performed urgently. Treatment should then be continued accordingly. If the pain does settle and does not recur for a number of days, despite gradual mobilization, the patient may be discharged home and be investigated as an out-patient.

Therapies

Interventional therapy depends on the angiographic findings. Left main stem coronary artery disease and triple-vessel coronary artery disease are indications for which bypass surgery has been shown to improve outcome. In other cases, symptoms will usually improve

after bypass grafting, although will often recur after a number of years. Balloon angioplasty may also be performed whereby a balloon, on the end of a catheter, is inserted percutaneously into an artery, and placed under X-ray control at the stenonic site. The balloon is then inflated to widen the lumen and a stent may be inserted afterwards to help keep the artery patent. The recurrence of symptoms is greater than after surgery, necessitating either repeat angioplasty or bypass grafting. It is essential to have cardiac surgical back-up if angioplasty is carried out.

Heart failure

The commonest cause of acute heart failure is pump failure due to ischaemia or infarction. However, other causes should be considered as many have specific treatments (Table 6.13). Some pathologies will result in high-output cardiac failure (e.g. thyrotoxic crisis, severe anaemia). The body's response to a fall in cardiac output is sympathetic induction of vasoconstriction and tachycardia. Paradoxically, this will increase the work-

TABLE 6.13   Heart failure: causes and treatment

Cause	Specific treatment
Myocardial infarction	Thrombolysis: consider early surgical revascularization
Drugs (e.g. beta-blockers, verapamil)	Specific 'antagonists' (e.g. β-agonists, calcium)
Dysrhythmias	Appropriate antidysrhythmic agents or pacemaker insertion
Valve dysfunction	Valve replacement, valvuloplasty (NB: antibiotics for endocarditis)
Ventricular septal defect	Surgery
Pericardial tamponade	Drainage
Constrictive pericarditis (e.g. TB)	Surgery
Haemorrhage and anaemia	Resuscitation and transfusion, correction of cause
Pulmonary embolus	Thrombolytics, embolectomy
Cardiomyopathy, myocarditis	Specific (e.g. immunosuppression)
Hypertension	Antihypertensives, treat cause if found
Thyrotoxic crisis	Iodine, propranolol, steroids, carbimazole
Wet beri-beri (i.e. vitamin B deficiency resulting in heart failure)	Vitamin B replacement

load, and thereby exacerbate the strain on a damaged heart. The BP will thus be initially maintained in the face of a falling cardiac output and may camouflage a barely adequate (or inadequate) cardiac output. Indeed, there may be an exaggerated vasoconstrictor response, which, with coexisting anxiety, may cause an initial elevation in BP, a further increase in LV afterload, and a greater reduction in cardiac output. Only when this vasoconstrictor reflex response fails will the blood pressure fall. When organ hypoperfusion coexists, this is termed cardiogenic shock.

The consequences of an inadequate cardiac output are clinically manifest through inadequacies of forward blood flow and increased retrograde venous congestion. Left-sided retrograde congestion results in an increase in left atrial and pulmonary venous pressures and increasing hydrostatic pressures within the lung, thereby forcing water from intravascular to interstitial compartments. When the lymphatics' absorptive capacity is exceeded pulmonary oedema with resulting dyspnoea and orthopnoea ensues. Gas exchange is impaired with resulting hypoxaemia. Right-sided retrograde congestion causes a raised CVP, hepatic congestion with elevated liver enzymes and bilirubin, and, eventually, progression to dependent oedema.

The combination of hypoxaemia, lactic acidosis, increased extravascular lung water, respiratory muscle fatigue (resulting from poor perfusion), and anxiety will cause tachypnoea and an increase in the work of breathing, accounting for up to 30% of total cardiac work. Either the left and/or right heart may be affected by the disease process. A worsening of lung disease may cause acute right ventricular decompensation. Myocardial ischaemia/infarction may affect predominantly one ventricle. The normal co-relationship between ventricular filling pressures no longer, holds. For example, with right ventricular infarction there may be high right-sided pressures (CVP) but low left-sided filling pressures (PAWP).

Ventricular compliance will also be affected; this worsens due to a variety of factors including myocardial ischaemia, increased afterload, and fluid overload. As a consequence, the ventricle becomes stiffer, altering the intraventricular pressure–volume relationship such that a higher filling pressure is required to achieve the same end diastolic volume (LVEDV). For the same filling pressure the LVEDV will thus be smaller and the stroke volume lower. Monitoring the patient using filling pressures alone (i.e. CVP and PAWP) is thus unhelpful.

Finally, the patient's fluid balance status in acute heart failure is often misjudged. The clinical or radio-logical presence of pulmonary oedema does not imply total body fluid overload. By the time they arrive to hospital the patient in acute pulmonary oedema may well be in negative fluid balance through a combination of sweating, mouth breathing, and inadequate fluid intake. The fluid is thus in the wrong compartment and requires redistribution rather than removal. The fall in cardiac output and intravascular volume leads to a drop in renal blood flow, stimulating the rennin–angiotensin–aldosterone system to produce still more vasoconstriction and oliguria.

With time, secondary hyperaldosteronism will promote fluid retention and an increase in circulating blood volume. The threshold of lymphatic drainage of pulmonary interstitial fluid will be raised and higher pulmonary arterial hydrostatic pressures will be tolerated. However, in the acute phase, the intravascular compartment is often contracted, a situation which may be further aggravated by fluid restriction and diuretic usage.

Assessment

Physical assessment:

- *Skin.* Cyanosis, pallor, and sweating may all be apparent. Inadequate forward blood flow resulting in organ hypoperfusion produces cold, shut-down peripheries. Peripheral oedema (leg or sacral) may be seen with right-sided heart failure.

- *Respiration.* The patient may be tachypnoeic, and may produce blood-stained frothy sputum as a result of pulmonary oedema. Wheeze ('cardiac asthma') may be a presenting feature.

- *General.* The patient may show signs of generalized weakness and fatigue.

- *Auscultation.* The apex beat of the patient's heart is often displaced, and a gallop rhythm (due to a third and/or fourth heart sound) may be heard on auscultation. In left heart failure end inspiratory crackles ('crepitations') may be heard at the lung bases.

Physiological assessment:

- *CVP* will be high with right-sided heart failure.

- *PAWP* will be elevated in left-sided heart failure.

- *Blood pressure* may be low, normal, or high.

- *Heart rate*: tachycardia will usually be evident unless bradycardia is the main cause of failure.

- *Renal function*: urine output may be reduced and renal dysfunction evident from blood urea and creatinine levels.

- *Lactic acidosis* is produced through insufficient tissue oxygen delivery and impaired hepatic uptake.

Neurological/psychological assessment:

- The patient may exhibit anxiety and distress. Mental obtundation may be seen as drowsiness, confusion, or agitation as a result of poor cardiac output and cerebral hypoperfusion.

Investigations

Urgent investigations include 12-lead ECG, chest X-ray, and appropriate blood investigations such as urea and electrolytes, haemoglobin, glucose, and cardiac enzymes. Troponin T or I should be measured if there is a suspicion of myocardial injury. A new marker, brain(B)-type natriuretic peptide (BNP), can also be measured. This is released into the bloodstream from the ventricle when it is excessively stretched. Although plasma BNP levels rise in other conditions such as pulmonary embolus, a high level is claimed to be diagnostic of heart failure and useful as a screening tool. The degree of elevation is a poor prognostic factor in chronic failure. Early studies also suggest it may be useful as a therapeutic endpoint for such patients.

Pulmonary oedema has a characteristic chest X-ray appearance with upper lobe blood diversion, increased fluid in the lymphatics (Kerley B lines) and the lung fissures, pleural effusions, and cardiomegaly. A 'bat's wing' appearance may be seen at the pulmonary hilum.

Echocardiography may show regions of the ventricular wall that either move poorly, irregularly, or not at all, or other causes such as pericardial tamponade or valvular dysfunction.

Priorities of care

- Basic resuscitation measures are aimed at restoring an adequate circulation as quickly as possible.

- Administration of high-flow, high-concentration oxygen.

- Preload and afterload reduction (by vasodilators, opiates, and, for intravascular overload, diuretics).

- Anxiolysis (opiates, e.g. diamorphine 2.5 mg IV repeated when required), reassurance, information, and comfort.

- If required, augmentation of cardiac output by inotropes or mechanical support including invasive or non-invasive mechanical ventilation, intra-aortic balloon pulsation (IABP) and ventricular support devices.

- After initial stabilization of the patient, further monitoring and investigations should be instituted.

Principles of care
Monitoring

This depends on the severity of the failure and usually consists of a minimum of continuous ECG monitoring, pulse oximetry, and frequent blood pressure monitoring. In progressively more severe cases, invasive arterial pressure monitoring, central venous pressure monitoring, and cardiac output monitoring will be required. Mixed venous saturation and wedge pressure can be obtained from pulmonary artery catheterization. Once adequate monitoring is in place, treatment can be titrated precisely to achieve adequate organ perfusion.

Rest

The heart can be 'rested' by reducing excessive degrees of preload and afterload, by reducing the work of breathing through mechanical ventilation, and by insertion of an IABP.

Optimizing intravascular fluid volume

The PAWP provides a rough guide to left ventricular filling. Abnormal elevations in PAWP (>18–20 mmHg) are seen in left heart failure and may indicate the need for preload reduction, albeit acknowledging that the decrease in ventricular compliance will increase filling pressures though not necessarily filling volumes. Patients with chronic heart failure will often run a high PAWP in the non-acute situation, sometimes >30 mmHg. Likewise, treatment with vasoconstrictors will further increase peripheral tone and reduce ventricular compliance, thereby elevating the PAWP still further for the same end diastolic volume. Thus, rather than routinely aiming for a target figure of 14–18 mmHg, the PAWP should be used in conjunction with stroke volume to monitor dynamic challenges such as a fluid challenge. Because of the potential alterations in ventricular compliance, and vasoconstriction induced by coexisting hypovolaemia (e.g. excessive diuretics) and inotropes, a fluid challenge should be contemplated even when the PAWP is 'normal' or even raised. No rise in stroke volume and a rise in PAWP >3 mmHg following a challenge suggests that optimal filling of the intravascular compartment has been achieved. The patient is very unlikely to decompensate with a single fluid challenge and the circulating volume should be optimized before introducing other drugs. A fall in blood pressure on a low vasodilator infusion dose suggests underfilling of the left ventricle. Even in patients with poor gas exchange a fluid challenge should not be withheld as the patient will generally die from organ hypoperfusion rather than hypoxaemia.

Supporting the cardiac output

Failing the above measures the heart can also be 'driven' by inotropes, although this should not be more than absolutely necessary to maintain adequate organ perfusion. No target figure of cardiac output exists. In general, the cardiac index (output indexed for body surface area) should exceed 2.2 1/min/m^2 (approx 3.5 1/min), but this is a very rough guide. More relevant is the worsening or improvement in base deficit and lactic acidaemia, the production of adequate urine, good cerebration, etc. The mixed venous oxygen saturation (S_vO_2) is a sensitive guide to the ability of the cardiorespiratory system to meet whole-body oxygen demands. In low-output states the tissues compensate for the decrease in oxygen delivery by extracting more oxygen and the S_vO_2 falls. In severe heart failure this can drop below 30%, indicating virtually maximal extraction with very little reserve held. Other than in sepsis, where a defect in tissue oxygen extraction often exists, the S_vO_2 is a sensitive indicator of the adequacy of tissue oxygen delivery. A mixed venous saturation of 60% is a useful goal in haemodynamic management.

Reducing ventricular afterload

The SVR is usually raised in heart failure and thus cardiac workload is increased. Reducing the afterload will reduce cardiac work. The cardiac output is usually augmented by vasodilatation, although further filling may be found necessary. Likewise, for right ventricular failure, manipulation of the pulmonary vascular resistance will allow optimization of right ventricular output.

Therapies

The standard textbook approach consists of oxygen, low-dose opiates, diuretics, and nitrates. These may be preceded or followed by inotropes depending on the presence or persistence of a low cardiac output/low blood pressure state. Diuretics cause an initial vasodilatation followed, 20–30 min later, by a diuresis. Although the vasodilatation is beneficial, the diuresis is not if the patient is not fluid overloaded. Falls in cardiac output following diuretic treatment of heart failure are well documented. Although symptomatic relief is quickly afforded with the initial vasodilatation and improvement in output, the ensuing diuresis may result in significant hypovolaemia with vasoconstriction, increased cardiac work, a fall in output, and reduced perfusion. This will lead to a metabolic acidosis and compensatory tachypnoea and oliguria. The tachypnoea and oliguria may be mistaken for worsening pump failure, resulting in the administration of additional, and larger, doses of diuretic, which compound the problem further.

Diuretic therapy should not be totally discounted. It does have a role in certain situations, notably true intravascular volume overload (e.g. excessive IV infusion), or total body fluid overload as may be often found with chronic heart failure. Furthermore, patients on long-term diuretic therapy will often require continuation to maintain an adequate diuresis. Cessation, if indicated, should be gradual. For those patients not on diuretics an effective diuresis may frequently be achieved by small intravenous doses (i.e. 10–20 mg).

Nitrates can be given rapidly either by oral or sublingual nitrolingual spray while an infusion is being prepared. Nitrates have both preload- and afterload-reducing properties which are dose dependent. Tolerance will develop by 24 hours, necessitating a higher dose to achieve a similar effect. A drop in blood pressure on a low-dose infusion is suggestive of hypovolaemia.

Once stabilized, the patient can be commenced on increasing doses of an ACE inhibitor. Nesiritide, a brain(B)-type natriuretic peptide analogue, is a new agent that has many similar properties to nitrates. It also has a natriuretic effect though, unlike nitrates, tolerance does not appear to be induced.

No drug used to increase cardiac contractility is a pure inotrope—all have additional vasodilator or vasoconstrictor properties to greater or lesser degrees. Falls in blood pressure are occasionally seen with dobutamine and, more commonly, with the phosphodiesterase inhibitor inodilators such as enoximone and milrinone. Reductions in dose, or fluid challenges, may be required to restore systemic blood pressure to satisfactory levels. The advantage of dobutamine over the currently available phosphodiesterase inhibitors is its much shorter half-life. Epinephrine, dopamine, and norepinephrine all possess vasoconstrictor properties. A balance has to be achieved between adequate vasoconstriction to maintain a reasonable coronary perfusion pressure and excessive vasoconstriction, which will increase cardiac work and myocardial oxygen consumption, possibly resulting in a fall in cardiac output. As norepinephrine and higher doses of dopamine have more of a vasoconstrictor effect than epinephrine, they should be generally used in heart failure states only in combination with dobutamine or a vasodilator. Levosimendan, a new calcium sensitizer agent, improves ventricular contractility and vasodilates peripherally without having a major impact on cardiac work.

CPAP or BiPAP reduce the work of breathing, improve oxygenation, and have beneficial effects on preload and afterload in heart failure. Mechanical ventilation, with or without the addition of PEEP, also reduces the work of breathing and allows the use of heavy sedation, thereby reducing demands placed upon the heart. It will also reduce right- and left-ventricular preload and left-ventricular afterload. In an overfilled state, cardiac output is augmented by the use of non-invasive or invasive mechanical ventilation; however a fall in output may be seen if the intravascular compartment is contracted.

Intra-aortic balloon counterpulsation and ventricular assist devices (see Chapter 8) can also be considered although their availability tends to be restricted to specialist centres. (See Table 6.14 for a summary of the management of heart failure.)

Indications for surgery are few. Some centres in the United States and Germany have shown significant improvements in outcome for post-infarction ventricular failure by salvaging ischaemic but not yet necrosed myocardium through either immediate angioplasty or surgery. A permanently damaged myocardium will not improve following revascularization. Other surgically remediable causes include papillary leaflet rupture of the mitral valve, aortic stenosis, and ventricular septal defect. Surgery may be required for uncommon pathologies such as constrictive pericarditis and hypertrophic obstructive cardiomyopanhy.

Pericarditis

Pericarditis is inflammation of the pericardium due to a variety of causes (see box).

CAUSES OF PERICARDITIS

- Infection: viruses (coxsackie, echo) or TB
- Myocardial infarction: either within 1–2 days, or Dressier's syndrome
- Malignancy
- Radiotherapy
- Trauma (including cardiac surgery)
- Uraemia
- Connective tissue disorders (e.g. SLE)

TABLE 6.14   Directed management of heart failure

Physiological derangement	Directed management
Vasoconstriction (indicated by low cardiac output, normal or high BP)	*Low PAWP or other evidence of hypovolaemia?*
	Colloid challenges to optimal stroke volume.
	BP high? PAWP high?
	Commence (or increase rate of nitrate infusion)
Low CO and BP despite optimizing fluid and nitrates	Consider:
	obstructive causes such as PE
	commence dobutamine or epinephrine ± more vasodilator
	intra-aortic balloon pump
	invasive/non-invasive mechanical ventilation
$S_vO_2 \leqslant 60\%$ ± signs of inadequate organ perfusion persisting despite optimization of ventricular filling and attempted normalization of afterload	Inotropes ± inodilators ± mechanical ventilation ± intra-aortic balloon pump ± ventricular assist device
Total body fluid overload, or intravascular volume overload	Diuretics: initially low doses, taking care not to cause hypovolaemia; increase as necessary.
	Haemofiltration: poor response to diuretics?
Poor urine output	Exclude hypovolaemia.
	Treat low-output state as above.
	Consider further elevation in mean systemic BP.
	Has an ACE inhibitor been administered? If so, consider stopping because of renovascular disease.
	Consider diuretics (initially at low doses) or haemofiltration

Assessment

Physical assessment:

- *Pain*: usually presents as a sharp, constant central chest pain eased by sitting forward and worsened by deep inspiration or coughing. It may radiate to the neck, arm, shoulder, or occasionally abdomen. It is not related to food nor eased by nitrates.

- *Auscultation*: may reveal a pericardial friction rub: a scratchy noise heard throughout the cardiac cycle caused by rubbing together of the inflamed surfaces.

- *Pulsus paradoxus*, a raised JVP, and muffled heart sounds may be present with severe constrictive pericarditis or a significant pericardial effusion.

Physiological assessment:

- *ECG*: classically reveals concave-upwards ST segment elevation in all leads with no reciprocal changes in the opposite leads.

- *Heart rate*: tachycardia may be evident.

- *Pyrexia* may be present.

(Pericardial tamponade may present with signs of poor forward flow and right heart congestion, or with cardiac arrest.)

Investigations

The chest X-ray (and echocardiograph) usually reveals no abnormality unless a pericardial effusion, constrictive pericarditis, or associated myocarditis is present. A significant pericardial effusion produces a globular cardiac contour on X-ray. Fluid in the pericardial space may be visualized by echo. In the case of constrictive pericarditis, small heart chambers and restricted filling are seen. Calcification may be visible in longstanding tuberculous pericarditis.

Principles of care

- Bedrest.

- Anti-inflammatory agents such as indomethacin.

- Treatment of the cause wherever possible.

Steroids are rarely indicated. Occasionally, surgery is needed when constrictive pericarditis causes haemodynamic compromise.

Pericardial tamponade

Significant pericardial effusions may require drainage (pericardiocentesis), either percutaneously or by open surgical drainage. The percutaneous approach is often done under echocardiography, fluoroscopic screening, or may be performed 'blind'. In this case, an ECG V lead may be attached to the needle to detect whether the myocardium is being penetrated (ST segment changes or multiple ventricular ectopics are often seen). The patient is laid resting semi-supine and after cleansing of the site and injection of local anaesthetic, a long, 18-gauge catheter connected to a syringe is introduced by the side of the xiphisternum under the costal margin and advanced in the direction of the scapula. When fluid is aspirated the catheter should be advanced no further. At this stage, a three-way tap can be attached and total drainage performed.

Alternatively, a guide wire may be advanced through the cannula into the pericardial space, the cannula removed, and a pigtail catheter placed over the guide wire. Specimens should be sent for culture and cytology where appropriate. Blood may be aspirated (haemopericardium), particularly after trauma, cardiac surgery, or malignancy. This differs from blood aspirated from within the heart chamber as it does not clot. If in doubt, the catheter may be transduced to see whether a characteristic right ventricular pressure waveform is seen. Further details on tamponade are given in Chapter 13.

Complications of needle pericardiocentesis include damage to the ventricle or a coronary artery, arrhythmias, or pneumothorax.

Infective endocarditis

Previously known as subacute bacterial endocarditis, this is an infection of the heart valves with or without vegetations, which may lead to destruction of the valve. Any bacteraemia may cause colonization of a heart valve. Recognized precipitating causes include dental manipulation, venous cannulation (iatrogenic or drug addicts), and surgery. Abnormal or prosthetic valves are more prone to colonization but half of all cases occur on previously normal valves. Left-sided heart valves are more commonly affected except in intravenous drug abusers who usually have right-sided heart valve lesions, particularly tricuspid. The commonest infecting organism is *Streptococcus viridans*, although others include enterococci (e.g. *S. faecalis*), *Staphylococcus aureus*, other bacteria, *Coxiella burnetti* ('Q fever'), fungi, and chlamydia.

Assessment

Physical assessment:

- The patient may demonstrate the physical features of acute heart failure (see earlier) or may present with embolic phenomena such as stroke.

- Vasculitis may also occur.
- There may be signs of chronic illness and infection (e.g. clubbing, splenomegaly, and weight loss).
- Auscultation may reveal heart murmurs.

Physiological assessment:

- Pyrexia is usually present.
- Chest X-ray is usually normal.
- ECG is usually normal

Endocarditis affecting chronically damaged or congenitally abnormal valves, or long-term implanted prosthetic valves, has a more insidious presentation with non-specific signs such as fever, malaise, weight loss, night sweats, and splenomegaly.

Investigations

- Repeated blood cultures should be taken.
- Echocardiography may reveal vegetations on the affected valves; however, these have to be large enough to be visualized (usually >3 mm). Transoesophageal echocardiography is a more sensitive technique for detection of vegetations. Bacterial and histological examination of any removed emboli may also aid diagnosis.

Priorities of care

- Treatment as for heart failure (see earlier).

Principles of care

- Conventional treatment should be applied to complications such as heart failure. However, embolic events are not usually treated with anticoagulants, particularly as infected emboli carry an increased risk of local aneurysm formation and potentially catastrophic bleeding.
- Antibiotic treatment has to be aggressive and prolonged (usually a minimum of 4–6 weeks). Depending on sensitivities, intravenous benzylpenicillin and gentamicin are usually given initially for streptococcal and enterococcal infections, whereas flucloxacillin and gentamicin are given for staphylococcal infections. Careful monitoring of drug levels must be performed. Other causative organisms, such as fungi or *Coxiella*, should be treated with the appropriate antifungals or antibiotics.
- Surgical removal of the damaged valve may be necessary though, if possible, this should be delayed until a course of antibiotics have been given.

- Rest is an important part of the patient's management.
- Education of the patient and information about the disease and preventive measures are important. Prophylaxis is very important in patients with known abnormal or prosthetic valves undergoing surgical or dental procedures.

Valvular heart disease: stenosis

Valvular stenosis predominantly affects the aortic and mitral valves.

Assessment

Aortic stenosis (AS) may present with angina, symptoms of heart failure, low output (including syncope: 'Stokes–Adams attacks'), or sudden death. Mitral stenosis (MS) usually presents with symptoms of heart failure including fatigue and breathlessness. Atrial fibrillation may also be a presenting feature of MS.

Investigations

Characteristic murmurs are heard for AS (ejection systolic murmur) and for MS (mid-diastolic rumbling murmur); their absence or prolongation may indicate increasing severity. The pulse pressure is usually narrow with AS. In MS, the chest X-ray may show an enlarged left atrium and radiological signs of pulmonary oedema; a bifid P wave (P mitrale) may be seen on the ECG. The definitive investigation for both valves is echocardiography where both the orifice area and the pressure gradient across the stenosed valve can be estimated non-invasively. Mural thrombi may also be seen, especially in cases of atrial fibrillation. Angiography may be needed, especially for AS where the coronary arteries may also be narrowed at their origin.

Principles of care

Heart failure is treated in conventional fashion, although digoxin and anticoagulation therapies are often used in concurrent atrial fibrillation for control of rate and prophylaxis against emboli. Valvotomy or balloon valvuloplasty may be attempted if the valve is still pliant, otherwise prosthetic replacement may be needed. This may be an emergency procedure when the heart is placed under considerable strain or decompensation occurs. Antibiotic prophylaxis against subacute bacterial endocarditis (SBE) should be taken during dental and surgical procedures.

Valvular heart disease: incompetence

Valvular incompetence may be due to either direct valve damage (e.g. endocarditis) or functional, i.e. secondary to dilatation of the ventricle. Regurgitant flow occurs, either back into the atria during systole with mitral and tricuspid incompetence, or back into the left ventricle during diastole with aortic incompetence.

Assessment

Incompetence results in a decrease in forward flow with symptoms of low output (e.g. fatigue) and an increase in retrograde congestion. This may result in breathlessness from pulmonary oedema for left-sided lesions, and hepatic congestion and peripheral oedema for right-sided lesions.

Investigations

Characteristic murmurs are heard for AR (high-pitched early diastolic murmur), MR (pan-systolic murmur), and TR (pan-systolic murmur, louder on inspiration). The chest X-ray may show cardiomegaly. A wide pulse pressure with a collapsing pulse is present with AR and a pulsatile liver with TR. Doppler echocardiography is again diagnostic.

Principles of care

Heart failure is treated in conventional fashion, although the valve should ideally be replaced before

---

CAUSES OF VALVULAR INCOMPETENCE

Aortic incompetence:

- Rheumatic heart disease
- Endocarditis
- Ankylosing spondylitis
- Marfan's syndrome
- Aortic dissection
- Syphilis

Mitral incompetence:

- Rheumatic heart disease
- Mitral valve prolapse
- Ruptured chordae tendinae or papillary muscle (after MI or trauma)
- Functional (due to dilated ventricle)
- Endocarditis
- Cardiomyopathy

Tricuspid incompetence:

- Rheumatic heart disease
- Functional (due to dilated ventricle)
- Endocarditis (especially drug abusers)

---

significant dysfunction has occurred. Antibiotic prophylaxis against SBE should also be given.

Cardiomyopathy/myocarditis

Cardiomyopathy is an idiopathic heart muscle disease not related to ischaemia. There are three types:

- congestive,
- hypertrophic (obstructed) HOCM hypertrophic obstructive cardiomyopathy,
- restrictive.

The causes of congestive and hypertrophic cardiomyopathy are unknown, although many cases of HOCM are congenital. Restrictive cardiomyopathy is due to stiffening of the endomyocardium; in the tropics it is mainly due to idiopathic fibrosis, while amyloid is the commonest cause in the UK.

Assessment

Physical assessment:

- Signs of heart failure (congestive).
- Simulating constrictive pericarditis (restrictive).
- Angina (HOCM).
- Syncope (HOCM).
- Palpitations may be experienced and a late systolic murmur may be heard due to obstruction of the left ventricular outflow tract (HOCM).
- Dyspnoea (HOCM).
- Sudden death can be a presenting feature of HOCM.

Physiological assessment:

- Heart rate: the pulse is jerky with a double apex beat (HOCM).

Investigations

Definitive diagnosis is usually made by echocardiography.

Principles of care

- Treatment as for heart failure.
- Angina may require beta-blockade and amiodarone may be needed for arrhythmias.
- Surgery (e.g. myomectomy) or transplantation may be necessary.
- Patients will require counselling and education regarding the disease and its prognosis

CAUSES OF OTHER TYPES OF HEART MUSCLE DISEASE

- Hypertension
- Haemochromatosis
- Alcohol
- Sarcoidosis
- Post-partum
- Friedrich's ataxia
- Diabetes
- Myotonic dystrophy
- Hyper- and hypothyroidism
- Radiation and cytotoxic drugs such as adriamycin

Other types of heart muscle disease

The symptoms are usually those of congestive cardio-myopathy with signs and symptoms of heart failure.

Myocarditis

The commonest cause of an acute myocarditis is viral, especially coxsackie virus. Other infections (e.g. diphtheria), rheumatic fever, connective tissue diseases (e.g. SLE), and drugs (e.g. cocaine) are also recognized as causing myocarditis.

The patient usually presents with symptoms of heart failure, angina, or dysrhythmias. Acute and chronic phase viral serology should be taken. Echocardiography usually shows dilated, poorly functioning ventricles.

Treatment is bedrest, and treatment of heart failure or angina, if present. The patient should be continuously monitored as arrhythmias can occur. Patients usually recover spontaneously but may progress to severe irreversible heart failure requiring cardiac transplantation.

Aortic aneurysm

A tear in the intimal lining of the aortic vessel wall allows blood to track into the media. The blood may track along the media dissection, either up or down the aorta, occluding branch vessels. Alternatively, rupture may occur through the outer adventitial layer. Atheroma is the commonest underlying pathology and this may be accelerated by hypertension and hyperlipidaemia. Congenital conditions such as Marfan's syndrome and other connective tissue disorders are also recognized. A major cause is direct trauma (see Chapter 13).

Assessment

Physical assessment:

- *Pain*: a tearing pain of abrupt onset in the chest or upper abdomen radiating through to the back is the classical mode of presentation.

- *Neurological symptoms*: syncope, headache, stroke, or paraplegia.

- *Pulses*: one or more of the major pulses may be absent or asymmetric.

- *Signs of acute aortic incompetence* may be present if the ascending aorta is involved. Angina may also be present due to occlusion of the origins of one or more coronary arteries.

Physiological assessment:

- Sudden cardiovascular collapse may occur.

- Blood pressure: there may be a discrepancy in systolic pressure between right and left arms of more than 15 mmHg.

Investigations

- Chest X-ray may reveal mediastinal widening.

- ECG is usually unremarkable, although ischaemic changes may be present.

- Echocardiography (particular from the trans-oesophageal approach) may be diagnostic although the definitive diagnosis is usually made by either CT scan or angiography—this will delineate the extent of the aneurysm (see Fig. 6.8).

Priorities of care

- Urgent resuscitation if there is cardiovascular compromise, including immediate transfer to the operating theatre if necessary.

- Pain relief (opiates are usually given).

- High-flow, high-concentration oxygen.

- If hypertensive, blood pressure should be reduced using an infusion of either sodium nitroprusside or labetalol commenced with the aim of reducing systolic blood pressure to below 100 mmHg if possible.

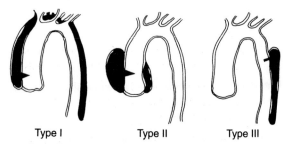

Fig. 6.8 Classification of thoracic aortic aneurysms.

Principles of care

+ Arterial cannula—for continuous blood pressure monitoring.

+ Bladder catheter—to measure urine output. Oliguria suggests that the lowering of blood pressure may be excessive while anuria is suggestive of aneurysmal involvement of the renal arteries.

+ It is important to reassure the patient and prevent unnecessary agitation.

The regional cardiothoracic unit should be contacted if a thoracic aortic aneurysm is suspected. The patient should be transferred promptly for any further investigations and surgery, as necessary. Ascending aortic aneurysms often require surgery while those involving the descending aorta are often managed conservatively in the first instance.

Pulmonary embolus

Detachment of part or all of a thrombus, usually from the deep veins of the legs or pelvis, or from within the right heart, passes into the pulmonary vasculature, blocking forward blood flow. The extent of flow obstruction depends on the size (or multitude) of clots, thereby giving rise to signs and symptoms of major (massive) or minor pulmonary embolism (PE). The patient may have recently undergone a long flight, surgery, or be undergoing a prolonged period of immobilization. There may be signs and symptoms of deep venous thrombosis.

Assessment

Physical assessment:

+ Major embolism: *respiration*—the patient will have acute dyspnoea from metabolic acidosis and hypoxaemia; *cardiovascular collapse*; *syncope*; *cyanosis*.

+ Minor embolism: *pain*—the patient will experience pleuritic pain; *respiration*—dyspnoea and haemoptysis will occur.

Physiological assessment:

+ Major embolism: *blood pressure*—hypotension; *heart rate*—tachycardia; *raised CVP*.

Investigations

+ Chest X-ray: pulmonary oligaemia (reduced blood vessel markings) may be seen in one of the lung fields.

+ ECG may show signs of right ventricular strain (S_1, Q_3, T_3, right-axis deviation, partial right bundle branch block, tachycardia).

+ Arterial blood gas analysis may show a low P_aO_2, ± a low P_aCO_2, and a metabolic acidosis. None of the above may be present with minor embolism though one or more wedge-shaped pulmonary infarcts may be seen on a chest X-ray.

+ A radioisotope ventilation/perfusion (V/Q) scan will provide an indication of the likelihood of PE by showing an area of lung (or multiple areas if multiple emboli are present) being ventilated but not perfused. However, a spiral CT scan with contrast or pulmonary angiography may be necessary for definitive diagnosis, especially if surgery is being contemplated.

Priorities of care

+ Resuscitation if cardiovascular collapse has occurred; fluid loading is the important first step in circulatory management, even though the CVP is usually elevated.

+ High-flow, high-concentration oxygen.

+ Adequate fluid loading.

+ Inotropes (epinephrine or dobutamine) if an inadequate response to fluid.

Principles of care

+ Mechanical ventilation may be necessary but gas exchange may worsen because of loss of preferential shunting of blood.

+ Early thrombolytic therapy should be considered for massive embolism where right heart strain is pronounced. Therapeutic regimens using once- or twice-daily low molecular weight heparins have been validated (PIOPED); however, the risk of a potentially catastrophic bleed outweighs the benefit in patients with non-decompensating emboli. The heparin should be continued until a therapeutic oral anticoagulant regimen is well established.

+ Positioning: the patient may prefer to lie flat to improve symptoms of dyspnoea by increasing their venous return.

+ Surgery: the role of surgery is controversial; embolectomy may be of benefit for single, centrally placed, massive clots.

Shock

Shock can be defined as a state of impaired tissue oxygenation (or cellular utilization of oxygen), resulting in a tissue oxygen debt. This shortfall produces a range of metabolic, biochemical, and physiological sequelae including a metabolic acidosis and decreased organ function (e.g. oliguria, confusion). Though hypotension is often present, shock can exist in the presence of a normal (or even elevated) blood pressure. On the other hand, the patient may have a low blood pressure without being shocked.

Classification of the major types of 'clinical' shock is summarized below. For further information please refer to the appropriate chapters mentioned. However, an alternative way of considering the pathophysiological mechanisms underlying shock is to consider the three components of tissue oxygen delivery, namely (1) cardiac output, (2) arterial oxygen saturation, and (3) haemoglobin concentration and, secondly, the ability of the cell to use oxygen—predominantly by the mitochondria to generate energy in the form of ATP. Shock can thus be due to one or more of the following:

- 'Circulatory hypoxia'—a cardiac output problem related to heart failure, hypovolaemia, pulmonary embolus, etc.
- 'Hypoxic hypoxia'—a problem with arterial oxygen saturation such as pneumonia, carbon monoxide poisoning.
- 'Anaemic hypoxia'—a low haemoglobin, e.g severe haemorrhage, haemolysis.
- 'Cellular dysoxia'—mitochondrial dysfunction due to sepsis, carbon monoxide poisoning, cyanide, etc.

Clinical forms of shock can be subdivided as in the following.

Cardiogenic shock

(See also the section in this chapter on heart failure.) This is the most severe manifestation of decreased (left or right) ventricular pump function. Usually as a result of extensive injury to the myocardium (e.g. ischaemia, myocarditis), but also due to other conditions (e.g. severe valvular regurgitation), the stroke volume and cardiac output are greatly reduced. There may also be a tachy- or bradyarrhythmia, occurring either as the primary cause or as a secondary response. Intracardiac filling pressures are usually increased. The body initially attempts to compensate for the decrease in cardiac output by vasoconstriction and diversion of blood away from 'non-essential' organs and tissues. However, at a certain point, these reflexes will fail and blood pressure falls, further compromising organ perfusion. In particular, underperfusion of the myocardium will impair cardiac contractility and promote further tissue damage. This may increase the size of any new infarction, causing yet further decreases in cardiac output. The usual appearance of cardiogenic shock is a low-pressure, low-output circulation with or without pulmonary oedema.

Inflammatory shock—including septic shock

(See aslo Chapter 12.) This occurs as a result of an extrinsic insult (e.g. infection, trauma, burns) triggering an exaggerated, generalized inflammatory response that leads to the clinical and pathological sequelae of organ dysfunction and failure. Sepsis (the systemic inflammatory response to infection) remains the most common single cause but 40–50% of patients do not have an identifiable septic focus nor a positive blood culture. The circulation is affected by this systemic inflammation through vasodilatation, vascular hypore-activity (decreased responsiveness to catecholamines such as norepinephrine), increased capillary leak, and myocardial depression. The classical manifestation of inflammatory shock is a low-pressure, high-output, 'hyperdynamic' circulation; however, excessive hypo-volaemia and myocardial depression may occasionally produce a low-pressure, low-output circulation.

Hypovolaemic shock

Hypovolaemia results from excessive fluid loss (e.g. haemorrhage, vomiting, diarrhoea, burns) or from inadequate fluid intake. This then leads to organ hypoperfusion. As with cardiogenic shock, the body initially attempts to compensate for the low-output state by vasoconstriction and redistribution of blood flow. The usual cardiovascular effects are tachycardia, hypotension, oliguria, decreased cardiac output, and a high SVR. Further details are given in Chapter 13 and the section on 'General principals of care' in this chapter.

Anaphylactic shock

An anaphylactic reaction is a potentially life-threatening, systemic response that occurs after re-exposure to an antigen. Anaphylactic shock usually occurs within seconds to minutes of exposure to the stimulus. The patient may present with rapid onset cardiovascular collapse, with or without myocardial depression, angio-edema, laryngeal obstruction, or severe bronchospasm. This can lead to death within minutes. A fuller explanation is given in Chapter 15, while anaphylaxis as a cause of hypotension is discussed in section on 'General principals of care' in this chapter.

Neurogenic shock

Patients with injury to the cervical or high thoracic cord may have reduced sympathetic outflow between T1 and L2 segments causing vasodilatation, hypotension, and bradycardia. Further details of this type of shock are given in the spinal injuries section of Chapter 13.

Obstructive shock

This occurs when an acute pathology (or decompensation of a chronic illness) causes obstruction to flow in a major vessel or within the heart. Examples include pulmonary embolus, tension pneumothorax, and pericardial tamponade.

Anti-arrhythmic drugs

Only those anti-arrhythmic drugs particularly relevant to the critically ill patient will be detailed in this chapter. Anti-arrhythmic drugs are categorized into four classes (I–IV), determined by their action on the electrophysiological mechanisms of the myocardial cell:

1. *Class I.* Class IA drugs lengthen the effective refractory period by: (1) inhibiting the fast sodium current and thus the speed of action potential; (2) prolonging the duration of the action potential.

   Class IB drugs inhibit the fast sodium current while shortening the duration of the action potential. This action is selective on diseased or ischaemic tissue and is thought to promote conduction block thereby interrupting re-entry (e.g. lidocaine, mexiletine, phenytoin).

   Class IC drugs possess three major electrophysiological effects: (1) powerful inhibition of His–Purkinje conduction with QRS widening; (2) marked inhibition of fast sodium channels with depression of speed of action potential; (3) shortened action potential in the Purkinje fibres only, leaving the surrounding myocardium unaltered (e.g. flecainide).

2. *Class II.* These agents include β-adrenergic antagonists. They also act on the β-receptors in the myocardium and block their effect (e.g. atenolol, labetalol, propanolol).

3. *Class III.* These agents lengthen the duration of the action potential and hence the effective refractory period. They also homogenize the pattern of the action potential throughout the myocardium. There is relatively little negative inotropic effect (e.g. amiodarone, sotalol, bretylium).

4. *Class IV.* These inhibit slow channel-dependent conduction through the AV node (e.g. adenosine, diltiazem, verapamil).

Amiodarone

This is a complex anti-arrhythmic drug sharing at least some of the electrophysiological properties of all four classes of anti-arrhythmics. Amiodarone lengthens the effective refractory period by prolonging the duration of the action potential. It also has a powerful class I effect, inhibiting inactivated sodium channels. It noncompetitively blocks α- and β-adrenergic receptors while a calcium antagonist effect may be responsible for the bradycardia and AV nodal inhibition that is sometimes associated with its use.

Indications

Control of ventricular tachyarrhythmias, recurrence of paroxysmal atrial fibrillation or flutter, paroxysmal supraventricular tachycardias, and Wolff–Parkinson–White arrhythmias.

Dosage

In life-threatening arrhythmias, amiodarone 300 mg IV may be given over 10–15 min followed by an infusion of 10–20 mg/kg/24 hours. The loading dose is essential because of the slow onset of full action. Otherwise, for less dangerous arrhythmias, 300 mg is infused through a central venous catheter over an hour followed by a further 900 mg over the next 23 hours. The daily dose is reduced thereafter.

Side-effects

In higher doses, pneumonitis may occur potentially leading to pulmonary fibrosis. Torsades de pointes may result from QT prolongation plus hypokalaemia. Amiodarone has a complex effect on the metabolism of thyroid hormones, the main action being inhibition of peripheral conversion of T_4 to T_3. It can cause phlebitis if infused peripherally. Nausea can occur in 50% of patients with cardiac failure.

Precautions

A pro-arrhythmic effect may occur if given with other drugs prolonging the Q-T interval. Amiodarone will prolong prothrombin time and may cause bleeding in patients on warfarin. It also potentiates the effect of digoxin.

Lidocaine (lignocaine)

This is a class IB agent that acts preferentially on the ischaemic myocardium and is more effective in the presence of a high plasma potassium level.

Indications

Emergency treatment of ventricular arrhythmias. Suppression of ventricular arrhythmias such as those associated with myocardial infarction and cardiac surgery.

Dosage

An initial loading dose of 100 mg IV is given followed by an infusion of 1–4 mg/min. This is gradually decreased after 24–30 hours. The dose should be decreased in the elderly where lidocaine toxicity develops rapidly.

Side-effects

Relatively few side-effects are seen, though high infusion rates may result in drowsiness, speech disturbances, and dizziness. If toxicity develops there may be seizures, agitation, or coma.

Precautions

Clearance of lidocaine via the liver may be reduced if the patient is receiving cimetidine, propanolol, or halothane. Lidocaine metabolites circulate in high concentrations and may contribute to toxic and therapeutic actions (Opie 1991). Drugs that induce hepatic enzymes, such as barbiturates, phenytoin, and rifampicin, may increase the dosage requirements.

Adenosine

This has multiple effects including opening of potassium channels and inhibition of sinoatrial and atrioventricular nodes. Opening of K^+ channels produces an indirect Ca^{2+} antagonist effect due to a change in polarity away from that required to open the slow Ca^{2+} channel

Indications

It is chiefly used in paroxysmal supraventricular tachycardia and is particularly effective in treating re-entrant tachycardias via the AV node.

It is also used as a useful diagnostic test to distinguish between VT and SVT with aberrant conduction. If it is effective in slowing the tachycardia, the arrhythmia is usually SVT with aberrant conduction. Occasionally, adenosine is effective in some types of VT.

Dosage

A rapid IV bolus of 3–6 mg is given initially; if not effective within 1–2 min a further IV bolus of 12 mg is given. The 12 mg dose may be repeated once. The effect is almost instantaneous but will last no longer than 10–30 s.

Side-effects

These include dyspnoea due to bronchoconstriction, and flushing and headache due to vasodilatory effects. Transient new arrhythmias may occur at the time of chemical cardioversion. Occasionally, the induced heart block may be prolonged.

Precautions

Adenosine should not be used in patients with asthma, second- or third-degree heart block, or sick sinus syndrome. The dose should be reduced if the patient is on dipyridamole therapy due to the inhibitory effect of dipyridamole on adenosine breakdown. Caffeine and theophylline will competitively antagonize adenosine.

Verapamil

This inhibits the action potential of the upper and middle nodal regions where depolarization is calcium-mediated. In is therefore able to terminate tachycardias of re-entry origin believed to be the cause of most paroxysmal supraventricular tachycardias. It increases AV nodal block as well as the effective refractory period of the AV node and will reduce the ventricular rate in atrial fibrillation or flutter.

Indications

It is used in supraventricular tachycardias and chronic atrial fibrillation or flutter where myocardial depression is not a problem.

Dosage

A slow bolus of 5–10 mg IV over at least 1 min can be repeated 10 min later if necessary. Calcium gluconate or chloride (5–10 ml, 10% solution) should be available for rapid administration (or pre-treatment) if there is a negative inotropic effect associated with the verapamil bolus.

Side-effects

These include hypotension and bradycardia. Its vasodilatory effects produce flushing, headaches, and dizziness. Rarely, there may be facial, epigastric, and gingival pain, hepatotoxicity, and transient mental confusion.

Precautions

Verapamil should not be give to patients with AV nodal disease, sick sinus syndrome, or myocardial depression. In should be given with caution if the patient has been treated with β-adrenergic blockers, or other anti-arrhythmics.

Magnesium sulphate

A low serum magnesium or a low intracellular magnesium content is associated with an increased risk of tachyarrhythmias. Trials have shown that infusions of magnesium are therapeutically effective. The actual mechanism by which it works has not yet been identified but could be direct inhibition of efflux of potassium from the cell, alteration of cellular calcium metabolism, decreasing peripheral vascular resistance, or stimulating a membrane-stabilizing enzyme (Zwerling 1987).

Indications

Recurrent ventricular arrhythmias have been terminated with the intravenous administration of magnesium sulphate. It is also used as a preventative measure in patients following AMI and in patients with heart failure, though no outcome benefit has been shown in large multicentre studies. However, the use of magnesium is considered a relatively safe intervention, which may be used when other anti-arrhythmic agents have failed or when there is reason to suspect magnesium depletion.

Dosage

The optimal dosage and frequency has still not been fully determined. An often-used dose is 10–20 mmol over 5–10 min (or, more rapidly in emergencies), followed by a further 20–40 mmol given over 5–10 hours.

Side-effects

Flushing, sweating, and a sensation of heat may occur with rapid IV injection.

Precautions

Serum magnesium levels should be monitored and kept below 2.7 mmol/l as higher levels are associated with bradycardia, prolonged PR intervals and AV block. Since magnesium is excreted via the kidneys, magnesium levels should be closely monitored in patients with renal impairment.

Drugs commonly used in the treatment of low cardiac output and/or hypotension

Inotropic drugs can be termed either positive or negative in relation to their effect on heart muscle. Positive inotropes increase the contractility of the myocardium and hence the stroke volume (e.g. epinephrine). Negative inotropes decrease the contractility of cardiac muscle (e.g. beta-blockers). Chronotropic drugs are those that increase heart rate (e.g. atropine).

The effect of the drugs used depends on their specific site of action. There include:

+ catecholamines, which work on the adrenergic receptor, of which there are two types alpha (α) and beta (β). These increase cyclic AMP levels and calcium levels within the heart or vascular smooth muscle cell;

+ dopaminergic receptors;

+ phosphodiesterase inhibitors such as milrinone (which also increase cardiac contractility by elevating cAMP levels, albeit through prevention of its breakdown);

+ calcium sensitizers (e.g. levosimendan) which augments the contractile apparatus of the muscle cell by enhancing the sensitivity of troponin to calcium.

An alternative option is to use a high-dose glucose–insulin–potassium infusion, which is thought to work by enhancing entry of glucose into the cells and accelerating glycolysis as an alternative energy source to compensate in part for mitochondrial dysfunction due to lack of oxygen.

Alpha-adrenergic receptors

There are two main types of alpha-receptor: α_1 and α_2. The principal effect of alpha-receptors is to cause vasoconstriction of vascular smooth muscle:

+ α_1-receptors are the postjunctional receptors of vascular smooth muscle.

+ α_2-receptors are found in the vascular smooth muscle of the skin and are also the pre-junctional receptors of nerve fibres. They inhibit the release of noradrenaline.

Beta-adrenergic receptors

There are two main types of beta-receptor: β_1 and β_2. The principal effects of beta-receptors are to cause vasodilatation and an increase in the rate of the heart and its contractility:

+ β_1-receptors are found in the sinoatrial node and myocardium and influence contractility and heart rate.

+ β_2-receptors are found in the arterioles of heart, liver, and skeletal muscle and in the smooth muscle of the bronchioles and cause vasodilatation.

Beta-blockers should be given with caution to patients with asthma or a history of obstructive airways disease, unless no alternative treatment is available, since there is a risk of inducing bronchospasm. The use of beta-blockers may also mask the compensatory physiological responses to hypoglycaemia and sudden haemorrhage (tachycardia and vasoconstriction), so particular care should be paid to diabetics and patients with blood loss. Beta-blockers may also compromise blood flow in patients with peripheral vascular disease. While caution should be applied to the use of beta-blockers in acute heart failure, large studies have shown a clear outcome benefit when given to patients with stable chronic heart failure.

β_2-Adrenergic agonists (e.g. salbutamol) depress plasma potassium and raise glucose levels, therefore these should always be monitored in patients receiving such drugs. The dosages of drugs should be titrated according to the patient's response and will require frequent or continuous monitoring of cardiovascular variables.

In general, begin at the lowest dose and increase gradually in increments according to their effect. Observe for side-effects, particularly arrhythmias and tachycardias. The infusions of these drugs should not be discontinued abruptly but the dose gradually decreased, observing for any deleterious effects.

Dopamine

The cardiovascular effects of dopamine depend on the dosage infused. At low dosage (1–3 mg/kg/min) it stimulates dopaminergic receptors, having a diuretic effect and vasodilating the splanchnic circulation. At a dosage of 5–10 mg/kg/min it stimulates mainly beta-receptors, causing an increase in cardiac output, contractility, and coronary blood flow. At this dosage it has little effect on heart rate and the blood pressure may in fact fall slightly due to the decrease in systemic vascular resistance. At higher doses (>10 mg/kg/min) the alpha-adrenergic effects predominate. There is increased peripheral vasoconstriction, which causes an increase in systolic blood pressure. These doses are approximate; some patients will react differently at lower doses.

Dopamine is administered as a continuous intravenous infusion via a flow-regulated pump. It should always be administered through a central vein due to its peripheral vasoconstrictor action. If extravasation occurs it can cause ischaemic tissue necrosis and skin sloughing. Side-effects include tachycardia, arrhythmias, angina, nausea, and vomiting.

Dobutamine hydrochloride

Dobutamine is a positive inotrope and a mild chronotrope. It is used to increase cardiac output in patients with low-output cardiac failure (e.g. myocardial infarction, cardiogenic shock, following cardiac surgery). It directly stimulates the β_1-receptors in the heart increasing rate and stroke volume. Systemic vascular resistance and left ventricular end diastolic pressure also decrease as it has some β_2 vasodilator properties.

It is administered as a continuous IV infusion (due to its short half-life of approximately 2 min), ideally centrally, but can be given via a peripheral vein if necessary. The dosage is 2.5–40 mg/kg/min titrated according to response.

Side-effects are dose related and include tachycardia, arrhythmias, headache, and chest pain. Hypotension can occur, predominantly due to its vasodilating effects. Dobutamine also increases AV conduction especially if the patient is hypovolaemic. Those with atrial fibrillation may develop rapid ventricular responses. Use with care in patients with myocardial infarction as an increased heart rate may precipitate angina and intensify ischaemia.

Down-regulation of the beta-adrenoreceptor may occur if dobutamine is continuously infused for longer than 72 hours; larger doses may be required to maintain the same effect.

Dopexamine hydrochloride

Dopexamine is an arterial vasodilator, a positive inotrope, and also causes splanchnic vasodilation. It is used to increase cardiac output in patients who have a raised systemic vascular resistance. It stimulates β_2-adrenergic and peripheral dopaminergic receptors, increasing cardiac output, heart rate, and reducing afterload. The vascular smooth muscle of the renal and mesenteric beds is also dilated, increasing blood flow to these areas.

Dopexamine is administered by continuous infusion, via a flow-regulated pump, into a central or large peripheral vein. Its half-life is 6–11 min. Dosage ranges from 0.5 to a maximum of 6 µg/kg/min. The dose should be increased in increments of 0.5–1 µg/kg/min at intervals of not less than 15 min.

Side-effects include tachycardia (dose-related), nausea, vomiting, tremor, and headaches. An increase in heart rate is the most common side-effect and may precipitate angina or intensify cardiac ischaemia.

Epinephrine (adrenaline)

Epinephrine is a positive inotrope and affects both alpha- and beta-receptors. It is the most potent alpha-receptor activator. Low doses produce predominantly beta effects while higher doses produce more alpha vasoconstricting effects. It increases heart rate, cardiac output, systolic blood pressure, and myocardial oxygen consumption. When administered as a bolus intravenously it causes a rapid rise in systolic blood pressure by increasing the strength of ventricular contraction, increasing heart rate, and causing constriction of the arterioles of the skin, mucosa, and splanchnic areas of circulation. However, when administered as an infusion there is often a decrease in peripheral resistance due to its action on beta-receptors of skeletal muscle. This vasodilator effect may predominate and any increase in blood pressure is a result of cardiac stimulation and increase in cardiac output. Peripheral resistance may rise or be unaltered owing to a greater ratio of alpha-to-beta activity in different vascular areas.

Although splanchnic blood flow is increased, renal blood flow can be decreased by up to 40%.

Epinephrine causes an increase in blood glucose as it decreases insulin secretion but increases glucagon secretion and the rate of glycogenolysis. It is also a bronchodilator but tends to increase the viscosity of secretions. It may also cause a profound metabolic acidosis due to accelerated aerobic glycolysis rather than secondary to ischaemia.

When administered as an infusion it should be given via a central vein as extravasation can cause local necrosis. Dosage is titrated according to response starting at 0.01 µg/kg/min by continuous infusion or 0.05–1 mg for bolus doses. Side-effects include tachycardia, palpitations, myocardial ischaemia, and headache.

Milrinone

Milrinone is a member of a new class of bipyridine inotropic/vasodilator agents with phosphodiesterase inhibitor activity. It is a positive inotrope and vasodilator, with little chronotropic activity and is different in structure and mode of action from either the digitalis glycosides or catecholamines.

Indications

Milrinone is used for the short-term intravenous treatment of patients with acute decompensated heart failure. In addition to increasing myocardial contractility, it improves diastolic function as evidenced by improvements in left ventricular diastolic relaxation.

The duration of therapy should depend upon patient responsiveness.

Side-effects

Supraventricular and ventricular arrhythmias can occur and it has been shown to increase ventricular ectopy, including non-sustained ventricular tachycardia. Milrinone produces a slight shortening of AV node conduction time, indicating a potential for an increased ventricular response rate in patients with atrial flutter/fibrillation which is not controlled with digitalis therapy.

Hypotension, headaches, hypokalaemia, nausea, vomiting, diarrhoea, tremor, and thrombocytopenia may also occur.

Precautions

Milrinone should not be used in patients with severe obstructive aortic or pulmonic valvular disease in lieu of surgical relief of the obstruction as it may aggravate outflow tract obstruction in hypertrophic subaortic stenosis.

Milrinone is excreted via the urine, and fluid and electrolyte changes and renal function should be carefully monitored during therapy. Improvement in cardiac output with resultant diuresis may necessitate a reduction in the dose of diuretic. Potassium loss due to excessive diuresis may predispose digitalized patients to arrhythmias. Therefore, hypokalaemia should be corrected by potassium supplementation in advance of or during use of milrinone.

Furosemide (frusemide) should not be injected into an intravenous line of an infusion of milrinone, as immediate precipitation will occur.

Dosage and administration

Milrinone is administered with a loading dose of 50 µg/kg given slowly over 10 min followed by a continuous infusion (maintenance dose) using a controlled infusion device (0.375–0.75 µg/kg/min).

The infusion rate should be adjusted according to haemodynamic and clinical response. Reductions in infusion rate may be necessary in patients with renal impairment.

Norepinephrine (noradrenaline)

Norepinephrine acts predominantly on alpha-receptors and increases blood pressure by increasing peripheral resistance. Cardiac output usually falls as a result. Hepatic, renal, and splanchnic flows are decreased but coronary blood flow is often increased due to the increase in diastolic pressure.

It decreases insulin secretion leading to an elevated blood glucose.

Norepinephrine is administered by continuous intravenous infusion via a flow-regulated pump. It should only be infused into a central vein. The dosage is titrated according to response starting at 0.01 µg/kg/min. Side-effects include arrhythmias, chest pain, and headache.

Levosimendan

This drug has two main mechanisms of action. It has a direct effect on the heart by increasing the sensitivity of troponin to calcium within the cardiomyocyte. For the same level of intracellular calcium (and thus the same level of cardiac work as the intracellular calcium level dictates the work of the cardiomyocyte), more actin–myosin cross-bridges are formed, producing an increased contraction. It also has a vasodilating action through its effects on opening the ATP-sensitive potassium channel in vascular smooth muscle, thereby causing relaxation.

The drug is usually given by a loading dose of 24 µg/kg over 10 min followed by an infusion in the range 0.05–0.2 µg/kg/min. However, as the loading dose is associated with an increased risk of hypotension, this can be omitted when given to hypotensive patients with low cardiac outputs.

Glucose–insulin–potassium (GIK)

This stratagem has been used for the last four or five decades as a means of increasing cardiac output. Although the precise mechanisms of action are not confirmed, it is postulated that increased substrate (glucose) provision and accelerated glycolysis augment cardiac efficiency and enhance contractility. A trial of 407 patients post-myocardial infarction (Diaz *et al.* 1998) randomized to either standard therapy, a low-dose GIK regimen (10% glucose solution containing 20 U insulin and 40 mmol KCl per litre infused at 1 ml/kg/hour) or a high-dose regimen (10% glucose solution containing 50 U insulin and 80 mmol KCl per litre infused at 1.5 ml/kg/hour) showed significant short-term outcome benefit in both GIK groups with this being maintained in the high-dose GIK group at 1 year.

Table 6.15 summarizes the drugs used in hypotension.

Intravenous drugs for hypertension

Sodium nitroprusside

Sodium nitroprusside acts directly on vascular smooth muscle causing predominantly arteriolar vasodilation.

It has an immediate effect but a short duration of action, therefore it is administered by continuous infusion. It should be administered via a flow-regulated pump and through a dedicated vein. Intra-arterial pressure monitoring is considered essential as sodium nitroprusside can cause profound hypotension. The cardiac output usually increases due to the decrease in systemic vascular resistance. The drug causes cerebral vasodilation and may increase intracranial pressure in normocapnic patients.

Dosage is 0.5-1.5 μg/kg/min initially and then adjusted according to response. The usual range is 0.5–8 μg/kg/min. Side-effects include headache, dizziness, nausea, palpitations, and retrosternal pain. When sodium nitroprusside is metabolized it forms cyanide ions and has the potential to produce cyanide toxicity. This is related more to the rate of the infusion than to the total dose given and the rate should not exceed 8 μg/kg/min. Ideally, it should not be given for more than 24–36 hours. A rising, and unexplained, metabolic acidosis may be due to cyanide accumulation.

The solution must be protected from the light. The drug is excreted renally but is removed by haemodialysis.

Glyceryl trinitrate and isosorbide dinitrate

Nitrates cause vasodilation of veins at lower doses. At higher doses, both arteries and veins are vasodilated; this can allow a smooth reduction in blood pressure. They will cause cerebral vasodilatation and may raise intracranial pressure. Duration of action is 2–5 min when given as an intravenous bolus. They should be administered via a volumetric pump and can be given into a peripheral vein.

Dosage is:

- glyceryl trinitrate: 5–200 μg/min
- isosorbide dinitrate: 2–83 μg/min.

Side-effects include headache, tachycardia, and nausea. Tolerance ('tachyphylaxis') will develop within 24 hours, requiring increasing doses to achieve the same effect.

Hydralazine

Hydralazine acts on vascular smooth muscle, predominantly arteriolar, causing peripheral vasodilation. It decreases systemic vascular resistance and can cause a compensatory tachycardia with an increased cardiac output. This tachycardia may precipitate pre-existing angina. It can be given as a repeated, slow bolus injection, or a continuous infusion via a volumetric pump.

TABLE 6.15 Summary of drugs used in hypotension

Drug	Primary action	CVS effect
Dopamine	Positive inotrope. Vasoconstrictor (high dose). Vasodilator (low dose)	↑ Cardiac output. ↑ SVR (high dose). ↓ SVR (low dose)
Dobutamine	Positive inotrope (NB: may vasodilate)	↑ Stroke volume. ↑ Cardiac output (heart rate). ↓ SVR
Dopexamine	Vasodilator. Positive inotrope	↑ Cardiac output. ↓ SVR
Epinephrine	Positive inotrope. Vasoconstrictor	↑ Cardiac output
Glucose–insulin–potassium	Positive inotrope	↑ Cardiac output
Levosimendan	Positive inotrope. Vasodilator	↑ Cardiac output. ↓ SVR
Norepinephrine	Vasoconstrictor. Some inotropic properties	↑ SVR

↑, increased; ↓, decreased.

Dosage is 20–40 mg when given as a bolus intravenously (and repeated as necessary), or as a continuous infusion at 200–300 µg/min initially and then 50–150 µg/min. It is incompatible with dextrose solutions as contact with glucose causes hydralazine to be rapidly broken down. Side-effects include nausea, vomiting, headache, tachycardia, palpitations, and flushing.

Phentolamine

Phentolamine acts by blocking alpha-adrenergic receptors. This causes vasodilation and a reflex tachycardia. It increases respiratory tract secretions, salivation, insulin secretion, and gut motility. Phentolamine is particularly useful when hypertension is due to a phaeochromocytoma, a reaction between foods containing pressor amines and monoamine oxidase inhibitors, or to clonidine withdrawal.

It can be given as a slow bolus injection or continuous infusion via a volumetric pump. Dosage is 5–10 mg when given as a bolus intravenously (and repeated as necessary) or as a continuous infusion at a rate of 5–60 mg over 10–30 min, and thereafter at 0.1–2 mg/min.

Side-effects include tachycardia, arrhythmias, dizziness, nausea, vomiting, and diarrhoea.

Labetalol

Labetalol acts by blocking both alpha- and beta-adrenoceptors, although beta-blockade predominates at higher doses. It blocks the alpha-adrenoceptors in the peripheral arterioles and therefore lowers systemic vascular resistance. The concurrent beta-blockade protects the heart from the reflex sympathetic drive that can be induced by this vasodilation. There is little change in cardiac output.

It can be administered as a repeated, slow bolus injection or as a continuous infusion via a volumetric pump. In a hypertensive crisis when the blood pressure needs to be reduced urgently 50 mg may be given as an intravenous bolus over at least 1 min. This may be repeated at 5-min intervals but not exceeding 200 mg in total. By intravenous infusion the rate is variable according to the cause of the hypertension and can be up to 160 mg/hour.

Side-effects include headache, rashes, difficulty in micturition, nausea, and vomiting. It can cause severe postural hypotension. There may be a small decrease in heart rate but severe bradycardia is unusual.

Propanolol

Propanolol is a beta-adrenoceptor antagonist. It is a negative inotrope, reduces heart rate, and increases peripheral resistance. It is administered as a slow bolus injection of 1–10 mg, repeated as necessary. Side-effects include bradycardia and bronchospasm. It may also block the sympathetic response to hypoglycaemia by impairing the gluconeogenetic response. Heart failure and heart block may be precipitated and peripheral vascular disease exacerbated.

Esmolol

Esmolol acts by beta-adrenoceptor blockade but has a very short half-life (9 min). It decreases cardiac output and heart rate. It is administered by continuous infusion, via a volumetric pump, at a rate of 50–150 µg/kg/min. Side-effects include bronchospasm, nausea and vomiting, and bradycardia.

Captopril

Captopril is an angiotensin-converting enzyme (ACE) inhibitor. ACE inhibitors act on the angiotensin–renin–aldosterone system causing mixed venous and arteriolar vasodilation.

Captopril lowers blood pressure by several mechanisms:

* inhibiting the conversion of angiotensin into the powerful vasoconstrictor angiotensin II,

* inducing natriuresis by reducing the secretion of aldosterone and increasing renal vasodilation,

* increasing peripheral vasodilation by stimulating the synthesis and release of prostaglandins.

Captopril can cause severe hypotension, particularly in patients with high renin states such as renal artery stenosis, hyponatraemia, or following vigorous diuretic therapy (e.g. in congestive heart failure). An initial test dose of 6.25 mg is usually given for this reason and its effect on blood pressure should be assessed prior to a regular prescription. After absorption from the stomach a response can occur within 15 min.

In hypertension, treatment is titrated according to the patient's needs and should be the lowest effective dose. The range is usually 12.5–50 mg twice daily. In the treatment of heart failure captopril is often given, up to a maximum dosage of 150 mg per day.

Renal function must be carefully monitored as the drug is excreted via the kidneys. It is effectively removed by haemodialysis. Side-effects include hyperkalaemia, angioedema, cough (due to increased sensitivity of the cough reflex), and altered immune function (neutropenia, skin rashes).

Test yourself

Questions

1. How can an elevated heart rate compromise cardiac output?

2. What is hypertensive encephalopathy?

3. What are troponins?

4. What is a cardiomyopathy? Name three types.

5. Captopril is an angiotensin-converting enzyme (ACE) inhibitor used in the treatment of hypertension. How does it work?

Answers

1. An elevated heart rate can compromise cardiac output by:
   increasing the amount of oxygen consumed by the myocardium;
   reducing the diastolic time, resulting in less time for perfusion of the coronary arteries;
   shortening the ventricular filling phase of the cardiac cycle, causing a decreased blood volume to be pumped on the next contraction.

2. Hypertensive encephalopathy can be caused by uncontrolled hypertension from any cause. In addition to organ damage, it is characterized by neurological signs resulting from reduced cerebral blood flow. There may be areas of cerebral infarction, haemorrhage, or transient ischaemia. Symptoms are initially severe headaches and nausea but can progress to deteriorating level of consciousness, seizures, and coma. If the hypertension is treated early, changes may be reversible but mortality is high.

3. Troponins are structural protein components of striated muscle. There are three types: troponin C, T, and I. Troponins T and I are found solely in cardiac muscle and are released following cardiac damage. They will not rise unless myocardial injury has occurred. Troponin I rises after 3–6 hours and peaks at about 20 hours. At 12 hours the sensitivity is generally good enough to exclude a myocardial infarct. Both troponins remain elevated for a much longer time than CK, AST or LDH. Troponin I is detectable in the blood for up to 5 days, and troponin T for 7–10 days following myocardial infarction. This allows a myocardial infarction to be diagnosed, or excluded, in a patient who presents late with a history of chest pain.

4. Cardiomyopathy is an idiopathic heart muscle disease not related to ischaemia. There are three types: congestive, hypertrophic (obstructed) HOCM = hypertrophic obstructive cardiomyopathy, restrictive.
   Causes of congestive and hypertrophic cardiomyopathy are unknown, although many cases of HOCM are congenital. Restrictive cardiomyopathy is due to stiffening of the endomyocardium; in the tropics it is mainly due to idiopathic fibrosis, while amyloid is the commonest cause in the UK.

5. ACE inhibitors act on the angiotensin-renin-aldosterone system causing mixed venous and arteriolar vasodilation. Captopril lowers blood pressure by several mechanisms:
   Inhibiting the conversion of angiotensin into the powerful vasoconstrictor angiotensin II.
   Inducing natriuresis by reducing the secretion of aldosterone and increasing renal vasodilation.
   Increasing peripheral vasodilation by stimulating the synthesis and release of prostaglandins.

References and bibliography

Abraham, A.S., Rosenmann, D., Kramer M., *et al.* (1987). Magnesium in the prevention of lethal arrhythmias in acute myocardial infarction. *Archives of Internal Medicine* **147**, 753–5.

Allen, B.J., Brodsky, M.A., Capparelli, E.V., *et al.* (1989). Magnesium sulfate therapy for sustained monomorphic ventricular tachycardia.. *American Journal of Cardiology* **64**, 1202–4.

Armstrong, R.F., Bullen, C., Cohen, S.L., *et al.* (1991). *Critical Care Algorithms*. Oxford University Press, Oxford.

Aviles, R.J., Askari, A.T., Lindahl, B., *et al.* (2002). Troponin T levels in patients with acute coronary syndromes, with or without renal dysfunction. *New England Journal of Medicine* **346**, 2047–52.

British Heart Foundation (2003). *What are Cardiac Troponins?* Factfile 08/2003.

Chatterjee, K., Swan, H.J.C., Kaushik V.S. *et al.* (1976) Effects of vasodilator therapy for severe pump failure in acute myocardial infarction on short-term and late prognosis. *Circulation* **53**, 797.

Des Jardins, T.R. (1988). *Cardiopulmonary Anatomy and Physiology: Essentials for Respiratory Care*. Delmar Publishers, New York.

DeSanctis, R.W., Doroghazi, R.M., Arsten, W.G., *et al.* (1987). Aortic dissection. *New England Journal of Medicine* **317**, 1060.

Diaz, R., Paolasso, E.C., Piegas, L.S. *et al.* on behalf of the ECLA (Estudios cardiologias Latinoamerica) Collaborative Group (1998). Metabolic modulation of acute myocardial infarction. The ECLA glucose-insulin-potassium pilot trial. *Circulation* **98**, 2227–34.

Editorial (1992). Thrombolysis for pulmonary embolus. *Lancet* **340**, 21.

Ebell, M.H., Flewelling, D., Flynn, C.A. (2000). A systematic review of troponin T and I for diagnosing acute myocardial infarction. *Journal of Family Practice* **49**, 550–6.

Forrester, J.S., Diamond, G. McHugh, T., *et al.* (1971). Filling pressures in the right and left sides of the heart in acute myocardial infarction. A reappraisal of central venous pressure monitoring. *New England Journal of Medicine* **285**, 190.

Ghani, M.F., Rabab, M. (1977). Effect of magnesium chloride on electrical stability of the heart. *American Heart Journal* **94**, 600–2.

Goldhaber, S.Z., Haire, W.D., Feldstein, M.L. *et al.* (1993). Alteplase versus heparin in acute pulmonary embolism: randomised trial assessing right ventricular function and pulmonary perfusion. *Lancet* **341**, 507.

Goldhaber, S.Z., Simons, G.R., Elliott, G., *et al.* (1993). Quantitative plasma D-dimer levels among patients undergoing pulmonary angiography for suspected pulmonary embolism. *Journal of the American Medical Association* **270**, 2819–22.

Gruppo Italiano per in Studio della Streptochinasi nell'Infarcto Miocardico. GISSI-2 (1990). A factorial randomised trial of alteplase versus streptokinase and heparin versus no heparin among 12490 patients with acute myocardial infarction. *Lancet* **336**, 65.

Hagen, P.J., Hartmann, I.J., Hoekstra, O.S., *et al.*; ANTELOPE Study Group (2003). Comparison of observer variability and accuracy of different criteria for lung scan interpretation. *Journal of Nuclear Medicine* **44**, 739–44.

Hampton, J.R. (1986). *The ECG in Practice*, 3rd edn. Churchill Livingstone, London.

Hope, R.A., Longmore, S.M.. Moss, P.A.U., *et al.* (1992). *Oxford Handbook of Clinical Medicine*, 2nd edn. Oxford University Press, Oxford.

Iseri, L.T., Freed, J., Bures, A.R. (1975). Magnesium deficiency and cardiac disorders. *American Journal of Medicine* **58**, 837–46.

ISIS-2 (1988). Randomised trial of intravenous streptokinase, oral aspirin, both, or neither among 17187 cases of suspected acute myocardial infarction: ISIS-2. *Lancet* **ii**, 349.

ISIS-4 (1995). A randomised factorial trial assessing early captopril, oral mononitrate, and intravenous magnesium sulphate in 58,050 patients with suspected acute myocardial infarction. *Lancet* **345**, 669–85.

Leak, D. (1986). Intravenous amiodarone in the treatment of refractory life-threatening cardiac arrhythmias in the critically ill patient. *American Heart Journal* **111**, 456–62.

Levick, J.R. (1991). *An Introduction to Cardiovascular Physiology*. Butterworth, London.

Nelson, G.I.C., Ahuja, R.C., Silke, B., *et al.* (1983). Haemodynamic advantages of isosorbide dinitrate over frusemide in acute heart failure following myocardial infarction. *Lancet* **i**, 730.

The PIOPED Investigators (1990). Value of the ventilation/perfusion scan in acute pulmonary embolism. Results of the prospective investigation of pulmonary embolism diagnosis (PIOPED). *Journal of the American Medical Association* **263**, 2753–9.

Opie, L.H. (1991). *Drugs for the Heart*, 3rd edn. W.B. Saunders, Philadelphia, PA.

Rasmussen, H.S., Aurup, P., Hojberg, S., *et al.* (1986). Magnesium and acute myocardial infarction: transient hvpomagnesaemia non induced by renal magnesium loss in patients with acute myocardial infarction. *Archives of Internal Medicine* **146**, 8724.

Rasmussen, H.S., Norregard, P., Lindeneg, O., *et al.* (1986). Intravenous magnesium in acute myocardial infarction. *Lancet* **1**(8475), 234–6.

Sasada, M.P., Smith, S.P. (1990). *Drugs in Anaesthesia and Intensive Care*. Castle House Publications, Tunbridge Wells.

Shechter, M. Hod, H., Marks, N. *et al.* (1990). Beneficial effect of magnesium sulfate in acute myocardial infarction. *American Journal of Cardiology* **66**, 271–4.

Singer, M. (1993) The management of acute heart failure: an iconoclastic view. *Care of the Critically Ill* **9**, 11.

Stein, P.D., Hull, R.D., Saltzman, H.A., *et al.* (1993). Strategy for diagnosis of patients with suspected acute pulmonary embolism. *Chest* **103**, 1553.

Sueta, C.A., Clarke, S.W., Dunlap, S.H., *et al.* (1994). Effect of acute magnesium administration on the frequency of ventricular arrhythmia in patients with heart failure. *Circulation* **89**, 660–6.

Swedberg, K., Held, P., Kjekshus, J., *et al.* (1992). Effects of the early administration of enalapril on mortality in patients with acute myocardial infarction. Results of the cooperative new Scandinavian enalapril survival study II (CONSENSUS H). *New England Journal of Medicine* **327**, 678–84.

Teo, K.K., Yusuf, S., Collins, R., *et al.* (1991). Effects of intravenous magnesium in suspected acute myocardial infarction: overview of randomised trials. *British Medical Journal* **303**, 1499–503.

The GUSTO Investigators (1993). An international randomised trial comparing four thrombolytic strategies for acute myocardial infarction. *New England Journal of Medicine* **329**, 673.

Timmis, A.D. (1985). *Cardiology*. Gower Medical Publishing, London.

Woods, K.L. (1993). Hypomagnesaemia and the myocardium. *Lancet* **341**, 155.

Woods, K.L., Fletcher, S., Roffe, C., *et al.* (1992). Intravenous magnesium sulphate in suspected acute myocardial infarction: results of the second Leicester Intravenous Magnesium Intervention Trial [LIMIT-2]. *Lancet* **339**, 1553–8.

Worsley, D.F., Alavi, A. (1995). Comprehensive analysis of the results of the PIOPED Study. Prospective Investigation of Pulmonary Embolism Diagnosis Study. *Journal of Nuclear Medicine* **36**(12), 2380–7.

Zwerling, H.K. (1987). Does exogenous magnesium suppress myocardial irritability and tachyarrhythmias in the nondigitalized patient? *American Heart Journal* **113**, 1046–53.

CHAPTER 7

Cardiac arrest and cardiopulmonary resuscitation

Chapter contents

Introduction

In the UK 40% of all hospital patients who have a cardiac arrest are initially resuscitated but only 17.6% survive to be discharged (Gwinnutt *et al.* 2000). This figure is similar in the USA with 44% initially resuscitated but only 17% surviving to discharge (Peberdy *et al.* 2003). Successful resuscitation is more likely with ventricular fibrillation or tachycardia (VF/VT) with an initial resuscitation rate of 71% and survival to discharge of 42% (Gwinnutt *et al.* 2000). Survival is also more likely in critical care areas. (BRESUS Study 1992, Dumot *et al.* 2001). This is possibly due to a combination of close observation, timely intervention, the type of arrhythmia, and the expertise associated with dealing with the critically ill. However, in view of the limited survival, the continuing focus should be on prevention of cardiac arrest itself in order to improve the patient's chances. More details of this are given in Chapter 1.

There is no doubt that personnel working in the critical care environment should be familiar with and skilled in cardiopulmonary resuscitation (CPR). Training should include aspects pertinent to resuscitation in the critical care area, such as the use of monitoring to give more information, or dealing with the ventilated patient who has a cardiac arrest.

It should be stressed at this point that the skills of basic life support are essentially practical ones which must be learnt and practised regularly using resuscitation training manikins in order to ensure retention. Research into proficiency in CPR has shown that up to 57% of qualified nurses were completely ineffective in performing basic life support (Wynne and Marteau 1987). Although this work was carried out among general ward nurses, similar studies in junior doctors have echoed this result (Skinner *et al.* 1985, Smith and Poplett 2002) and the need for continuous updating and practice of these skills cannot be overemphasized. This chapter will outline the pathophysiology associated with cardiac arrest, discuss the overall management, and examine in detail the techniques and drugs used for CPR. Finally, the care of the patient and his or her family following successful and unsuccessful resuscitation will be discussed.

Definition

Cardiac arrest is defined as the absence or severe reduction of cardiac output resulting in inadequate perfusion of vital organs and causing cerebral and myocardial ischaemic damage. This is associated with the following arrhythmias:

◆ ventricular fibrillation (VF)

◆ ventricular tachycardia (VT)

◆ asystole

◆ pulseless electrical activity (PEA).

Other arrhythmias (see Chapter 6), may also produce a severe reduction or absence of cardiac output and in this instance should be treated as cardiac arrest. (Note: ventricular tachycardia is not always associated with a severe reduction or loss of cardiac output, see Chapter 6.)

Pathophysiology

The events following cardiac arrest consist of:

1. Loss of oxygen supply to the tissues due to loss of blood flow.

TABLE 7.1	Arrhythmias associated with cardiac arrest			
	Ventricular fibrillation(VF)	**Pulseless ventricular tachycardia (VT)**	**Asystole**	**Pulseless electrical activity (PEA)**
Definition	Sudden loss of co-ordinated electrical activity leading to random contraction of individual myocardial fibres	A repetitive electrical discharge from a ventricular ectopic focus	Complete absence of electrical activity	Organized electrical activity but no effective myocardial contraction takes place
ECG trace	Rapid irregular activity without rate or recognizable shape	Rapid, wide QRS complexes (rate 150–220 bpm)	No recognizable activity although occasional agonal (dying) beats may be seen	QRS complexes are present
Arterial pressure waveform	None	None or very low	None	None or very low pressure

2. Rapid depletion of high-energy phosphates, such as adenosine triphosphate (ATP), in the myocardial cells. These are not replenished due to the lack of oxygen supply and absence of aerobic metabolism.

3. Failure of pacemaker activity, impulse conduction, and myocardial contractility due to lack of ATP.

4. Complete loss of electrical activity.

It is possible for electrical dysfunction to be the primary event in which case the order of events will commence with item 4.

Ventricular fibrillation occurs early in cardiac arrests unless the primary cause is electrical dysfunction (see Table 7.2). However, most of the primary rhythms found in in-hospital cardiac arrests are non-shockable, i.e. asystole or PEA (Gwinnutt *et al.* 2000, Peberdy *et al.* 2003). The ventricular fibrillation will rapidly degenerate into a small-amplitude waveform (the so-called 'fine' VF) and finally to electrical standstill (asystole).

In spite of what may appear to be good pulse volume and blood pressure the actual cardiac output associated with external chest compressions (ECC) is only 20–30% of normal (Peters and Ihle 1990). This is because pressure does not directly equate with blood flow. The 'pulse' felt during CPR is more likely to be a pulse pressure wave transmitted down the arteries from chest compression. It is therefore more readily felt in atherosclerotic arteries which are less elastic and therefore likely to transmit the pressure to a greater extent.

TABLE 7.2	Factors associated with sudden ventricular dysrhythmias	
Drug toxicity	Digoxin (often precipitated by hypokalaemia and hypomagnesaemia)
	Amphetamines
	Tricyclic antidepressants
	Adrenergic drugs
	Cocaine
Electrolyte disturbance	Hypokalaemia
	Hypomagnesaemia
	Hypercalcaemia
External factors	Unsynchronized cardioversion attempt
	Exacerbating factors of myocardial ischaemia (hypoxaemia, carbon monoxide poisoning, hypoperfusion due to hypovolaemia, ventricular failure, rapid tachycardia)
	Electrocution

Thus, the pulse cannot be relied upon as a marker of adequacy of CPR.

These marginal levels of cardiac output produced by ECC mean that inadequately oxygenated tissues will convert to anaerobic glycolysis with the production of lactic acid and the development of metabolic acidosis. This is compounded by the respiratory acidosis which may have built up from the period without ventilation. Once adequate ventilation occurs the arterial pH returns to normal but the venous pH remains low due to high mixed venous CO_2 levels associated with poor pulmonary perfusion (Weil *et al.* 1986).

The peripheral blood vessels are initially vasoconstricted by the release of high levels of catecholamines (up to 300 times normal levels). This is followed by a fall in systemic vascular resistance (SVR) due to loss of blood flow and vasodilatation due to hypoxia, lactic acidosis, hypercapnia, and ischaemia.

There is then thought to be a down-regulation of response to catecholamines by α-receptors in the vasculature due to overstimulation from the high initial endogenous catecholamine release (Lindner 1991). Further response may then be limited to high levels of catecholamines and to α$_2$-receptors. This vasodilatation produces a rapid equilibration of arterial and venous pressures.

Assessment

The clinical signs of cardiac arrest are:

♦ Absence of pulse: this should be felt for at least 5–10 s (usually the femoral or carotid, as central pulses are less likely to be affected by vasoconstriction and are most easily felt).

♦ Loss of consciousness.

♦ Minimal or absent respirations.

♦ ECG exhibiting any of the arrhythmias listed in Table 7.1 accompanied by loss of the arterial waveform.

♦ Recognition of cardiac arrest in the ICU is facilitated by ECG and haemodynamic monitoring which is usually already in place on the patient. Alarms will alert the nurse immediately and intervention can be swift. (Note: monitors are not infallible if the patient is otherwise well and has a palpable pulse, check for disconnection of leads or damping/kinking/blockage of the arterial cannula or tubing.)

Although some authorities have previously recommended assessing the pupillary response to light, this is not a reliable method of determining loss of cardiac output. It takes between 45 s and 1 min for pupils to become fixed and dilated and they can be affected by other drugs commonly used in the ICU such as opiates (pupillary constriction in high doses), and atropine or adrenaline/epinephrine (pupillary dilatation).

Aims of treatment

1. Establish and maintain an airway.

2. Provide adequate ventilation with 100% oxygen or as near as possible.

3. Support organ perfusion with external chest compressions until spontaneous cardiac output is restored.

4. Restore spontaneous cardiac output and stabilize the patient.

The overall aim of intervention is the return of an adequate spontaneous circulation with minimal cerebral dysfunction. Resuscitation can only really be consid-

TABLE 7.3 Factors likely to affect outcome following cardiac arrest out of hospital (Herlitz et al. 2003)	
Factors associated with decreased likelihood of survival	Age >70 years
	Atropine required in emergency department
	Chronic treatment with diuretics
Factors associated with increased likelihood of survival	VF/VT as first recorded rhythm
	Witnessed arrest
	Bystander initiated CPR
	Conscious on admission to hospital
	Sinus rhythm on admission to hospital
	Lidocaine given in emergency department

TABLE 7.4 Factors likely to affect outcome following cardiac arrest in hospital (Gwinnutt *et al.* 2000)	
Factors associated with decreased likelihood of survival	Epinephrine (adrenaline) use
	Out of hours resuscitation (17:00–09:00)
	Multiple defibrillation attempts
	Second cardiac arrest
	Arrest on the ward
Factors associated with increased likelihood of survival	VF/VT as initial rhythm
	Circulation restored in <3 min
	Age <70 years

ered successful if the patient is able to return home with intact cerebral function. The probability of an unsuccessful outcome increases with the length of time taken to restore cardiac output (Tables 7.3 and 7.4).

Life Support techniques in the Critical Care Environment

These are based on the guidelines of the Resuscitation Council (UK) (2000), but are specifically applied to the critical care situation.

Confirm cardiac arrest

In the previously conscious patient, the first step to achieving this is by shouting the patient's name or 'Are you all right?' and shaking them. In many cases, in the critical care environment this is unnecessary or inappropriate, either because ECG and arterial blood pressure monitoring make cardiac arrest obvious or because the patient is unresponsive for other reasons such as sedation. The critical care nurse will be aware from both the ECG trace and the loss of arterial pressure that there is a serious problem and will immediately summon assistance.

Summon assistance

This is the next most important step. There should be no hesitation in using the cardiac arrest buzzer or shouting loudly even if the exact situation is uncertain. Commencing basic life support without ensuring there is the back-up of advanced life support is only likely to decrease the chances of resuscitation.

Precordial thump

> If ECG monitoring indicates VF or VT and immediate defibrillation is not available, a precordial thump should be attempted. If this is delivered within 30 s after cardiac arrest it may convert VF back to a perfusing rhythm (Resuscitation Council (UK) 2000).

The precordial thump should be taught and practised during resuscitation training. It is essentially a blow on the lower third of the patient's sternum using the lateral aspect of a closed fist. The degree of force should not be excessive, enough for a sharp blow obtained using the weight of a swing from the elbow. The sudden blow of mechanical energy acts like the electrical energy associated with a defibrillatory shock and dissipates the chaotic electrical system in ventricular fibrillation sufficiently for sinus rhythm or some other pacemaker activity to return. It has also been shown to be effective in pulseless ventricular tachycardia. There is a small risk of exacerbating a ventricular arrhythmia, in particular deteriorating a ventricular tachycardia to asystole (Bossaert and Koster 1992) but this is outweighed by the potential benefit of terminating the arrhythmia swiftly.

Defibrillation

> The faster ventricular fibrillation and/or tachycardia is terminated, the better the outcome for the patient.

Although this does not form part of basic life support it is a priority which should be considered immediately in the critical care environment. The chances of successful defibrillation are optimal within the first 90 s before global hypoxia has occurred (Resuscitation Council (UK) 2000) and the chance of successful defibrillation declines by 7–10% for each minute the arrhythmia persists. If defibrillation is successful within this time there is also an increased likelihood of long-term survival. In most ICUs, access to a defibrillator is not a problem and defibrillation should be the first response if the patient is in ventricular fibrillation. Nurses remain in a difficult position in some hospitals where defibrillation is not considered part of the nursing role. However, if nurses are adequately trained to defibrillate there is no reason why they should not carry this out. Immediate defibrillation can save valuable time and may influence the patient's ultimate outcome. If defibrillation cannot be carried out immediately then basic life support should be commenced. The ability of the heart to respond to resuscitative measures and the consequent survival rate deteriorate with delay in initiating cardiac compression. The number of joules (units of energy) and technique of defibrillation will be discussed in detail later in the chapter.

Airway control

Non-intubated patients

> If there is no artificial airway of any kind then the patient's own airway must be assessed for patency and kept open.

The suggested manoeuvre for opening the airway is the use of the head tilt and chin lift or jaw thrust (Fig. 7.1),

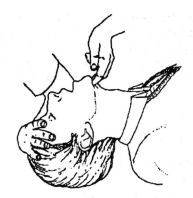

Fig. 7.1 Opening the airway. (Reproduced with permission from Handley A.J. and Swain A. (ed.) (1994). *Advanced Life Support Manual*, 2nd edn. Resuscitation Council, UK.)

which should pull the base of the tongue away from the back of the throat.

This means placing two fingers of one hand under the point of the chin and the other hand over the forehead. The head is then tipped back pulling the chin upwards. The airway should be cleared of any obvious obstruction using a Yankauer sucker. Well-fitting dentures should be left in place to improve the seal around the mouth for ventilation but loose-fitting or broken dentures should be removed. An oropharyngeal airway, such as a Guedel airway, is useful in maintaining the patient's airway and can be inserted once the airway is clear.

An alternative airway is the laryngeal mask airway (LMA). This is a conventional endotracheal tube at one end, which has an inflatable elliptical cuff at the other. The LMA is placed through the patient's mouth into the pharynx until the cuff is at the level of the larynx. When inflated, this cuff forms an airtight seal around the posterior perimeter of the larynx allowing ventilation of the patient. The technique of insertion is more easily taught than endotracheal intubation but it may not be as effective in preventing aspiration and its place in resuscitation has yet to be established.

SIZES OF LARYNGEAL MASK AIRWAYS AND CUFF INFLATION VOLUME

- Cuff size 3: inflation volume 20 ml (air)
- Cuff size 4: inflation volume 30 ml (air)
- Cuff size 5: inflation volume 40 ml (air)

Intubated patients

These are patients with endotracheal tubes and tracheostomies, already in place.

> If there is any doubt about the patency of the endo-
> tracheal or tracheostomy tube a suction catheter
> should be inserted to check for and, if possible,
> remove any occlusion.

If there is an immovable obstruction or doubts about
the position of the tube in the trachea it should be
removed as a manner of urgency. This should only be
done by nurses in the unlikely event that there are
no medical staff available. The patient should be re-
intubated as quickly as possible but may be maintained
in the short term by bag and mask ventilation.

If the tube is patent, the patient should be ventilated
on 100% O_2 during the arrest and until stabilization is
achieved.

Breathing

> In the cardiac arrest situation *the patient should be ven-
> tilated with as near to 100% oxygen as possible* in order
> to maximize arterial PO_2.

If the patient is not intubated, there are a number of
ways that ventilation can be carried out. The most basic
is mouth-to-mouth ventilation which requires no equipment but will only deliver expired air to the patient. It
is not recommended in the critical care situation partly
because of the risks to the carer but mostly because it is
inefficient in terms of oxygen delivery. Expired air has
an oxygen concentration of only 16% which will provide little in the way of oxygen to meet the needs of the
patient even if it is delivered properly.

In the critical care environment, 100% oxygen is
readily available and the patient should be ventilated
via a bag and tight-fitting anaesthetic mask. The manual
resuscitation bag (MRB) used for ventilation should not
be a rebreathing bag as this will increase P_aCO_2 if used
for any length of time. A bag with a one-way valve, such
as a self-inflating bag-valve-mask with a reservoir
attached, is more suitable for resuscitation. Bag-valve-
mask ventilation is a skill that requires considerable
practice on training manikins and it can be done very
poorly by novices. A two-person technique is likely to
be more effective (Resuscitation Council (UK) 2000),
with one person holding the mask in place while the
other ventilates with the bag.

Positioning of the patient's head and neck is important. When maintaining the airway without intubation
the patient should have no pillow under the head and
the neck should be flexed with the head tipped back

(see Fig. 7.1). While ventilating the patient via the
mask, the head tilt is maintained by lifting the lower
jaw forward at the angle using the fingers while the
thumbs secure the seal of the mask to the face.

Whichever method of ventilation is used the patient
should initially be given two slow breaths sufficient to
cause the chest to rise. It is vital that chest movement is
observed as it is the only indicator that the airway is
patent and that tidal volume is sufficient. The volume
of air used to inflate the lungs should be sufficient to
cause the chest to rise.

Each of the initial breaths should last for 1–1.5 s
(Melker 1985) so that the chest is seen to rise and fall
between breaths. If breaths are given too rapidly there
is an increased likelihood of inflation of the stomach
with possible regurgitation and aspiration of stomach
contents.

When the anaesthetist is ready to intubate a pillow
can be placed under the patient's shoulders and occiput
to facilitate placement of the tube in the trachea.
Intubation should be preceded by at least 15 s of high-
concentration oxygen.

If the patient is already intubated and ventilated then
either the ventilator can be turned to 100% oxygen or
the patient can be manually ventilated on 100% oxygen
using a self-inflating bag. If there is any doubt at all
about the efficacy of the ventilator then it is safest to
switch to the self-inflating bag and investigate any
problems of ventilation. However, if high airway pressures are required to inflate the lungs then mechanical
ventilation is generally more effective than manual
efforts, providing settings are appropriate and correct
position of the tube is assured.

Pneumothorax should be considered if airway pressures have increased acutely in the ventilated patient
who has a cardiac arrest.

Circulation

External cardiac compressions should not be interrupted unless the patient is to be defibrillated or when
rhythm change indicates the need for pulse check.

It is very unlikely that there will only be a single
person resuscitating in the ICU so it is probable that
external chest compressions (ECC) will be started at the
same time as airway clearance and ventilation is being
carried out. Therefore, single-person resuscitation will
be discussed only briefly.

The technique of ECC must be carried out with the
patient flat on his/her back and on a firm surface. If the
patient is in a chair, the floor is the nearest and easiest
place. If the patient is on a special pressure support bed

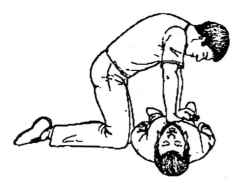

Fig. 7.2 Position for chest compression. (Reproduced with permission from Handley A.J. and Swain A. (ed.) (1994). *Advanced Life Support Manual*, 2nd edn. Resuscitation Council, UK.)

the nurse responsible for his/her care should be familiar with the emergency button to flatten or harden the bed.

Compressions are carried out using the heel of one hand placed on the lower third of the sternum in the midline, with the other hand placed on top. Location of the correct position is by placing the middle finger of one hand on the xiphisternum, the index finger above this, and then the heel of the other hand next to the index finger. The arms should be straight and the shoulders above the patient's sternum (see Fig. 7.2). Compressions should continue at a rate of 100/min (with a ratio of 15 compressions to two breaths when the patient is not intubated) and should only be interrupted as directed by the need for defibrillation, intubation, or pulse checks. Any interruption will reduce the coronary perfusion pressure produced by the compressions and there will be some delay before this is restored.

The sternum should be depressed 4–5 cm (1.5–2 inches) in the adult. The compressions can be asynchronous with ventilations if the patient is intubated because the ET tube cuff will prevent the force of compression expelling the breath and inflating the stomach.

The ratio is 15 compressions to two breaths for synchronized support unless the patient is intubated when asynchronous support with ECC at 100 compressions/min with ventilation at around 12 breaths/min will be used.

It is helpful if the person carrying out ECC counts aloud so that synchronization with ventilation in the non-intubated patient is possible and to assure the team leader than ECC is being carried out. If ECC is discontinued for any reason the count should continue with the word 'off' interposed between each number (i.e. 'one-off, two-off, three-off, four-off', etc.). This reminds the team leader that the patient has no circulatory support during this time.

Advanced life support techniques

Properly performed basic life support will keep the patient alive for up to 20–30 min but will not reverse the problem causing the initial arrest. Advanced life support includes the use of defibrillation, drugs, and other supportive measures to increase the efficacy of basic life support and to deal with the problem causing cardiac arrest.

Points to remember (see Fig. 7.3):

1. Adrenaline (epinephrine) should be given as 10 ml of 1 in 10 000 dilution (= 1 mg). The volume of fluid ensures that most of the adrenaline will enter the circulation even without a flush whereas 1 mg in only 1 ml fluid (1 in 1000 dilution) is likely to remain within the IV cannula.

2. ECC should continue at a rate of 100 compressions/min immediately following any intervention except between each of the grouped direct current (DC) shocks in the repeated cycles. The first three DC shocks should be given within 60 s. Otherwise ECC should not be interrupted for more than 30 s as the maximum achievable perfusion pressure will take some time to re-establish.

3. Between administration of each drug, ECC should continue for at least 2 min to ensure adequate circulation of the drug.

4. If IV access is impossible then endotracheal administration of twice the recommended doses of adrenaline (epinephrine), amiodarone, or atropine should be carried out as appropriate.

5. If IV access is peripheral, a large volume of flush (at least 20 ml) should be administered following administration of drugs and the limb should be massaged towards the trunk to assist the returning circulation.

6. It is vital that any shockable rhythm is not missed (fine VF can be misinterpreted as asystole): check the gain control (adjusts the size of the waveform on the monitor), lead connections, and electrode attachment on the patient.

7. External temporary pacing can be used in ventricular standstill, where P waves are still visible. This is an easy and fast method of pacing without the accompanying problems of transvenous or oesophageal systems. It is a system of pacing via electrode pads which are placed

Advanced Life Support Algorithm for the management of cardiac arrest in adults

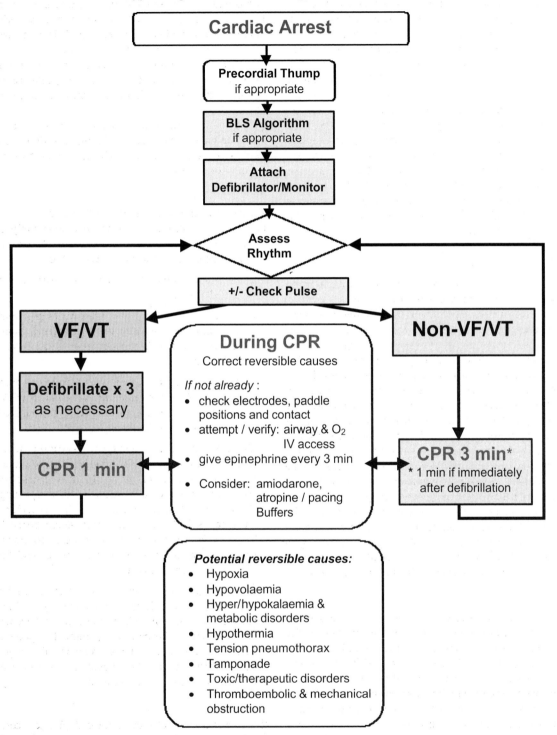

Fig. 7.3 Resuscitation Council (UK) universal treatment algorithm for the management of cardiac arrest in adults. BLS – Basic life support; CPR – cardiopulmonary resuscitation; VF/VT – ventricular fibrillation/ventricular tachycardia.

anteriorly over the precordium and posteriorly just below the scapula and to the left of the vertebrae. These pads allow excellent conduction of electrical current with an even dispersion over a wide area. This reduces the discomfort associated with the electrical stimulus. The pacemaker is connected and set at 80 to 100 beats on 100 mA current. This level may alter according to the pacemaker in use and to the patient's pacing threshold. To find the patient's threshold the level of current is adjusted upwards until QRS beats accompanied by a pulse are obtained (pacing capture) or the maximum is reached. Once capture is achieved the current level is then set to 10–20 mA higher than the patient's threshold. The patient should be paced at a fixed rate while ECC continues to avoid interference. ECC is only discontinued when there is a palpable pulse with pacing.

Defibrillation

All qualified and appropriately trained nursing and medical personnel working in intensive care should be able to manually defibrillate a patient. The improved resuscitation success rate with fast response defibrillation of VF means that it is now essential that all nursing and medical personnel responsible for acutely ill patients are trained and able to defibrillate (Chamberlain 1989; Resuscitation Council (UK) 2000). Automated external defibrillators (AED) are now commonly used both in hospital and throughout many other sites where large numbers of people are present, such as railway stations, airports, and large institutions. Their use is not common in the critical care environment where the need for more flexible defibrillation systems including cardioversion means that manual defibrillators are generally more useful.

Defibrillation is the passage of a current of electricity through the fibrillating heart. This will depolarize the cells and allow them to repolarize uniformly to organized contractions using standard conduction pathways and allowing normal pacemakers to regain control.

The defibrillator

The defibrillator stores and delivers pre-set amounts of DC electrical energy via two paddles placed on the patient's chest. The energy is measured in joules. Until recently, all defibrillators delivered a single directional monophasic waveform (current flowed in one direction from one electrode to the other). Recently defibrillators have been developed which produce biphasic waveforms. These deliver a current that flows firstly in one direction and then reverses to the opposite direction for the remainder of the electrical discharge. The advantage of these waveforms is that they are associated with a decreased defibrillation threshold and a lower level of energy needed to successfully defibrillate. There is also a longer refractory period which may help to block further recurring fibrillation.

In order to monitor ECG via the paddles some defibrillators require setting to 'paddles' while others automatically monitor via paddles until altered to an ECG lead.

Defibrillation can be delivered using either paddles with conducting (gel) pads or through multifunction 'hands-free' adhesive pads which can be used both to defibrillate and pace.

Safety aspects

The electrical energy delivered by defibrillation is potentially lethal if it strikes a bystander so a number of precautions are essential prior to defibrillation. The person defibrillating is responsible for the safety of others:

- A warning to 'stand clear' should be clearly stated prior to defibrillation.

- Ensure no other person is in contact with the patient or any conducting surfaces such as the metal frame of the bed or the IV infusion stand, just before defibrillation.

- Pressure should be applied to the paddles when placed firmly against the skin to avoid possible arcing (passage of current from paddle-to-paddle or paddle-to-patient's skin, through air).

- Electrode pads are highly effective electrical conductors and are used to provide an efficient conduction path to the patient This directs the path of the electrical current and reduces the risk of current passing through less efficient conduction pathways such as air or bare skin. Gel conduction pads should be used. These pads will dry out causing increased transthoracic impedance after 30 min and should be changed (Deakin *et al.* 2000).

- Remove any metal or foil objects on the patient's chest or upper body. They will preferentially conduct the electrical current and, in so doing, will become very hot causing burns to the patient. The patient will also receive a reduced amount of charge. Glyceryl trinitrate patches should also be removed because of their explosive capability.

Defibrillation technique

If the patient is not already monitored, place gel conduction pads in the positions shown in Fig. 7.4 and apply the defibrillator paddles to the chest.

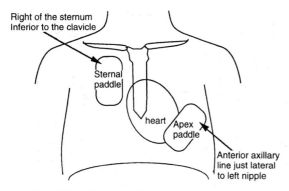

Fig. 7.4 Paddle positions for defibrillation.

Ascertain the patient's heart rhythm and unless it is certain asystole or pulseless electrical activity (PEA), charge the defibrillator to 200 joules (J) or biphasic equivalent. Press firmly on the paddles, warn all personnel to stand clear (check this visually), confirm VF (or VT) again on the monitor, and depress both paddle buttons simultaneously to discharge the shock. If the defibrillator is a fast charging model then immediately recharge and repeat defibrillation at 200 J or biphasic equivalent providing the patient remains in VF/VT. There may be a short period of spurious asystole (Resuscitation Council (UK) 2000); however, if this continues and there is either asystole or PEA then the paddles should be replaced in the machine and a pulse check carried out. If there is no pulse, then ECC should be recommenced for 1 minute initially without any drugs.

If the patient is still in VF/VT the shock should be immediately repeated, followed by a 360 J shock or biphasic equivalent if this is unsuccessful. Further management should then follow the advanced life support algorithm (Fig. 7.3).

FACTORS WHICH WILL REDUCE IMPEDANCE

- Firm pressure of approximately 10 kg (25 lb) per paddle.

- Use of conducting gel pads.

- Multiple shocks (i.e. more than two and fewer than five in succession with a short time interval between discharges).

- Increased delivered energy.

- Increased paddle surface area.

- Application of shocks during the end expiratory phase of respiration.

Transthoracic impedance, or the resistance of the chest to conduction of the electrical current, is an important and variable factor in delivering the peak amount of current to the myocardium. Bone is a very poor conductor of electricity and should be avoided. Reduction of impedance will assist the delivery of peak current and all possible steps should be taken to do so.

An alternative paddle position, which may be useful in the obese patient who has increased transthoracic impedance, is the anterior–posterior position. For this, the patient is rolled on to his/her side and one pad is placed over the left precordium next to the base of the sternum while the other is placed in the same position posteriorly to the left of the spine. This can only be safely achieved if a hands-free pad system is in use for defibrillation.

Hands-free defibrillation pads are now available for most types of defibrillator (they are always used for AEDs)—the advantages are safety for the operator, improved contact with the patient, and speed.

Mechanism of external cardiac compression (ECC)

The cardiac output produced by good external cardiac compression is only 20–30 % of normal (1.2–1.5 1/min) and the cerebral blood flow is only 15% of normal if CPR is carried out immediately the arrest occurs. Cerebral blood flow during CPR diminishes with the time taken to commence ECC. This is obviously a fairly inefficient method of maintaining circulation and there is a great need to find ways to improve it.

The mechanism of ECC is important for two reasons: (1) depending on the method of blood flow either the rate of ECC or the duration of each compression will have an effect on the cardiac output and (2) methods of improving the blood flow generated will differ according to the mechanism.

There are two proposed mechanisms by which blood flow is generated during ECC. The first is the 'cardiac pump' theory, which was proposed by Kouwenhoven *et al.* (1960) when they first described external cardiac compressions (Fig. 7.5).

PATIENT FACTORS REDUCING THE SUCCESS OF DEFIBRILLATION

- Acidosis

- Hypoxia

- Electrolyte imbalance

- Hypothermia

- Drug toxicity

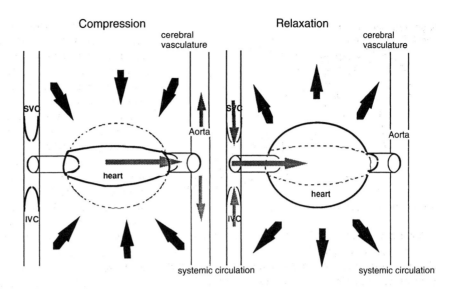

Fig. 7.5 Model of the cardiac pump theory.

This theory suggests that ECC produces compression of the heart itself between the lowered sternum anteriorly and the vertebrae posteriorly. The compression increases pressure inside the heart and blood is forced out through the aorta and pulmonary artery. Back-flow through the venae cavae and the pulmonary veins is prevented by the presence of intracardiac and venous valves. Atrioventricular filling would then take place during relaxation as the drop in pressure would draw blood back into the heart. Again, retrograde flow would be prevented by venous valves. If this theory is correct then an increased rate of CPR will improve cardiac output as each compression will only deliver a set amount of blood (i.e. that contained within the heart inself).

The second mechanism is the 'thoracic pump' theory, which suggests that the whole thorax acts as a pump during ECC (Fig. 7.6).

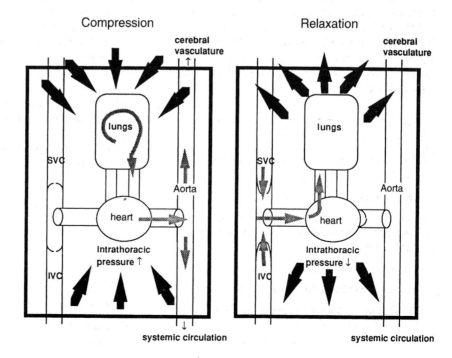

Fig. 7.6 Model of the thoracic pump' theory.

The compression raises intrathoracic pressure resulting in blood flow from the lungs (which act as a large capacity reservoir) into the left side of the heart. This forces blood already in the heart out through the aorta. Retrograde flow from the lungs is prevented by partial closure of the pulmonary valve, venae cavae valves, and by collapse of the veins themselves which are then resistant to flow. Atrioventricular filling then takes place during relaxation as the release of pressure in the intrathoracic space would draw blood mainly from the superior vena cava through the right side of the heart to fill the pulmonary vessels. If this theory is correct then increased depth and time of compression and increased intrathoracic pressure is likely to increase the cardiac output because an increased volume of blood will be squeezed from the lungs. This would also explain the improvement in cardiac output seen with asynchronous ventilation and compression.

In both mechanisms, the cause of flow is increased pressure with cardiac and venous valves ensuring one-way flow. The normal arterial resistance to flow is not present due to the loss of vasoactive peripheral tone during hypoxia, ischaemia, and acidosis (see above). Arterial and venous pressures rapidly equilibrate and forward blood flow (arterial to venous) must therefore be generated by a pressure differential between the mean aortic and the mean right atrial pressure.

Most research supports the thoracic pump' theory because:

1. The tricuspid and mitral valves are open during ECC.

2. During chest compression with a flail segment (see Chapter 13), the arterial pressure does not increase until the segment is stabilized (by intermittent positive pressure ventilation).

3. Consciousness during VF can be maintained by encouraging repeated coughing which also increases intrathoracic pressure and can maintain an arterial pressure of up to 100 mmHg.

Rate and duty cycle

Duty cycle refers to the duration of compression as a fraction of the total compression/relaxation movement in ECC.

Research into the length of the duty cycle and rate of compressions has shown that maximum systolic flow is obtained with a compression rate of around 100/min and a 50% duty cycle. Unfortunately, this can be subject to other variables such as blood volume and distribution, vascular resistance, force of chest compression, and drugs. The recommended rate is now 100 ECC/min (Resuscitation Council (UK) 2000)

TABLE 7.5 Potentially reversible causes of PEA

Potential cause of PEA	Response
Hypoxia	Check air entry, tracheal tube placement, oxygen supply, etc.
Hypovolaemia	Ensure fluid replacement is adequate/attempts to control haemorrhage are instigated
Hypo/hyperkalaemia and other metabolic disorders	IV calcium chloride for hyperkalaemia, hypocalcaemia, and hypermagnesaemia
Hypothermia	Institute methods of rewarming such as warm air devices, warmed IV and NG fluids, bladder, peritoneal, and gastric lavage with warm (40 °C) fluid. Extracorporeal circulation such as cardiopulmonary bypass
Tension pneumothorax	Decompression with needle thoracocentesis
Tamponade	Needle pericardiocentesis/cardiothoracic surgical intervention
Toxic/therapeutic disorders	Drug screen and appropriate antidotes
Thromboembolic and mechanical obstruction (most commonly pulmonary embolus)	Thrombolysis or cardiothoracic surgical intervention

Pulseless electrical activity

If there is an ECG rhythm which is normally associated with a cardiac output but the patient remains pulseless, then the underlying cause this failure must be identified and corrected. See Table 7.5.

Management of cardiac arrest

The high stress and need for immediate response associated with cardiac arrest make it one of the most potentially disorganized situations liable to occur within the ICU. In order to avoid the ineffective chaos that can ensue, all personnel should be trained in advanced cardiac life support and management of the arrest should follow structured lines. Training should include simulated cardiac arrests with feedback and debriefing managed in a constructive way.

One person *only* should be designated 'team leader' at a cardiac arrest. Decisions on interventions should be made by this person and all information pertaining to the situation should be passed to them. They should not take a practical role (unless it is essential) but, if possible, remain slightly detached with an overview of all that is

CAUSES OF CARDIAC ARREST IN THE ICU PATIENT

- Hypovolaemia
- Myocardial infarction
- Hypoxaemia
- Myocardial ischaemia
- Pneumothorax
- Intrinsic cardiac instability (arrhythmias)
- Brainstem CVA
- Hypothermia (<28 °C)
- Drugs (e.g. verapamil)
- Anaphylaxis
- Iatrogenic (e.g. disconnection from or failure of the ventilator)
- Metabolic imbalance (e.g. calcium, magnesium, potassium phosphate)

going on. Management of cardiac arrest requires an optimum number of people. Too many will increase the confusion and may physically impede necessary personnel reaching the patient. Too few will mean unnecessary delays in instituting interventions. It has been shown that survival decreases with increasing numbers of personnel attending the arrest (BRESUS Study 1992).

Most authorities suggest between three and five people. The Royal College of Physicians recommends a minimum of two doctors, usually a medical registrar and an anaesthetist, as well as one other member who may be a technician, or another doctor. In most cases, a nurse who has specialist knowledge or training is included on the team. In the ICU this will generally be the nurse caring for the patient, who will form the all-important link between knowledge of the patient and his/her condition and the specialist knowledge provided by the team. A back-up nurse can provide assistance as necessary. This back-up should reflect the experience and skills of the nurse assigned to the patient. A junior nurse will require experienced back-up, while an experienced nurse can be assisted by a junior who can learn from the experience. The nurse-in-charge should be fully aware of the situation but may not necessarily need to remain with the patient provided the back-up is appropriate.

Roles during cardiac arrest

Nurse 1 (the nurse caring for the patient)

Diagnose cardiac arrest, alert other team members, initiate CPR, inform other team members of the history and preceding events, record events and interventions, protect the patient's dignity and rights where possible, speak to the family with the doctor.

Nurse 2 (back-up)

Bring emergency equipment, prepare defibrillator and defibrillate if appropriate, draw up drugs and infusions, record events and interventions, take over CPR from nurse 1 when required.

Team leader

(The senior doctor attached to the ICU, otherwise the duty medical registrar or, if no senior medical staff are present, the nurse-in-charge.) Reaffirm arrest diagnosis and arrhythmia, direct overall resuscitation, decide on interventions, assess response, may defibrillate if appropriate, may obtain central venous access if appropriate, prescribe drugs, ensure CPR is being done correctly and that ECC is rotated so that fatigue is not a problem, call in outside help if necessary, decide on endpoint if resuscitation is unsuccessful, speak to the family.

Anaesthetist

Intubate if necessary, secure airway, obtain central venous access, ventilate or attach to ventilator and, if necessary, assist with ECC.

Agents used in resuscitation

Oxygen

The poor levels of cardiac output produced by ECC mean that anything less than 100% oxygen saturation of haemoglobin will limit the amount of oxygen delivered to the tissues. In order to ensure full saturation, 100% oxygen should be given as soon as possible and 100% oxygen saturation should be maintained following successful resuscitation to help the patient to clear the tissue oxygen debt that will have built up during CPR.

Vasopressors (α-receptor agonists)

The principal drug used to support CPR is adrenaline (epinephrine). It has mixed α- and β-receptor actions (see Chapter 6) but it is predominantly the alpha effects which are responsible for supporting resuscitation. The alpha effect consists primarily of vasoconstriction which increases aortic diastolic blood pressure and coronary and cerebral perfusion. The β-receptor action has chronotropic and inotropic effects on the myocardium and a vasodilator effect on the coronary arteries.

Disadvantages associated with its use are:

- Increase in myocardial oxygen demand in VF (probably related to increased frequency and amplitude of fibrillatory contractions).

♦ Impairment of subendocardial blood flow (probably by increasing the muscular tension which compresses coronary vessels).

The recommended dose is 1 mg IV (10 ml of 1:10 000 solution) every 3 min of CPR (14 µg/kg/3 min). There has been no evidence to support an improved outcome from the use of high dose (5 mg every 5 min (70 µg/kg/5 min)) epinephrine (Resuscitation Council (UK) 2000).

Vasopressin

This is a naturally occurring hormone (antidiuretic hormone) that works as a powerful vasoconstrictor by stimulating smooth muscle V_1 receptors. It improves coronary perfusion pressure and *in vitro* studies have shown it to be associated with better blood flow to vital organs, delivery of cerebral oxygen, chances of resuscitation, and neurological outcome than epinephrine (Wenzel *et al.* 2004).

A recent large study (Wenzel *et al.* 2004) comparing two doses of 40 IU vasopressin with two doses of 1 mg epinephrine in 1186 patients suffering out-of-hospital cardiac arrests found no difference in survival to discharge in patients with VF/VT. However, patients in asystole were more likely to survive to hospital admission (29.0% versus 20.3% in the epinephrine group; $P = 0.02$) and to hospital discharge (4.7% versus 1.5%, $P = 0.04$). Even so, survival in this group is not large.

Vasopressin is more effective in an acidotic environment which may explain its relative success in the asystolic group.

It is thought there may be a place for vasopressin in resuscitating asystolic patients and possibly in conjunction with epinephrine in the VF/VT group.

Atropine

Atropine effectively blocks vagal influence on the heart at the level of the sinoatrial nodal pacemaker. It enhances the rate of discharge of the sinus node and decreases atrioventricular conduction time. It is most effective in cases of asystole caused by toxic effects of choline esters (e.g. methacholine, carbachol), anticholinesterases (e.g. neostigmine, pyridostigmine), or other parasympathomimetic drugs (e.g. pilocarpine). It has not been established whether it has any effect in other causes of asystole. There are no known disadvantages associated with its use in the asystolic arrest.

The recommended dose is 3 mg IV given once only.

Amiodarone

Amiodarone is a potent ventricular and supraventricular anti-arrhythmic. It works by prolonging the duration of the action potential, equalizing the length of repolarization in all myocardial cells, and increasing the effective refractory period. It is used for atrial fibrillation and flutter, prevention of ventricular fibrillation and tachycardia, and for arrhythmias in Wolff–Parkinson–White syndrome. During resuscitation it should be considered if VF/VT persists after the first three shocks have been administered. It can also be used as a stabilizing agent following defibrillation.

The initial dose is 300 mg (diluted to 20 ml in 5% glucose) or 5 mg/kg IV. It can be given peripherally in the arrest situation but wherever possible should be given through a central line, followed by an infusion of 10–20 mg/kg/24 hours.

Magnesium

Magnesium has been shown to suppress myocardial irritability and prevent tachyarrhythmias *in vitro* but clinical evidence of this remains inconclusive. The actual mechanism by which it works has not yet been identified but could either be by direct inhibition of the efflux of potassium from the cell, alteration of cellular calcium metabolism, decreasing peripheral vascular resistance, or stimulating a membrane-stabilizing enzyme (Zwerling 1987).

However, use of magnesium is considered a relatively safe intervention which may be used when other antiarrhythmic agents have failed, in torsade de pointes (ventricular tachycardia with an axis that changes continuously from positive to negative), or when there is reason to suspect magnesium depletion.

The usual dose is 1–2 g or 4–8 mmol (2–4 ml of 50% magnesium sulphate) which can be repeated after 10–15 min. Side effects are extremely rare.

Lidocaine (lignocaine)

Lidocaine is a membrane-stabilizing antidysrhythmic. It primarily inhibits retrograde conduction and re-entry mechanisms by equalizing the action potential duration of individual cells so that they are less likely to depolarize before the myocardium as a whole (see Chapter 6). It may alter the defibrillatory threshold by stabilizing the arrhythmia thereby making defibrillation more difficult.

A disadvantage associated with its use is a potential increase in the defibrillatory threshold.

The recommended dose is 100 mg IV bolus. This is given either as 10 ml 1% lidocaine or 5 ml 2% lidocaine.

It is not recommended in the algorithm for VF/VT (Fig. 6.3) by the Resuscitation Council (UK) but should be considered if amiodarone is not available. The initial bolus dose is only effective for approximately 10 min and should be followed by a further bolus dose or an infusion. Following successful resuscitation from VF or VT, a lignocaine infusion of 2–4 mg/ min may be commenced.

Sodium bicarbonate

Sodium bicarbonate is now only recommended if proven pH is below 7.1 or in tricyclic overdose (Resuscitation Council (UK) 2000).

Sodium bicarbonate was originally used during CPR to reverse metabolic acidosis. It was given as a first-line response to cardiac arrest but is now regarded as a second-line drug to be considered in arrests lasting longer than 10–15 min. Research has shown an increase in venous CO_2 levels following administration of sodium bicarbonate ($NaHCO_3$) and it may actually exacerbate intracellular and respiratory acidosis. In the blood, bicarbonate (HCO_3^-) combines with hydrogen ions (H^+) to form H_2CO_3 which dissociates into H_2O and CO_2. This CO_2 diffuses rapidly into cells and combines with H_2O to form H_2CO_3 (carbonic acid). The HCO_3 does not diffuse into the cell as rapidly and therefore cannot buffer the intracellular acid. Paradoxical intracellular acidosis is thereby increased despite a decrease in extracellular acidosis. This is particularly apparent in the CSF due to the free diffusibility of CO_2 through the blood–brain barrier where increased acidosis has marked impairment on cerebral blood flow.

Other problems associated with sodium bicarbonate are:

- Increased plasma osmolality following infusion and the ensuing cerebral damage related to serum osmolality of greater than 350 mOsmol/l.
- Arterial alkalosis causing a shift in the oxyhaemoglobin dissociation curve to the left resulting in decreased availability of oxygen to the tissues.
- Arterial alkalosis may also increase cerebral vascular resistance thus reducing cerebral blood flow.
- Arterial alkalosis may reduce the effectiveness of vasopressors.

Its use is correctly restricted to prolonged arrests (>10–15 min) where the acidosis is severe, and in hyperkalaemia or anaphylaxis with bronchoconstriction where epinephrine may be potentially ineffective because of marked acidosis.

The dose is 50 mmol (50 ml of 8.4% solution) which can be repeated as necessary.

Calcium

Calcium is essential in myocardial excitation—contraction coupling, in increasing contractility, and in enhancing ventricular automaticity during asystole. In the past, calcium was administered in the arrest situation for the above effects but evidence to support this is lacking. Unfortunately, there are other effects associated with calcium which are potentially more deleterious to outcome, namely:

- Prevention of reperfusion of ischaemic areas of the brain and heart due to vascular spasm related to intracellular calcium overload and impairment of oxidative phosphorylation of the mitochondria.
- Cytoplasmic calcium accumulation is associated with cell death.
- Inhibition of calcium accumulation following an ischaemic episode preserves myocardial function.

There is some experimental evidence that cerebral blood flow and neurological recovery following global ischaemia may be promoted by calcium antagonists but this has yet to be confirmed.

Calcium is recommended for use only in highly specific circumstances where hypocalcaemia or blockage of calcium channels may be the cause of the arrest. This includes hypocalcaemia, hyperkalaemia, hypermagnesaemia, and untoward reaction to calcium channel blockers such as verapamil.

The dose is 10 ml of 10% calcium chloride. Calcium chloride is used in preference to calcium gluconate because the number of free calcium ions produced is three times greater for the same volume of drug (2.25 mmol in 10 ml 10% calcium gluconate to 6.8 mmol in 10 ml 10% calcium chloride).

Intravenous fluids

It is usual to set up a crystalloid solution, such as 0.9% sodium chloride, to provide a flush for IV drugs and dilution if necessary. If hypovolaemia is suspected then colloid or O rhesus-negative blood (for severe blood loss) may be infused.

Care should be taken to ensure that drugs are actually reaching the circulation and if there is any doubt an alternative IV access should be used. Ideally, there should be central venous access as poor peripheral circulation makes it unlikely that drugs given peripherally will have a chance to circulate. (Note: the intracardiac route for drugs is no longer recommended as there is little advantage to it. The high level of complications and the difficulty of insertion make it a dangerous proposition without real added benefit.)

Care of the successfully resuscitated patient

It is usual for patients in the post-arrest period to be admitted to the ICU. The exceptions may be the patient

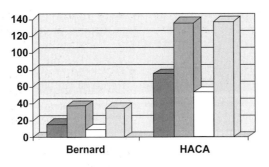
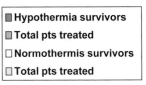

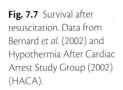

Fig. 7.7 Survival after resuscitation. Data from Bernard *et al.* (2002) and Hypothermia After Cardiac Arrest Study Group (2002) (HACA).

in the coronary care unit whose ventricular fibrillation responds immediately to defibrillation or the patient who has an end-stage disease where intensive care is not appropriate. Immediately post-arrest, the patient remains unstable and extremely vulnerable to further problems. The decision to transfer to intensive care should be made by the team leader in consultation with the ICU staff and the medical staff responsible for the patient.

Even with the most effective cardiopulmonary resuscitation, the patient will have suffered a period of relative ischaemia which will have the greatest effect on those organs most dependent on a continuous supply of oxygen. The cerebral tissues are particularly susceptible due to their high energy requirements and the minimal substrate reserves for anaerobic metabolism. There is, therefore, a high risk of cerebral damage which is exacerbated by hyperglycaemia and acidosis. Certain interventions will protect the cerebral tissues from further injury related to the return of blood flow (re-perfusion injury; see Chapter 10) and may reduce the damage already present.

Hypothermia post-arrest

A number of studies have shown the protective effect of hypothermia on the brain following cardiac arrest (Sterz *et al.* 2003). This is thought to be due to the increase in tolerance of anoxia associated with a lower metabolic rate, which is particularly important in the brain.

POTENTIAL COMPLICATIONS OF THERAPEUTIC HYPOTHERMIA

 ◆ Pneumonia

 ◆ Sepsis

 ◆ Cardiac arrhythmias

 ◆ Coagulopathy

Sterz *et al.* (2003)

Two studies recently reported increased survival (Bernard *et al.* 2002, Hypothermia After Cardiac Arrest Study Group 2002 (HACA)) and a higher rate of neurological recovery (Bernard *et al.* 2002) (Fig. 7.7). The patients received cooling to between 32 and 34 °C for 24 hours following VF/VT arrest (HACA 2002) or to 33 °C for 12 hours if still unconscious after return of spontaneous circulation post VF/VT arrest (Bernard *et al.* 2002).

Sterz *et al.* (2003) propose that patients are cooled as fast as possible to 33 °C for 24 hours and then rewarmed in not less than 8 hours to at least 36 °C. Measurement of body temperature should be by a reliable method such as Foley catheter probes. Patients should receive muscle relaxants to prevent shivering. Expected complications should be monitored for and where possible prevented.

Treatment following resuscitation

1. Mechanical ventilation to achieve normocapnia. Some authorities recommend short-term hyperventilation to reduce PCO_2 (usually to 3.5–4.0 kPa). This causes cerebral vasoconstriction and reduces cerebral blood volume which may help to limit any increase in intracranial pressure, but may also increase cerebral ischaemia. Its use remains controversial.

2. Maintenance of an adequate cardiac output and normotension to avoid further ischaemia and preserve cerebral perfusion pressure (see Chapter 10).

3. Adequate oxygenation to avoid hypoxaemia.

Treatment following the return of spontaneous circulation

The nurse should:

1. Check that the patient's ventilation is adequate and that there is air entry to both lungs.

2. Attach a pulse oximeter if this is not already in place and confirm that the patient is ventilated on 100% oxygen.

3. Check the blood pressure either with a sphygmomanometer or using the arterial trace.

4. Obtain an arterial blood gas sample and measure blood gases, electrolytes, blood glucose, and haemoglobin.

5. Confirm with medical staff whether the patient is to be kept ventilated and administer sedation as prescribed if necessary.

6. Obtain a chest X-ray to check for: fractured ribs, pneumothorax, possible aspiration, position of central venous lines, ET tube, and NG tube.

7. Take a 12-lead ECG.

8. Measure CVP and urine output.

More specific responses (e.g. insertion of a pulmonary artery catheter) will be necessary according to the individual patient's needs and treatment will probably have to be changed frequently at first to accommodate changes in the patient's condition.

When the patient is stable, intravenous catheters placed during the cardiac arrest should be assessed and replacement considered in view of the non-sterile circumstances in which they were inserted.

Once the patient is stable, full attention can be turned to the patient's family. Although they should have been updated during the cardiac arrest they will still require a full explanation of what has happened. If the patient arrested on the ward and has been transferred to critical care then the family will require details of what this entails. It is often helpful to have a nurse from the ward who knows the patient's family present to provide a known point of contact for them. A senior member of the medical staff and a nurse should explain what has occurred, giving as much information as the family can absorb. Much of it will require repetition due to the distressed state they are in and care must be taken to avoid jargon and emotive terms such as 'shocked out of VF'.

Complications of resuscitation

The technique of ECC can produce some complications and an awareness of this possibility should be maintained when assessing the patient post-resuscitation. These include fractured ribs, flail chest, and pneumothorax, all of which should be excluded on chest X-ray and examination. The possibility of aspiration of gastric contents during resuscitation should also be considered.

Ethics of resuscitation

The main concern for all those associated with resuscitating patients is that inappropriate cardiopulmonary resuscitation will simply prolong the act of dying rather than offering a chance of survival. Resuscitation attempts do not allow a peaceful and dignified death. They can remove the family and loved ones from the scene and guarantee a technical, intervention-dominated approach to what may be the patient's final minutes. Resuscitation is a valued and appropriate response if the patient has a chance of recovery and there is no end-stage terminal disease underlying the arrest, but if it is carried out in the wrong circumstances then it has little benefit for the patient or family.

There are two situations where assessment is difficult. The first is the resuscitation of 'out of hospital' victims whose medical history and circumstances are unknown to the team. In this case, resuscitation is always attempted. The second is the hospital inpatient who has an end-stage chronic disease or malignancy but who has not been assessed by the medical team for a 'do not attempt resuscitation' (DNAR) decision in spite of clearly being unsuitable for resuscitation. Resuscitation will still be initiated by junior staff who do not have the seniority to make any other decision. Following resuscitation, the patient may then require intensive care and unless senior medical staff are called in to assess the patient, they may be admitted inappropriately to the ICU.

There is little that can be done about the first situation but the frequency of the second situation can be limited by the awareness and responsibility of senior medical staff. Discussion of prognosis and DNAR orders at an appropriate stage in the patient's terminal illness, either with the patient themselves or with them and their family, is important. Advance directives or 'living wills' may also be brought into the discussion as they can provide a clear record of the patient's wishes (Institute of Medical Ethics Working Party 1993). All staff should be familiar with local policies on DNAR decisions. All regular members of the caring team should also be involved in the discussion. An informed decision which is communicated to all personnel caring for the patient will prevent inappropriate resuscitation attempts.

Resuscitation can produce four results:

◆ complete recovery
◆ partial recovery
◆ prolonged survival
◆ death.

The two extremes of complete recovery or death do not involve the moral problems associated with the grey areas of partial recovery and prolonged survival. Patients who are still decorticate, decerebrate, or flaccid and unresponsive to stimulation 24 hours after arrest have only a 7% chance of wakening. In one study, no patient with these findings on the third or fourth day after arrest survived (Snyder and Tabbaa 1987, cited in Abramson 1990). The worst possible scenario is to leave a patient in the so-called 'persistent vegetative state' where all higher neurological function is lost and the patient remains alive but functioning purely on brainstem reflexes (see Chapter 10). These patients may end up in the ICU post-arrest and the problem of how far to continue treatment then ensues. Assessment of neurological function is extremely difficult with no clearly identifiable marker of neurological dysfunction at this level. There is no simple formula that can be applied and each patient has to be assessed as an individual by the team as a whole. It is also appropriate to discuss the situation with the family. However, they should never be made to feel that withdrawal of treatment is their decision, due to the enormous potential for guilt that this could evoke. Ultimately, the decision must be made by the ICU consultant in conjunction with the patient's own consultant and the intensive care team.

Test yourself

Questions

1. List the differences between an arrest situation on the ward and an arrest situation in the critical care area.

2. What are the priorities in an arrest situation where the rhythm is defibrillation-responsive?

3. Your ventilated patient develops high airway pressures, low oxygen saturations, a tachycardia, and hypotension. This is then followed by loss of cardiac output, but a tachycardia remains on the monitor. What is this and what would you suspect is the cause of it? How is it treated?

4. Review a patient you have cared for recently where a DNAR order has been made. What do you think are the reasons for this decision? Do you feel they are the right reasons? What is the chance of surviving to be discharged home for a patient who has an arrest in the ICU?

Answers

1. Immediate access to skilled assistance and equipment. After the initial pulse check to ensure that the problem is not with the arterial line, cardiac output can be visualized on the monitor.

   Patients are often already intubated and ventilated, and mechanical ventilation can continue (on 100% O_2) providing this is not the cause of the problem.

Arrests are infrequent and rarely unexpected (unless in a coronary care or cardiac surgical unit).

2. Defibrillation

   Airway patency and breathing

   Identifying a cause

3. Pulseless electrical activity

   Tension pneumothorax

   Needle thoracocentesis followed by a chest drain

References and bibliography

Abramson, N.S. (1990). Cardiac arrest and the brain. In: *Update in Intensive Care and Emergency Medicine* (ed. J.L. Vincent), Vol 10, pp. 603–11. Springer, Berlin.

Anderson, F.D. (1988). Issues in the postresuscitation period. *Critical Care Nursing Quarterly* **10**, 51–61.

Baskett, P.J.F. (1986). The ethics of resuscitation. *British Medical Journal* **293**, 189–90.

Bossaert, L., Koster, R. (1992). Defibrillation: methods and strategies. *Resuscitation* **24**, 211–25.

Bernard, S.A., Gray, T.W., Buist, M.D., *et al.* (2002). Treatment of comatose survivors of out-of-hospital cardiac arrest with induced hypothermia. *New England Journal of Medicine* **346**, 557–63.

BRESUS Study (Tunstall Pedoe, H., Bailey, L., Chamberlain, D.A., *et al.*) (1992). Survey of 3765 cardiopulmonary resuscitations in British hospitals: methods and overall results. *British Medical Journal* **304**, 1347–51.

Chamberlain, D.A. (1989). Advanced life support. *British Medical Journal* **299**, 446–8.

Cheney, R. (1988). Defibrillation. *Critical Care Nursing Quarterly* **10**, 9–15.

Dumot, J.A., Burval, D.J., Spring, J., *et al.* (2001). Outcome of adult cardiopulmonary resuscitations at a tertiary referral center including results of limited resscitations. *Archives of Internal Medicine* **161**. 1751–8.

Deakin, C.H., Petley, G.W., Drury, N.E., *et al.* (2000). How often should defibrillation pads be changed? 1)The effect of evaporative drying. *Resuscitation* **45**, S45.

Gwinnutt, C.L., Columb, M., Harris, R. (2000). Outcome after cardiac arrest in adults in UK hospitals: effect of the 1997 guidelines. *Resuscitation* **47**, 125–35.

Herlitz, J., Bång, A., Gunnarsson, J., *et al.* (2003). Factors associated with survival to hospital discharge among patients hospitalized alive after out of hospital cardiac arrest: change in outcome over 20 years in the community of Göteborg, Sweden. *Heart* **89**, 25–30.

Hypothermia After Cardiac Arrest Study Group (2002). Mild therapeutic hypothermia to improve the neurologic outcome after cardiac arrest. *New England Journal of Medicine* **346**, 549–56.

Institute of Medical Ethics Working Party (1993). Advance directives: partnership and practicalities. *British Journal of General Practice* **43**, 16971.

Iseri, L.T., Freed, J., Bures, A.R. (1975). Magnesium deficiency and cardiac disorders. *American Journal of Medicine* **58**, 837–46.

Kouwenhoven, W.B., Jude, J.R., Knickerbocker, G.G. (1960). Closed chest cardiac massage. *Journal of the American Medical Association* **173**, 94–7.

Lindner, K.H. (1991). Vasopressor therapy in cardiopulmonary resuscitation. In: *Update in Intensive Care and Emergency Medicine* (ed. J.L. Vincent), Vol. 10, pp. 18–24. Springer, Berlin.

Melker, R.J. (1985). Recommendations for ventilation during cardiopulmonary resuscitation: time for a change? *Critical Care Medicine* **13**, 882–3.

Peberdy, M.A., Kaye, W., Ornato, J.P., *et al.* (2003). Cardiopulmonary resuscitation of adults in the hospital: a report of 14 720 cardiac arrests from the National registry of cardiopulmonary resuscitation. *Resuscitation* **58**, 297–308.

Peters, J., Ihle, P. (1990). Mechanics of the circulation during cardiopulmonary resuscitation. Pathophysiology and techniques (Parts I and II). *Intensive Care Medicine* **16**, 11–27.

Planta, I., Weil, M.H., Planna, M., *et al.* (1991). Hypercarbic acidosis reduces cardiac resuscitability. *Critical Care Medicine* **19**, 1177–81.

Resuscitation Council (UK) (2000). *Advanced Life Support Manual*. Resuscitation Council (UK), London.

Royal College of Nursing (RCN) (1992). *Resuscitation: Right or Wrong*. RCN, London.

Royal College of Physicians (RCP) (1987). *Resuscitation from Cardiopulmonary Arrest. Training and Organisation*. RCP, London.

Saunders, J. (1992). Who's for CPR? *Journal of the Royal College of Physicians* **26**, 254–7.

Schleien, C.L., Berkowitz, I.D., Traystman, R., *et al.* (1989). Controversial issues in cardiopulmonary resuscitation. *Anesthesiology* **71**, 133–49.

Skinner, D.V., Camm, A.L., Miles, S. (1985). CPR skills of preregistration house officers. *British Medical Journal* **290**, 1549.

Smith, G., Poplett, N. (2002). Knowledge of aspects of acute care in trainee doctors. *Postgraduate Medical Journal* **78**, 335–8.

Sterz, F., Holzer,M., Foine,F., *et al.* (2003). Hypothermia after cardiac arrest: a treatment that works. *Current Opinion in Critical Care* **9**, 205–10.

Weil, M.H., Rackow, E.C., Trevino, R., *et al.* (1986). Difference in acid–base state between venous and arterial blood during cardiopulmonary resuscitation. *New England Journal of Medicine* **315**, 153–6.

Wenzel, V., Krismer, A.C., Arntz, H.R., *et al.* (2004). A comparison of vasopressin and epinephrine for out-of-hospital cardiopulmonary resuscitation. *New England Journal of Medicine* **350**, 105–13.

Wynne, G. (1990). Revised guidelines for life support. *Nursing Times* **86**, 70–5.

Wynne, G., Marteau, T. (1987). Race against time. *Nursing Times* **83**, 16–17.

Zwerling, H.K. (1987). Does exogenous magnesium suppress myocardial irritability and tachyarrhythmias in the nondigitalized patient? *American Heart Journal* **113**, 1046–53.

Cardiac surgery

Introduction

This chapter is intended to give an overview of the care of patients undergoing cardiac surgery from an intensive care perspective. Cardiac transplantation will be covered briefly. It will concentrate on:

- The physiological consequences of cardiopulmonary bypass.

- Surgical procedures.

- Care of the patient following surgery.

- Complications following cardiac surgery.
- Mechanical cardiac assist devices.

Preparation of the patient prior to surgery

The seminal works of Hayward (1975) and Wilson-Barnett (1984) have illustrated the influence that patient preparation and teaching can have on the response to hospitalization and surgery. It can reduce anxiety prior to operation and moderate the physiological response to post-operative stress. This is particularly important in the preparation of patients for cardiac surgery, where anxiety may already be high due to the perceived high-risk nature of the operation.

Preparation and provision of information should start from the time of the surgeon's decision that surgery is required. The patient is informed of the risks involved as well as the likely benefits. Pre-admission information has been shown to be significantly more effective for retention of knowledge, positive patient mood, and improved response to regaining independence post-operatively (Cupples 1991). Many patients visit the cardiac surgery unit 2 weeks prior to surgery for the pre-operative work-up. This is an ideal opportunity to prepare them and provide information in the form of booklets, videos, and one to one counselling sessions.

Elements of pre-operative preparation

1. Patients and family are seen by a nurse from the intensive care who will explain:

   - what happens to the patient during the course of their stay and the likely time span,
   - what sensations they may feel and what they may hear and see,
   - how the presence of the endotracheal tube will affect them and an explanation of alternative forms of communication,
   - the role of the intensive care nurse,
   - the function of the intensive care equipment,
   - visiting arrangements and direct line telephone number.

   (All this information should be backed up by written details which will allow the patient to refer back to any point requiring clarification or reminder.)

2. Patients and family are offered the opportunity to visit the ICU and become more familiar with the environment.

GUIDELINES FOR GIVING PRE-OPERATIVE INFORMATION

Establish the patient's understanding and discuss:

1. The patient will wake in the ICU:
   he/she may hear before being able to move or respond

2. The endotracheal tube will cause:
   an inability to talk
   a need for suctioning and associated sensations
   a need for alternative methods of communicating

   The likely length of time it will be in place and the possibility of an extension of this should be discussed.

3. The ventilator may still be attached:
   what it does
   what it feels like
   the importance of relaxing and letting it do the work.

4. Alarms and buzzers:
   what they mean
   what they sound like.

5. Pain:
   where it will be
   what it will feel like
   what can be done for it (positioning, support, analgesia)
   how to let the nurse know the patient has pain.

6. ICU nurse:
   always nearby: watching and monitoring progress.

7. Physiotherapy:
   pain relief will be given prior to any physiotherapy
   the patient to inform the nurse if this is insufficient
   need for deep breathing and coughing after extubation
   need for leg exercises while in bed
   early mobility.

8. Chest drains:
   what they are
   what they do
   when they will be removed (pain relief prior to removal).

   Always check the patient has understood. Ask if he/she has any other questions.

3. Assessment of the patient's and family's understanding of the operation.

4. Assessment of the patient's physical and psychological status and identification of any problems likely to have an effect in the post-operative phase.

Anatomy and physiology

Figure 8.1 shows the heart and coronary arteries. Figure 8.2 is a longitudinal section of the heart showing the valves.

Surgical procedures

Coronary artery bypass graft

Coronary artery disease is a major cause of morbidity and mortality in the western world. Statistical data from the British Heart Foundation (BHF)report that death rates from coronary artery disease in the UK are still amongst the highest in the world with the highest incidence in the UK occurring in Scotland and the north of England.(British Heart Foundation 2003)

The development of ischaemic heart disease is multifactorial and prevention through education is obviously the most important healthcare intervention. Until these initiatives reduce the incidence of coronary artery disease, it is likely that demand for coronary artery surgery will remain high. In some types of atherosclerotic narrowing, angioplasty provides a degree of revascularization and is becoming an alternative in specific groups of patients (see below).

The most common type of cardiac surgery performed in the UK is coronary artery bypass grafting (Society of Cardiothoracic Surgeons (SCTS) 2002). The aim is to improve the patient's prognosis and alleviate other

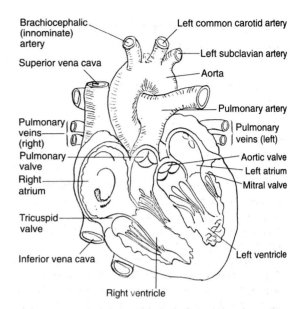

Fig. 8.2 Longitudinal section of the heart showing the valves and major vessels.

symptoms associated with atherosclerotic narrowing of the coronary arteries (ischaemic heart disease). Coronary artery bypass grafting involves grafting either a piece of saphenous vein from the leg or the internal thoracic (mammary) artery, to a point on the coronary artery distal to the atherosclerotic lesion, providing an alternative route for blood flow past the vessel obstruction.

Surgery is established therapy for patients with left main stem, triple vessel (left anterior descending, right, and circumflex coronary artery) disease. It is also indicated for narrowing of the proximal left anterior descending (LAD) artery, angina, and poor left ventricu-

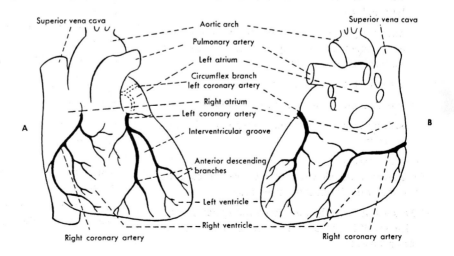

Fig. 8.1 The heart, showing coronary arteries: A, anterior view; B, posterior view.

FACTORS ASSOCIATED WITH RISK OF HEART DISEASE

- Cigarette smoking
- Hypercholesterolaemia
- Obesity
- Hypertension
- Familial history
- Diabetes mellitus
- High sugar or fat diet

  Note: females attain the same risk as males after the menopause (American Heart Association)

INDICATIONS FOR EMERGENCY CORONARY ARTERY SURGERY

- Continued unstable angina with maximum medical treatment.
- Failed angioplasty with acute symptoms.

RISK FACTORS FOR UNDERGOING CARDIAC SURGERY

- Hypertension
- Smoking
- Peripheral vascular disease
- Cerebrovascular disease
- Repeat coronary artery surgery
- Chronic obstructive airway disease (COAD)
- Three-vessel disease
- Female gender
- Renal impairment
- Left main stem disease
- Ejection fraction <30%
- Emergency surgery
- Age >70 years

Keogh (2003)

lar function if symptoms are present and persist despite maximal drug therapy (ACC/AHA 1999).

Surgery is considered for any patient who does not respond symptomatically to maximal medical therapy or who has unstable angina which does not settle with optimal conservative treatment. The benefits in terms of improving prognosis are less certain except in cases of triple vessel, proximal LAD, and left main stem disease.

Surgery will not cure atherosclerotic disease; there is a recognized incidence of graft occlusion and continuing coronary artery atheroma (see Table 8.1). However, surgery has been shown to improve quality of life in this group of patients.

Improvement in quality of life associated with coronary artery surgery is achieved by:

- Greater relief from angina.
- Less limitation of activity.

- Better exercise tolerance.
- Less need for beta-blockers, nitrates, and additional medication.

The severity of symptoms is not always a reflection of the severity of disease. Exercise testing and coronary angiography are the best methods of determining suitability for surgery. Assessment by coronary angiography establishes

- Location and severity of coronary occlusion(s).
- Rate of flow through vessel distal to lesion(s).
- The functional status of the left ventricle.
- The function of aortic and mitral valves..

Mortality for patients undergoing cardiac surgery is calculated on the basis of various risk factors (see box).

A number of assessment scores exist to calculate the risk, e.g. Parsonnet and Euroscore. Those with poor left ventricular function (commonly, ejection fraction <30%) have an increased risk of mortality with or without surgery. The functional limitation expressed by the ejection fraction is classified as normal, mild, moderate, or severe.

TABLE 8.1 Graft survival (from Loop *et al.* 1986)

	Conduit patency		
	At 1 yr	At 5 yr	At 10–12 yr
Saphenous vein	80–88%	82%	55%
Left internal thoracic (mammary) artery to left anterior descending	98%	97%	96%

Ejection fraction = percentage of ventricular end diastolic volume ejected during systole (normal = 67 ± 8%)

Surgical technique

The vessel forming the graft may be either a vein (usually the long saphenous vein) or the internal mammary/thoracic artery (IMA/ITA) (see Fig. 8.3 and box). If the vein is used, it must be carefully harvested from the leg and tested for patency by filling with normal saline or heparinized blood. Care must be taken to ensure that the vein is 'the right way round' and that any valves do not obstruct the flow of blood.

The proximal end of the vein or arterial graft is attached to the aorta and the distal end to a point on the coronary artery distal to the occlusive lesion. Grafts can be simple with end-to-side anastomosis (end of vessel to side of coronary artery), or sequential with a side-to-side anastomosis (side of vessel to side of coronary artery) followed by an end-to-side anastomosis to another artery.

If the IMA/ITA is used, it is usually dissected and mobilized as a pedicled graft (i.e. the proximal end remains attached to the subclavian artery) to the coronary artery. This involves opening the pleura, freeing the IMA/ITA, and cauterizing off the intercostal artery branches. IMA grafts can also be either simple or sequential and can be either left (to the left coronary artery) or right (to the right or circumflex coronary artery).

The IMA has been shown to be superior in terms of long-term patency and degree of subsequent atherosclerosis compared with saphenous grafts.(Loop *et al.* 1986)

VESSELS USED FOR GRAFTS

Venous conduits:

- long or short saphenous,
- cephalic,
- umbilical.

Arterial conduits:

- internal thoracic,
- radial,
- right gastroepiploic,
- inferior epigastric,
- splenic,
- lateral costal.

Valve replacement

Elective valve repair or replacement is usually carried out for moderate or severe degrees of dysfunction (Table 8.2 and box).

Currently there is approximately a 4.8% mortality depending on the valve and pathology (Society of Cardiothoracic Surgeons of Great Britain and Ireland 2000–2001). Risk to the individual with endocarditis, a re-operation, or requiring multiple valve replacement is greatly increased. Although valve disease and dysfunction can involve any intracardiac valve, the lower

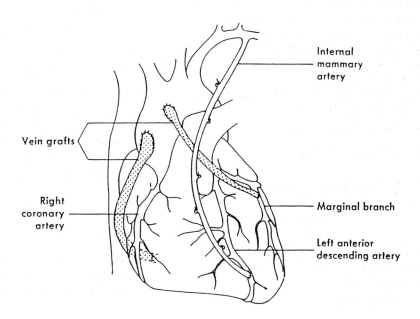

Fig. 8.3 Grafts to the heart can be arterial or venous conduits.

TABLE 8.2	Clinical effects of valve dysfunction		
Disorders requiring valve surgery	**Causes**	**Dysfunction**	**Effects**
Mitral stenosis	Rheumatic heart disease, bacterial endocarditis, calcification	Forward flow through the stenotic valve is impeded by fibrosed and contracted valve leaflets, commissures and chordae tendinae	High left atrial pressures produce left atrial dilatation, pulmonary hypertension, and right heart failure. Poor left ventricular filling produces low cardiac output and systemic blood flow
Mitral regurgitation	*Acute*: endocarditis, chest trauma, myocardial infarction. *Chronic*: rheumatic heart disease, calcification, myxomatous degeneration, left ventricular dilatation	*Chronic*: retrograde flow from ineffective valve closure is due to the disease process causing thickening and contracture of cusps preventing closure. Ventricular dilatation stretches the valve so that the cusps do not meet. *Acute*: retrograde flow is due to erosion or perforation of cusps or chordae by infection, and rupture of papillary muscle or chordae by trauma or myocardial infarction	*Chronic*: high left atrial pressures produce left atrial dilatation and, late on in the disease, pulmonary hypertension, and right heart failure. *Regurgitation of ventricular outflow* produces low cardiac output with ventricular hypertrophy and dilatation. *Acute*: insufficient time for compensatory mechanisms means that cardiac output falls dramatically, pulmonary oedema develops rapidly, and shock ensues
Aortic stenosis	Rheumatic fever, calcification of bisuspid valve (a common congenital cause)	Forward flow through the valve is impeded by fibrous contractures and commissure fusion as a result of the disease process	*Impeded ventricular outflow* produces low cardiac output and decreased coronary perfusion. *Ventricular hypertrophy* increases ventricular volume and pressure. This is reflected backwards and increases left atrial pressures with eventual pulmonary hypertension and right heart failure. *Angina* due to myocardial ischaemia occurs as a result of poor coronary perfusion and increased myocardial oxygen demand from ventricular hypertrophy. *Syncope* (fainting) occurs when cardiac output cannot increase to meet increased bodily demands (e.g. exercise) and cerebral perfusion is compromised
Aortic regurgitation	*Chronic*: rheumatic fever, aneurysm of the ascending aorta. *Acute*: blunt chest trauma, ruptured ascending aortic aneurysm, infective endocarditis	*Chronic*: aneurysm causes annular dilatation so cusps are unable to meet, disease process thickens and retracts cusps, thus retrograde flow of blood occurs during systole. *Acute*: ruptured ascending aortic aneurysm dilates and damages the valve. Infection erodes and ruptures the cusps	*Chronic*: cardiac output decreases and left ventricular volume and pressure increase. *Blood regurgitates* back from the aortic root during diastole leading to widened pulse pressure. *Left ventricular hypertrophy and dilatation* occur and eventual increases in left atrial pressure and pulmonary pressures lead to right heart failure. *Acute: left ventricular failure* develops rapidly with acute development of pulmonary oedema

DISORDERS REQUIRING VALVE SURGERY

- Trauma (rare).
- Chronic rheumatic heart disease, calcification, myxomatous degeneration, left ventricular dilatation.
- Rheumatic fever, calcification of bicuspid valve (a common congenital cause).
- Chronic rheumatic fever, aneurysm of the ascending aorta.
- Chronic calcification, rheumatic heart disease, bacterial endocarditis.
- Acute: endocarditis, myocardial infarction.

FACTORS ASSOCIATED WITH INCREASED RISK IN VALVE SURGERY

- Pathology of valve dysfunction (e.g. infection).
- Left ventricular dysfunction.
- Hepatic dysfunction (indicating advanced disease).
- Repeat operation.
- Emergency operation.

pressures in the right side of the heart usually mean that tricuspid and pulmonary valve dysfunction are less significant. Surgery is more commonly performed on aortic and mitral valves (Society of Cardiothoracic Surgeons of Great Britain and Ireland 2000–2001), less frequently on the tricuspid valve, and rarely on the pulmonary valve. Mitral stenosis is sometimes repaired by valvotomy particularly in the child where replacement at an early age will require larger valves as the child grows.

Surgical technique

The technique of valve replacement utilizes cardiopulmonary bypass in the same way and for the same reasons as coronary artery bypass grafts (CABGs), i.e. to provide a period of time without myocardial contraction, allowing the surgeon to operate.

A median sternotomy incision is made. The approach to the mitral valve is through the left atrium and the approach to the aortic valve is via the ascending aorta. The dysfunctioning valve is removed with preservation of the posterior valvular apparatus and the site of the annulus is measured. A mechanical or tissue valve of the appropriate size is sutured to the annulus or a valvotomy/valve repair is performed, the heart is de-aired, and bypass is gradually weaned.

Cardiopulmonary bypass

Most cardiac surgery currently requires the cessation of myocardial contractions. During this time some form of myocardial protection is necessary. Circulatory flow and oxygenation must then be supported by an alternative mechanism. This mechanism is cardiopulmonary bypass (Fig. 8.4). Recently some CABGs have been performed without instigation of cardiopulmonary bypass (the 'off-pump' procedure) but this technique is relatively new.

The cardiopulmonary bypass machine consists of a reservoir, one or more pumps, an oxygenator, heat exchanger, bubble trap and filter.

Oxygenator

The membrane oxygenator consists of gas-permeable microporous polypropylene or silicone membranes which separate the blood flow from the gas flow. Venous blood is filtered and pumped through the sheets or hollow fibres of the membrane. Movement of

FACTORS DETERMINING VALVE REPLACEMENT WITH EITHER A MECHANICAL OR TISSUE/BIOPROSTHETIC VALVE

Mechanical valve

- Patients <65 yr for aortic valve replacement, and <70 yr for mitral valve replacement.
- Patients requiring warfarin therapy because of risk factors for thromboembolism.
- Low rate of structural deterioration, especially in younger patients.

Bioprosthetic (porcine or pericardial) valve

- Patients >65 yr of age who need aortic valve replacment and do not have risk factors for thromboembolism.
- Patients with likely compliance problems with warfarin therapy.
- Lack of need for antithrombotic therapy.

American Heart Association (2000)

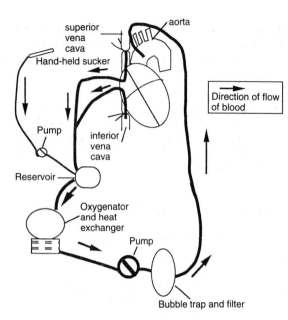

Fig. 8.4 Diagram showing the cardiopulmonary bypass circuit.

gas across the membrane is governed by partial pressures and the solubility of the gas. Alteration of the concentration of oxygen in the gas flow will alter arterial oxygen tension while variation in the rate of flow is used to regulate carbon dioxide levels.

Pump mechanisms

There are two types of pump, occlusive and non-occlusive which maintain a constant output. An occlusive roller pump results in pulsatile flow which provides pressure and flow. The roller pump uses a head which almost occludes a flexible silicone portion of the bypass circuit in a circular motion thus compressing and forcing blood forwards.

The non-occlusive centrifugal pump results in non-pulsatile flow and provides flow and finite pressure. This is the most frequently used type of pump in the UK.

Priming

The bypass circuit is primed with a 1.5–2 litre volume of either electrolyte solution such as Ringer's lactate solution, colloid, or blood (Lilley 2002). The electrolyte solution produces a reduction in viscosity of the patient's blood which decreases intracapillary sludging related to the non-pulsatile low rate of flow. Complement activation is also decreased. The large added volume of fluid required to maintain a satisfactory circulation via the pump may mean considerable fluid retention by the patient. This is usually eliminated by the patient within 48 hours post-operatively, but can be

the source of a number of fluid management problems if the patient has poor renal, pulmonary, or ventricular function.

Before attachment to the patient, the venous and arterial ends of the circuit are connected to form a closed system and the priming fluid is pumped round. This de-airs the circuit and gives time for the heat exchanger to raise the priming solution to a uniform temperature of 35–37 °C.

Initiating bypass

Prior to initiation, the patient is anticoagulated to an activated clotting time (ACT) of about 400 s using 300–400 IU/kg of heparin. The arterial cannula is then placed in the aorta (most commonly) and the arterial side of the bypass circuit is attached. Venous cannulae are then inserted either into the superior and inferior venae cavae or into the right atrium. All venous blood is then siphoned into the venous reservoir and the arterial pump is started to return oxygenated blood to the aorta. At the same time the patient may be cooled to 24–32 °C using the heat exchanger. Once the patient reaches the desired temperature, the ascending aorta is clamped and fibrillatory arrest is induced.

Myocardial protection methods

1. *Cardioplegia method.* This method is used worldwide. It is performed using blood or crystalloid hyperkalaemic solution which is administered antegrade or retrograde once the aortic cross clamp is applied.

2. *Non-cardioplegia method.* Intermittent aortic cross clamp and fibrillation. The heart is actively put into ventricular fibrillation using a continuous current to the heart. At completion of each individual bypass graft the heart is defibrillated back to sinus rhythm using low-voltage DC internal paddles.

In longer procedures cold cardioplegic arrest may be used. This produces a hyperkalaemic hypothermic, diastolic arrest at 7 °C. The solution is infused directly into the coronary arteries. One litre of the cardioplegic solution provides myocardial protection for approximately 30–35 min and during the ischaemic period of aortic cross-clamping. The infusion will need to be repeated in 500–600 ml aliquots. Cardioplegic arrest of up to 60 min is usually well tolerated but prolongation will cause tissue acidosis, subendocardial necrosis, and compromised cardiac performance.

Withdrawal from cardiopulmonary bypass

Once surgery is completed, the patient is rewarmed to 37 °C using the heat exchanger. Air is vented from the heart chambers and aortic root, and the aortic cross-clamp is removed. The coronary arteries are perfused and the myocardium is warmed by the circulating blood. A cardiac rhythm may resume spontaneously or ventricular fibrillation may occur which requires defibrillation. Occasionally, pacing may be necessary to initiate an effective rhythm. Pulmonary ventilation is restarted and the rate of cardiopulmonary bypass reduced. While blood is passing through both the pulmonary circulation and the bypass circuit the patient's response is assessed. If the cardiac function is adequate,

bypass is discontinued and the cannulae removed. Heparinization is then reversed with protamine sulphate and the chest wall is closed.

Protective mechanisms employed during bypass

1. *Hypothermia*. Every 7 °C reduction produces a 50% reduction in tissue oxygen demand. This allows lower rates of flow for bypass, and provides protection for cerebral tissue. Localized myocardial cooling protects the heart during cross-clamp time.

TABLE 8.3 Functional physiological differences during cardiopulmonary bypass and their effects on the patient

Function	Effect	Patient problem
Non-pulsatile low-pressure flow	Activates baroreceptors invoking release of ADH and the renin–angiotensin response	Fluid retention. Movement of blood from venous reservoirs such as the splanchnic bed
	Increased circulating catecholamines and increased SVR	Peripheral vasoconstriction, increased likelihood of hypertension post-operatively
	Altered glucose transport across cell membrane	Mild hyperglycaemia
Blood contact with foreign surfaces: tubing, oxygenator, filters, and roller pumps	Complement activation and release of other vasoactive substances leading to increased vascular permeability	Fluid shift into interstitial space, loss of circulating blood volume
	Platelet activation of intrinsic clotting pathway and release of vasoactive substances	Risk of microemboli
	Platelet damage with induced thrombocytopenia and altered function	Reduction in platelet adhesion and decrease by 50–70% of platelet numbers. Increased risk of post-operative bleeding
Hypothermia	Increased SVR	Peripheral vasoconstriction
	Decrease of normal tissue oxygen requirements	
	Increased blood viscosity but compensated for by haemodilution	
	Impairment of cellular transport mechanisms and pancreatic islet cell release of insulin	Hyperglycaemia
	Possible mild depression of cardiac output and a transient sinus bradycardia	A reduced cardiac output and a slower heart rate may occur which corrects as the patient warms. There may be oliguria due to decreased renal perfusion
Haemodilution	Improved capillary flow during hypothermia due to decreased viscosity and decreased shear rates for red blood cells	Reduced haemoglobin and haematocrit
	Increased fluid load, much of which may move into the interstitium due to the effects of vasoactive substances (see above)	Patient may remain fluid-overloaded post-operatively. Polyuria post-operatively
Absence or reduction of pulmonary ventilation	Reduced alveolar distension is insufficient to activate surfactant	Increased risk of atelectasis
Absence of pulmonary perfusion	Sequestration of blood in pulmonary microcirculation and breakdown of capillary walls	Increased risk of microthrombi, pulmonary shunting, and interstitial oedema

2. *Anticoagulation* prevents coagulation arising from contact with foreign surfaces.

3. *Haemodilution.* Avoidance of extreme intravascular-interstitial fluid shifts during bypass due to an almost isotonic perfusate, with a reduction in blood viscosity will reduce peripheral vascular resistance and improve capillary perfusion, particularly during hypothermia. It will also reduce sludging of blood components around the bypass circuit and decreases the likelihood of microemboli.

Table 8.3 shows the physiological effects on the patient of cardiopulmonary bypass intervention.

Closure of the chest and completion of surgery

Pacing wire placement should also be identified/confirmed by the documentation and ECG if the patient is actively being paced.

If pacing is thought to be required post-operatively, epicardial pacing wires will be placed on the ventricle and brought out through the chest wall conventionally to the left of the sternal incision. If atrial pacing wires are also required these will be placed on the epicardial surface of the atria and externalized to the right of the sternal incision.

In many centres, the pericardium is closed to assist right ventricular function.

Chest drains are placed in the pericardial space and in the mediastinum. They are externalized through separate incisions.

A pleural drain or drains may be necessary if the pleural space is entered during the procedure.

Haemostasis is achieved and sternal closure using stainless steel wires or sutures is carried out. The skin is closed and dressings applied.

Care of the patient following surgery

During closure of the chest and transfer from theatre the patient may become less stable. A degree of urgency is therefore necessary in ensuring that the patient is attached to the ventilator, baseline observa-

---

MINIMUM BYPASS FLOW RATES

- 2.4 1/min/m² to maintain oxygenation at 37 °C.

- 1.2 l/min/m² to maintain oxygenation at 25 °C.

Note: uncertainty remains as to what constitutes optimal local blood flow, particularly with regard to cerebral flow.

PREPARATION OF BED SPACE FOR RECEIVING THE PATIENT

- Carry out safety checks and equip bed space (see Chapter 3).

- Colloid such as hexastarch, gelofusine, etc.

- Labels for drains, drain bottles, and infusions.

- Ready access to drugs including sedatives, analgesics, vasodilators, inotropes, potassium, furosemide (frusemide).

---

tions and assessment are carried out, and any haemodynamic or respiratory problems are dealt with promptly.

Immediate interventions

(Note: these can be performed by two nurses to allow speedy assessment of the patient.)

1. Connect monitoring—priorities are the arterial line, CVP, and ECG (check readings and inform medical staff immediately if there are any problems).

2. Attach the patient to the ventilator after checking the required tidal volume, respiratory rate and F_iO_2 settings with the anaesthetist.

3. Auscultate the patient's chest for air entry (see Chapter 4) to confirm ET tube placement, and check for any evidence of pneumothorax, lung collapse, and possible build up of secretions.

4. Label chest drains and bottles, and mark the level of drainage. Check suction on pre-vacuumed bottles, or attach to suction.

5. Measure urine meter contents and discard into collection bag.

6. Attach maintenance fluid (e.g. electrolyte solutions such as Hartmanns) and check existing drug infusions for dilution and rate.

7. Remove rectal probe and go with core temperature probe; adjust bed clothing to ensure adequate covering for rewarming. Use may be made of warming blankets such as the Bairhugger or space blankets.

8. Attach a peripheral temperature probe.

9. Assess the patient for conscious level and signs of pain (see Chapter 10).

10. Check arterial blood gas, electrolytes, and haemoglobin at about 10–15 min after patient is attached

to the ventilator unless the patient's condition requires earlier measurement.

11. Perform a 12-lead ECG. Chest x-ray is not always routine but may be requested.

Fast track patients

Patients with short bypass times, uncomplicated surgery, and no co-morbidity are often 'fast tracked'. In this case, they are given a specific short-acting anaesthetic agent and initially follow the normal post-operative course. However, they will then be extubated at between 4 and 6 hours, mobilized to a chair, and transferred to a high-dependency setting on the day of surgery (Flynn *et al.* 2004).

Complications following cardiac surgery

Patients are usually transferred directly to a critical care area following surgery where they are closely monitored and ensuing problems can be dealt with promptly. This is a period of stabilization and rapid recognition of any problems with immediate intervention will often prevent major complications arising subsequently.

Haemodynamic instability

Problem: hypotension

Hypotension due to either hypovolaemia, arrhythmias, poor left ventricular contractility, or tamponade. Consider iatrogenic hypotension due to drugs such as vasodilators, beta-blockers, or sedatives as a possible cause.

The goal is to maintain a systolic blood pressure >90 mmHg but this may be altered by the individual

---

GOALS OF POST-CARDIAC SURGERY CARE

- Maintain good levels of oxygenation and carbon dioxide.
- Haemodynamic stability and adequate organ perfusion.
- Maintain haemostasis.
- Rewarming without significant problems.
- Prevent/reduce atelectasis.
- Prevent/reduce cerebral dysfunction.
- Provide adequate analgesia.
- Maintain fluid and electrolyte balance.
- Appropriate and problem-free extubation.

---

patient's operative course. If the patient has had saphenous vein grafts, low perfusion pressures during diastole may result in collapse of the non-muscular vein wall, and this may cause occlusion if prolonged. More importantly, low mean arterial pressures will reduce vital organ perfusion, such as to brain and kidneys, increasing the risk of organ damage.

Management of hypotension

If CVP or PA pressures are low, rapid volume replacement is given usually as a bolus of fluid. The pressures are rechecked and according to the patient response, more fluid is given as necessary.

If CVP or PA pressures increase by >3mmHg. following 200 ml fluid replacement, and hypotension continues, intervention is aimed at improving myocardial contractility with inotropes (see Chapter 6 for details).

If the patient has concurrent arrhythmias, intervention is also aimed at treating these (see below).

Cardiac tamponade is discussed as a separate problem.

Problem: hypertension

Hypertension due to either a previous history of hypertension, increased catecholamine release following cardiopulmonary bypass (see above for details), pain and anxiety, adverse drug reaction, hypothermia, or unknown aetiology. Hypertension is a common problem in those suffering from atherosclerotic disease and can be serious post-operatively. High systolic pressures may cause leakage and bleeding at suture sites and even rupture of graft anastomoses.

The goal is to maintain the systolic pressure at <140 mmHg although this may need to be lower in patients with bleeding problems or friable graft tissue. Different surgeons may stipulate different upper limits of systolic pressure.

Management of hypertension

In is important to exclude causes such as pain or anxiety before using vasodilator therapy. Patient comfort and level of analgesia should be assessed regularly and pain relieved as per unit policy. Hypovolaemia should be corrected prior to the use of vasodilators and further fluid may be needed as vasodilatation occurs.

Glyceryl trinitrate (GTN) is the usual first choice for reducing blood pressure, but in some circumstances other drugs such as sodium nitroprusside are preferred. Both of these drugs are delivered as an intravenous infusion which is titrated to maintain systolic blood pressure between 100 and 140 mmHg.

Unless there is a previous history, hypertension is usually short-lived and vasodilators can be weaned off by the following day. In some cases, oral drugs, such as ACE inhibitors, beta-blockers, or calcium antagonists, may be necessary to control blood pressure for a longer period.

Arrhythmias

A number of factors contribute to an increased likelihood of arrhythmias in the post-operative period. These are:

TABLE 8.4 Causes and management of specific arrhythmias

Arrhythmia	Cause	Problem	Management
Sinus tachycardia	Hypovolaemia, catecholamine release (from surgery, from pain and anxiety), possible side-effect of inotropic drugs	Decreased ventricular diastolic filling time compromises cardiac output. Increased myocardial oxygen demand increases cardiac work. Decreased coronary artery perfusion time reduces coronary artery flow	First, correction of any underlying cause (i.e. give fluid if hypovolaemic, analgesia if in pain, etc.). Review any inotropic support if necessary
Ventricular ectopics	Electrolyte imbalance (principally potassium), hypoxia, surgical trauma, myocardial ischaemia, catecholamine release, occasionally mechanical irritation from chest drains or pulmonary artery catheter if used	Increased risk of ventricular arrhythmias, reduced cardiac output due to poor filling time for premature beat	Correct any underlying cause. Keep the serum potassium above 4.5 mmol/l. If ectopics are frequent or close to previous complexes then magnesium, lidocaine, or amiodarone (if there is depressed myocardial function) may be considered
Ventricular tachycardia and fibrillation	Hypoxia, myocardial ischaemia, electrolyte imbalance, myocardial irritability from surgical trauma	Loss of cardiac output	Immediate defibrillation with DC shock of 200 J externally or 5–10 J internally
Supraventricular tachycardias (SVT)	Myocardial irritability post-surgical trauma, myocardial ischaemia, possible side-effect of inotropic drugs	Decreased ventricular diastolic filling time with reduced cardiac output. Increased myocardial oxygen demand increases cardiac workload. Decreased coronary artery perfusion time reduces coronary artery flow	Correct any underlying cause, including hypovolaemia. Keep the serum potassium above 4.5 mmol/l. Amiodarone verapamil, adenosine, magnesium, and DC cardioversion may all be considered
Atrial fibrillation and flutter	In patients following valve surgery long-standing atrial dilatation and stretching induces atrial fibrillation, hypoxia, poor coronary perfusion and myocardial ischaemia	Loss of 'atrial kick' (top-up filling of the ventricle during atrial systole), if the ventricular rate is also rapid then problems as for SVT	Amiodarone is the usual first-line therapy, but digoxin may be useful. Keep the serum potassium above 4.5 mmol/1. DC cardioversion if the ventricular rate is rapid and blood pressure is compromised
Bradyarrhythmias (junctional rhythm, atrioventricular blocks and bundle branch blocks)	Depression of the conduction system cells by cardioplegia, myocardial ischaemia, injury to nodes and conduction pathways by surgical intervention, sutures, or oedema. More common in valve surgery due to the proximity of the aortic and mitral valves to the conduction system	Possible decreased cardiac output, increased ventricular filling which may overload the compromised ventricle	Atropine bolus (usually 500 μg to a max of 3 mg) If an epicardial pacing wire is *in situ* pacing would initially be used. A transvenous pacing wire may be inserted if necessary
Sinus bradycardia	Pre-operative use of beta-blockers, increased vagal tone	As above	If the cardiac output is compromised then management is as above

1. The myocardium is more irritable due to handling and surgical trauma.

2. Electrolyte imbalances (especially potassium and magnesium) induced by cardioplegia, fluid shifts, and renal dysfunction.

3. Conduction defects are more common in valve replacement surgery and VSD closure due to the proximity of surgery to the conduction system. Atrial fibrillation is common in mitral valve disease.

4. The heart is less able to cope with added stress due to the underlying pathology.

Management

The causes and management of specific arrhythmias are outlined in Table 8.4.

Cardiac tamponade

Compression of the myocardium occurs when blood (or other fluid) accumulates around the heart. This impedes venous return and reduces contractility by restricting ventricular filling, thus reducing stroke volume and cardiac output. Stroke volume is dependent on preload, afterload, and myocardial contractility (this is discussed fully in Chapter 7).

Following cardiac surgery, tamponade is most likely to occur as a result of blockage of the pericardial chest drain through clotting. If drains are patent and recent brisk bleeding has not suddenly ceased then tamponade is unlikely. Most patients have their pericardium left open to decrease the risk of tamponade (see Fig. 8.5 for the effects of cardiac tamponade).

Management

Support of cardiac output using fluid resuscitation with or without inotropes is necessary until surgical intervention has decompressed the heart. In the acute tamponade (where circulation is compromised), surgery will be carried out at once at the patient's bedside (see below for details) However, if time allows, patients are less likely to suffer complications if they are returned to theatre.

Alteration in fluid and electrolyte balance

Total body fluid increases during cardiopulmonary bypass due to pump priming fluid, haemodilution, increased antidiuretic hormone (ADH) secretion, and activation of the renin–angiotensin-aldosterone response to low perfusion. However, much of this fluid is actually interstitial rather than intravascular due to alterations in capillary membrane permeability by vasoactive substances. These substances are released

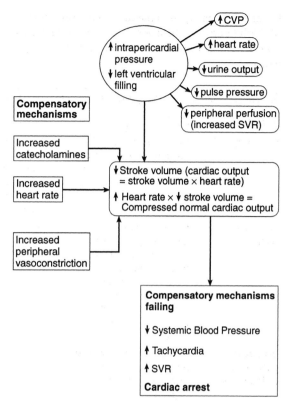

Fig. 8.5 The effects of cardiac tamponade.

possibly as a response to contact with the foreign surfaces of the bypass circuit or to organ hypoperfusion. There may also be a reduction in colloid osmotic (oncotic) pressure due to haemodilution, which will contribute to loss of fluid into the extravascular spaces. The patient may have a positive fluid balance of up to 5 litres and as much as 20% of this may be extracellular. In spite of this extravascular excess, it is still possible for the patient to have an intravascular volume deficit which must be corrected in order to prevent a decreased cardiac output and hypotension. This deficit can be further affected by vasodilatation during warming and blood loss.

Sodium levels may be raised due to multiple causes, including the effect of the renin–angiotensin-aldosterone response (see Chapter 9) during bypass, renal dysfunction, and alterations to the sodium cell membrane pumps. It is therefore usual to give glucose 5% or Hartmanns as crystalloid replacement fluid postoperatively.

Hypokalaemia is a frequent problem due to haemodilution, use of diuretics, and the renin–angiotensin-aldosterone response (see Chapter 9).

Occasionally, hyperkalaemia is a problem if the patient develops acute renal failure or receives large amounts of cardioplegia.

In some units, magnesium is given routinely as there may be significant losses due to diuresis and levels may fall due to haemodilution.

Management

Intravascular fluid volume is maintained using colloid or blood according to the level of the patient's haemoglobin. In most units, haemoglobin is maintained at a level >7g/dl (National Blood Users Group 2001).

Crystalloid infusions are generally kept to a maintenance level to avoid further extravascular fluid loading.

The CVP, PA pressure, and non-invasive devices such as oesophageal Doppler are used to monitor intravascular volume status. Colloid/blood is given to maintain blood pressure and urine output as required.

Sodium and potassium levels are monitored regularly and potassium is given via central venous access to maintain levels greater than 4.5 mmol/l.

Bleeding

Bleeding post-operatively occurs as a result of either incomplete surgical haemostasis or coagulopathy. The main causes of coagulopathy post-cardiopulmonary bypass are:

1. *Inadequate heparin reversal.* The heparin antagonist protamine sulphate is usually administered at the end of cardiopulmonary bypass. The dose given is based on the ACT. This may be inaccurate or insufficient in view of 'heparin rebound'.

2. *The phenomenon of 'heparin rebound'.* Heparin that has been sequestrated in the tissues during cardiopulmonary bypass is mobilized during warming and vasodilatation. This has a delayed anticoagulant effect and further protamine may be necessary.

3. *Consumption of clotting factors and platelets during bypass.* Cardiopulmonary bypass can cause mechanical destruction of platelets due to activation by contact with a foreign surface. Normally, the platelet count falls to 50–70% of baseline on initiation of cardiopulmonary bypass but returns to normal within 24 hours due of release of platelets from the spleen into the circulation. Consumption of clotting factors is also a problem during bypass and this can be accentuated by haemodilution post-bypass.

4. *Platelet dysfunction.* Circulating platelets may be damaged due to the effects of passage through roller pumps and filters. Pre-operative use of platelet inhibitory drugs, such as aspirin and dipyridamole, may further add to the effect. Post-operative platelet counts are usually low but platelets are not usually replaced unless the patient is actively bleeding or the platelet count falls below 50 000/mm^3.

Management

Protamine is given in the first instance if the ACT is prolonged (>160 s). Tranexamic acid (an antifibrinolytic agent) is also used to support clotting. Clotting factors in the form of fresh frozen plasma are given to replace those consumed.

If the platelet count is low (<50 000/mm^3), if there is active bleeding, or if the patient has recently been taking non-steroidal anti-inflammatory drugs, platelets are transfused.

Hypertension is controlled to decrease the risk of bleeding (see above).

Some advocate that a positive end expiratory pressure (PEEP) of between 10 and 15 cmH$_2$O should be added. The theory behind this is that increasing intrathoracic pressure will: (a) occlude small oozing blood vessels if this is the cause and (b) decrease venous return in hypertensive patients thus reducing blood pressure. Its efficacy has non been fully established and it is not common practice in many units.

If bleeding continues at >100 ml/hour for 4 hours despite correction of coagulopathy or at >400 ml over 1 hour then the patient is usually taken back to theatre for re-exploration.

Pulmonary dysfunction

Post-operative pulmonary complications tend to occur in patients with a prior history of respiratory dysfunction. It is therefore important to ascertain any risk factors during pre-operative assessment. Arterial blood gases are not routinely taken pre-operatively, but provide a useful baseline in the high-risk patient. Patients who smoke are more likely to have thick, tenacious sputum and atelectasis, and therefore require more physiotherapy, humidification, and suction over the post-operative period. The period of apnoea during bypass can cause alveolar collapse and retention of secretions. This is partly due to the period without ventilation and partly due to the decreased release of surfactant which is activated by alveolar distension. The sequestration of blood in the pulmonary microcapillaries can cause microthrombi and potential shunting. It may also contribute to interstitial oedema which occurs as a result of bypass complement activation causing capillary leak.

Management

It is usual to ventilate patients for a period of time postoperatively to allow the high levels of narcotic analgesia and anaesthesia to wear off, and to promote re-expansion of alveoli. Some fit, stable patients can be extubated immediately without ill-effect; however, the majority of patients appear to benefit from a period of mechanical ventilation. This allows adequate levels of analgesia to be given without fear of compromising respiration and reduces cardiac work during optimization of the circulation and rewarming.

Some units recommend the use of 5 cmH$_2$O PEEP during this period to aid opening of collapsed alveoli.

Once the patient is awake and cooperative, weaning to a spontaneous ventilatory mode is carried out, and the patient's ability to breathe spontaneously is assessed. Clinical assessment of respiratory function and arterial blood gases give the best guidance; once these are within normal limits the patient is extubated. Following extubation, it is essential that the patient continues to breathe deeply and cough in order to prevent collapse of the lung bases and sputum retention. Adequate analgesia should be given to permit this and to allow turning and movement. The patient should be encouraged to hold his chest on either side of the sternal incision with his hands to give support during coughing.

Alternatively, splinting with a pillow may be of benefit. Frequent intervention by nursing staff in encouraging deep breathing and coughing is a vital part of post-operative support as is chest physiotherapy. Early mobilization is also encouraged.

Cerebral dysfunction

Protection of cerebral function during the low perfusion pressures of cardiopulmonary bypass is promoted by hypothermia (reduction of cerebral O$_2$ requirements) and haemodilution (improved capillary flow at low temperatures). However, post-operative neurological sequelae include short-term memory loss, poor concentration, focal deficits, confusion, cerebrovascular accidents, and acute psychosis.

In general, cerebral dysfunction is multifactorial involving factors such as inadequate perfusion and microembolism of air or particulate matter (Newman and Harrison 2002).

The risk of cerebral dysfunction increases with increasing age, diabetes, pre-existing carotid or cerebrovascular atherosclerotic disease, and the presence of calcified material that may break loose during manipulation (Stygall et al. 2000).

Management

Identification of those at risk and frequent neurological assessment will allow early detection of neurological dysfunction. Maintenance of blood pressure and oxygenation to ensure cerebral perfusion and tissue oxygenation is an important part of nursing observation.

Renal dysfunction

There is an increased risk of renal failure associated with cardiopulmonary bypass. This is due to decreased renal blood flow during bypass, hypotension, hypoperfusion, and free haemoglobin resulting from red blood cell damage and cellular debris damaging the tubules. Increased risk factors include bypass time and pre-existing renal dysfunction. Haemolysis of red blood cells may occur during bypass and haematuria may be seen.

Patients may be polyuric post-operatively as the excess fluid associated with the pump priming is removed. Oliguria can also occur as a result of high levels of ADH secreted in response to the low perfusion pressure and non-pulsatile flow of cardiopulmonary bypass. The renal vasoconstrictor effect is potentiated by high catecholamine levels and renin–angiotensin–aldosterone release. Hypovolaemia, hypotension, and a low cardiac output in the peri-operative period may all contribute to oliguria.

Management

Correction of contributory factors, such as hypovolaemia, hypotension, and poor cardiac output, is the first step. Dopamine is no longer used to promote renal perfusion alone; however, it may be given as inotropic support, according to local practice. Once the contributory factors are corrected, if the patient remains oliguric then small doses of diuretic, such as furosemide (frusemide) (10–20 mg), may be required to stimulate urine output. This is often necessary in patients on long-term diuretic therapy.

Pain and anxiety

Pain is an individual and subjective experience. The level of pain perceived by patients following cardiac surgery will vary according to understanding, culture, pain threshold, and perception of the pain experience. Factors that affect perception of the pain experience include anxiety and fatigue. Whatever the level, all patients will experience some pain following surgery related to either the sternal incision and rib spreading, the chest drains, or the leg wound if they have a saphenous vein graft. Patients who have an internal mammary artery graft may experience increased pain and discomfort due to the need for further incisions into the parietal pleura and greater stretching of the intercostal muscles (Trehan *et al.* 2000).

Pain from the surgical incision should be differentiated from ischaemic chest pain, e.g. by 12-lead ECG.

Pain is an important factor in initiating the sympathetic response of increased catecholamine production, vasoconstriction, raised blood pressure, and tachycardia. Vasoconstriction and tachycardia will increase cardiac work and decrease coronary artery perfusion time which can compromise the post-operative recovery of cardiac function. Pain relief is therefore an important (as well as humane) intervention and should be a major priority of nursing care.

Once chest drains are removed patients usually experience considerably less pain at rest (Milgrom *et al.* 2004).

Management

Physiological indicators of pain and distress, such as raised blood pressure, tachycardia, and sweating, are the criteria used to assess pain levels when the patient first returns from theatre. Occasionally the patient may still be fully or partially paralysed from the intraoperative muscle relaxant, which may in itself invoke these physiological responses. Later, as the anaesthetic wears off, patients may be able to respond sufficiently to indicate whether they have pain or not. Once the patient is able to respond, the use of a visual analogue scale is helpful so that patients can rate their pain and efficacy of the analgesia can be evaluated.

Intervention

Opiates are the analgesic of choice in the immediate post-operative phase. The secondary effect of suppression of respiratory drive may aid comfort whilst on mechanical ventilation until patients are stable and ready to be weaned.

Following extubation, oral analgesia is then preferred as these are easier to administer and carry less risk of respiratory depression. However, intravenous opiates are still required prior to chest drain removal (Carson *et al.* 1994). Usually, patients are able to take oral analgesia as soon as they can comfortably drink following extubation. The choice of analgesic depends on individual unit policy.

Patient-controlled analgesia is a method used in some units to ensure that patients receive the levels of analgesia they require, when they wish. This can be of benefit in the post-operative period. Some studies have suggested that the use of relaxation techniques and music therapy may relieve anxiety which can affect patients' perception of their pain (Barnason *et al.* 1995).

Evaluation

One of the most important and often the most neglected nursing aspect of pain relief is the need to evaluate and record the effectiveness of analgesia (Tittle and McMillan 1994, Puntillo 1994, Gujol 1994, Gelinas *et al.* 2004). Again, this is best using a visual analogue scale and asking the patient to rate their pain. Unless they are obviously asleep and comfortable, further questioning of the intubated patient once analgesia has had time to take effect will indicate whether pain has been relieved.

Psychological disturbance and intellectual dysfunction

Symptoms range from short-term memory loss and poor concentration to anxiety and depression. In the extreme situation, post-cardiotomy psychosis may occur. This has been described as a range of behaviour in the post-operative period varying from confusion and disorientation to visual and auditory hallucinations, delusions, and paranoia (Quinless *et al.* 1985).

A number of patients will experience short- and long-term cognitive changes. Long-term changes can be more subtle (Selnes *et al.* 1999).

Factors, such as length of perfusion time, hypotension, and prolonged anaesthesia have been associated with an increased incidence of post-cardiotomy psychosis.

Management

One of the most important aspects of management is giving the patient pre-operative information about the phenomenon so that they are potentially able to recognize and cope with the problems involved. The transient nature of these phenomena should be emphasized. The patient's family should also be warned about this, and the possibility of depression and anxiety in the post-operative period. In the true psychotic state, patients do not have insight into their perception of reality and management requires antipsychotic agents and reorientation over a prolonged period.

Emergency reopening of the chest

This procedure is carried out for the following reasons:

1. The patient deteriorates and does not respond to fluid challenge and inotropes.

2. There is a sudden substantial blood loss (>500 ml drained in minutes).

If possible, the patient is returned to theatre but even a short journey can be hazardous for an unstable patient.

Sudden loss of cardiac output will also require chest opening and internal (manual) cardiac compression. This is because differentiation between left ventricular dysfunction and cardiac tamponade can be difficult as both will cause reduced cardiac output and systemic blood pressure with increased heart rate and central venous pressure. Pulmonary artery wedge pressure and left atrial pressure are also raised.

Chest reopening may be necessary to determine whether the problem is tamponade or ventricular dysfunction. External cardiac compression is fairly inefficient in the patient with a sternal split and it is difficult to maintain adequate tissue perfusion in the presence of cardiac tamponade. There may also be added trauma caused by the force of massage leading to disruption of suture lines or possible damage to grafts or valves themselves.

Sudden arterial bleeding may occur from suture-line leakage or complete rupture of the anastomosis. If the rate of bleeding exceeds the capacity of the drains then tamponade will add to the hypovolaemic low-output problem.

Management

In the first instance, the patient's cardiac function should be supported with colloid, blood infusion ± inotropes as appropriate.

Any other contributory factors should be excluded or corrected. These include hypoxaemia due to hypoventilation, pneumothorax, or inadequate oxygen delivery and metabolic acidosis due to the above or to poor cardiac function. Chest drains should be milked or irrigated to make sure they are clear.

Chest reopening in the ICU

Although this is an emergency, it is important that the atmosphere remains calm. Initially, the equipment necessary for the procedure should be brought to the patient's bedside (see box). Having made the decision to reopen the patient's chest in the ICU, the surgeon will start to scrub up. The necessary equipment is brought to the bedside and the area cleared as far as possible. If necessary, patients in adjoining bed areas may be moved to allow sufficient space at the bedside. The area should be effectively screened.

Procedure

The surgeon may attempt to relieve tamponade immediately by opening the sternal incision at the base of the xiphoid process and dissecting the substernal space up to the edge of the pericardium with his finger. It may be possible to release the pressure by drainage of a collection of blood in this area sufficient to stabilize the patient for return to theatre. If this is not possible, or the patient does not respond, then re-entry into the chest must be carried out in the ICU.

The skin and soft tissue sutures are divided and the sternal wires cut with wire cutters. The ribs can then be spread using a retractor and the heart exposed. If the pericardium was closed during surgery it is reopened. Access to the heart for internal cardiac compression is then possible and the circulation can be well supported while a bleeding point is located.

CAUSES OF VENTRICULAR DYSFUNCTION

Mechanical:

+ kinked or occluded bypass grafts

+ malfunctioning valve prosthesis.

Functional:

+ coronary vasospasm

+ ischaemic mitral regurgitation.

Metabolic:

+ hypoxaemia

+ acidosis.

Internal cardiac compression is far more efficient for maintaining coronary perfusion, cerebral blood flow, and mean systemic arterial pressure than external cardiac massage (Grishkin 1988).

The patient may have to go back onto cardiopulmonary bypass in order to correct the problem. This will occur in theatre with the surgeon supporting the circulation by internal cardiac compression during transfer.

Once the problem has been corrected, the patient may require an intra-aortic balloon pump or left ventricular assist support until his /her cardiac function recovers from the insult.

DISADVANTAGES OF CHEST REOPENING IN THE ICU

+ Increased risk of wound infection

+ Poor lighting and limited equipment

+ Often performed in emergency by junior surgeons

+ Absence of trained theatre staff to assist

THE TECHNIQUE OF INTERNAL (MANUAL) CARDIAC COMPRESSION

1. The ventricles are compressed between the palms of the hands.

2. The heart is compressed between the palm of one hand and the undersurface of the sternum (left anterior thoracotomy approach only).

The heart should be kept in its anatomical position to avoid kinking of the venae cavae and arteries.

Survival following chest reopening is related to the underlying cause. Fairman and Edmunds (1981) found that 60% of patients who had chest reopening performed for bleeding or tamponade survived. There is insufficient data available to identify the morbidity for patients who required chest re-opening for circulatory support for ventricular dysfuntion.

Mechanical cardiac assist devices

Intra-aortic balloon pump

The intra-aortic balloon pump (IABP) was first introduced clinically in 1967 by Kantrowitz and associates. It is designed to improve coronary artery perfusion by inflating during diastole and to reduce left ventricular afterload by deflating during systole.

Description

A central catheter with a polyurethane balloon (between 30 and 50 cm^3 depending on patient size), approximately 25 cm (10 inches) long. The insertion may be sheathed or sheathless. The balloon is inserted into the femoral artery, either percutaneously or directly during cardiac surgery, and advanced into the descending thoracic aorta. Correct positioning of the balloon in the thoracic aorta is important. Optimal positioning is approximately 2 cm below the left subclavian artery and as high above the femoral bifurcation as is possible. The distal end of the balloon is then proximal to the renal arteries.

During insertion, there is a risk of liberating embolic particles into the circulation so limb perfusion and neurological function should be monitored closely.

The catheter of the balloon is attached via a Luer lock fitting to the console of the pump. The pump shuttles helium (or carbon dioxide) under pressure through the catheter into the balloon which is inflated. The helium is then sucked out of the balloon by the creation of a vacuum by the pump. This mechanism allows for a very fast response to triggers for inflation and deflation. Some types of balloon also have a central lumen which allows monitoring of aortic pressures from the tip of the balloon.

Triggers for the pump cycle

1. The standard trigger mechanism is the R wave of the patient's ECG. This will cue inflation of the balloon following systole. Timing of inflation and deflation requires adjustment and will be discussed below.

2. Systolic arterial pressure may be used if the R wave is unable to trigger properly.

3. Pacing spikes may also be used to trigger inflation.

COMPONENTS OF THE IABP

♦ Intra-aortic balloon

♦ Monitoring system

♦ Trigger mechanism

♦ Gas drive system

---

4. Some pumps have an automatic facility for use during cardiac arrest or to provide pulsatile flow during cardiopulmonary bypass.

Indications for use of the IABP

The two most common uses for the IABP are support of the failing heart in cardiogenic shock and weaning from cardiopulmonary bypass.

The role of the IABP is to provide short-term support allowing the heart to recover from the myocardial infarction, cardiac surgery, or coronary angioplasty. It cannot be considered as a long-term solution although there are cases of use for as long as 46 days (Lazar *et al.* 1992).

Contraindications for use of the IABP

1. *Aortic valve incompetence.* The most obvious contraindication to the IABP is an incompetent aortic valve. If the aortic valve allows regurgitation of blood flow, this will be compounded by balloon inflation during diastole adding to ventricular work.

INDICATIONS FOR USE OF THE IABP

1. Cardiogenic shock.

2. Weaning from cardiopulmonary bypass.

3. Refractory ventricular failure.

4. Unstable refractory angina.

5. Impending infarction.

6. Mechanical complications due to acute myocardial infarction (i.e. ventricular septal defect, mitrial regurgitation, or papillary muscle rupture).

7. Ischaemia related to intractable ventricular arrhythmias.

8. Cardiac support for high-risk general surgical patients.

9. Support and stabilization during coronary angiography and angioplasty.

10. Intra-operative pulsatile flow generation.

---

2. *Aortic aneurysm.* The movement of the balloon in the aorta would be likely to dislodge aneurysmal debris leading to emboli and possibly, rupture of the aneurysm.

3. *Previous aortofemoral or aortoiliac bypass grafts.* Insertion of the balloon would be impossible.

4. *Severe peripheral vascular disease.* Insertion of the balloon would be difficult and there would be an increased risk of occlusion of the vessel and dislodgement of emboli.

Underlying physiology

In the failing heart, maintenance of cardiac output requires an increased myocardial oxygen demand. This increased demand cannot be met by existing coronary artery perfusion and tissue hypoxia occurs. Tissue hypoxia is particularly apparent in the myocardial tissues due to the low level of oxygen extraction reserve.

The normal level of oxygen saturation in the coronary sinus (venous blood drained from the heart) is 30–40% which leaves little room for increasing oxygen extraction as a method of compensation. Cardiac output continues to fall and a degenerative spiral of cardiogenic shock develops.

The main goals of therapy for a failing left ventricle are to:

♦ decrease left ventricular workload and

♦ improve coronary artery perfusion.

Both of these goals can be achieved mechanically using the intra-aortic balloon pump (IABP).

Decreased left ventricular workload

A major determinant of left ventricular workload is afterload. Afterload is defined as the amount of wall tension which must be generated by the ventricle to raise intraventricular pressure sufficiently to overcome impedance to ejection. Production of the force required to overcome afterload consumes the greatest amount of oxygen during the cardiac cycle. Thus, decreasing impedance will reduce left ventricular workload and myocardial oxygen consumption.

Impedance to ejection is generated by the aortic valve, the aortic end diastolic pressure, and vascular resistance. The aortic valve provides a fairly constant beat-to-beat impedance to ejection and cannot be manipulated. The aortic end diastolic pressure and the vascular resistance can be manipulated to decrease afterload.

The IABP decreases aortic end diastolic pressure by deflating the aortic balloon immediately prior to systole. This lowers aortic end diastolic pressure and therefore reduces impedance to left ventricular ejec-

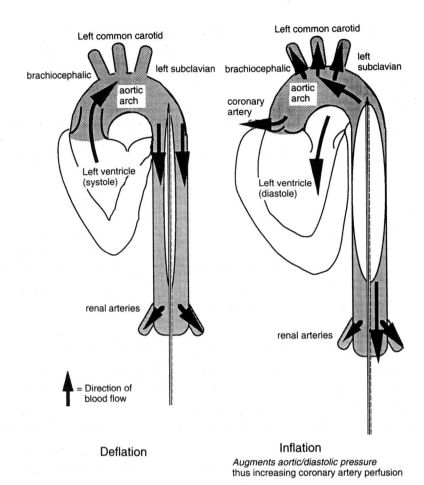

Fig. 8.6 IABP effects of inflation and deflation.

Deflation

Inflation
Augments aortic/diastolic pressure thus increasing coronary artery perfusion

tion. Left ventricular workload is reduced, left ventricular emptying is increased, and myocardial oxygen consumption is decreased (see Fig. 8.6).

Improved coronary artery perfusion

Coronary artery perfusion pressure is the difference between aortic diastolic pressure and myocardial wall tension. Myocardial wall tension is greatly reduced during diastole and 80% of coronary blood flow occurs at this time. Reduction of afterload allows increased left ventricular emptying which means that myocardial wall tension during diastole is reduced allowing increased coronary flow.

> Coronary artery perfusion pressure = aortic diastolic pressure − myocardial wall tension.

The IABP increases coronary artery perfusion by inflating the aortic balloon during diastole. This increases aortic end diastolic pressure and retrograde coronary artery flow, thereby increasing coronary artery perfusion.

Timing

The precise timing of inflation and deflation is an important factor in optimizing the support provided by the IABP. If inflation occurs too early then it will cause impedance to aortic blood flow. If it occurs too late, it will reduce the amount of augmentation. If deflation occurs too early then augmentation will be limited, and if it occurs too late it will act as an additional impedance to aortic blood flow.

Timing of inflation and deflation is judged from the arterial pressure waveform (see Fig. 8.7):

- *Inflation* should occur on the closure of the aortic valve which is seen on the arterial waveform as the dicrotic notch.

- *Deflation* should occur just before the aortic valve opens or during isovolumetric contraction of the ventricle.

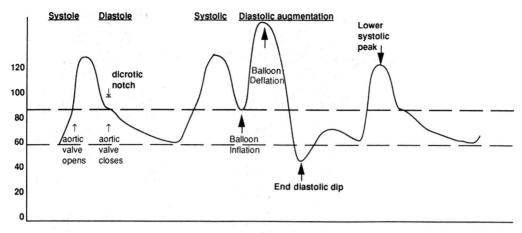

Fig. 8.7 Timing inflation and deflation from the arterial pressure waveform. (Arterial or aortic waveform with IABP on 1:2 assist.). *Arterial or aortic waveform analysis.* In order to obtain a clear comparison of augmented and unaugmented pressures the IABP cycle should be set to 1:2 and the frame either frozen or a recording obtained. The patient can then continue on 1:1 while the waveform is analysed.

(1) Identify the dicrotic notch—inflation should occur at this point on the augmented waveform producing a sharp V shape. This denotes optimal timing of inflation producing maximal augmented volume.

(2) Compare systolic and augmented diastolic upstroke—the upstrokes should be parallel to each other and steeply inclined. This gives an indication of the speed of increase in aortic root pressure and thus the effectiveness of increased coronary artery perfusion.

(3) Compare systolic and augmented diastolic peaks—the augmented peak should be equal to or higher than the systolic. The greater the peak in diastolic pressure the greater the increase in aortic root pressure.

(4) Check the end diastolic dip—this should fall swiftly with a decreased end diastolic pressure. Correct timing of deflation immediately prior to systole produces a steep drop in end diastolic pressure and reduction of the impedance to the next systolic ejection. This represents the degree of afterload reduction.

(5) Review the following systolic peak—this should be lower than the unassisted systolic peak. This is because less work is required to overcome resistance to ejection. However, this may not be the case in non-compliant (atherosclerotic) vasculature.

Timing errors

Errors which cause the most harm are *early inflation* and *late deflation*. These actually increase myocardial oxygen consumption and workload, adding to the limitations of the failing heart:

♦ *Early inflation.* The balloon inflates before aortic valve closure, acting as an impedance to blood flow and increasing afterload. The augmentation upstroke will occur before the dicrotic notch and very close to the systolic peak.

♦ *Late inflation.* The balloon inflates after the dicrotic notch limiting the diastolic augmentation and reducing assistance to coronary artery perfusion. The waveform between systole and augmented diastole may lose its sharp V shape and look more like a U.

♦ *Early deflation.* The balloon deflates before diastole is finished thereby producing a steep fall following diastolic augmentation. Augmentation falls sharply and reduction in afterload is less evident leading to increased ventricular work.

♦ *Late deflation.* The balloon remains inflated, acting as an impedance to ventricular ejection and increasing ven-

tricular work. The waveform may appear widened following diastolic augmentation and there is no evidence of the end diastolic dip.

Problem-solving

1. Decreased augmentation

This can be due to:

1. Balloon leak or need for balloon refill (evident by decreased augmentation pressure and loss of end diastolic dip). The need for balloon refill is due to the gradual diffusion of helium through the balloon membrane and leakage at tubing connections.

2. A change in patient dynamics.

Management:

♦ Check that the automatic balloon refill programme (if present) is functioning. The balloon is automatically refilled every 2 hours.

♦ Manually refill the balloon if necessary.

♦ If a balloon leak has occurred a loss in effectiveness will be evident and return of blood back up the catheter may be seen. Medical staff should be informed at once as the balloon will need removal.

• If the patient has a tachycardia >120 bpm or decreased intravascular volume, balloon augmentation and effectiveness will be reduced. Switching the timing of assist to a 1:2 beats ratio may improve augmentation during tachycardia. Decreased intravascular volume should be corrected.

2. Dampened waveform

This can be due to:

1. Air in the transducer or system.

2. An excessive length of pressure monitoring tubing.

3. Build-up of clot at the tip of the monitoring cannula.

Management:

• Check transducer and flush system, removing any obvious air bubbles and reducing the length of the pressure line to the minimum required for safety.

• Fast flush the line for several seconds.

3. Deterioration in haemodynamic status

This can be due to:

1. The patient—tachycardia, decreased intravascular volume, decreased systemic vascular resistance, or any other factor liable to affect normal functioning haemodynamic status.

2. The IABP—balloon leak or need for refill, inappropriate timing for any change in cardiac rhythm. The balloon loses approximately 1–2 ml of gas per hour by diffusion across the membrane.

Management:

• Correct patient-related problems as per usual protocols.

• Manually refill the balloon and check tubing between balloon and console for any signs of blood leakage (this will occur if there is a leak in the balloon). (See below for management of balloon leak.)

4. Balloon leak

This can be due to:

1. Friction with atheromatous plaque in the aorta.

2. A faulty balloon. There will be a reduction in the effectiveness of the balloon and eventually blood may leak into the catheter and track back to the connecting tubing.

Management:

• Decrease balloon inflation frequency to a minimum and notify the medical staff immediately. There is a risk of gas embolus, the severity of which depends on the gas used to inflate the balloon. Carbon dioxide is

much more soluble than helium and therefore less likely to be a serious problem unless the leak is very large. The balloon will have to be replaced as soon as possible.

5. Malpositioning of the balloon

The balloon may become displaced during patient movement and the efficiency of augmentation may be decreased. If displacement is upwards it is possible for the left subclavian artery to become occluded. If displacement is downwards it is possible for the renal arteries to become obstructed.

Management:

• The left radial artery should be palpated hourly and the colour and temperature of the limb checked to ensure adequate circulation.

• Any acute loss of urine output may indicate displacement of the balloon.

• The position of the balloon should be confirmed on X-ray and checked by a doctor. If necessary, repositioning should be carried out.

Problems related to the patient with an IABP

1. Potential impairment of peripheral circulation

The presence of the balloon catheter in the femoral artery will cause a reduction in blood flow to the limb. In some cases, thrombosis of the vessel has occurred and emergency embolectomy has been required.

Management:

• The patient's lower limbs should be examined hourly and compared for colour, temperature, and peripheral pulses.

• It is usual for the patient to be prescribed an intravenous heparin infusion to maintain the ACT > 150 s throughout the period of balloon insertion.

• Avoidance of hip flexion of the cannulated leg will reduce the risk of blood flow obstruction.

• Inflation and deflation should continue unless the balloon is about to be removed. Total balloon immobility will increase the likelihood of thrombus formation and should never last longer than 30 min (Joseph and Bates 1990). If necessary, the balloon can be maintained on minimum augmentation until it can be removed.

2. Restricted movement contributing to atelectasis and pressure area problems

The patient's position is restricted by the need to avoid hip flexion which may obstruct the gas supply to the balloon or the blood flow round the catheter to the patient's leg. His/her mobility is restricted by attachment to the balloon catheter and other cannulae.

Management:

- The patient can turn from side-to-side as well as lie supine and should be encouraged to do so. The limiting factor is keeping the degree of hip flexion to a minimum.

- The patient can sit up to an approximate 30° angle and this should be encouraged to allow deep breathing and expansion of the lower lobes of the lung.

- The patient is highly susceptible to pressure area problems, requiring as much support as necessary to reduce the risk of skin breakdown as well as 2-hourly position changes.

3. Bleeding and coagulopathy

The need for heparinization to avoid thrombus formation around the balloon and in the patient's leg distal to the balloon catheter means that bleeding may become a problem.

Management:

- The ACT should be checked regularly, usually 24-hourly, unless there are major problems obtaining anticoagulation when bolus doses of heparin may be used and ACT or formal clotting studies should be checked shortly after administration. The patient should be observed for any sign of coagulopathy such as bleeding around cannulae sites, mucosa, gums, and evidence of petechiae.

4. Fear of dependency and possible disconnection

Patients may be aware of the presence of the balloon pump and require information from the nursing and medical staff about its role and the length of time it will remain in place. This is a stressful situation so information will require repetition and simplification if it is to be taken in. The patient may develop a dependence on the balloon pump and require frequent reassurance when being weaned from it.

5. Infection

The patient is vulnerable to further infection due to his/her illness and the number of invasive cannulae which bypass the normal body defence mechanisms.

Management:

- Careful asepsis is essential, as with all critically ill patients.

- Catheter and cannulae sites should be checked for redness and swelling.

- Dressings which are non-occlusive should be changed if they become wet or soiled.

- Semi-occlusive transparent membrane dressings should be dressed as necessary.

(For further details see Chapter 3.)

Weaning from the IABP

Prior to attempted weaning of the balloon pump the patient should be stable and requiring only low levels of vasopressor or inotropic support. Ideally, they should show evidence of adequate cardiac function, good peripheral perfusion, and adequate urine output.

Weaning can be commenced either by reducing the ratio of assisted beats or reducing the augmentation of the balloon (the volume of inflation/deflation). The ratio of assist is usually reduced initially to 1:2 then 1:3 (down to 1:8 on certain pumps) and so on provided that the patient remains stable with adequate cardiac function, peripheral perfusion, and urine output. Where possible, cardiac output measurement will provide optimum monitoring of the response to weaning. The minimum amount of time between each reduction should be 30 min although it is usually longer.

The balloon augmentation is usually reduced by 10–20% using the same criteria for patient tolerance.

Removal of the IABP

Depending on whether the balloon was placed surgically or percutaneously the patient will either return to theatre or have the balloon removed in the ICU. Heparinization is discontinued before balloon removal but bleeding may be prolonged from the percutaneous insertion site. This will require manual pressure for up to 30 min and a high-pressure dressing following this. In some centres, a Fogarty catheter is passed proximal to the aortic bifurcation and distal to the popliteal artery to clear any clot that may be present and to prevent emboli.

Following balloon removal the site should be inspected hourly for signs of further bleeding and the peripheral circulation assessed for signs of occlusion.

Ventricular assist devices

These are mechanical devices which work in conjunction with the patient's own ventricle although they are capable of providing total cardiac output if necessary. They can support either or both ventricles.

Indications

The majority of these devices are used as a temporary bridge to allow time to set up cardiac transplantation. However, some are used to support patients who cannot be weaned from cardiopulmonary bypass after surgery, and patients in cardiogenic shock following myocardial infarction.

Description
The assist device consists of:

1. A blood sac which acts as a prosthetic ventricle.

2. Valves to provide unidirectional flow.

HAEMODYNAMIC INCLUSION CRITERIA (FROM RUZEVICH 1991)

- MAP < 60 mmHg
- LA and/or RA pressure > 20 mmHg
- Urine output <20 ml/hour
- Cardiac index <2.0 1/min/m²

This is despite maximum drug support, optimal preload, and IABP if appropriate.

HAEMODYNAMIC EXCLUSION CRITERIA (FROM RUZEVICH 1991)

1. Significant complicating illness (other than cardiovascular problem):
   - chronic renal failure or post-operative renal failure
   - severe cerebrovascular disease
   - metastatic disease
   - severe hepatic disease
   - significant blood dyscrasia
   - severe pulmonary disease.
2. Uncontrollable haemorrhage.
3. Massive air embolization.
4. Massive haemolysis.
5. Transfusion reaction.
6. Technically unsuccessful operation:
   - immediate paravalvular leak
   - left ventricular outflow obstruction
   - residual atrioventricular valve
   - regurgitation.
7. Acute cerebral damage resulting in either or both, fixed pupils and a flat electroencephalogram.

---

3. A power source to provide the blood flow. This is usually pneumatic for short-term devices, requiring bulky lines and a compressor which limit patient movement. Long-term devices which are implantable currently use electrical power from a rechargeable battery.

Insertion
Cannulation of the appropriate side of the heart is required. These are usually standard cardiopulmonary bypass cannulae which are placed in the right atrium and pulmonary artery for right ventricular assist and in the left atrium and aorta for left ventricular assist. Biventricular assistance is possible with cannulation of both sides of the heart.

Implantable devices
These devices are limited to left ventricular support and are generally used as a bridge to transplantation.

The pump is placed in the patient's abdomen with a conduit made from Dacron inserted into the left ventricular apex for inflow and another Dacron conduit inserted into the aorta for outflow. External connections for power and drive control are still necessary but are considerably less bulky than the pneumatic drive lines necessary for non-implantable devices.

Advantages:
- decreased risk of infection
- decreased risk of thrombus formation,
- increased patient mobility.

Disadvantages:
- cost
- supports single ventricle only
- difficult no insert
- requires apex cannulation.

Artificial hearts
These have rarely been used in the UK and most experience is from the US and France.

The total artificial heart (e.g. Jarvik) is designed to replace the patient's own heart. The patient's own heart is removed and the prosthetic ventricles are attached to the atrial cuff remnants on the inflow. The aorta and pulmonary artery are attached to the ventricular outflow.

Indications
Artificial hearts are occasionally used for temporary support following rejection of a cardiac transplant.

They may also be indicated in left ventricular tumour or massive thrombus.

Problems associated with the patient on a ventricular assist device

1. *Bleeding and coagulopathy.* Heparin is used to prevent coagulation in the short term. Bleeding may occur as a result of coagulopathy or due to use of cardio-pulmonary bypass prior to use of the device. Use of centrifugal pumps and the haemopump device may cause haemolysis.

2. *Infection.* The patient is highly vulnerable due to his/her critical state and transplantation cannot occur until clear of systemic infection. Sources may be systemic or via the pneumatic drive lines through the skin.

3. *Mechanical failure.* With improvement in device reliability this is rarely a problem.

The best survival rates are for the use of left ventricular assist devices (6% survived to transplant and 54% survived overall); however, such patients are carefully selected.

Cardiac transplantation

Since the first human-to-human transplantation was carried out in 1967 the overall survival rate has increased to 80% for 1 year and to 63% at 5 years (UK Transplant Activity 2001). A major factor in this has been the use of immunosuppressive agents, particularly ciclosporin to prevent rejection. About 3000 transplants are performed annually, with the vast majority being in the US.

The majority of adult patients who receive a cardiac transplant have either ischaemic heart disease or end-stage cardiomyopathy. About 52% of recipients are in the 50–64 year age group and less than a quarter of these are women (Massad 2004).

INDICATIONS FOR CARDIAC TRANSPLANT

- Any end-stage heart disease with a limited prognosis (i.e. <50% survival at 1 year): e.g. cardiomyopathy, left ventricular dysfunction with ejection fraction <20%.

- Congenital heart disease not amenable to surgical palliation or correction.

- Cardiogenic shock or low cardiac output state with reversible end-organ dysfunction requiring mechanical support (e.g. IABP).

- Low cardiac output state or refractory heart failure requiring inotropic support.

Selection of recipient

This is usually undertaken using experience of absolute and relative contraindications, relative need, and matching with the donor.

Absolute contraindications

1. *High (>15 mmHg) transpulmonary pressure gradient* (difference between the mean pulmonary artery pressure and the mean left atrial pressure). High pulmonary vascular resistance increases right ventricular afterload causing a risk of right ventricular failure in the donated heart.

2. *Active systemic infection.* Immunosuppression post-organ donation will drastically reduce any resistance and mortality will greatly increase.

3. Positive HIV antibodies.

4. *Malignancy.* Immunosuppression will allow rapid spread of any pre-existing malignancy.

5. *Irreversible hepatic and renal failure.* There is increased morbidity and ciclosporin is both hepato- and nephrotoxic.

6. Recent substance abuse.

7. Peripheral vascular disease.

8. *Peptic ulceration.* Corticosteroids used in immunosuppression will exacerbate the problem.

9. *Advanced peripheral or cerebral vascular disease.* Increased morbidity may limit the benefit of a transplant.

10. *Psychologically unstable and socially unsupported,* with or without dependence on alcohol or drugs.

Factors, such as age and diabetes, are relative contraindications and each patient should be assessed on an individual basis.

Donor selection

Full details of preparation for organ donation can be found in Chapter 10.

Once criteria are fulfilled the donor is taken to theatre for organ removal. The donor heart is preserved by infusion of cold cardioplegia solution and placed in cold normal saline surrounded by ice. Total ischaemic time should be less than 4 hours.

Care of the patient post-cardiac transplantation

On the whole, care is similar to that described for any patient following cardiac surgery; however, there are a few differences.

Important changes in the patient following cardiac transplantation include:

1. *Denervation.* The donor heart has the nerve supply severed so control by the autonomic nervous system is lost. Loss of vagal influence means that the resting heart rate is higher than normal (>100 bpm) and variations due to respiration are not present. Similarly, manoeuvres used to influence the heart via vagal stimulation, such as carotid sinus massage or the Valsalva manoeuvre, will have no effect.

   The heart has an atypical response to metabolic demands, thus tachycardia may not appear as an immediate response to hypovolaemia and exercise initiates only a slow response in cardiac output. In the same way, the heart is slow to respond to discontinuation of these demands and tachycardia may continue for some time. Orthostatic hypotension may also occur as a result of this.

   Pain in response to myocardial ischaemia is no longer transmitted to the brain and the patient will not experience angina. It is therefore necessary to have regular stress testing and angiography.

2. *Presence of two sinoatrial nodes.* The posterior walls of the patient's own right and left atria remain *in situ* including the sinoatrial node. The transplanted heart also has a sinoatrial node and two P waves are visible on the ECG.

3. *Immunosuppression and infection.* Rejection is a major problem following transplantation. The main immunosuppressants used are ciclosporin A or FK506 (tacrolimus), azathioprine or mycophenolate mofetil, and corticosteroids. These are started in the pre-operative period and, with the exception of corticosteroids, will continue throughout the patient's life.

   Infection is thus a major problem for transplant patients and asepsis must be scrupulous for all interventions. Patients are nursed in protective isolation during their initial recovery.

The major causes of death post-heart transplant are infection, right-sided heart failure and pulmonary hypertension, multisystem organ failure, acute cellular rejection, coronary artery vasculopathy, and malignancy.

References and bibliography

ACC/AHA guidelines for coronary artery bypass surgery: executive summary (1999). *Circulation* **100**, 1464–80.

ACC/AHA Task Force on practice guidelines (2000). Management of patients with valvular heart disease.

Allen, J.K. (1990). Physical and psychosocial outcomes after coronary artery bypass graft surgery: review of the literature. *Heart and Lung* **19**, 49–54.

American Heart Association. Menopause and the risk of heart disease and stroke. www.americanheart.org

Barnason, S., Qimmerman, L., Nieveen, J. (1995). The effect of music interventions on anxiety in the patient after coronary artery bypass grafting. *Heart and Lung* **24**, 124–32.

Butchart, E.G. (1990). Surgery for heart valve disease. *Hospital Update* **15**, 963–76.

British Heart Foundation (2003). *Statistical Database Summary.* www.bhf.org.uk

Carson, M.M., Barton, D.M., Morrison C.G., *et al.* (1994). Managing pain during mediastinal chest tube removal. *Heart and Lung* **23**, 500–5.

Cupples, S.A. (1991). Effects of timing and reinforcement of pre-operative education on knowledge and recovery of patients having coronary artery bypass graft surgery. *Heart and Lung* **20**, 654–60.

Duebener, L.F., Hagino, I., Sakamoto, T., *et al.* (2002). Effects of pH management during deep hypothermic bypass on cerebral microcirculation: Alpha-stat versus pH stat. *Circulation* **106**(12, Suppl. 1), I103–I108.

Fairman, R.M., Edmunds, L.H. (1981). Emergency thoracotomy in the surgical intensive care unit after open cardiac operation. *Annals of Thoracic Surgery* **32**, 386–91.

Flynn,M., Shepherd,W., Holmes,C., *et al.* (2004). Fast-tracking revisited: routine cardiac surgical patients need minimal intensive care. *European Journal of Cardiothoracic Surgery* **25**, 116–22.

Gelinas, C., Fortier, M., Viens, C., *et al.* (2004). Pain assessment and management in critically ill intubated patients: a retrospective study. *American Journal of Critical Care* **13**, 126–35.

Girling, D.K. (1990*a*). Cardiopulmonary bypass: part 1. *Hospital Update* **15**, 799–804.

Girling, D.K. (1990*b*). Cardiopulmonary bypass: part 2. *Hospital Update* **15**, 875–81.

Grishkin, B.A. (1988). Open-chest resuscitation. *Critical Care Nursing Quarterly* **10**, 17–24.

Gujol, M.C. (1994). A survey of pain, assessment and management practices among critical care nurses. *American Journal of Critical Care* **3**, 123–8.

Hayward, J. (1975). *Information: a Prescription Against Pain.* Royal College of Nursing, London.

Joseph, D.L., Bates, S. (1990). Intra-aortic balloon pumping: how no stay on course. *American Journal of Nursing* **90**, 42–7.

Keogh, BE. (2003). *Risk Stratification in Adult Cardiac Surgery.* NHS Information Authority. www.nhsia.nhs.uk

Large, S.R., Schofield, P.M. (1991). Heart transplantation. *Hospital Update* **16**, 808–16.

Lazar, J.M., Ziady, G.M., Dummer, J., *et al.* (1992). Outcome and complications of prolonged intraaortic balloon counterpulsation in cardiac patients. *American Journal of Cardiology* **69**, 955–8.

Ley, S.J., Miller, K. Skov, P., *et al.* (1990). Crystalloid versus colloid fluid therapy after cardiac surgery. *Heart and Lung* **19**, 3140.

Lilley, A. (2002). The selection of priming fluids for cardiopulmonary bypass in the UK and Ireland. *Perfusion* **17**, 315–19.

Loop, F.D., Lytle, B.W., Cosgrove, D.M., *et al.* (1986). Influence of the internal-mammary-artery graft on 10-year survival and other cardiac events. *New England Journal of Medicine* **314**, 1–6.

Massad, M.G. (2004) Current trends in heart transplantation. *Cardiology* **101**, 79–92.

Meighan Rimar, J., Rubin, A. (1988). Emergency reopening of a median sternotomy for pericardial decompression and cardiac massage. *Critical Care Nurse* **8**, 92–101.

Milgrom, L.B., Brooks, J.A., Qi, R., *et al.* (2004). Pain levels experienced with activities after cardiac surgery. *American Journal of Critical Care* **13**, 116–25.

National Blood Users Group (2001). *A Guideline for Transfusion of Red Blood Cells in Surgical Patients.*

Newman, S.P., Harrison, M.J.G. (2002). Coronary-artery bypass surgery and the brain:persisting concerns. *The Lancet Neurology* **1**, 119–25.

Puntillo, K.A. (1994). Dimensions of procedural pain and its analgesic management in critically ill surgical patients. *American Journal of Critical Care* **3**, 116–22.

Quinless, F.W., Cassese, M., Anherton, N. (1985). The effect of selected pre-operative intraoperative, and post-operative variables on the development of postcardiotomy psychosis in patients undergoing open heart surgery. *Heart and Lung* **14**, 334–41.

Raymond, M., Conklin, C., Schaeffer, J., *et al.* (1984). Coping with transient intellectual dysfunction after coronary bypass surgery. *Heart and Lung* **13**, 531–9.

Robertson, J.M., Buckberg, G.D., Vinten-Johansen, J., *et al.* (1983). Comparison of distribution beyond coronary stenosis of blood and assanguinous cardioplegic solutions. *Journal of Thoracic Cardiovascular Surgery* **86**, 80–6.

Ruzevich, S. (1991). Heart assist devices: state of the art. *Critical Care Nursing Clinics of North America* **3**, 723–32.

Selness, O.A., Goldsborough, M.A., Borowicz, L.M., *et al.* (1999). Neurobehavioural sequelae of cardiopulmonary bypass. *The Lancet* **353**, 1601–6.

Society of Cardiothoracic Surgeons of Great Britain and Ireland (2000–2001). *National Adult Cardiac Surgical Database.*

www.scts.org/doc/890 (From the Society of Cardiothoracic Surgeons of Great Britain and Ireland. *UK Cardiac Surgical Register* (2000–2001) Report. Surgical activity and unit results. http://www.ctsnet.org/file/SCTS2000pages46–59.pdf)

Society of Cardiothoracic Surgeons of Great Britain and Ireland (2001). *Valvular Surgery.* www.scts.org/doc/890 (From the Society of Cardiothoracic Surgeons of Great Britain and Ireland. *UK Cardiac Surgical Register* (2000–2001) Report. Surgical activity and unit results. http://www.ctsnet.org/file/SCTS2000pages46–59.pdf)

Society of Cardiothoracic Surgeons of Great Britain and Ireland (2002). http://www.scts.org/doc/890 (From the Society of Cardiothoracic Surgeons of Great Britain and Ireland. *UK Cardiac Surgical Register* (2000–2001) Report. Surgical activity and unit results. http://www.ctsnet.org/file/SCTS2000pages46–59.pdf)

Stygall, J., Kong, R., Walker, J.M., *et al.* (2000). cerebral microembolism detected by transcranial doppler during cardiac surgical procedures. *Stroke* **31**, 2508–10.

Tittle, M., McMillan, S.C. (1994). Pain and pain-related side effects in an ICU and on a surgical unit: nurses' management. *American Journal of Critical Care* **3**, 25–30.

Trehan, N., Malhotra, R., Mishra, Y., *et al.* (2000). Comparison of ministernotomy with minithoracotomy regarding postoperative pain and internal mammary artery characteristics. *The Heart Surgery Forum* **3**, 300–6.

UK Transplant Activity (2001). www.uktransplant.org.uk

Weber, K. M. (1990). Cardiac surgery and heart transplantation. In: *Critical Care Nursing: A Holistic Approach* (ed. C.M. Hudak, B.M. Gallo, J.J. Benz), pp. 259–85. Lippincott, Philadelphia, PA.

Weiland, A.P., Walker, W.E. (1986). Physiologic principles and clinical sequelae of cardiopulmonary bypass. *Heart and Lung* **15**, 34–9.

Wilson-Barnett, J. (1984). Alleviating stress for hospitalised patients. *International Review of Applied Psychology* **33**, 493–503.

CHAPTER 9

Renal problems

Chapter contents

Introduction

The kidney performs a wide variety of physiological functions. It plays a crucial role in the maintenance of acid–base, electrolyte, and fluid balance, and in the excretion of metabolic waste products. The physiological consequences of renal dysfunction can be widespread and devastating.

While some patients admitted to the CCU with renal problems are already in established renal failure, others can also be at high risk of development of renal failure following admission. This may occur as a result of direct renal trauma (including urological surgery), inadequate perfusion states, such as heart failure and massive haemorrhage, or as a consequence of multi-system disease involvement, such as systemic lupus erythematosus. The preservation of renal function and the early detection of dysfunction are integral to the care of any critically ill patient.

Functional anatomy and physiology

The main functions of the kidneys are shown in Table 9.1. The kidney achieves these functions by filtration, reab-

TABLE 9.1   Functions of the kidney
Production of urine
Excretion of waste products
Control and maintenance of fluid balance
Maintenance of acid–base balance
Control and maintenance of electrolyte balance
Renin production
Erythropoietin production
Control of calcium reabsorption and vitamin D hydroxylation

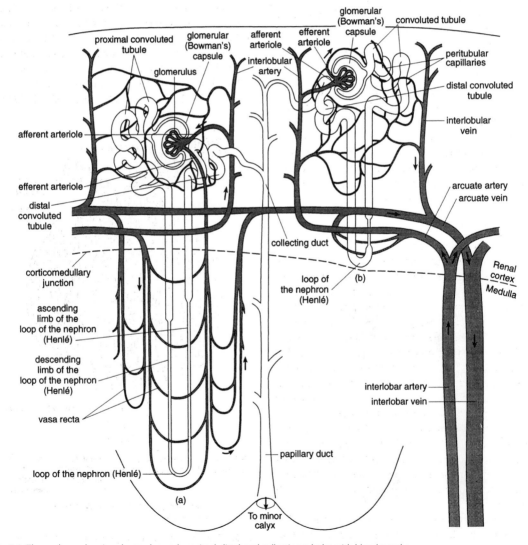

Fig. 9.1 The nephron, showing glomerulus, and proximal, distal, and collecting tubules with blood supply.

sorption, and secretion. Additionally, there are two other homeostatic mechanisms that are integral to kidney function, namely the renin-angiotensin-aldosterone (RAA) and antidiuretic hormone (ADH) pathways.

The nephron

The functional unit of the kidney is the nephron. There are approximately 1 million nephrons per kidney. Nephrons can be further defined as being either cortical, with their glomeruli in the cortex and short loops of Henle, or juxtamedullary, with glomeruli in the juxtamedullary region and long loops of Henle reaching down into the medulla.

Each nephron consists of a glomerulus, a glomerular capsule, a proximal convoluted tubule, a loop of Henle (descending and ascending limbs), a distal convoluted tubule, a collecting duct, and the accompanying vasculature (Fig. 9.1).

Blood supply

Blood enters the kidney via the renal arteries which are branches of the aorta. Each kidney receives approximately 625 ml/min of blood; this constitutes, in total, 25% of the cardiac output. The renal arteries divide into the interlobar arteries which further divide into arcuate arteries, then into interlobular arteries, and finally into afferent arterioles. Blood flow in the renal cortex is greater than in the renal medulla.

The glomerulus

The afferent arterioles feed the glomeruli which are enclosed within the glomerular capsule. The glomerulus is often described as a 'tuft' of capillaries; this arrangement allows a large surface area to be available for filtration. The capsule is double walled; the outer wall is known as the parietal layer and the inner as the visceral layer. The two are separated by the capsular space. The visceral layer of the capsule and the endothelial layer of the glomerulus constitute the endothelial–capsular membrane, which rests on a layer of contractile mesangial cells. Modified cells, known as juxtaglomerular cells, are situated around the afferent and efferent arterioles. Parts of the distal tubules lie in close proximity to their originating arterioles; these tubule cells are known collectively as the macula densa. The juxtaglomerular cells and macula densa together form the juxtaglomerular apparatus which secretes renin.

Blood entering the glomerulus from the afferent arteriole is filtered by the endothelial–capsular membrane. The membrane is impermeable to molecules greater than 4 nm in size (molecular weight of 70 000 daltons (Da)).

Filtration also depends on the molecular shape, electrostatic charge, and opposing pressures within the glomerulus and capsule. Blood in the glomerulus creates a hydrostatic pressure (~60 mmHg) which tends to force fluid out of the afferent vessels. This hydrostatic pressure is opposed by the pressure within the capsular space (~20 mmHg) and the osmotic pressure exerted by the blood in the glomerulus (~30 mmHg). The filtration pressure is therefore equal to:

60 mmHg – 20 mmHg – 30 mmHg = 10 mmHg.

If the glomerular pressure should fall (e.g. during haemorrhage) to a level where it is equal to the sum of the capsular pressure and the osmotic pressure, then no filtration will occur. As a compensatory mechanism in the event of a decrease in glomerular filtration rate (GFR), chloride reabsorption by the macula densa cells of the distal tubules is increased, resulting in dilatation of the afferent arterioles and an increase in blood flow and thus GFR. The presence of reabsorbed chloride can

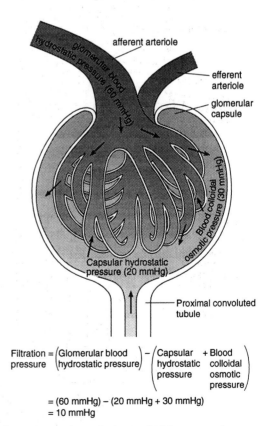

Filtration = (Glomerular blood pressure hydrostatic pressure) – (Capsular hydrostatic pressure + Blood colloidal osmotic pressure)

= (60 mmHg) – (20 mmHg + 30 mmHg)
= 10 mmHg

Fig. 9.2 Bowman's capsule, showing fluid dynamics producing filtration pressure.

promote renin secretion which will cause efferent arteriolar constriction, thus increasing glomerular pressure and hence GFR (Fig. 9.2).

Blood which is not filtered through the membrane leaves the glomerulus via the efferent arterioles. The efferent arterioles in the cortical region of the kidney divide to form peritubular capillaries around the convoluted tubules. The juxtaglomerular efferent arterioles also form peritubular capillaries but, in addition, form a network of thin-walled vessels known as the vasa recta which reach down into the renal medulla. The peritubular capillaries and the vasa recta eventually join to form the interlobar veins and, finally, the renal veins. Fluid which is filtered across the endothelial-capsular membrane is known as filtrate and enters the next part of the nephron, the proximal convoluted tubule. The filtrate at this stage has an osmolality of 300 mOsmol/l.

> **Osmolality** is the osmotic pressure of a solution expressed in osmoles or milliosmoles per kilogram of water.

In the proximal tubule various solutes are reabsorbed (both actively and passively) into the surrounding peritubular capillaries, reducing the filtrate by some 75–80%. As sodium (a positively charged ion) is reabsorbed, leaving the tubules and moving into the peritubular capillaries, the blood within those capillaries becomes positively charged. Chloride (a negatively charged ion) follows, moving from the filtrate into the capillaries to achieve an electrostatic balance. The presence of sodium and chloride in the peritubular capillary blood increases its osmolality. Water then moves from the filtrate in the proximal tubule into the blood by osmosis (Table 9.2).

TABLE 9.2 Solutes reabsorbed in the proximal tubule

Sodium (80%)
Water (80%)
Phosphate
Chloride
Glucose
Bicarbonate
Potassium
Sulphate (100%)
Amino acids
Low molecular weight proteins

> **Osmosis** is the movement of a pure solvent (e.g. water) through a semi-permeable membrane from a solution that has a lower solute concentration to one that has a higher solute concentration.

> **Diffusion** is the process by which particulate matter in a fluid moves from an area of higher concentration to an area of lower concentration resulting in an even distribution of particles.

The proximal tubule is always permeable to water and therefore has no control over water moving out of the tubule. This is referred to as obligatory reabsorption. Water reabsorption, 80% of which occurs in the proximal tubule, is therefore controlled by sodium movement. After leaving the proximal tubule the filtrate enters the loop of Henle where more sodium, chloride, bicarbonate, and glucose are reabsorbed into the peritubular blood. The ascending limb of the loop is impermeable to water. Chloride ions are actively reabsorbed, moving from the filtrate into the interstitial fluid and then into the peritubular capillaries. The blood in the capillaries becomes negatively charged and, in order to equalize this, sodium follows chloride passively. This results in the filtrate becoming less concentrated, its osmolality now being approximately 100 mOsmol/l. Conversely, the interstitium surrounding the loop becomes hyperosmolar, in the region of 1200 mOsmol/l. The filtrate then enters the distal convoluted tubule where further solute reabsorption occurs, making the filtrate even more dilute. Various substances, including creatinine and drugs, are secreted by the distal tubules into the filtrate for excretion. The final part of the nephron is the collecting duct, running through the renal medulla, which takes the filtrate, now called urine, to the ureters.

The distal tubules and the collecting ducts are sites of action for both the RAA and ADH mechanisms (Figs 9.3 and 9.4). The RAA pathway controls sodium reabsorption from the distal tubules and collecting ducts. Sodium reabsorption is dependent on its concentration in the extracellular fluid. Because water accompanies sodium, extracellular volume is also affected. The RAA mechanism can therefore manipulate sodium levels and blood volume. Although 80% of water reabsorption is obligatory via osmosis from the proximal tubule, ADH can control reabsorption of water from the distal tubules and collecting ducts.

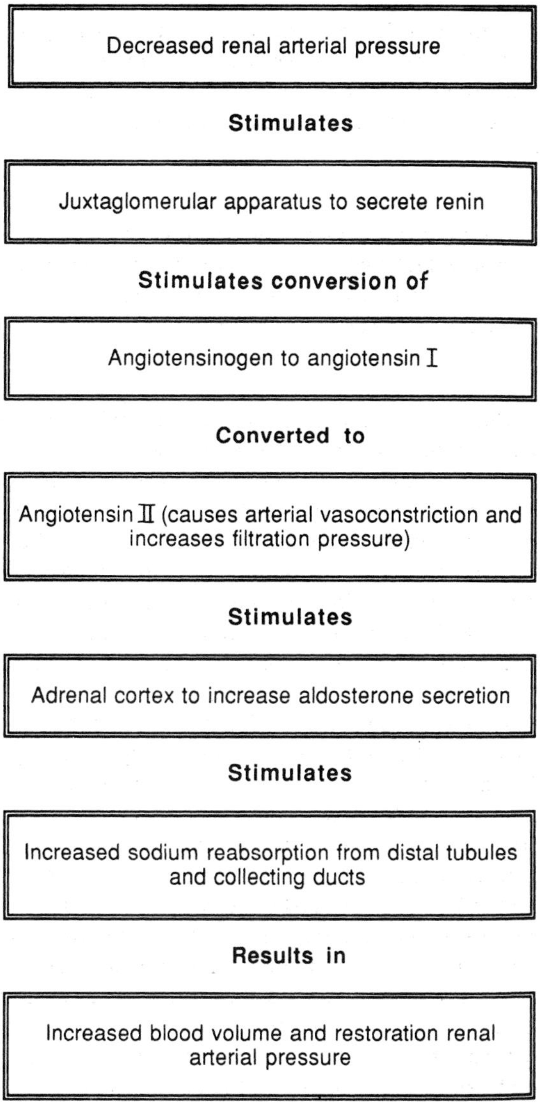

Decreased renal arterial pressure

Stimulates

Juxtaglomerular apparatus to secrete renin

Stimulates conversion of

Angiotensinogen to angiotensin I

Converted to

Angiotensin II (causes arterial vasoconstriction and increases filtration pressure)

Stimulates

Adrenal cortex to increase aldosterone secretion

Stimulates

Increased sodium reabsorption from distal tubules and collecting ducts

Results in

Increased blood volume and restoration renal arterial pressure

Fig. 9.3 The renin–angiotensin–aldosterone (RAA) mechanism.

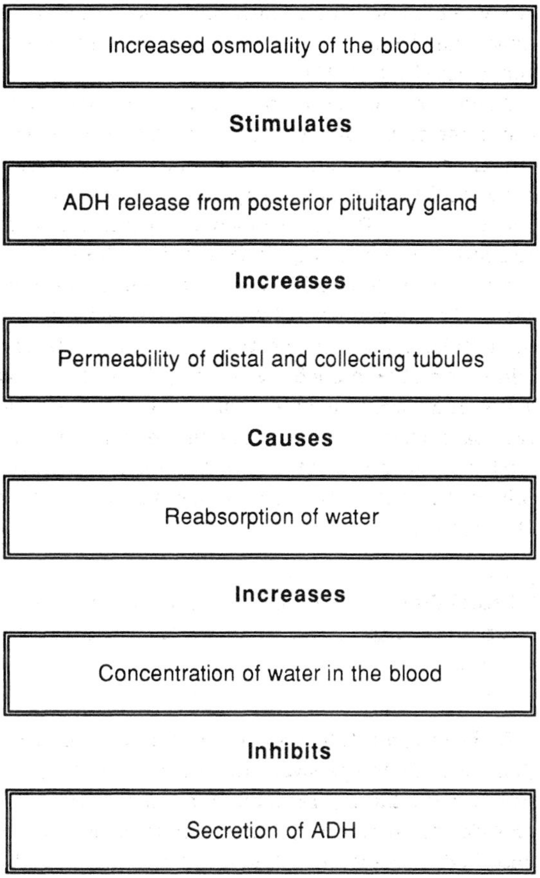

Increased osmolality of the blood

Stimulates

ADH release from posterior pituitary gland

Increases

Permeability of distal and collecting tubules

Causes

Reabsorption of water

Increases

Concentration of water in the blood

Inhibits

Secretion of ADH

Fig 9.4 Antidiuretic hormone (ADH) mechanism.

Concentrating abilities of the kidney

In the process of reabsorbing solutes, the filtrate becomes progressively more dilute during its passage through the nephron. The impermeability of the ascending limb of the loop of Henle to water and the control over water reabsorption by ADH in the distal tubules and collecting ducts further ensures a dilute filtrate by the end of the nephron. The reabsorption of solutes results in the interstitium becoming more concentrated, particularly in the medulla of the kidney. However, there are physiological circumstances, such as dehydration, where excretion of waste products in a dilute urine is not desirable. This concentrating ability depends upon the maintenance of a hyperosmolar medullary interstitium. As previously mentioned, chloride and sodium reabsorption in the ascending limb of the loop of Henle increases the solute concentration in the interstitium which is carried down into the medulla by blood flow in the vasa recta. The osmolality of the medulla is further increased by the movement of sodium and chloride out of the collecting ducts. ADH can promote the movement of water out of the collecting ducts. This results in a high urea concentration within the ducts. Urea then moves, by diffusion, out of the ducts and into the surrounding interstitium. The concentration of urea in the interstitium is greater than in the loop of the nephron and so urea moves into the loop, again by diffusion. When the filtrate (containing the diffused urea) reaches the ascending limb of the loop and the distal tubule, water but not urea is removed under the control of ADH, resulting in further concentration of urea in the collecting ducts. The counter-current mechanism also maintains medullary osmolality.

In practical terms, the loop of Henle consists of two parallel tubes with fluid flowing in opposite directions—'counter-current flow'. The descending limb, being impermeable to solutes and permeable to water, allows the movement of water by osmosis into the relatively more concentrated interstitium, thus increasing the concentration of the filtrate. This pattern continues and accumulates through the descending limb, reaching an osmolality of 1200 mOsmol/l. Sodium and chloride move from the ascending limb into the interstitium of the medulla. As this part of the loop of Henle is impermeable to water, the filtrate becomes progressively less concentrated, being 200 mOsmol/l at the cortex. The accompanying vasa recta are similar to the loop in that there are ascending and descending limbs. Indeed, it is partly this arrangement that keeps the medulla concentrated. As blood moves (within the vasa recta) towards the medulla, solutes enter the blood from the interstitium.

When the now concentrated blood moves into the ascending vasa recta and moves back towards the cortex, the solutes diffuse back into the interstitium. The counter-current mechanism partly depends on a sluggish blood flow within the vasa recta. If that flow increases (e.g. during haemodilution or volume expansion), medullary osmolality is disrupted, decreasing water absorption and resulting in a dilute urine.

Acid–base balance

An acid is a substance that can provide hydrogen ions (H^+) and a base (an alkali) is a substance that can accept hydrogen ions. Even in extremely acidic solutions, the concentration of H^+ ions is small and therefore relative values are inconvenient to use. The pH scale is a measurement of the H^+ ion concentration and is a negative logarithm of the H^+ concentration. A change of one pH unit therefore represents a 10-fold change in the H^+ concentration in opposing directions. Thus if the H^+ concentration rises, the pH falls and if the H^+ concentration falls, the pH rises.

The pH of blood is maintained between the narrow limits of 7.36 and 7.44 by buffers available in the blood, lungs (see Chapter 4), and kidneys. An increase in arterial blood pH above 7.43 constitutes an alkalosis and a pH below 7.37 an acidosis. The alkalosis or acidosis can be respiratory, metabolic, or mixed in origin (Table 9.3) (see also Chapter 4 for respiratory alkalosis–acidosis). In addition to the changes in pH, abnormal bicarbonate values also accompany metabolic acidosis (<21 mmol/l) and metabolic alkalosis (>28 mmol/1).

TABLE 9.3	Causes of metabolic acidosis and alkalosis
Metabolic acidosis	Acute and chronic renal failure
	Ingestion of acids (e.g. salicylates)
	Severe loss of small bowel or biliary fluid
	Tissue ischaemia or necrosis
	Diabetic ketoacidosis
	Drugs, poisons (e.g. cyanide, phenformin)
Metabolic alkalosis	Excessive sodium bicarbonate infusion
	Excessive ingestion of alkali
	Loss of gastric acid (e.g. excess vomiting or nasogastric drainage)
	Infusion of excessive citrate
	Liver failure

Blood buffers

Blood buffers can exercise a rapid response to changes in pH but their effects last for a relatively short time. The most important buffer in the extracellular fluid is bicarbonate (HCO_3^-) buffering hydrogen ions to form carbonic acid (H_2CO_3). Carbonic acid easily dissociates into water (H_2O) and carbon dioxide (CO_2). The carbon dioxide can then be eliminated by the lungs:

$$HCO_3^- + H^+ \leftrightarrow H_2CO_3 \leftrightarrow H_2O + CO_2.$$

Plasma proteins can also act as buffers, but this contribution is relatively small compared with the bicarbonate system. Haemoglobin is important as it is present in erythrocytes which are prime sites for carbonic acid formation and is thus immediately available to buffer hydrogen ions from carbonic acid.

Stewart's strong ion theory of acid–base balance

An alternative theory has been proposed to explain the mechanisms of acid–base balance. In contrast to the conventional Henderson-Hasselbalch approach, Stewart's theory suggests that three independent variables determine pH in plasma by changing the degree of water dissociation into hydrogen ions. These three variables are the strong ion difference (SID), the PCO_2 and the charge from weak acids (A_{TOT}). Strong ions are those that are fully dissociated in biological solutions; in humans these are principally sodium (Na^+) and chloride (Cl^-). Other less important strong ions are potassium (K^+), magnesium (Mg^{2+}), calcium (Ca^{2+}) and sulphate (SO_4^{2-}). A decrease in the SID, an increase in PCO_2 and an increase in A_{TOT} will all have an acidifying effect on the plasma (Skellet et al. 2000).

Renal component in acid–base balance

A low blood pH will stimulate the tubular cells to secrete hydrogen ions into the filtrate. To maintain electrostatic balance, sodium (Na^+) diffuses from the filtrate into the tubular cells where it combines with bicarbonate to produce sodium bicarbonate ($NaHCO_3$). This bicarbonate is then absorbed into the blood and acts as a systemic buffer. In conjunction with the excretion of excess hydrogen ions, the kidney thus attempts to counteract acidosis. Similar processes occur with ammonia and phosphate (see Fig. 9.5).

Acute renal failure

Two types of acute renal failure should be distinguished (Renal Association 2002):

1. Failure of the kidneys alone, with other organ systems functioning normally to begin with.
2. Multiorgan failure.

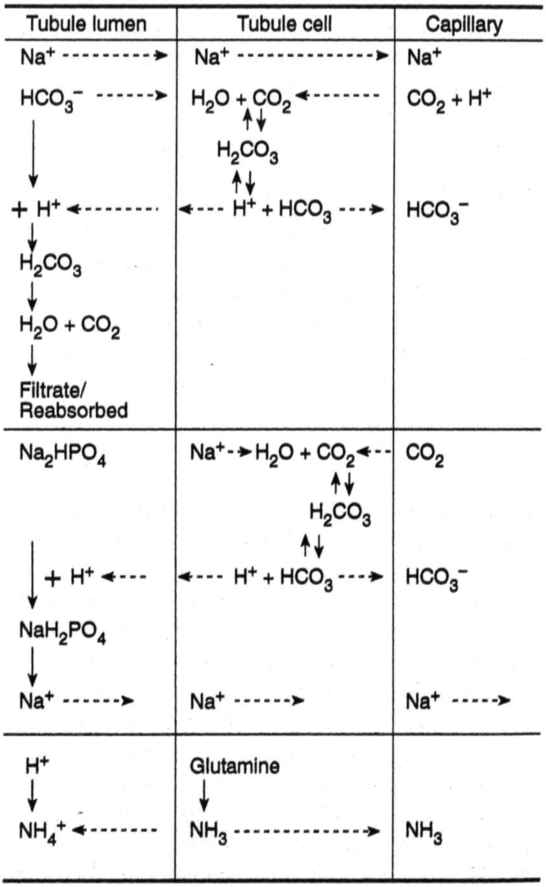

Fig. 9.5 Diagrammatic representation of renal control of acid–base balance with bicarbonate, phosphate, and ammonia.

The majority of renal failure seen in critical care is associated with multiorgan failure. Acute renal failure occurs in approximately 30% of critically ill patients. The mortality in patients who develop renal failure through hypoperfusion is much higher than those patients who receive toxic doses of pharmacological therapy (Galley 2000). The mortality rate in those with renal failure alone is <5% and those with multiorgan failure is >40% (Renal Association 2002).

The role of sepsis in the development and subsequent course of acute renal failure has been extremely well documented; indeed, one study demonstrated that sepsis was the major cause of death in 52% of patients with acute renal failure (Beaman and Adu 1992). These daunting figures serve to emphasize the need for awareness of the precipitating causes of acute renal failure and, thereafter, early detection and treatment.

Definitions

The terminology surrounding acute renal failure can be quite confusing and the following should help clarification:

- *Acute renal failure.* The sudden development of renal insufficiency, leading to uraemia and loss of electrolyte control in a previously well patient.

- *Oliguria.* A urine volume of less than 0.5 ml/kg/hour in an adult.

- *Pre-renal acute renal failure.* This is also termed 'reversible renal hypoperfusion' which arises as a result of renal hypoperfusion from hypovolaemia and/or a low cardiac output and/or a low perfusion pressure. It is reversible on restoration of renal blood flow and/or systemic blood pressure, thus possibly preventing the development of established renal failure.

- *Acute tubular necrosis.* A term frequently used in the clinical setting to describe a form of acute reversible renal failure. This definition often inaccurately reflects histological findings.

- *Non-oliguric acute renal failure.* Acute tubular necrosis, where there is uraemia and loss of electrolyte control though no coexisting oliguria.

Causes of acute renal failure

The cause of acute renal failure is frequently multifactorial. However, it is useful to classify the causes into three main groups (see also Tables 9.4, 9.5, and 9.6):

1. pre-renal
2. renal (intrinsic)
3. post-renal.

TABLE 9.4	Pre-renal causes of acute renal failure

Cause	Examples
Hypovolaemic causes	Hypovolaemia, burns, gastrointestinal losses, renal losses, third space losses such as sepsis, pancreatitis
Cardiogenic causes	Arrhythmias, heart failure, valvular dysfunction
Obstructive causes	Pericardial tamponade, pulmonary embolism

TABLE 9.5	Intrinsic causes of acute renal failure

Acute tubular necrosis	Unrelieved pre-renal causes
	Acute haemorrhage
	Haemoglobin/myoglobin
	Pancreatitis
	Septic abortion
	Eclampsia
	Post-operative
	Cardiogenic shock
	Burns
	Nephrotoxins (e.g. radiographic contrast, heavy metals, organic solvents, aminoglycosides, amphotericin)
	Systemic lupus erythematosus
Cortical necrosis	Snake venom
	Nephrotic syndrome
	Renal artery occlusion/emboli
	Renal vein thrombosis
	Disseminated intravascular coagulation
	Acute pyelonephritis
	Hepatorenal syndrome
	Glomerulonephritis
	Polyarteritis nodosa
	Post-streptococcal infection
	Goodpasture's syndrome
	Wegener's granulomatosis
	Infective endocarditis
	Henoch–Schönlein purpura
Acute interstitial nephritis	Penicillins, e.g. methicillin, ampicillin, benzylpenicillin
	Cephalosporins, e.g. cephalexin
	Sulphonamides
	Rifampicin
	Diuretics: thiazides furosemide
	Non-steroidal anti-inflammatory drugs, e.g. indomethacin, diclofenac
	Phenytoin

TABLE 9.6	Post-renal causes of acute renal failure

Intra-ureteral	Calculi
	Papillary necrosis
	Crystals (e.g. uric acid)
	Tumour
	Blood clot
Extra-ureteral	Retroperitoneal fibrosis
	Tumour
	Aneurysm
Bladder obstruction	Prostatic hypertrophy
	Bladder tumour
	Blood clot
	Calculi
	Functional neuropathy
Urethral obstruction	Stricture
	Meatal stenosis
	Phimosis

Note: **Intra-abdominal pressure**—any cause of increased abdominal pressure including ascites may result in abdominal pressure that exceeds renal perfusion pressure causing deterioration in renal function (Sizer and Cottam 2003).

Mechanisms of acute renal failure

A sudden and sustained fall in renal blood flow leads to a fall in glomerular filtration rate (GFR) resulting in a reduction in urine output and a decrease in urea and creatinine clearance (Blakeley and Smith 2003). At this stage, because tubular function and concentrating ability are maintained, rises of urine osmolality, urea, and creatinine and a fall in urinary sodium are seen. If renal perfusion is restored at this point established renal failure can be avoided. However, if renal perfusion is not restored, the GFR further decreases, along with the urine output, with progressive tubular damage. Concentrating ability is lost with a resulting loss of sodium reabsorption.

Despite a decrease in renal perfusion and GFR, there are some patients who present with 'non-oliguric renal failure', maintaining an adequate urine output. The reasons for this remain unclear; however, it has been postulated that improved fluid therapy and the increased use of high-dose loop diuretics may contribute. The prognosis is improved for non-oliguric renal failure when compared with oliguric renal failure (Beaman and Adu 1992).

There are a number of theories to explain the events occurring at nephron level following an ischaemic insult to the kidney. Some or all of the following may coexist in acute renal failure.

Tubuloglomerular feedback

During periods of renal hypoperfusion, cortical blood flow is proportionally reduced in relation to medullary blood flow; this is felt to be a protective mechanism for the medulla which normally operates on the verge of hypoxia. This action will also decrease the oxygen demand necessary for solute reabsorption as the GFR drops. If this mechanism fails, medullary ischaemia occurs and the solute reaching the macula densa will activate the tubuloglomerular feedback mechanism. Chloride ions in particular are thought to play an activating role. A further consequence of this is vaso-constriction which, in turn, further reduces GFR (Schrier *et al.* 1990).

Reduced glomerular permeability

Local stimuli (including angiotensin II, thromboxane, and histamine) cause glomerular mesangial cell contraction which serves to reduce the area available for filtration and permeability.

'No reflow' phenomenon

Endothelial cell swelling resulting from the ischaemic injury prevents reperfusion of the microcirculation despite the restoration of renal blood flow. The efferent arterioles of the cortical glomeruli supply blood to the medulla. These arterioles divide and form the vasae rectae, which in themselves are resistance vessels with the ability to control medullary blood flow. The ascending vessels have very thin walls and are susceptible to compression by local swollen tubules.

Tubular obstruction

Obstruction of the tubules by debris causes a rise in intratubular pressure until glomerular filtration stops.

Filtrate 'back-leak'

The damaged tubular basement membrane allows filtrate to escape and the GFR is further reduced. The role of mediators produced in the kidney is becoming increasingly recognized. It is known that some prostaglandins (PGI_2 and PGE_2) will act beneficially by promoting vasodilatation and mesangial cell relaxation and inhibiting platelet aggregation. Conversely, thromboxane (TxA_2) will cause vasoconstriction and glomerular cell contraction (reducing filtration surface area), and will promote platelet aggregation (Schieppati and Remuzzi 1990).

Nitric oxide (NO), formerly known as endothelium-derived relaxant factor (EDRF), has been shown to regulate blood flow in resistance vessels (including the vasa recta) to promote vasodilatation. Physiological antagonists to NO are the endothelins which promote vaso-constriction. In response to ischaemia endothelins are thought to cause mesangial cell contraction (Neild 1990).

The effects of reperfusion of previously ischaemic tissue are increasingly becoming understood. The restoration of oxygen delivery, the accumulation of calcium and the correction of acidosis promotes phospholipid activity and oxygen radical formation. This results in cell membrane damage, a rise in intracellular calcium, a reduction in ATP synthesis, and a reduction in mitochondrial respiration, all of which contribute to cell death. This may also in part explain a continuing deterioration in renal function despite restoration of renal blood flow.

Investigation and diagnosis of acute renal failure

Any investigation or diagnostic method should, in the first instance, concentrate on distinguishing the cause of the renal failure (pre-renal, intrinsic, or post-renal) to enable prompt and appropriate treatment. The patient

TABLE 9.7 Investigations of acute renal failure

Urine	Urinalysis
	Urine microscopy, culture, and sensitivity
	Electrolytes, osmolality, urea, and creatinine
	Creatinine clearance
	Urine/plasma ratios of urea, sodium, and osmolality
	Myoglobinuria
Blood	Full blood count
	Coagulation screen
	Electrolytes, urea, creatinine, calcium, phosphate, magnesium, glucose
	Arterial blood gases
	Liver function tests
	Creatine kinase
	Autoantibodies (e.g. ANCA for Wegener's granulomatosis, polyarteritis nodosa or antiglomerular basement antibody for Goodpasture's syndrome)
Radiological	Plain abdominal and chest X-ray
	Renal ultrasound
	Urography
	Isotope renography
	CT scan
Other	12-lead ECG
	Renal biopsy

TABLE 9.8	History and physical examination
History	Taken from patient, family members, case notes, the referring team. *Including*:
	(1) Coexisting diseases (e.g. diabetes, heart failure, hypertension, vascular disease)
	(2) Any potentially nephrotoxic medication (e.g. non-steroidal anti-inflammatory drugs, aminoglycosides)
	(3) History of trauma
Physical examination	*For*: (1) Signs and symptoms of uraemia (e.g. drowsiness, coma, nausea, vomiting, pruritis)
	(2) Bruising, possibly indicating platelet dysfunction
	(3) Signs of metabolic acidosis hyperventilation or 'air hunger'
	(4) Pericarditis
	(5) Joint pain
	(6) Signs of fluid overload (e.g. raised jugular venous pressure, peripheral, and pulmonary oedema)

may present with pre-renal failure which, with rapid detection and treatment, could prevent progression to established renal failure (Table 9.7).

A history should be taken and physical examination performed (see Table 9.8). For diagnosis and further management it is vital that the chronological sequence of events is ascertained. Coexisting diseases, which may have a causative or exaggerating effect, may be discovered. The patient may be taking medication which might affect the kidney or its vascular supply (e.g. angiotensin-converting enzyme (ACE) inhibitors such as enalapril or captopril). Physical examination could reveal signs and symptoms of uraemia, anaemia, coagulopathy, and fluid overload, all indicative of renal dysfunction.

Urinary investigations

The simple 'stick test' will reveal pH and specific gravity values, glucose, ketones, bilirubin, urobilinogen, protein, and blood. The presence of protein may indicate an underlying glomerulonephritis or interstitial nephritis. The presence of blood may indicate haemoglobin or myoglobin in the urine (i.e. intravascular haemolysis or rhabdomyolysis, respectively).

The urine can be examined directly for red and white blood cells or the urinary sediment after centrifugation for casts and crystals.

MICROSCOPIC EXAMINATION OF URINE

- *Acute nephritis*: white blood cells and white blood cell casts.
- *Acute tubular necrosis*: tubular epithelial cells and casts.
- *Glomerulonephritis*: granular and red cell casts.

Creatinine clearance using a 24-hour collection of urine and a plasma sample can be used to make an assessment of GFR. It is calculated as follows (normal GFR = 120 ml/min):

$$GFR = \frac{\text{creatinine concentration (urine) (mmol/l)} \times \text{urine volume (ml/min)}}{\text{creatinine concentration (plasma) } (\mu\text{mol/l})}$$

Table 9.9 indicates urinary values for oliguria secondary to either renal or pre-renal causes. Caution must be exercised when interpreting such values if the patient has pre-existing renal disease and/or has received diuretics, as these can affect tubular concentrating ability and urinary electrolyte excretion.

In the clinical setting, the differentiation between the patient in pre-renal and established renal failure is not always as well defined as Table 9.9 would suggest. Many patients fall between the two categories, especially those with non-oliguric renal failure.

Blood investigations

The blood urea can be raised in the absence of a reduction in GFR from:

- increased protein catabolism, as seen in burns, fever, and after surgery;
- from increased protein intake (e.g. gastrointestinal bleeding with increased reabsorption of amino acids;
- dehydration.

Therefore, uraemia is a less reliable indictor of renal function than creatinine concentration. Creatinine pro-

TABLE 9.9	Diagnostic urinary indices for oliguria	
Test	**Pre-renal**	**Renal**
Specific gravity	>1020	1010
Osmolality (mOsmol/kg)	>500	250–300
Sodium (mmol/l)	<15	>40
Urea (mmol/l)	>250	<160
Urine:plasma osmolality ratio	>1.3:1	<1.1:1
Urine:plasma urea ratio	>10:1	<4:1
Urine:plasma creatinine ratio	>40:1	<20:1

duction is related to lean body mass except in rhabdomyolysis. Therefore, the plasma creatinine is reduced in the very young, the elderly, and in those with alcoholism and chronic wasting diseases. Blood urea and creatinine levels have limitations in diagnosing renal dysfunction in that plasma creatinine concentrations reach the upper limit of normal after 50% of renal function is lost and then doubles for each further 50% loss of renal function (Short and Cumming 1999). It is important to remember that GFR declines with age and, if accompanied by a reduction in muscle mass, the serum creatinine can remain within normal values.

Blood gas analysis will often reveal a metabolic acidosis, with a reduced bicarbonate, a significant base deficit, and a low pH value. Approximately 95% of the total body potassium is intracellular. Together with other cations (e.g. calcium and magnesium), potassium is responsible for maintaining osmotic pressure in the intracellular fluid compartment. In the extracellular fluid compartment, potassium is instrumental in neuromuscular and cardiac function. Hyperkalaemia is frequently seen in acute renal failure due to the accumulation of hydrogen ions within the cells, forcing potassium out of the cells to maintain ionic balance.

Calcium levels tend to fall as the phosphate level rises in acute renal failure. In health, the kidneys produce 1α-hydroxylase which converts 25-hydroxycholecalciferol into 1,25-dihydroxycholecalciferol This, in turn, promotes reabsorption of calcium from bone and decreases urinary calcium excretion. See Table 9.10 for a summary of blood investigations in acute renal failure.

Radiological investigations

These include the following:

- *Renal ultrasound.* Useful for estimating renal size or detecting an obstruction. Probably the most common and useful radiological investigation of acute renal failure in the CCU.

- *Urography.* Renal size and presence of an obstruction, suspected trauma.

- *Isotope renography.* Renal function, size, vasculature, and outflow.

- *Computed tomography (CT) scanning.* If retroperitoneal disease is suspected. Often used as an alternative to arteriography or venography.

- *Plain abdominal X-ray.* Detection of renal calculi.

- *Renal biopsy.* If the acute renal failure is unexplained and a histological diagnosis is required. Renal biopsy is not advised if the patient only has one kidney. Any coagulation abnormalities must be corrected prior to biopsy and the patient monitored closely for 24 hours for signs of bleeding.

Priorities of care

As with any patient, the three main priorities are those of: Airway, Breathing, and Circulation.

Airway

The patient's conscious level may deteriorate in the presence of uraemia. Neurological observations should

TABLE 9.10	Blood investigations in acute renal failure	
Test	**Normal value**	**Value in acute renal failure**
Full blood count	Haemoglobin (Hb): 12—18 g/dl	Hb normal or low with anaemia or dilutional effect
	White blood cells (WBC): (4–11) × 10⁹/litre	WBC normal or raised if accompanying infection/ inflammation
Platelet count	(150–400) × 10⁹/litre	Normal (but function may be decreased or low, e.g. in systemic lupus erythematosus)
Sodium	132–144 mmol/l	Normal, high, or low
Potassium	3.3–4.7 mmol/l	Normal, high, or low
Urea	2.5–6.6 mmol/l	Raised
Creatinine	55–120 µmol/l	Raised
Phosphate	0.8–1.4 mmol/l	Usually raised
Glucose	Fasting <5.5 mmol/l	Normal
Osmolality	285–295 mOsm/l	Usually raised
Magnesium	0.75–1.0 mmol/l	Variable
Calcium	2.12–2.62 mmol/l	Normal or low

be performed when the patient is admitted to the critical care unit to provide a baseline, and recorded frequently thereafter. The patient may lose the ability to maintain a patent airway. Although airway adjuncts, such as nasopharyngeal and oropharyngeal (Guedel) airways, have their uses the patient will probably require endotracheal intubation.

Breathing

The patient's respiratory status may be affected by pulmonary oedema from fluid overload, coexisting pulmonary insufficiency (e.g. acute respiratory distress syndrome), or the neuronal effects of uraemia. If the patient is severely acidotic, 'Kussmaul' breathing (see Chapter 4) may be observed with the patient breathing rapidly and deeply. This may occur in the patient with or without a patent airway and may eventually necessitate intubation and ventilation if the acidosis cannot be corrected and the patient tires.

On admission, the patient's respiratory rate and pattern of breathing should be documented and recorded regularly thereafter. Continuous pulse oximetry is a simple and immediate form of assessing oxygenation in addition to arterial blood gas estimation and should also be monitored. The patient's pulmonary secretions should be noted, in particular to detect pulmonary oedema, pulmonary haemorrhage (in the presence of coagulopathy), or 'pulmonary–renal syndromes', such as Wegener's or Goodpasture's.

Circulation

ECG and blood pressure monitoring should be standard. A method of measuring ventricular filling pressures is also essential to gauge volume load. As a minimum, a central venous catheter should be inserted and, if available, other forms of monitoring cardiac output such as the oesophageal Doppler. The insertion of any intravascular lines should be performed under strict aseptic conditions to prevent infection.

Bleeding in uraemic patients is most commonly due to defects in platelet adhesion or aggregation (Liesner

TABLE 9.11 Agents used in the treatment of hyperkalaemia

Treatment of hyperkalaemia	Timing of effect
Glucose/insulin	Immediate effect
Intravenous calcium	Immediate effect
Renal replacement therapy	Immediate effect
Sodium bicarbonate	Immediate effect
Calcium resonium	Delayed effect

and Machin 1997); prior to intravascular catheter insertion, the bleeding and clotting times should be investigated and treated as appropriate. One dose of DDAVP (l-desamino-8-D-arginine vasopressin; desmopressin) can be given to improve platelet function transiently in the presence of uraemia if surgery or an invasive procedure is required. An adequate circulating volume should be maintained at all times, together with an effective perfusion pressure.

Peaked T waves may be seen on the ECG suggesting hyperkalaemia, although this may be present without this sign. Hyperkalaemia and any destabilizing arrhythmias should be treated swiftly. Untreated hyperkalaemia can lead to ventricular arrhythmias. Hyperkalaemia can be treated with calcium resonium 30 g (orally or rectally); this non-absorbable ion exchange resin removes potassium from the circulation but it does not have a rapid effect (see also Table 9.11). For more immediate control of the effects of hyperkalaemia, 10 ml of 10% calcium chloride can be given to stabilize the myocardial cell membrane. This is followed by 50 ml of 50% glucose containing 10–12 units of soluble insulin infused over 30–60 min and repeated as necessary. Insulin promotes intracellular movement of potassium, thereby lowering the blood level. If the patient is not anuric/oliguric and fluid overloaded, sodium bicarbonate (100 ml aliquots of 8.4% solution) may be useful as it will also lower the blood potassium level and provide symptomatic relief from the metabolic acidosis. However, ongoing treatment of the acid–base derangement is normally achieved with a form of renal replacement therapy.

Principles of care

Monitoring urine output

A deteriorating urine output is usually the first indicator of a potential renal problem. In an adult, an hourly volume of 0.5 ml/kg/h is the minimum acceptable volume. If the patient does not have a urinary catheter *in situ* then catheterization should be performed and a catheter left in place and connected to a drainage bag for further monitoring of urine volumes. The drainage bag tubing should be supported or fixed to the patient's leg to prevent drag on the urethra. A fluid balance chart to record intake and output on an hourly basis should be maintained.

If a urinary catheter is already in place the possibility of catheter blockage should be excluded by bladder irrigation. If necessary, the catheter should be replaced. If the patient is anuric, the presence of a urinary catheter may cause infection and it should be removed. Likewise, it is essential that in patients with nephrostomy tubes, ureteric stents, or urostomies, the possibility of obstruction is ruled out.

If the patient has been admitted post-urological surgery or post-renal trauma, the possibility of blood and blood clots causing an obstruction, or an anastomotic leak/ureteric rupture must be strongly suspected. If the patient is oliguric and circulating fluid volume has been optimized, the fluid intake should be restricted to replace urine output plus insensible losses only. This is acceptable in the critically ill patient for only a short period of time as intense fluid restriction precludes provision of adequate nutrition; renal replacement therapy is often implemented for this reason.

Care should be taken when administering hypertonic solutions, such as sodium bicarbonate, mannitol, or 10–50% glucose, if the patient is oliguric. The hypertonicity will draw extravascular fluid into the circulation and the patient may become intravascularly fluid-overloaded.

Avoidance of pre-renal renal failure

If the urine output is less than 0.5 ml/kg/h and the urinary catheter is patent, there may be a pre-renal cause of oliguria.

It is essential that the patient has an adequate circulating blood volume. The presence of tachycardia, hypotension, and cool peripheries may indicate that extra fluid is required. If so, the patient should be administered aliquots of colloid, 200–300 ml at a time (see section on fluid challenge in Chapter 6). The patient's ventricular filling pressures (determined by either the central venous pressure and/or the pulmonary artery wedge pressure, as available) or the stroke volume and cardiac output should be measured before and after each bolus of fluid. If, 5–10 min following the bolus of fluid, the filling pressure rises more than 3 mmHg and remains at that level then the patient probably has an adequate circulation. However, if there is no change or only a small increase then the optimal filling pressure may not have been achieved. Further fluid should be administered as appropriate.

AVOIDANCE OF PRE-RENAL RENAL FAILURE

- Adequate circulating volume and organ perfusion pressure.
- Adequate cardiac output.

When the patient has a pulmonary artery catheter, oesophageal Doppler, or other flow monitor, the stroke volume and cardiac output can be used to determine the optimal filling pressure (see Chapter 6). The urine output should be reassessed in the light of an adequate circulating volume; if there is no improvement and the patient remains tachycardic, ± hypotensive, and peripherally cool, attempts should be made to increase the cardiac output with a suitable inotropic or vasodilating agent (see Chapter 6). Cardiac output studies during this phase are useful to determine the effect of any inotropes administered. It is vital that attention be paid to the maintenance of an optimum cardiac output and circulating blood volume during all stages of the patient's illness.

Diuretic therapy

If the patient has a good circulating volume and an adequate cardiac output but remains oliguric, diuretics can be given in an attempt to promote a diuresis. The two classes of diuretics that can be given in this situation are:

- loop (e.g. furosemide (frusemide)) and
- osmotic (e.g. mannitol).

It has not been shown that either type of diuretic improves renal function but they can promote a diuresis. Mannitol may have a beneficial role in myoglobinuria, radiological contrast media-induced renal failure, and nephrotoxicity (Corwin and Bonventre 1988). However, the administration of mannitol can increase the extracellular fluid volume and may cause pulmonary oedema.

The administration of furosemide is also not without risk. If a diuresis is promoted, the fluid and solute loss can cause hypovolaemia and exacerbation of poor renal perfusion. Although furosemide may increase the urine output, there is no evidence that it increases survival (Corwin and Bonventre 1988). There is some evidence that these two agents may have a more effective role in the patient who is 'at risk', rather than in the patient who is in established renal failure (Lazarus 1990) (see Table 9.12 for the actions of mannitol and furosemide).

The administration of a diuretic may promote a diuresis and the development of established oliguric renal failure may be avoided. The patient may enter into a phase of non-oliguric acute renal failure, in which adequate volumes of urine are produced but renal function deteriorates as urine quality is poor. Investigations, as outlined in the section on acute renal failure, must be performed, a diagnosis made, and appropriate management strategies determined. It is often at this point when the renal failure is established and is no longer reversible that patients are admitted to the critical care unit.

TABLE 9.12	Actions of mannitol and furosemide
Mannitol	May reduce cell swelling and decrease tubular cell injury
	May increase extracellular volume and therefore cardiac output
	May decrease blood viscosity and systemic oncotic pressure resulting in an increase in GFR
	May increase intratubular flow, preventing obstruction
	May cause vasodilatation of glomerular capillaries, perhaps by increasing prostaglandin production
Furosemide	May increase intratubular flow, preventing obstruction
	May cause vasodilatation of glomerular capillaries
	May inhibit tubuloglomerular feedback increasing GFR
	May decrease transport related oxygen consumption

TYPICAL DOSAGES OF MANNITOL AND FUROSEMIDE IN RENAL FAILURE

- Mannitol: 500 mg/kg (i.e. 5 ml/kg of 10% solution or 2.5 ml/kg of 20% solution).
- Furosemide: 20–100 mg bolus followed by an infusion of 2 mg/min up to a maximum of 500 mg.

Nutrition

The patient in acute renal failure is often extremely catabolic and the implementation of nutrition should be a priority as muscle mass is quickly broken down to provide an energy source. Enteral nutrition is preferable with fewer complications (e.g. metabolic or feeding line-related sepsis); it also maintains gut integrity and may help to prevent translocation of bacteria and endotoxins.

There are no real differences for renal failure patients from the general rules of nutrition in the critically ill patient. Nutritional therapy should not depend on the severity of renal failure but should correct general nutritional deficiencies. It is suggested that calorific intake should not exceed 30–35 kcal/kg/day which should meet energy requirements. In addition, renal replacement therapy allows the adaptation of individual patients' needs (Kierdorf 1995, Alvestrand 1996).

It may be useful to calculate the patient's requirements with a metabolic computer (see Chapter 11). Protein requirements rarely exceed 14 g of nitrogen per day, except in the patient with burns. Extra protein losses occur with peritoneal dialysis and amino acid losses with haemofiltration, and this should be allowed for in the feeding regimen.

Electrolyte and trace elements should be titrated and supplied according to blood levels and not simply given as a routine. The B group vitamins are water soluble and can be removed during dialysis and haemofiltration. They should therefore be supplemented regularly.

Skin integrity

The risk of tissue breakdown and the development of decubitus ulcers are high in this group of patients. Renal failure has often been caused by a state of hypoperfusion, where intense peripheral vasoconstriction occurs as a compensatory mechanism. In addition, these patients often require inotropic support which can further decrease blood supply to the skin and underlying tissue.

Lengthy periods of time spent inserting lines, investigating, and fluid resuscitating often require the patient to remain in one position which can aggravate the situation even further.

The patient should be examined and assessed for risk of developing pressure sores as soon as possible following admission. This should be documented, along with a preventative strategy or a treatment programme appropriate to the risk or the sore involved. It may be necessary to use a pressure-relieving mattress or bed if the patient is particularly vulnerable or is too cardiovascularly unstable to withstand frequent changes of position. Care should also be taken with skin underlying ECG electrodes, lines, and endotracheal tapes as it can quickly break down in the presence of poor skin perfusion. The patient may experience skin irritation arising from azotaemia (high blood levels of nitrogenous waste products). Care should be taken that the patient does not scratch him/herself causing disruption of skin integrity and supra-added infection.

Renal replacement therapy

The indications for commencing a form of renal replacement therapy (RRT) are not absolute and considerable leeway is possible. General indications are as follows:

- metabolic acidosis (e.g. pH <7.3 and falling).
- hyperkalaemia (e.g. >6 mmol/l and rising),
- fluid overload or to create space for nutrition,
- severe uraemic symptoms (confusion, pericarditis, nausea, vomiting, etc.),

◆ urea >30 mmol/l and rising, creatinine > 300 μmol/l and rising.

The overall aims of any form of renal replacement therapy are:

◆ To relieve fluid overload, restore, and maintain fluid balance.

◆ To remove waste products (i.e. urea and creatinine).

◆ To correct and maintain metabolic and electrolyte balance.

Types of renal replacement therapy

◆ Slow continuous ultrafiltration (SCUF)

◆ Continuous arteriovenous haemofiltration (CAVH)

◆ Continuous venovenous haemofiltration (CVVH)

◆ Continuous venovenous haemodiafiltration (CVVHD)

◆ Continuous venovenous haemodialysis (CVVHD)

◆ Intermittent haemodialysis (IHD)

◆ Peritoneal dialysis (PD)

◆ Continuous ambulatory peritoneal dialysis (CAPD)

◆ A combination of IHD and haemofiltration

Basic physiological principles common to all renal replacement therapies

Diffusion

Diffusion is the movement of solutes across a semi-permeable membrane from an area of high concentration to an area of low concentration. A concentration gradient is therefore always necessary for diffusion to occur. Molecules with a smaller molecular weight will move across a semi-permeable membrane more readily than those with a larger molecular weight. A semi-permeable membrane has a defined pore size and any molecule exceeding this will not be able to pass through. Diffusion will be affected by the resistance offered by the membrane; this is related to the thickness, size, and shape of the pores. Diffusion is utilized in peritoneal dialysis, haemodialysis, and haemodiafiltration (see Fig. 9.6).

Ultrafiltration

This is a method of convective transport. It can be defined as the bulk movement of water together with permeable solutes through a semi-permeable membrane. Water molecules are small and can pass through all semipermeable membranes. The driving force for ultrafiltration can be either an osmotic gradient or hydrostatic pressure (see Fig. 9.7):

Diffusion

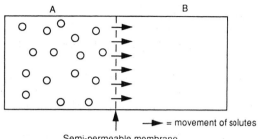

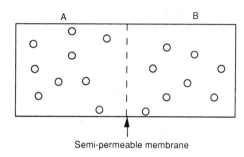

Fig. 9.6 The movement of solutes across a semi-permeable membrane.

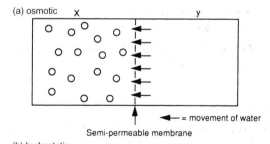

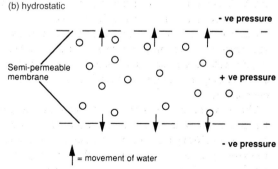

Fig. 9.7 Ultrafiltration: (a) osmotic; (b) hydrostatic.

1. *Osmotic ultrafiltration.* Water will be drawn across a semi-permeable membrane from a hypotonic solution into a hypertonic solution. The osmotic 'pull' is generated by the concentrated solute in the hyper-

tonic solution. Osmotic ultrafiltration is utilized in peritoneal dialysis.

2. *Hydrostatic ultrafiltration*. Water is forced across a semi-permeable membrane by a hydrostatic pressure exerted across the membrane. Hydrostatic ultrafiltration is utilized in haemofiltration and haemodialysis.

The *ultrafiltration coefficient* (KUF) indicates the permeability of the semi-permeable membrane. The KUF is defined as the number of millilitres of fluid per hour that will be transferred across the membrane per mmHg pressure gradient across the membrane.

Extracorporeal methods of renal replacement therapy

The majority of ICUs are now able to offer a vascular form of renal replacement therapy, including arteriovenous and venovenous methods. Haemodialysis and haemofiltration share some common principles and these will be discussed prior to addressing the techniques individually.

Buffers

To enable effective treatment of the metabolic acidosis which frequently accompanies acute renal failure, a buffer must be provided either in the dialysate fluid or in the replacement fluid (haemofiltration only). Lactate is commonly used as the buffer for haemofiltration: it is metabolized by the liver to bicarbonate. Acetate is another buffer, but there is insufficient evidence evaluating the use of acetate-buffered solutions and limited support for its use compared with lactate- and bicarbonate-buffered solutions (Schetz *et al.* 2002). Bicarbonate itself can also given as a buffer in haemodialysis.

Artificial membranes

There is a wide choice of artificial kidneys/filters available, all of which have differing membrane properties.

There are two main groups of membranes:

1. *Cellulose membranes*: cuprophane, cellulose hydrate, cellulose acetate.

2. *Synthetic membranes*: polycarbonate, polysulfone, polyamide, polyacrylonitrile.

The cellulose membranes have traditionally been used for chronic haemodialysis (HD), having a relatively low permeability with a cut-off at approximately 5000 Da. The cuprophane membrane in particular has been associated with complement activation, cytokine generation, and white cell and platelet activation, all of which can lead to pulmonary and other organ dysfunction (Bihari and Beale 1992). The synthetic membranes are, on the whole, not associated with such disturbances. Polyacrylonitrile, in particular, is a highly biocompatible and permeable membrane with a cut-off of approximately 35 000 Da.

The artificial kidney itself can either be of a hollow fibre or a flat plate design. Most haemofiltration kidneys are hollow fibre.

TABLE 9.13 Vascular access in renal replacement therapy

Access	Use	Comment
Separate artery and vein cannulation	Non-blood pump method	Commonly femoral approaches used. Renders patient immobile, blood flow obstructed if legs bent
Arteriovenous shunt (e.g. Schribner). Radial artery cephalic vein or post tibial artery/long saphenous vein	Pumped and non-pumped methods	Provides good blood flow
		Cannot be changed, along with other patient lines if sepsis suspected
Double lumen: jugular vein access	Pumped methods	Provides good blood flow
		Position often uncomfortable for patient
		Can be difficult to fix to the skin due to position
Double lumen: subclavian vein approach	Pumped methods	Provides good blood flow
		Allows greater patient mobility
		Potential insertion complications: pneumothorax brachial plexus injury thrombosis/ stenosis
Double lumen: femoral vein approach	Pumped methods	Provides good blood flow if legs kept straight
		No proven increased risk of infection
		Can be a difficult site to expose for observation

Vascular access

Any of the 'spontaneous' extracorporeal methods of renal replacement therapy (i.e. those without a blood pump in the circuit) require the vascular access to be arterial in origin so as to supply sufficient pressure to drive blood around the circuit and provide an adequate filtration pressure (Table 9.13). However, these are no longer frequently used.

Once a blood pump has been incorporated, blood flow is not dependent upon arterial pressure and access may be gained from a vein. This is the most common and safest method of renal replacement therapy for the critically ill patient.

For relatively short-term use in the CCU, a 'double-lumen cannula' is commonly used. This is a Y-shaped cannula inserted into a large vein (e.g. femoral, internal jugular, or subclavian vein). One arm of the Y allows

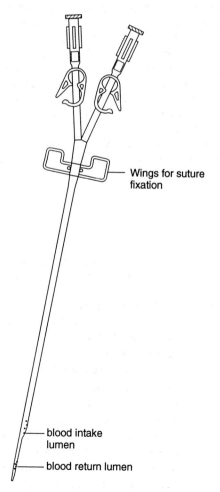

Wings for suture fixation

blood intake lumen

blood return lumen

Fig. 9.8 Double-lumen vascular cannula for venovenous haemo(dia)filtration.

blood to be drawn away from the patient while the other arm allows blood to be simultaneously pumped back into the patient further up the vein to prevent recirculation (Fig. 9.8).

Anticoagulation

Most forms of extracorporeal circulation require anti-coagulation to help prevent platelet and coagulation system activation as a response to contact with a foreign surface (i.e. the circuits and filter). Ineffective anti-coagulation will cause clotting in the artificial kidney. Although filter clotting is time-consuming, expensive, and decreases overall efficiency, it does not directly present a hazard to the patient other than loss of blood in the circuit volume (approximately 150–200 ml) and consumption of clotting products. However, the infusion of too much anticoagulant can be extremely dangerous and the patient's coagulation status should be monitored. Any signs of bleeding from vascular access sites, the gastrointestinal tract, or mucosal membranes should be viewed with suspicion and investigated.

There are methods during intermittent HD that allow for anticoagulation-free dialysis. This is occasionally successful for continuous techniques such as haemo-filtration and is highly dependent on the individual patient's endogenous coagulant status.

There are a number of tests used to assess anti-coagulation during renal replacement therapy:

1. *Activated clotting time* (ACT). Blood is added to a tube containing siliceous earth which accelerates the clotting process. A machine (e.g. Haemochron) is then used to automatically tilt/rotate the tube and to detect clot formation. During HD, ACT is normally maintained at 200–250 s (baseline = 120–150 s). During haemofiltration the ACT would normally be maintained at approximately 150–220 s (same baseline as above).

2. *Whole blood partial thromboplastin time* (WBPTT) The clotting process is accelerated by the addition of 0.2 ml of actin FS reagent (Thrombofax) to 0.4 ml of blood. This is set in a heating block at 37°C for 30 s and then tilted every 5 s until a clot forms. During HD the WBPTT would be maintained at the baseline value +40–80%, approximately 120–140 s. During haemofiltration, a baseline value +50% would be maintained.

3. *Lee–White clotting time*. In this method, 0.4 ml of blood is added to a glass tube which is inverted every 30 s at room temperature until a clot forms. A baseline would be 4–8 min with a desired value of 20–30 min. This is the least accurate or desirable method of assessing anticoagulation status.

4. *Activated partial thromboplastin time* (APTT). A test used to measure the time taken in seconds for a fibrin clot to form in a plasma sample after an optimal amount of calcium chloride, a partial thromboplastin reagent (phospholipid), and a contact factor activating agent have been added to the sample. The APTT should be checked 4–6 hours after starting a heparin infusion. Aim for 1.5–2.5 times the control.

Types of anticoagulant

Heparin is the most frequently used anticoagulant. However, it is a difficult agent to titrate, particularly because its effects vary so dramatically between individuals. The half-life of heparin can range from 45 s to 4.5 hours for no predictable reason.

The most common type of heparin used is mixed molecular weight unfractionated heparin which is not cleared across artificial membranes fully due to its high negative charge and protein binding. There has been increased interest in low molecular weight heparin which, in theory, presents fewer haemorrhagic risks to the patient. However, use of low molecular weight heparin is considerably harder to monitor, requiring an anti-Factor Xa assay which, in most hospitals, is not performed as an urgent/emergency procedure. As a consequence, it is rarely used.

The dose of heparin required during haemofiltration is less than in HD. Commonly, doses of 5–10 IU/kg/hour are infused proximal to the filter. If the patient has adverse reactions to heparin (e.g. thrombocytopenia) or is at risk from bleeding (e.g. post-surgery), epoprostenol (PGI$_2$) or alprostadil (PGE$_1$) can be infused instead at 2.5–10 ng/kg/min. These prostaglandins act by inhibiting platelet aggregation (see Chapter 14). This allows the rate of heparin infusion to be decreased to $\leq$250 IU/hour or stopped completely. If the patient develops heparin-induced thrombocytopenia syndrome (HITS) *all* heparin must be stopped, including that in flush lines. Low molecular weight heparin may be used as an alternative but this does not completely remove the risk of HITS. Heparin-bonded circuits are being developed but are currently very expensive.

There has been increasing interest in the use of citrate regional anticoagulation. Citrate acts by chelating ionized calcium in the extracorporeal circuit (Monchi *et al.* 2004). If the citrate is added proximal to the filter, the ionized calcium binds to the citrate and thus plasma levels fall sufficiently to prevent clotting as calcium is a necessary co-factor for this to occur. Citrate also has the advantage of being metabolized by the liver to bicarbonate. However, the patient may require calcium replacements infused directly in order to counteract the effects of hypocalcaemia. Monitoring of APTT, ionized calcium level, pH, and sodium levels is necessary.

Direct thrombin inhibitors include hirudin and a newer substance, argatroban. These have yet to be fully evaluated (Davenport and Mehta 2002). The major problem with this group of drugs is the lack of agents that can reverse their action, the duration of which is further prolonged in renal failure (up to several days). These is thus the risk of prolonged bleeding.

Haemofiltration

Principles

Haemofiltration is a convective process in which there is mass movement of plasma water and solutes across a highly permeable membrane. The blood on one side of the membrane exerts a hydrostatic pressure (from the presence of a pump in the circuit or the patient's arterial pressure). This pressure allows plasma water and solutes to move across the membrane by hydrostatic ultrafiltration to become the 'filtrate'. The constant draining of the filtrate compartment ensures a negative pressure on the other side of the membrane, thus maintaining a pressure gradient. Much of the protein as well as cellular constituents of blood are prohibited from moving across the membrane due to their molecular size.

The process is not selective and the removal of waste products can only be achieved by the removal of an accompanying load of water and other solutes. The volume of filtrate removed can be over 2 l/hour; to maintain cardiovascular stability, fluid must be replaced concurrently up to the desired fluid balance. The fluid used as replacement should be isotonic and should also aim to replace the solutes lost as filtrate that would otherwise be selectively reabsorbed by the normal kidney (Table 9.14).

Dose-dependent haemofiltration

Currently 1–2 litre exchanges are performed in clinical practice. Some experts recommend that in critically ill patients ultrafiltration rates should be prescribed according to body weight of up to 35 ml/kg/hour which may be associated with lowered mortality rates (Ronco *et al.* 2000).

The amount of filtrate removed in most newer haemofiltration machines can be controlled through a volumetric pump distal to the artificial kidney.

Advantages of dose-dependent haemofiltration

♦ Haemofiltration allows continuous control of uraemia and fluid balance which promotes cardiovascular stability.

TABLE 9.14 Typical constituents of haemofiltration replacement fluid

Description	Standard solution	Low-lactate solution	Bicarbonate for severe acidosis
Fluid volume (litres)	5	5	5
Sodium (mmol/l)	142	140	110.5
Potassium (mmol/l)	0	0	0
Calcium (mmol/l)	2	1.75	1.84
Magnesium (mmol/l)	0.75	0.75	0.53
Chloride (mmol/l)	103	115	115.3
Lactate (mmol/l)	44.5	30	3.16
Glucose (g/l)	0	1.1	0

- It does not require the utilization of specialist renal staff or equipment/water supplies.

- It can be performed in the critical care unit, negating the need to transfer critically ill patients to renal centres.

Disadvantages of dose-dependent haemofiltration

- The efficiency is low—a haemofiltration removal rate of 1 l/hour equates to a creatinine clearance of 16 ml/min. However, for most patients this is adequate unless they are highly catabolic (Wendon *et al.* 1989).

- In view of its low efficiency, haemofiltration is a continuous process and thus restricts the patient's mobility and necessitates constant patient-centred activity which can disrupt rest and sleep patterns.

- Anticoagulation has to be continuous, albeit at a relatively lower dose.

- Removal and consequent administration of large volumes of fluid is nurse-intensive and open to potential error.

Types of haemofiltration

Haemofiltration can be spontaneous, where blood flow through the extracorporeal circuit depends on the patient's arterial pressure, or it can be assisted with the inclusion of a blood pump in the circuit. Most critical care units use commercial haemofiltration machines for venovenous haemofiltration (or haemodiafiltration) as this ensures an automated and safe system. However, it is vital that any nurse responsible for haemofiltration is able to understand the principles on which the automated system is based. If not, then inadvertent errors may be made and trouble-shooting of problems will be limited.

Continuous arteriovenous haemofiltration

Continuous arteriovenous haemofiltration (CAVH) usually refers to a spontaneous method where arterial access and venous return is used. However, CAVH can also refer to a pumped method where, for whatever reason, separate arterial and venous cannulation (or an arteriovenous shunt) is utilized. CAVH is much less frequently used now, as the lack of pressure alarms in the circuit and the limitations associated with dependence on arterial pressure make the technique both inefficient and unsafe.

Continuous venovenous haemofiltration

Continuous venovenous haemofiltration (CVVH) refers to a pumped method which uses either a double-lumen cannula sited in a large vein or two separate venous cannulae for blood access and return. Once a blood pump has been included in the extracorporeal circuit,

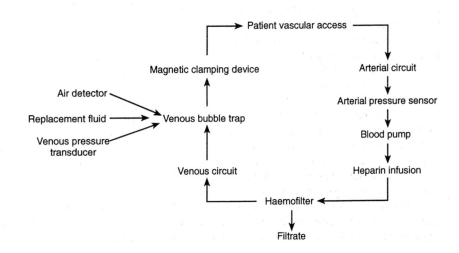

Fig. 9.9 Continuous venovenous haemofiltration (see text).

the alarm and monitoring devices common to dialysis machines must also be incorporated (see Fig. 9.9). CAVH is a relatively simple and inexpensive process but is totally dependent on the patient's systolic blood pressure to maintain an adequate blood flow and, therefore, an adequate filtration rate. In these patients, CVVH is preferred because far higher filtration rates can be maintained with the use of a blood pump. Whether CAVH or CVVH are used, the inadequacies, increased workload, and potential dangers of concurrent removal and replacement of fluid and solutes remain.

Continuous venovenous haemodiafiltration (CVVHD)

CVVHD requires a dialysate solution run through the artificial kidney, in a counter-current direction to the blood and on the opposite side of the membrane. Filtration still occurs because a pressure gradient still exists (albeit to a lesser degree) but, in addition, diffusion can be utilized to facilitate the removal of solutes. This decreases the need to remove such vast volumes of fluid in order to achieve the same result.

The dialysate used is commonly the same as the replacement fluid or, occasionally, peritoneal dialysis fluid. The main disadvantage of using peritoneal dialysis fluid is that glucose can diffuse into the blood causing hyperglycaemia and it is not generally recommended. The flow rate of the dialysate can be up to 2 l/hour, depending on the clearance of solutes desired.

High volume haemofiltration

Ronco and Bellomo (2000) advocate the benefits of increasing ultrafiltration rates during continuous haemofiltration therapy. This involves increasing the ultrafiltration rate from 1–2 l/hour to 3–4 l/hour. Alternatively, it can also be performed by maintaining the usual ultrafiltration rate over night but increasing rates to as much as 6 l/hour for limited periods during the day. These higher filtration rates have been associated with improved removal of inflammatory mediators in the septic patient (Ronco and Bellomo 2000). This practice is not widespread as not all critically ill patients can sustain the higher clearance rates and it is time-consuming, labour-intensive, and expensive.

Assisted haemo(dia)filtration techniques

A number of commercially available machines are available from different manufacturers for haemofiltration, their modes of operation differ but they are all based on the same principles. The machines provide a safe and accurate method of renal support, but must be set up and used by adequately trained personnel as the risk of user errors and patient complications are high.

EXAMPLE 1 CALCULATING REPLACEMENT VALUES

Intake:

Enteral feed: 120 ml

Omnopon: 5 ml

Insulin: 2 ml

Total: 127 ml

Output:

Wound drain: 50 m

Filtrate: 1500 ml

Total: 1550 ml

The time cycles are hourly and the patient is prescribed to have a neutral balance at the end of each cycle. To achieve this, 1423 ml of replacement fluid should be given over the same time cycle (1550–127 ml).

EXAMPLE 2

Intake:

Parenteral feed: 100 ml

Adrenaline: 5 ml

Fentany: 15 ml

Insulin: 3 ml

Total: 113 ml

Output:

Nasogastric tube: 50 ml

Filtrate: 1800 ml

Total: 1850 ml

The time cycle is hourly and the patient is prescribed to have a balance of –100 ml at the end of each cycle. The amount of replacement fluid to be given is:

1850 – 113 = 1737 ml (to achieve neutral balance)

1737 – 100 = 1637 ml (to achieve a negative balance of 100 ml/hour).

Fluid balance

Some haemofiltration machines operate on specific time cycles over a number of hours, others operate on an hourly basis. Whichever time unit is used, the patient's intake (nutrition, drugs, and infusions) must be balanced against any losses, including the filtrate. A target fluid balance (either positive or negative) is determined on the basis of clinical assessment of intravascular and total body fluid volume status. Most machines incorporate pumps for replacement fluid and dialysate fluid, as well as the blood pump and filtrate pump. Spontaneous methods would utilize a separate volumetric pump.

Fluid balance recordings must be documented clearly to avoid confusion and checked carefully to avoid accidental hypo- or hypervolaemia. If a form of haemodiafiltration is used, the volume of dialysate infused must be subtracted from the total filtrate volume to obtain the actual filtrate volume.

Haemodynamic monitoring

Continuous ECG and blood pressure monitoring are essential, primarily to detect signs of hypovolaemia (i.e. tachycardia and hypotension). If significant hypovolaemia occurs, an increase in the core–peripheral temperature gap and decreased cardiac filling pressures (e.g. central venous pressure, pulmonary artery wedge pressure) would also be observed.

Relative hypovolaemia can be observed when instigating haemofiltration as the patient has to become accustomed to an additional circulation (the extracorporeal circuit). Prior to use, the haemofiltration circuits have to be primed (usually with heparinized saline) to remove air, to coat the circuit with heparin, and to flush the artificial kidney. There are two options when commencing the procedure. One is to attach the patient to both ends of the circuit which results in the patient receiving the prime solution remaining in the circuits (approximately 80 to 200 ml). This may not be desirable if the patient is severely overloaded. The second option is initially to attach the arterial end of the circuit only, allowing the patient's blood to move into the circuit and expelling any prime solution before attaching the venous circuit. This method can lead to relative hypovolaemia due to the patient losing blood into the circuit without receiving any back until the prime has been lost and the venous limb attached. If this method is used a colloid solution must be immediately available to be infused if hypovolaemia becomes apparent.

When the technique is established, hypovolaemia may occur if the patient's fluid requirements change. Critically ill patients experience fluid shifts and periods of vasoconstriction and vasodilatation, all serving to alter fluid status. The original fluid balance aims may not now be tolerated by the patient and should be reassessed. It should be borne in mind that any signs of hypo- or hypervolaemia could be caused by inaccurate fluid balance

recordings and calculations should always be checked to guard against this.

Pre-filter or post-filter attachment of replacement fluid.

Replacement fluids can be administered prior to or after the filter during continuous renal replacement therapy. However, pre-filter administration is said to affect solute clearance as it will dilute the amount of blood (and therefore solutes) passing through the kidney at the set blood flow per minute. The advantages are that pre-filter fluid administration may prolong filter life, reduce anticoagulation requirements, and may be considered in patients with frequent filter clotting. (Schetz 2002).

Arrhythmias can occur, as with haemodialysis, due to hypo/hyperkalaemia or hypovolaemia. Serum potassium values should be checked at least 4-hourly, especially with haemofiltration alone. If employing haemodiafiltration, electrolyte balance is less likely to present a problem as serum levels can equilibrate with the dialysate fluid. Therefore, if the dialysate fluid contains 4.5 mmol/l of potassium and the serum potassium falls below that value, potassium will diffuse across the artificial membranes into the blood until the serum potassium has reached 4.5 mmol/l. If the patient's potassium should rise above 4.5 mmol/l the reverse would happen. The same principle applies to all serum constituents which can diffuse across the artificial membranes. Notably, sodium losses during haemofiltration can exceed sodium intake and additional sodium may have to be infused. In haemodiafiltration, the sodium levels can be maintained by diffusion from the dialysate.

The patient's central temperature should be monitored and maintained at >36°C. The effect of circulating blood outside the body where it rapidly cools will reduce the patient's body temperature, as can the infusion of large volumes of replacement fluid. Replacement fluid should be warmed (i.e. via a blood-warming device) prior to infusion. If required to maintain temperature, the dialysate fluid can also be warmed prior to use. Some machines incorporate a blood-warming device. Conversely, in the pyrexial patient, infusion of unwarmed replacement fluid can be used with therapeutic benefit. It is important to remain aware that an underlying pyrexia may be masked by the cooling effect of continuous haemofiltration and haemodiafiltration.

Nursing interventions
Rest and sleep

One significant disadvantage of continuous haemofiltration and haemodiafiltration is that the nurse's attention is focused around the patient continuously, night and day. This is unavoidable, but steps should be taken to allow the patient adequate periods of rest and sleep. If desired, the technique can be stopped during the night but this has to be weighed against the cost and nursing time implications of changing circuitry every 24 hours.

Psychological care

The sight of seemingly large volumes of blood in an extracorporeal circuit is often taken for granted by the critical care staff but can be frightening for both patient and relatives. This should be anticipated and the necessary steps taken to reduce any anxiety. The possibility of haemofiltration as a treatment should be introduced to the patient and relatives prior to its commencement. If there has not been any previous discussion, the 'sudden' appearance of yet another piece of machinery can be viewed by the relatives as treatment which was not anticipated and as an 'emergency' (i.e. introduced as a result of a sudden deterioration in condition). It must be emphasized that giving the patient and relatives prior warning not only maintains their confidence in the critical care staff but also helps to minimize anxiety.

Changing the circuit

There are no specific guidelines regarding the frequency of changing circuits. Circuit or filter changes should be governed by manufacturer's advice and local hospital infection control policy (Clark *et al.* 2002) or if there is:

1. a significant reduction in performance;

2. known or suspected bacteraemia;

3. evidence of a large clot in the filter or bubble trap which traps and consumes platelets and may provide a medium for bacterial growth.

Ideally, the decision to change the circuit should be made while it is still possible to return the volume of blood within the circuit back to the patient. This is done by disconnecting the arterial circuit from the patient and attaching it to a bag of normal saline (0.9% sodium chloride). The saline is then allowed to run through the circuit pushing the blood back into the patient via the venous circuit which remains attached. If the circuit has been changed because of clotting, the reason for clotting must be investigated prior to the connection of a new circuit. If inadequate anticoagulation was the cause (as detected by coagulation tests), the rate of heparin infusion should be increased, perhaps accompanied by more frequent coagulation tests. Clotting in the venous bubble trap and artificial kidney may be detected by pressure increases in the venous pressure monitor (Table 9.15).

A pumped method of renal support is usually preferable to gain a more constant blood flow and therefore an improved control of uraemia. Spontaneous methods can be severely hampered in hypotensive patients, even if the pressure gradient across the semi-permeable membranes in the artificial kidney has been enhanced by lowering the level of the filtrate collecting vessel or applying suction to the filtrate collection point. In pumped methods, the blood flow must be maintained at greater than 100 ml/min to avoid clotting in the artificial kidney. While the speed of blood flowing through the circuit is important, so is the consistency of that speed. If, for example, the vascular access is a femoral vein cannula and the patient is bending his/her legs, the flow of blood from the femoral vein will be intermittent and this can precipitate clotting in the artificial

TABLE 9.15 Problems associated with haemofiltration

Problem	Cause	Action
Filtrate volumes in excess of ability to concurrently replace fluid	Can be experienced with new circuits, usually settles down after 3–4 hours	The filtrate outflow line can be partially clamped. Blood flow rate can be reduced but should be maintained above 100 ml/min
Filtrate volumes decreasing	Inadequate blood flow (slow blood pump speed, obstructed access)	In pumped methods: (a) check blood pump speed (>100 ml/min), (b) check vascular access
	Clotting in the artificial kidney	Clotting: see below
Clotting of the circuit	Low blood flow, intermittent blood flow (from poor access), cool blood, inadequate anticoagulation, inadequate priming technique, low blood antithrombin III level	It is possible to continue with some clot present provided: (a) sufficient volumes are produced for control of uraemia, (b) clots are not encouraging further clinically significant platelet adherence (as detected by a continuing low serum platelet count and spontaneous bleeding from line sites), (c) that the patient is not bacteraemic (clots in the kidney would provide a good medium for bacteria). If indicated, the circuit should be changed

kidney. The arterial pressure monitor will detect significant decreases in blood flow from the vascular access. If the flow is severely obstructed, air can be seen being sucked into the arterial circuit by the blood pump. If the circuits are being changed frequently and vascular access is thought to be the problem, it is sensible to review the site of access. Often, when moving the patient, blood flow can be interrupted because of cannula movement. The effects of this can be reduced by slowing the blood pump speed for the duration of the

Anticoagulation in Haemofiltration

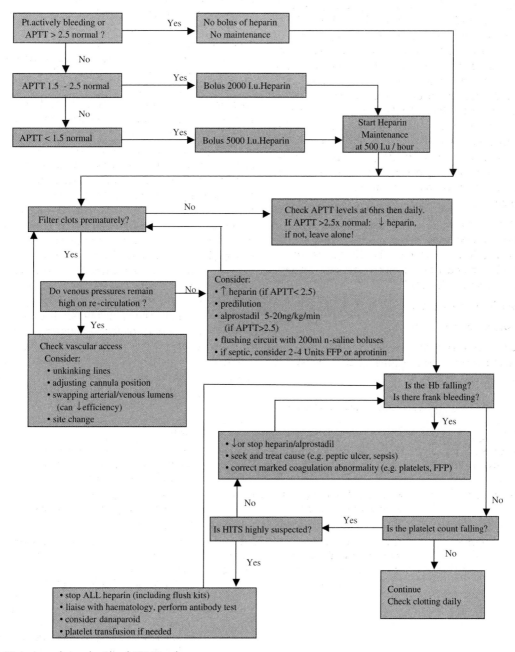

Fig. 9.10 Anticoagulation algorithm (UCLH Trust).

move on the pretext that a constant blood flow, although at a slower speed, is preferable to no blood flow.

If clotting occurs soon after connecting the patient with no other obvious problem or alarm status, it is likely that the priming technique has been inadequate. One of the most important functions of priming is to flush the artificial kidney of any sterilizing and stabilizing materials and to open up the pores in the semipermeable membranes. If this has not been achieved, at best there will be poor diffusive function of the membrane and, at worst, it will clot prematurely. Additionally, if clotting is a continual problem, it may be that the patient has a low plasma level of antithrombin III; this will disrupt the pathway through which heparin works. Options in this case include giving antithrombin III (which is expensive) or fresh frozen plasma which will replace a certain amount of antithrombin III. A less effective alternative is to use prostacyclin to anticoagulate. Failure to establish the cause of repeated clotting of the artificial kidney and circuits can be expensive, time-consuming, and, most importantly, allows only intermittent control of uraemia. Many units now use protocols to guide the management of anticoagulation during renal replacement therapy (Fig. 9.10).

Monitoring of anticoagulation

If unfractionated heparin is being administered, coagulation screens (systemic APTT or ACT) should be taken post-filter (Davenport and Mehta 2002).

Safety

The importance of constant nursing attendance cannot be overemphasized. While the machines, cannulae, and circuits are now purpose-built, the consequences of disconnection somewhere in the extracorporeal circuit can be dire. The spontaneous methods of haemofiltration, although simple, do not incorporate any alarm systems and extra vigilance is called for. Undetected disconnection can lead to exsanguination and/or air embolism. If air has been entrained, the patient should be placed in a head down position and, if possible, on the left side. The rationale for this positioning is that air will always move to the top of any fluid medium and the priority is to prevent air entering the pulmonary circulation.

The vascular access should be in easy view and inspected regularly. The circuits should be supported to avoid undue tension being placed on the cannula(e). Arteriovenous shunts should be kept warm and unkinked to guard against clotting of the shunt; periods of hypotension will also promote clotting in the shunt. The circuits and the haemofiltration machine should be positioned to avoid being an obstacle to other necessary pieces of equipment, especially emergency items. The need to reach something quickly could result in the inadvertent removal of circuits and cannulae.

Infection

Critically ill patients who have acute renal failure are immunocompromised to a greater or lesser degree. Extra caution must be exercised when priming circuits and replacing bags of replacement fluid or dialysate fluid. Strict asepsis must be adhered to when inserting and re-dressing lines. There is evidence to suggest that the skin is the most common source of microorganisms in catheter-associated bacteraemias. The vascular access must be sutured into position and, to avoid undue movement, be dressed with an adherent material. A suitable dressing should be transparent for ease of viewing. If a local site infection is suspected, a swab should be taken for microbiological analysis and the catheter removed and replaced at a different site in an aseptic manner. If a septic focus is suspected, blood cultures should be sent with the catheter tip to the microbiology department.

Drug removal

In addition to waste products and other solutes, therapeutic drugs can also be removed by the artificial kidney. There are considerable data referring to drug removal during haemodialysis but less so with haemofiltration. During renal replacement therapy the dose of drug administered should be on the assumption that the GFR is 10–50 ml/min and 10 ml/min for a patient who has not been commenced on renal replacement therapy (Blakeley and Smith 2003). This is less of a problem in haemodialysis as, unless absolutely necessary, the giving of drugs can be avoided during the 3–4 hour dialysis session. In haemofiltration, unfortunately, this is not the case. It is known that protein-bound drugs are far less likely to be removed by the artificial kidney in view of the size of the drug–protein complex. It is important to remember this when titrating vasoactive drugs, sedatives, muscle relaxants, or analgesics when the patient's requirements may seem unusually high. Plasma levels of aminoglycoside antibiotics (e.g. gentamicin), and other drugs which can be monitored (e.g. digoxin and aminophylline) should be regularly checked to ensure therapeutic levels.

Intermittent haemodialysis (IHD)

Principle

Blood is pumped into an extracorporeal circuit where it is anticoagulated prior to passage through an artificial kidney or dialyser. This contains multiple hollow fibres or sheets which form the semi-permeable membranes.

Within the artificial kidney a dialysate fluid is pumped on the opposite side of the semi-permeable membrane to the blood and in a counter-current direction. Waste products move from the blood, across the membrane, into the dialysate by diffusion.

Blood flows of up to 600 ml/min can be achieved during haemodialysis. While the clearance of small molecules depends on the concentration gradient across the membrane, their clearance can also be improved by increasing the counter-current dialysate flow rate, which is commonly set at up to 500 ml/min. Water is removed by ultrafiltration and this can be achieved by the exertion of a pressure across the semipermeable membrane (the so-called 'transmembrane pressure', TMP). The TMP can be exerted in two ways: first, by the partial occlusion of the dialysate inflow line with the dialysate pump on the outflow line; and secondly, by generating a positive pressure in the blood compartment.

The dialysate is usually supplied in concentrated form and needs to be diluted with water. Proportionators mix the correct volume of water with the correct amount of dialysate concentrate and are either incorporated within each dialysis machine or are situated centrally in a unit and then pumped to individual machines.

Vast quantities of water, in the range of 120 litres per session, are required and it must be sterile and specially treated, either by reverse osmosis or ion exchange resins. There are systems available which allow the spent dialysate to be recycled by passing it through a sorbent cartridge. This method utilizes 6 litres as opposed to 120 litres of water per session. It is, however, a relatively expensive option.

Advantages of haemodialysis

◆ The most effective method of clearing waste products.

◆ Uses an intermittent technique, and only requires anticoagulation during the procedure.

◆ The patient can be mobile between dialysis sessions.

TYPICAL DIALYSATE COMPOSITION

◆ Sodium: 140 mmol/l

◆ Potassium: varying concentrations

◆ Calcium: 1.6 mmol/l

◆ Magnesium: 0.75 mmol/l

◆ Chloride: 100 mmol/l

◆ Acetate: 35 mmol/l

◆ Dextrose: varying concentrations

◆ The intermittent nature incurs lower demands on nursing time.

◆ The closed-circuit system ensures less risk to staff from hepatitis B or C, or HIV infection (though these are becoming more common with continuous systems).

Disadvantages of haemodialysis

◆ Nursing staff need to be specifically trained in the technique.

◆ During a 2–4-hour period of HD, enough fluid has to be removed to allow nutrition and other infusions to be given throughout the following 24–72 hours between dialyses.

◆ The patient may require a negative fluid balance at the end of dialysis, necessitating rapid and significant fluid shifts leading to potential haemodynamic instability in the critically ill patient.

◆ Haemodialysis provides only episodic control of uraemia.

◆ Hypoxaemia, hypotension, and complement activation are associated with cheaper types of membrane and buffer solutions, all of which are undesirable in the critically ill patient.

◆ The equipment and water supply required can be expensive.

Nursing interventions

Many nursing interventions are focused on the detection and early treatment of complications. The dialysis machine incorporates numerous monitoring and alarm systems which must be observed, recorded, and acted on accordingly.

Complications

In addition to responding to the monitoring and alarms facilities provided by the dialysis machine, the patient must also be observed for the development of potential complications.

Hypotension

Hypotension in the patient receiving haemodialysis can be related to a variety of causes. It is commonly caused by hypovolaemia from the rapid and excessive removal of fluid. The use of acetate as the buffer is also known to precipitate vasodilatation and hypotension. The critically ill patient receiving haemodialysis should have continuous blood pressure monitoring by either invasive or non-invasive methods to allow early detection of hypotension.

Cardiac arrhythmias

Arrhythmias, commonly due to hyper- or hypokalaemia or to hypovolaemia can occur during dialysis. Tachycardias may occur as compensatory mechanisms in the event of hypovolaemia and hypotension. The patient should have continuous ECG monitoring.

Hypoxaemia

In is known that certain dialyser membranes can cause hypoxaemia, in particular the cuprophane membrane. The causes are thought to be cytokine activation, oxygen removal, and shunting. Continuous pulse oximetry, supported by arterial blood gas monitoring, if indicated, should be performed during dialysis.

Muscle cramps, nausea, and vomiting

The aetiology of cramps, nausea, and vomiting is largely unknown yet they are experienced by many patients receiving haemodialysis. The critically ill patient, who may be sedated, could present with signs of restlessness, agitation, and tachycardia. The possibility of cramps or nausea should be considered. Common predisposing factors to cramps are hypotension, dehydration, and a low plasma sodium. Hypotension itself is a potent cause of nausea.

Disequilibrium syndrome

This is a rare yet serious potential complication of haemodialysis. It is thought to be caused by the rapid removal of urea and 'uraemic toxins' during dialysis which results in a much decreased concentration of these substances in the plasma when compared with the cerebrospinal fluid (CSF). The osmotic gradient now existing between plasma and CSF allows water to move into the CSF and the brain tissue. The patient can present with headache, vomiting, restlessness, convulsions, and even coma. The severely uraemic patient should not experience a reduction in plasma urea of greater than 30% in the first instance to avoid this complication.

Acute haemolysis

This can be caused by overheated, hypotonic, or contaminated dialysate fluid. The patient may complain of back pain, tightness in the chest, and dyspnoea. Blood in the venous circuit may take on a 'port wine' appearance in colour. If haemolysis is not detected early, hyperkalaemia can result from the release of potassium from the haemolysed red cells.

Plasma estimations of sodium, potassium, urea, and creatinine should be taken before and after dialysis, in addition to a coagulation screen. If possible, the patient should be weighed (perhaps on a 'weigh bed') before and after each session to estimate fluid status.

Peritoneal dialysis (PD)

Principles

Waste products from the body diffuse across the peritoneum (the semi-permeable membrane) into a dialysate fluid. Flow rates of 70–100 ml/min can be achieved across the peritoneum. Fluid is removed by osmotic ultrafiltration, the osmotic pull provided by varying concentrations of glucose in the dialysate. The higher the concentration of glucose, the stronger the osmotic pull and the more fluid is removed. Blood electrolytes can be manipulated by alteration of the electrolyte levels in the dialysate; diffusion again being the mode of transport. This form of dialysis may be used in children and in long-term patients with diabetes, but it is not as efficient at dialysis at removing large molecular weight molecules (Currie and O'Brien 2001)

A catheter, commonly a Tenckhoff catheter, is placed into the peritoneal cavity. This is a sterile procedure, performed using local anaesthetic. The catheter is positioned either in the midline, approximately 3 cm below the umbilicus, or to either side of the abdomen, usually lateral to the border of the rectus muscle. Prior to insertion, the bladder should be emptied and an examination performed to exclude any organ enlargement in order to prevent accidental perforation.

Dialysate fluid is infused via the catheter into the peritoneum. Diffusion of waste products and ultrafiltration of water occurs across the peritoneal membrane, into the dialysate which is then drained out via the catheter. The degree of diffusion and ultrafiltration can be controlled by altering the time that the dialysate remain in the peritoneal space, the so-called 'dwell time'. For the purposes of acute PD a typical pattern of treatment would be hourly cycles, 10 min for the dialysate to run in, 30 min dwell time, and 20 min for the dialysate to run out. The more rapidly these cycles are repeated, the more diffusion is enhanced. The volume of fluid infused depends upon the size of the peritoneal cavity and how much can be tolerated by the patient. One litre is frequently used and tolerated. There are three concentrations of glucose generally available—1.36%, 2.27%, and 3.86%—the latter achieving the greatest osmotic pull and so the greatest water removal. Automatic cycling machines are available which save considerable nursing time.

Advantages of peritoneal dialysis

◆ It is relatively simple and inexpensive and can be performed by relatively unskilled nurses.

Disadvantages of peritoneal dialysis

◆ It has questionable control of uraemia, especially in the catabolic patient, and is contraindicated in the

CONCENTRATION OF PERITONEAL DIALYSIS FLUID AVAILABLE

The dialysate solution usually contains glucose as the osmotic gradient

- 1.36% per cent, weak
- 2.27% per cent, medium
- 3.86% per cent, strong.

Also contained in the solutions are sodium, potassium, calcium. and lactate.

Currie and O'Brien (2001)

presence of abdominal trauma, abdominal sepsis, or post-abdominal surgery.

- It carries a risk of peritonitis.
- The presence of dialysate fluid in the peritoneum can cause abdominal distention and restrict diaphragmatic movement.
- Protein can be lost across the peritoneum, which may be difficult to replace.

Nursing interventions

The peritoneal dialysate fluid must be warmed prior to infusion to prevent hypothermia. Blood glucose levels must be checked regularly as these can rise due to the diffusion of glucose from the dialysate into the body. If concentrated dialysate fluids are used, the blood sugar levels must be checked more frequently. Potassium (2–4 mmol/l) is often added to the dialysate to regulate body potassium. One of the most common operational problems with PD is that of dialysate outflow failure.

TABLE 9.16 Outflow problems in peritoneal dialysis

Cause	Action
Kinking of the catheter	Re-establish good catheter position and secure place
Decreased bowel motility	Use of laxatives, suppositories, enemas, and diet
Obstruction by fibrin plugs or strands	Add heparin to the dialysate 200–500 IU/litre
Obstruction by fibrin not responsive to heparin	Infuse streptokinase into the catheter (750 000 IU diluted in 30–100 ml normal saline). Clamp the catheter for 2 hours then reassess drainage
Peritonitis	Add appropriate antibiotics to dialysate

The dialysate fluid removed should at least equal, if not exceed, the volume infused; failing this, steps should be taken to rectify the situation (Table 9.16).

Strict asepsis must be adhered to when changing the dialysate bags or when disconnecting the circuit for any reason. Care must be taken to avoid infection of the catheter site. This can be achieved by preventing undue movement of the catheter by stabilization and by using aseptic technique when cleaning the site and changing the dressing. The patient should be observed for signs of abdominal pain which can indicate either peritonitis or over-distension from too great a dialysate volume per cycle. If the patient is self-ventilating, care must be taken to position the patient such that the presence of dialysate fluid in the abdomen does not restrict diaphragmatic movement. The respiratory rate should be checked at regular intervals.

Haemofiltration, haemodiafiltration, and haemodialysis, are the most common forms of renal replacement therapy in the critical care area today. There are some other techniques which are combinations of haemodialysis and haemofiltration (e.g. continuous ultrafiltration with periods of dialysis, CUPID). A purpose-built machine and circuits are used. Fluid removal is performed gently over the 24-hour period then, using the same set-up, dialysis can be performed periodically. The principles of management are as for dialysis and haemofiltration (Milne 1986).

Disorders associated with acute renal failure

Rhabdomyolysis

The association between acute renal failure and skeletal muscle damage was first described by Bywaters and Beal in 1941 (see Better 1990). It is a condition which combines pre-renal, nephrotoxic, and obstructive causes of acute renal failure.

The damaged muscle can release substances with significant clinical consequences (see box). The released phosphate chelates with calcium and this can cause hypocalcaemia. Hyponatraemia and hypovolaemia can also accompany this condition due to increased leakage of salt and water.

Management of rhabdomyolysis

The principal aims in management are:

1. prevention of acute renal failure;

2. correction of electrolyte imbalances; and

3. prevention of further muscle necrosis.

THE CAUSES OF RHABDOMYOLYSIS

- Direct trauma, crush injury, burns
- Muscle compression from prolonged immobility (surgery, coma)
- Metabolic illness (diabetic metabolic decompensation)
- Hypokalaemia, hypophosphataemia
- Myxoedema
- Myositis
- Temperature extremes
- Toxins—alcohol, solvents, carbon monoxide, drug abuse (e.g. heroin, ecstasy)
- Muscular dystrophies
- Excessive muscle activity (e.g. prolonged seizures)

SUBSTANCES RELEASED BY MUSCLE

- Potassium → hyperkalaemia
- Hydrogen ions → acidosis
- Phosphate → hyperphosphataemia
- Creatine → high creatine kinase level
- Myoglobin → myoglobinuria

Myoglobin (an iron-containing pigment found in skeletal muscle) has nephrotoxic effects, especially in the presence of volume depletion and acidosis. Early and aggressive volume replacement combined with alkalinization of the urine (pH > 7) should be implemented as soon as possible. Alkalinization aids renal excretion of myoglobin and protects the kidney against oxidant damage. Myoglobin can also obstruct the renal tubules and, in addition to the maintenance of a good circulating volume, mannitol and/or furosemide can be used to ensure a high urine throughput. Care should be taken to maintain patency of the urinary catheter, especially if the urine contains large amounts of myoglobin. The associated hyperkalaemia is often resistant to dextrose and insulin therapy; it may be the overriding initial indication for renal replacement therapy (haemodiafiltration). These patients are also known to be highly catabolic and nutrition must be introduced at an early stage.

Special attention must be paid to any area of musculoskeletal damage. The patient may present with compartment syndrome in which a muscle compartment has been compressed resulting in a restricted neurovascular supply to the extremity distal to the injury and muscle necrosis. Urgent fasciotomy is indicated if compartment syndrome is present otherwise massive muscle and nerve damage may ensue. Compartment pressures can be monitored using a needle connected by tubing to a manometer; fasciotomy should be contemplated if pressures exceed 20–25 mmHg. Any extremities which are affected should also be observed frequently for the presence of pulses and impaired circulation (e.g. pallor, temperature difference) as well as swelling and pain. Fasciotomy should be urgently performed if any of these are noted.

Hepatorenal syndrome

Hepatorenal syndrome (HRS) is a recognized syndrome in which renal failure accompanies liver failure, especially cirrhosis. The pathogenesis is not fully understood; however, the kidneys on examination appear normal and the resulting renal dysfunction appears to be in part due to decreased blood flow because of vasoconstriction of the renal cortical vessels. Patients with acute liver failure as a result of hepatitis or paracetamol poisoning are also known to develop HRS.

HRS is characterized by the presence of a low urinary sodium (<10 mmol/l) and increased urinary osmolality in the absence of proteinuria. Sodium and water conservation are intact, unlike acute renal failure with coexisting liver disease where urinary sodium is >20 mmol/1. The management of this condition includes renal replacement therapy, appropriate strategies for treatment of the liver failure, and control of ascites (see Chapter 11). Small case series suggest that N-acetylcysteine and/or vasopressin (or analogues such as terlipressin) may also offer some outcome benefit for this high-mortality condition.

Glomerulonephritis

The term 'glomerulonephritis' encompasses a large number of renal disorders. Patients can present with varying clinical features that can often be difficult to relate to histological findings. Circulating immune complexes that trigger inflammatory and complement reactions cause over 95% of cases of glomerulonephritis. In less than 5% of cases an inflammatory response set up by circulating immunoglobulins is thought to cause the condition. Some specific forms of glomerulonephritis may be encountered in the critical care setting and these are described below.

Goodpasture's syndrome

This is an autoimmune disease seen more frequently in young men. It is often accompanied by haemoptysis, anaemia, proteinuria, and renal failure. Bilateral lung opacities are seen on chest X-ray and the pulmonary involvement can necessitate intubation and ventilation. Steroids and plasmapheresis are the mainstays of treatment. It is diagnosed by a positive titre of anti-glomerular basement membrane antibody in the blood.

Vasculitis

Vasculitis is often seen in polyarteritis nodosa, which may present with variable features including asthma, fever, skin rashes, hypertension, neuropathy, and abdominal pain. Renal failure can develop rapidly with haematuria, proteinuria, and nephrotic syndrome. Treatment is with steroids, cyclophosphamide, and plasmapheresis. Diagnosis is by histology or a raised P-ANCA test. (P-ANCA is the P form of antineutrophil cytoplasmic antibody).

Vasculitis can also accompany Wegener's granulomatosis, a disease affecting the respiratory tract and kidney with vasculitic lesions. Again, steroids, cyclophosphamide and plasmapheresis are used as treatments. Diagnosis is by histology or a positive titre to the C-form of antineutrophil cytoplasmic antibody (C-ANCA) in the blood.

Systemic lupus erythematosus

Systemic lupus erythematosus (SLE) is a systemic disease that can affect the kidneys and cause renal failure. Females are affected more than males with variable presenting features often including fever, rashes, and arthritis. Cerebral, hepatic, and myocardial involvement and thrombotic events can also be seen and may be the reason for admission into critical care. Diagnosis is by positive titre to double-stranded DNA antibody in the blood, and treatment consists of steroids and immunosuppressants.

References and bibliography

Alvestrand, A.(1996). Nutritional aspects in patients with acute renal failure/multiorgan failure. *Blood Purification* **14**,109–14.

Beaman, M., Adu, A. (1992). Acute renal failure. In: *Care of the Critically Ill Patient* (ed. J. Tinker and M. Zapol), 2nd edn, pp. 515–30. Springer, Berlin.

Better, O.S. (1990). Acute renal failure and crush injury. In: *Acute Renal Failure in the Intensive Therapy Unit* (ed. D. Bihari and G. Neild), pp. 215–21. Springer, Berlin.

Bihari, D. and Beale, R. (1992). Renal support in the intensive care unit. *Current Science* 272–8.

Blakeley, S., Smith, G.(2003). Acute renal failure and renal replacement therapy in the ICU. *Anaesthesia and Intensive Care Medicine* 108–11 (www.frca.co.uk/article.aspx?articleid=100367).

Clark, W., Leblanc, M., Levin, N. (2002). The Acute Quality Dialysis Initiative—part IV: Membranes for CRRT. *Advances in Renal Replacement Therapy* **4**, 265–7.

Corwin, H.L., Bonventre J.V. (1988). Acute renal failure in the intensive care unit. Part 2. *Intensive Care Medicine* **14**, 86–96.

Currie, A., O'Brien, P. (2001).Renal replacement therapies. *Pharmaceutical Journal* **266**, 666–70.

Davenport, A., Mehta, S. (2002). The Acute Quality Dialysis Initiative—part IV: Access and anticoagulation in CRRT. *Advances in Renal Replacement Therapy* **9**, 273–81.

Galley, H.F. (2000). Can acute renal failure be prevented. *Journal of the Royal College of Surgeons of Edinburgh* **45**, 44–50.

Kierdorf, H.P. (1995). The nutritional management of acute renal failure in the intensive care unit. *New Horizons* **3**, 699–707.

Lazarus, J.M. (1990). Prophylaxis of acute renal failure in the intensive care unit. In: *Acute Renal Failure in the Intensive Therapy Unit* (ed. D. Bihari and G. Neild), pp. 280–309. Springer, Berlin.

Liesner, R.J., Machin, S.J.(1997). ABC of clinical haematology: platelet disorders. *British Medical Journal* **314**, 809–12.

Milne, A.D. (1986). Continuous ultrafiltration with periods of dialysis. *Care of the Critically Ill* **1**, 168–76.

Monchi, M., Berghmans, D., Ledoux, D., *et al.* (2004). Citrate vs.heparin for anticoagulation in continuous venovenous hemofiltration:a prospective randomized study. *Intensive Care Medicine* **30**, 260–5.

Neild. G.H. (1990). Endothelial and mesangial cell dysfunction in acute renal failure. In: *Acute Renal Failure in the Intensive Therapy Unit* (ed. D. Bihari and G. Neild), pp. 77–89. Springer, Berlin.

Renal Association (2002). *Treatment of Adults and Children with Renal Failure: Standards and Audit Measures*, 3rd edn. Royal College of Physicians of London and the Renal Association, London.

Ronco, C., Bellomo, R. (2000). Technical requirements for high volume hemofiltration. *International Journal on Haemofiltration and Blood Purification Techniques* (www.invivo.net/hemofiltration/journal/texts/hvhf.html).

Ronco, C., Bellomo, R., Homeld, P., *et al.* (2000). Effects of different doses in continuous venovenous hemofiltration on outcomes in acute renal failure: a prospective randomised trial. *Lancet* **356**, 26–30.

Schetz, M.R., Leblanc, M., Murray, P.T. (2002). The Acute Quality Dialysis Initiative—part VII: Fluid composition and management. *Advances in Renal Replacement Therapy* **4**, 265–7.

Schieppati, A., Remuzzi, G. (1990). Eicosanoids and acute renal failure. In: *Acute Renal Failure in the Intensive Therapy Unit* (ed. D. Bihari and G. Neild), pp. 115–29. Springer, Berlin.

Schrier, R.W., Abraham W.T., Hensen, J. (1990). Strategies in management of acute renal failure in the intensive therapy unit. In: *Acute Renal Failure in the Intensive Therapy Unit* (ed. D. Bihari and G. Neild), pp. 193–214. Springer, Berlin.

Short, A., Cumming, A. (1999).ABC of intensive care: renal support. *British Medical Journal* **319**, 41–4.

Sizer, E., Cottam, S. (2003). Clinical aspects of hepatic problems. *Anaesthesia and Intensive Care Medicine* 42–3 (www.frca.co.uk/documents/4_2_42.pdf)

Skellet, S., Mayer, A., Durward, A., *et al.* (2000). Chasing the base deficit: hyperchloraemic acidosis following 0.9% saline fluid resuscitation. *Archives of Disease in Childhood* **83**, 514–16.

Wendon, J., Smithies, M., Sheppard, M., *et al.* (1989). Continuous high volume venous—venous haemofiltration in acute renal failure. *Intensive Care Medicine*, **15**, 1–6.

Neurological problems

Introduction

There is limited scope within the confines of one chapter to cover all the neurological conditions that the intensive care nurse might meet. However, important aspects of neuroscience nursing and some of the more common conditions are covered. A brief overview of related basic anatomy and physiology is also included as revision for the reader.

An understanding of neurological conditions and their consequences, and the ability to effectively monitor and detect changes in a patient's condition are crucial to patient outcome. Improving ICU care, in combination with good medical and nursing management, can prevent secondary brain injury and has been shown to improve outcome in this group of patients. While this chapter focuses mainly on the acute nursing and medical management, it should be recognized that rehabilitation for these patients starts as soon as possible, even in the acute stages of intensive care, and this requires a multidisciplinary approach.

Anatomy and physiology

The bony cranial vault, three layers of protective membranes (the meninges), and the cerebrospinal fluid (CSF) all physically protect the brain.

Meninges

The three layers of meninges are (see Fig. 10.1):

1. *Dura mater* (Latin for 'hard mother'). The dura is the outermost layer and is made of tough fibrous connective tissue with an outer (periosteal) and an inner (meningeal) component. The two layers are fused except where they separate to form the dural venous sinuses and at the level of the foramen magnum where the inner layer only continues to form a tube-shaped sac around the spinal cord. The dural layer extends into the cranial cavity to form the falx cerebri (between the two hemispheres) and the tentorium cerebelli (between the cerebellum and the occipital lobes). While neural tissue itself does not generally sense pain, the dura does.

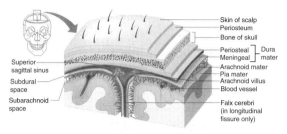

Fig. 10.1 The meninges of the brain. Reprinted from Marieb, E.N. (2003) *Essentials of Human Anatomy and Physiology*, 7th edn, with permission from Pearson Education.

2. *Arachnoid mater* (from the Greek word meaning spider). The arachnoid is the middle of the three meninges and adheres closely to the inner surface of the dura mater. It is a thin, avascular, spider-web-like membrane. It contains arachnoid villi—protrusions of arachnoid membrane into the superior sagittal sinus. The arachnoid villi act as one-way valves for the flow of CSF from the subarachnoid space to the venous sinuses.

3. *Pia mater* (Latin for 'tender mother'). The pia is the innermost layer and is composed of thin connective tissue. Unlike the dura and arachnoid layers which closely follow the contours of the cranial vault, the pia mater follows the contours of the brain. As a result, the space between the arachnoid and pial layers (the subarachnoid space), which contains cerebrospinal fluid, is not uniform, with the larger spaces called subarachnoid cisterns.

Cerebrum

The cerebrum is divided into two cerebral hemispheres (Fig. 10.2). Outermost on each hemisphere (2–4 mm thick) is the cerebral cortex, or grey matter, which consists of nerve cell bodies. The cerebral cortex is necessary for conscious awareness, thought, memory, and intellect. All sensory input has to reach the cerebral cortex (mostly via the thalamus) to be consciously perceived and interpreted and passed on to the cortical motor areas for the appropriate response. Certain important areas of grey matter are also found deeper in the brain tissue, such as the thalamus and basal ganglia (see below).

The white matter beneath the grey matter consists of the axons that project from the cell bodies and carry messages between them. Many axons are surrounded by a layer of lipid or myelin sheath that acts as an electrical insulator, allowing rapid transmission of impulses. Ascending fibres taking sensory information to the cor-

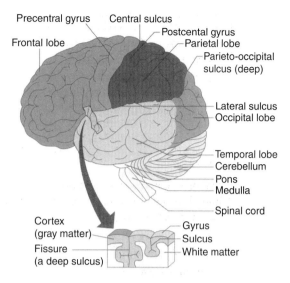

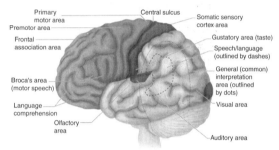

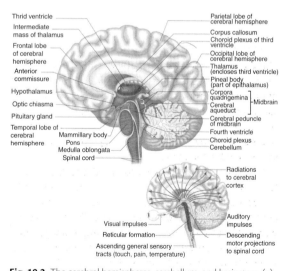

Fig. 10.2 The cerebral hemispheres, cerebellum, and brainstem. (a) Left lateral view of major structural areas. (b) Functional areas of the cerebral hemisphere. (c) Midbrain structures, cerebellum, and brainstem. Reprinted from Marieb, E.N. (2003) *Essentials of Human Anatomy and Physiology*, 7th edn, with permission from Pearson Education.

tex and descending fibres controlling movement cross over, or decussate, from one side to the other. Thus each cerebral hemisphere mostly perceives sensations and controls the movements of the opposite side of the body. In the majority of individuals, cortical areas in the frontal, parietal, and temporal lobes of the left hemisphere are responsible for the comprehension and expression of language. The left hemisphere is therefore said to be dominant for language.

Each hemisphere is divided into four lobes

1. The *frontal lobe* is concerned with executive functioning. It contains important areas—the primary motor cortex, pre-motor cortex, and supplementary motor cortex and Broca's area for speech in the dominant hemisphere.

2. The *parietal lobe* deals mainly with functions connected with movement, orientation, and calculation and contains the primary somatosensory cortex and association cortex.

3. The *temporal lobe* is concerned with sound, speech comprehension (dominant hemisphere), and some aspects of memory, and contains the primary auditory cortex and auditory association cortex (also known as Wernicke's area in the dominant hemisphere).

4. The *occipital lobe* is made up almost entirely of visual processing areas with the primary visual cortex and visual association cortex.

Cerebellum

The cerebellum (from Latin diminutive form of cerebrum meaning 'little brain') modulates and regulates motor function. It is primarily concerned with coordination of movements on the same side. The integrity of the cerebellum is important for smooth, accurate, coordinated motor tasks and the maintenance of a stable posture.

Thalamus

The thalamus is an area of grey matter deep within the brain that acts as a relay station, modifying and directing incoming information to the appropriate area of the cerebral cortex for further processing. The cerebral cortex in turn can modify the activity of the thalamus, thus influencing the messages sent.

Hypothalamus

The hypothalamus has been established as the master pacemaker driving circadian rhythms in physiology and behaviour through autonomic and neuroendocrine modulation via the pituitary gland. The hypothalamus plays an important role in thermoregulation.

Basal ganglia

The basal ganglia control motor output for the body, head, and eyes and work in conjunction with the supplementary motor area of the frontal lobes to plan movements prior to their initiation.

Brainstem

The brainstem, comprising the midbrain, pons, and medulla, has attachments for cranial nerves III to XII (see Table 10.1) and contains part of the reticular formation that controls level of consciousness, the cardiovascular system and the respiratory system. In addition, ascending and descending fibres pass through the brainstem *en route* to the thalamus and the spinal cord.

Communication within the central nervous system

Nerve cells, or neurons (Fig. 10.3), are the structural and functional units of the nervous system. The functions of the neuron are to receive and integrate incoming information from sensory receptors or other neurons and transmit information to other neurons or effector organs. They generate and conduct electrical changes in the form of nerve impulses and communicate chemically with other neurons at points of contact called synapses.

TABLE 10.1 Cranial nerves

Cranial nerve	Main function(s)
Olfactory (sensory)	Smell
Optic (sensory)	Vision
Oculomotor (mixed—primarily motor)	Movement of eyelid and eyeball, pupil size and shape
Trochlear (mixed—primarily motor)	Movement of eyeball
Trigeminal (mixed)	Chewing, facial sensation
Abducens (mixed—primarily motor)	Movement of eyeball
Facial (mixed)	Facial expression, activates salivary and lacrimal glands, supplies taste buds of anterior tongue
Vestibulocochlear (sensory)	Hearing and balance
Glossopharyngeal (mixed)	Swallowing, gag reflex
Vagus (mixed)	Swallowing, speech, control of visceral organs
Accessory (mixed—primarily motor)	Movement of head and shoulders
Hypoglossal (mixed—primarily motor)	Swallowing

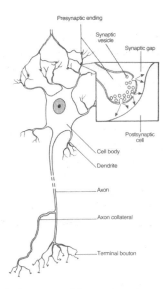

Fig. 10.3 The basic structure of the neuron and synapse. Reprinted from Crossman, A.R. and Neary, D. (1998) *Neuroanatomy: an Illustrated Colour Text*, with permission from Elsevier.

TABLE 10.2	Neurotransmitters
Neurotransmitter	**Details**
Acetylcholine (ACh)	ACh is the transmitter between neurons and striated muscle and at autonomic ganglia and produces an excitatory effect. Blockage of acetylcholine receptors (AChR) in skeletal muscles at the neuromuscular junction occurs after administration of non-depolarizing neuromuscular blocking drugs (e.g. atracurium, vecuronium) and in the disease myasthenia gravis (see later)
Glutamate	Glutamate is widespread throughout the CNS and has an excitatory effect. It is important for learning and memory and is implicated in epilepsy and excitotoxic cell death after brain injury
γ-Aminobutyric acid (GABA)	GABA has a high concentration in the thalamus, hypothalamus, and occipital lobes and is the most common inhibitory neurotransmitter. Some drugs enhance the action of GABA (such as anti-anxiety drugs) and some of the drugs used to control epilepsy work by modifying the balance between glutamate and GABA effects
Dopamine (DA)	DA is found mainly in the midbrain and basal ganglia and exerts a mostly inhibitory effect. It is involved in emotional responses and subconscious movement of skeletal muscles and is implicated in Parkinson's disease, addiction, and schizophrenia
Noradrenaline (NE)	NE is released at some neuromuscular and neuroglandular junctions and is mostly excitatory. It is highly concentrated in the brainstem and is involved in arousal, dreaming, and regulation of mood. Changes in noradrenaline levels are implicated in depressive illness
Serotonin (5-hydroxytryptamine (5-HT))	Serotonin is concentrated in the brainstem and is mostly excitatory. It is involved in inducing sleep, sensory perception, temperature regulation, and control of mood. Like noradrenaline, serotonin is implicated in depressive illness

The release of a neurotransmitter substance at these synapses is the essential link between neurons.

A neuron's chemical and physical environment influences both impulse conduction and synaptic transmission. Alkalosis (an increase in pH above 7.45) results in increased excitability of neurons, while acidosis (a decrease in pH below 7.35) results in progressive depression of neuronal activity.

The other major cells within the central nervous system (CNS) are the neuroglial cells (from the Greek word meaning glue) that provide support, insulation, and nourishment to neurons. Unlike neurons, the neuroglial cells do not have a direct role in information processing but they take on a number of supporting roles essential for the normal functioning of neurons. There are four types of neuroglial cells. Oligodendroglia form the myelin sheath around neuronal axons, which is important for the propagation of the nerve impulse (in the peripheral nervous system myelin is made by Schwann cells). Astrocytes form tight junctions between neurons and the blood supply and therefore are essential to the 'blood–brain barrier'. Ependymal cells form the inner surface of the ventricles and central canal of the spinal cord. Microglia have a phagocytic role when there is injury to the CNS.

Neurotransmitters

A large number of transmitter substances have been identified within the CNS (Table 10.2). These neurotransmitters forge lines of communication between brain cells and are localized in certain parts of the brain. They can excite, inhibit, or enhance the actions of post-synaptic neurons. These include acetylcholine (ACh), various amino acids (glutamate, γ-aminobutyric

TABLE 10.3	Neuropeptides
Neuropeptide	**Details**
Substance P	Substance P is found in sensory nerves, spinal cord pathways and parts of the brain associated with pain
Enkephalins	Enkephalins are the body's own natural painkillers and are several times more potent than morphine
Endorphins	Endorphins are concentrated in the pituitary gland and, like enkephalins, have morphine-like properties to suppress pain. Both enkephalins and endorphins inhibit pain impulses partly by suppressing substance P

acid (GABA) and catecholamines (noradrenaline, dopamine, serotonin).

Peptides

A large number of peptides are also stored and released at synapses (Table 10.3). These neuropeptides modulate the release and effects of other transmitters and include substance P, enkephalins and endorphins.

Ventricular system

The ventricular system consists of two C-shaped lateral ventricles (one in each hemisphere), a narrow slit-like third ventricle (bounded on either side by the thalamus and hypothalamus) and a fourth ventricle (between the cerebellum and the brainstem at the level of the pons and medulla) (Fig. 10.4).

In adults, approximately 150 ml of CSF is in circulation, half around the brain and half around the spinal cord. CSF is constantly produced by the choroid plexus of the ventricles and fills the ventricular and subarachnoid spaces (about 500 ml is produced daily). CSF is reabsorbed through the arachnoid villi in the sagittal sinus into the venous system. CSF cushions and protects the brain, acts as a pathway for nutrients and chemical mediators, and affects cerebral blood flow and pulmonary ventilation via pH levels.

Cerebral circulation

Arterial blood supply

Arterial supply is via two arterial systems, the right and left internal carotid arteries, which supply the anterior two-thirds of the cerebral hemispheres, and the vertebrobasilar system, which supplies the posterior regions of the hemispheres, the brainstem, and the cerebellum (Fig. 10.5). The anastamoses of the internal carotid system and the vertebrobasilar system (at the anterior and posterior communicating arteries) form the circle of Willis.

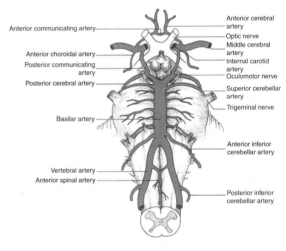

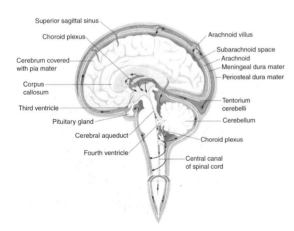

Fig. 10.4 The ventricular system. Reprinted from Marieb, E.N. (2003) *Essentials of Human Anatomy and Physiology*, 7th edn, with permission from Pearson Education.

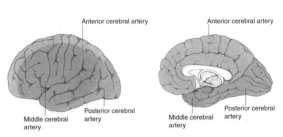

Fig. 10.5 (a) Cerebral arterial blood supply (circle of Willis). (b) Cortical distribution. Reprinted from Crossman, A.R. and Neary, D. (1998) *Neuroanatomy: an Illustrated Colour Text*, with permission from Elsevier.

Venous drainage

Venous drainage comprises a series of external and internal veins, which drain into the venous sinuses, formed by folds of the dura mater (Fig. 10.6). The sinuses have no valves and therefore venous drainage is dependent on gravity. Superficial cerebral veins in the subarachnoid space drain the cerebral cortex and white matter and empty into the intracranial venous sinuses. The upper part of each hemisphere drains into the superior sagittal sinus, the middle part drains into the cavernous sinus and the lower part drains into the transverse sinus.

Spinal cord

The spinal cord is continuous with the medulla oblongata of the brainstem and is surrounded and protected by the vertebral column and three layers of membrane (the meningeal layer of the dura, the arachnoid, and the pia mater). The spinal cord is almost divided into two symmetrical halves by anterior and posterior grooves and in the centre is the small central canal, which is a continuation of the cerebral ventricular system. In contrast to the cerebrum and cerebellum, in the spinal cord the grey matter (consisting of nerve cell bodies) is innermost, and the white matter (containing ascending and descending nerve fibres) is on the outside.

Many functions within the spinal cord can operate in an automatic or reflex action. However, when information is conveyed to specific areas of the brain via the ascending nerve fibres, the brain can exert a controlling influence over these spinal mechanisms via the descending nerve pathways.

Neurological assessment

Despite continued developments in neuromonitoring, clinical observation of the patient remains the most sensitive measure of neurological function. Impaired consciousness is an expression of dysfunction of the brain as a whole and changes in conscious level provide the best indication of the development of complications following brain injury.

Components of consciousness

Consciousness is a state of general awareness of oneself and the environment. It has two components, arousal and awareness, and these correspond to two brain structures, the reticular activating system (RAS) and the cerebral cortex respectively (see Fig. 10.2). Consciousness depends on the interaction between the neurons in the reticular activating system in the brainstem and the neurons in the cerebral cortex. The content of consciousness is determined by the neurons in the cerebral cortex while the neurons in the reticular activating system are responsible for the primitive state of arousal.

Arousal

Simply being awake is a primitive state managed by the RAS. The RAS consists of neurons that extend through the central core of the brainstem, with projections upwards to the cortex and downwards to the spinal cord. It receives auditory impulses, visual impulses, and impulses from the ascending sensory tracts, and, because of its connections, it is ideal for governing arousal of the brain as a whole.

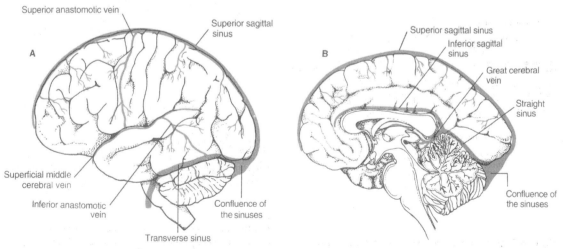

Fig. 10.6 Cerebral venous drainage: (a) lateral view, (b) sagittal view. Reprinted from Crossman, A.R. and Neary, D. (1998) *Neuroanatomy: an Illustrated Colour Text*, with permission from Elsevier.

Unless inhibited by other brain areas, e.g. sleep-inducing areas, reticular neurons send a continuous stream of impulses to the cerebral cortex, maintaining the cortex in an alert, conscious state. The RAS is the physical basis of consciousness. It is selective, forwarding only essential information to the cortex and filtering out unnecessary information. Certain drugs have a direct effect on the RAS—it is depressed by alcohol, sleep-inducing drugs and tranquillizers, and some mood-enhancing drugs, e.g. LSD, can remove the filter system in the RAS causing heightened sensory arousal.

Awareness

Awareness is the more sophisticated part of consciousness, requiring an intact cerebral cortex to interpret the sensory input from the RAS and respond accordingly.

Assessing consciousness

Consciousness cannot be measured directly and can only be assessed by observing a person's behaviour in response to different stimuli. The response the patient gives indicates the level at which the sensory information has been translated within the CNS.

Levels of sensation

Sensory impulses terminating in the spinal cord can generate spinal reflexes without involving the brain, e.g. the brain-dead patient whose legs move when a peripheral painful stimulus is applied to them. The sensation is translated by the spinal cord and it is the spinal cord that generates the reaction. Sensory impulses reaching the lower brainstem cause subconscious motor reactions, e.g. non-purposeful decorticate (flexor) and decerebrate (extensor) motor responses. Impulses that reach the thalamus can be identified as a specific sensation (touch, pain, etc.) and localized crudely in the body, e.g. the patient flexing to painful stimuli. Only when sensory information reaches the cerebral cortex do we experience precise localization, e.g. the patient localizing to a painful stimulus. The sensory cortex identifies and localizes the source and the motor cortex acts to remove the noxious stimulus.

Neurological assessment

Neurological assessment must include:

- assessment of conscious level (Glasgow Coma Scale)
- limb assessments
- pupil size and reaction to light
- vital signs.

The Glasgow Coma Scale

Prior to the development of the Glasgow Coma Scale in 1974, level of consciousness was described in terms such as stupor, semi-coma, and deep coma, but these terms were not clearly defined and there was a great deal of inconsistency when assessment was carried out by different observers. The Glasgow Coma Scale was designed to standardize observations using a simple system based on clearly definable criteria that could be reproduced objectively and reliably by a range of medical and nursing personnel. It defined conscious level in terms of three modes of behaviour: eye opening, verbal response, and motor response. In each category, it assesses the response generated by different stimuli, with the increasing stimulus required to elicit a response indicating a decrease in the level of cerebral functioning. Each response is also given a score—the minimum a patient can score is 3 and the maximum is 15 (Table 10.4). The best response is recorded in each category therefore it provides a global assessment only.

The Glasgow Coma Scale is universally used to assess conscious level in the acute phase of brain injury and should be charted as a graph to enable easy identification of a change in the patient's condition. It is more accurate in assessing altered levels of consciousness due to cerebral trauma than medical causes of coma.

TABLE 10.4 The Glagow Coma Scale

Eye opening	Score	Verbal response	Score	Motor response	Score
Spontaneous	4	Orientated	5	Obeys commands	6
To speech	3	Confused	4	Localizes to pain	5
To pain	2	Inappropriate words	3	Flexes to pain	4
None	1	Incomprehensible sounds	2	Abnormal flexion	3
		None	1	Extension	2
				None	1

ASSESSMENT OF EYE OPENING

- *Spontaneous*: observed before you approach the patient or speak to him/her.
- *To speech*: call the patient's name.
- *To pain*: apply pressure to the side of the finger. (Central stimulus to supraorbital nerve will cause grimacing and eye closure.)
- *None*: ensure painful stimulus is adequate.

Eye opening

Eye opening looks at the arousal mechanisms and control of the eyes in the brainstem.

Even when brain damage is severe all patients who survive will eventually open their eyes (usually within 2–4 weeks). Spontaneous eye opening merely indicates that the arousal mechanisms in the brainstem are active but does not necessarily mean that the patient is aware.

Verbal response

Verbal response assesses two elements of cerebral functioning, comprehension and transmission of sensory input and the ability to articulate a reply. An orientated response shows a high degree of integration within the nervous system.

Motor response

Motor response is the most important prognostic aspect of the Glasgow Coma Scale after traumatic brain injury.

ASSESSMENT OF VERBAL RESPONSE

- *Orientated*: knows time, place, person. (Should know who he/she is, where he/she is and why he/she is there and know the month, year, season. If the patient answers one or more component wrongly then he/she must be recorded as confused.)
- *Confused*: talking in sentences but disorientated to time and place. (Patient attends to questioning but shows disorientation.)
- *Inappropriate words*: utters occasional words rather than sentences. (These are often abusive words elicited by noxious stimuli rather than spontaneous.)
- *Incomprehensible sounds*: groans or grunts.
- *None*: if the patient has an ET tube or tracheostomy T is recorded in this section.

ASSESSMENT OF MOTOR RESPONSE

- *Obeys commands*: 'Hold up your arms.' 'Stick out your tongue.' (If asking the patient to squeeze your hand beware of the reflex hand grasp in unconscious patients.)
- *Localizing to pain*: apply a painful stimulus to the supraorbital nerve until a response is observed. If the patient responds by bringing h/her hand up purposefully to the chin or above, this is localizing. (If there is trauma to the eyes, use the trapezius pinch.)
- *Flexing to pain*: elbow bending is recorded as flexing to pain.
- *Abnormal flexion to pain*: elbow flexion is accompanied by a spastic flexion of the wrist.
- *Extending to pain*: straightening of the elbow is recorded as extending to pain.
- *None*: ensure the stimulus is adequate.

In this category the *best* response is recorded as an indication of the functional state of the brain as a whole. In addition, only the response of the *upper limbs* is recorded as these are more reliable than lower limb responses that could be purely spinal reflexes.

If the patient does not obey commands motor activity has to be assessed by applying a central painful stimulus (pressure on the supraorbital nerve) and observing the response. The stimulus must be applied in a standard way and maintained until a maximum response is obtained. If applying pressure to the supraorbital nerve is inappropriate, e.g. the patient has eye swelling or orbital fractures, then the next recommended central stimulus is trapezius pinch. If there is no response to central stimulus then a peripheral stimulus should be applied.

Limb responses

A difference in responsiveness in one limb compared with the other indicates focal brain damage. Hemiparesis or hemiplegia usually occurs in the limbs on the opposite side to the lesion (due to decussation of nerve fibres in the medulla). However, it may also affect the limbs on the same side as the lesion due to pressure on the contralateral hemisphere (Kernohan's notch syndrome—a false localizing sign).

Pupillary response

Pupillary response to light is dependent upon intact afferent (optic nerve) and efferent (oculomotor nerve) function transmitting the light impulse from the retina to the midbrain and hence the pupillary musculature. A dilating pupil indicates an expanding lesion on the same side (ipsilateral since the oculomotor nerve does not decussate) and is an important localizing sign. Pupillary pathways are relatively resistant to metabolic insult and, therefore, the presence or absence of the light reflex is the single most important sign potentially distinguishing structural from metabolic coma:

- Pupils should be assessed for size, shape, equality, and reaction to light.

- Bilaterally fixed and dilated pupils in a patient whose motor response is flexion or localizing suggests the recent occurrence of a seizure (or homatropine eye drops).

- Muscle relaxants do not affect pupil reaction, and in the patient who is paralysed and sedated for ventilation it is the only clinical sign of raised ICP that can be tested. Since pupil abnormalities are a late sign of intracranial complications these patients require ICP monitoring.

- Damage to the cervical cord or brachial plexus can cause inequality of the pupils due to Horner's syndrome.

Vital signs

Temperature

Temperature regulation may be disrupted due to damage to the hypothalamus. In the acute phase of brain injury hyperthermia should be treated since it will exacerbate cerebral ischaemia and adversely affect outcome.

Heart rate

ECG changes may occur in the acute stage following cerebral insult as a result of catecholamine release (the transient 'sympathetic storm'). These can include peaked P waves, prolonged QT interval, heightened T waves, ST segment elevation or depression:

- Bradycardia (HR < 50 bpm) is present in the later stages of raised ICP (compensatory phase—Cushing's response) or when there is an associated cervical injury.

- Tachycardia (HR > 100 bpm) is present in the terminal stage of raised ICP.

- Arrhythmias are seen particularly in posterior fossa lesions or when there is blood in the CSF.

Blood pressure

In a normal brain a fall in blood pressure does not cause a drop in cerebral perfusion pressure since autoregulation results in cerebral vasodilation to protect brain tissue. However, following cerebral insult, when autoregulation may be impaired, hypotension may lead to brain ischaemia. Hypotension (defined as a systolic BP < 90 mmHg) has been uniformly identified as the most predominant factor in secondary brain injury and has the highest correlation with morbidity and mortality:

- Hypotension is rarely attributable to cerebral injury itself, although it can occur in children. In severe injury it will occur as a terminal event when the regulatory mechanisms in the medulla are no longer functioning due to inadequate perfusion and will be accompanied by tachycardia.

- When hypotension and tachycardia are seen together the possibility of extracranial haemorrhage should be investigated.

- Hypotension and bradycardia are seen in associated cervical spine injury due to autonomic dysfunction.

- Hypertension is associated with a rising ICP and is part of the Cushing's response—rising BP with a widening pulse pressure, bradycardia, and decreasing respirations. This is a late response that may not appear in some patients and is invariably preceded by a drop in GCS.

Respiration

Respiratory complications are common following cerebral insult and patients often require advanced respiratory support even in the acute stage:

- The cerebral hemispheres regulate voluntary control over the muscles used in breathing.

- The cerebellum synchronizes and coordinates muscular effort.

- The brainstem regulates the automaticity of breathing.

Initially an acute rise in ICP will cause slowing of respiratory rate indicating loss of all cerebral and cerebellar control of breathing, with respiratory function at only brainstem level. As ICP continues to rise the rate becomes rapid indicating that the brainstem too is affected.

Appropriate use of neurological assessment

The recording of neurological observations is only indicated when a patient has an injury or illness affecting the central nervous system. When the injury or illness involves the brain, observations must include Glasgow Coma Scale, pupil, and limb assessments. When it involves the spinal cord, then limb assessments only need to be recorded (C1–T6, upper and lower limbs; T7 and below, lower limbs only). This applies even in high cervical spine surgery. The only exceptions are when there has been additional foramen magnum decompression or transoral access to the odontoid peg. In these cases, the Glasgow Coma Scale should also be documented in the first 12 to 24 hours post-surgery to detect haematoma formation or swelling which might cause compression of the brainstem or impede drainage of the fourth ventricle and lead to hydrocephalus. After this initial post-operative period limb assessments only are required.

The Glasgow Coma Scale was designed for the acute phase of brain injury when the patient's condition may fluctuate and there is a risk of secondary complications. It is not always an appropriate tool in chronic neurological conditions. Once the patient has passed the acute phase, when neurological observations need to be recorded less than every 4 hours, then the appropriateness of using the Glasgow Coma Scale should be questioned.

Intracranial dynamics and possible changes following brain injury

Most of the evidence for the changes in intracranial dynamics that can occur following brain injury is derived from studies in traumatic brain injury (TBI). However, in practice we can use some of the findings to guide the intensive care management of patients with other brain insults where raised intracranial pressure is a component (e.g. subarachnoid haemorrhage, encephalitis).

Volume–pressure relations

The Monro–Kellie hypothesis states that the sum of the intracranial contents of blood (10%), brain (80%), and cerebrospinal fluid (CSF) (10%) is constant. Since the skull is considered as an enclosed and rigid container, an increase in the volume of any one of the intracranial components must be offset by a decrease in one or more of the others or it will lead to a rise in intracranial pressure (ICP). Under normal circumstances, a small increase in brain volume will be compensated by translocation of CSF and venous blood to the spinal CSF space and to extracranial veins, respectively. However, once these compensatory mechanisms have been exhausted even a small increase in volume will result in substantial ICP increases. Compliance (the change in volume for a given change in pressure) provides an index of compensatory reserve, with low values suggesting a diminished reserve (Fig. 10.7).

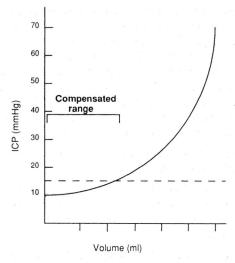

Fig. 10.7 Volume–pressure curve.

After injury the brain's ability to react to volume changes may be impaired by several factors, including the failure of autoregulatory mechanisms (see below), disruption of the blood–brain barrier (BBB) and oedema. The point at which a critical volume is reached is dependent not only on the individual but also on the speed of expansion.

Intracranial pressure (ICP)

ICP is defined as the CSF pressure within the lateral ventricles, and the normal range in adults is 0–10 mmHg, with lower ranges (up to 7 mmHg) in children. The volume of the intracranial components must be in a state of dynamic equilibrium to keep ICP constant. ICP rises transiently in response to actions such as coughing and sneezing without any adverse effect as compensatory measures quickly reduce ICP before any damage is caused by compromised blood flow. The duration of

TABLE 10.5 Causes of raised ICP

Brain	Tumour
	Abscess
	Oedema
Blood	Haemorrhage
	Haematoma
	Restricted venous return
	Increased cerebral blood flow
CSF	Over-secretion (rare)
	Impaired circulation
	Impaired absorption

ICP > 20 mmHg strongly correlates with increased morbidity and mortality. Table 10.5 shows somw cause of raised ICP.

Cerebral perfusion pressure (CPP)

CPP is the driving force for the delivery of blood (and therefore the delivery of oxygen and glucose) to the brain and is an estimate of the adequacy of the cerebral circulation. CPP represents the blood pressure gradient across the brain, and in its simplified form can be calculated as the difference between the incoming mean arterial blood pressure (MAP) and the opposing ICP on the arteries (CPP = MAP – ICP). In the healthy brain intrinsic autoregulatory mechanisms (see below) protect brain tissue from damage when there are brief changes in MAP or ICP.

After severe injury changes in either MAP or ICP will alter CPP. In the initial stages following TBI low BP rather than high ICP is the most frequent cause of inadequate CPP.

Cerebral blood flow (CBF)

The brain has little ability to store the precursors of metabolism and therefore neuronal function is critically dependent on CBF to meet its metabolic demands. The brain requires a constant supply of blood to provide oxygen and glucose and, within limits, the vessels of the cerebral circulation can respond to meet these needs.

The amount of blood delivered to the brain is highly regulated and is determined by several factors discussed below.

Pressure autoregulation

Autoregulation is the intrinsic ability of cerebrovascular smooth muscle to maintain a relatively constant CBF over a wide range of perfusion pressures (50–150 mmHg). The cerebral vessels change diameter inversely with changing perfusion pressures. As CPP rises the vessels constrict to prevent damage to smaller vessels from higher pressures, and as CPP falls the vessels dilate so that blood flow is kept constant. In hypertensive patients the autoregulatory pressure limits are higher (i.e. the autoregulation curve is shifted to the right).

After injury this autoregulatory response may be disrupted with CBF and CPP dependent on systemic circulation. In addition, the injured brain may require the CPP to be above normal to maintain CBF, and may be slower than normal to react to pressure changes. A shift to the right, increasing the lower and upper limits of autoregulation, occurs with chronic hypertension and sympathetic activation (e.g. shock or stress), and a shift to the left, reducing the lower and upper limits, occurs with hypoxia, hypercarbia, and vasodilators. Acute hypertension, i.e. a rapid increase in perfusion pressure to above the upper autoregulatory limit, may result in cerebral oedema secondary to increased microvascular pressures.

Metabolic regulation

Blood flow and metabolism in the normal brain are tightly coupled to ensure that cellular demands are matched by CBF. Although the exact mechanisms involved are not fully determined, it is proposed that concentrations of extracellular ions, such as hydrogen, calcium, and potassium, and of metabolic products, such as adenosine, thromboxane, and prostaglandins may act as local vasoregulators to match local blood flow to local metabolic demands. The normal cerebral metabolic rate for oxygen consumption ($CMRO_2$) is 3 ml/100 g/min.

Following injury, metabolic regulation can be disrupted. Oxygen extraction rate increases up to 100% when CPP decreases below 50% in order to maintain a stable $CMRO_2$. Flow metabolism is important in regional, rapid control of blood flow, whereas other mechanisms, e.g. pressure autoregulation, involve global, slower control. When blood flow and metabolism are no longer coupled, CBF is not reduced in areas of de-

---

CEREBRAL BLOOD FLOW

- Normal CBF 50–60 ml/100 g/min (750 ml/min for the entire brain,15% of total resting cardiac output).

- Global CBF remains stable but regional increases of 50 to 100% may occur locally during normal neuronal activity.

- Oxygen supply to the brain is about 80% of total body oxygen consumption.

- Each day the brain requires 1000 litres of blood flow to obtain 71 litres of oxygen and 100 g of glucose.

- Cessation of CBF causes unconsciousness within 5–10 s due to lack of delivery of oxygen to the brain cells.

- If CBF < 25–30 ml/100 g/min mental confusion and loss of consciousness will occur.

- If CBF < 15 ml/100 g/min measurable electrical activity (EEG) is absent.

- If CBF < 8 ml/100 g/min cellular alteration and cell death occur.

pressed metabolism, leading to a state of *luxury perfusion* (decreased oxygen extraction fraction).

Chemical regulation

Alterations in arterial oxygen partial pressure (P_aO_2) and arterial carbon dioxide pressure (P_aCO_2) can have a profound effect on CBF. Moreover, the effects of hypoxaemia and hypercapnia are additive, therefore a poorly ventilated and marginally oxygenated patient will have a dramatic increase in CBF.

1. *Oxygen.* CBF changes with arterial O_2 content to maintain the appropriate tissue O_2 tension for cerebral metabolism. The precise chemical mediator for this response is not known. However, adenosine, a metabolic product, is thought to play an important role in this response. CBF is not affected until the P_aO_2 falls below 7 kPa. At this point cerebral vasodilatation begins and CBF increases. At very high P_aO_2 levels (>40 kPa) there may be a slight decrease in CBF. Mild hypoxia (P_aO_2 < 7kPa) is associated with a two-fold increase in CBF, while severe hypoxia is associated with a five-fold increase in CBF. Hypoxia (P_aO_2 < 8 kPa) has been shown to be the second most influential cause of secondary brain injury, after hypotension, and worsens outcome.

2. *Carbon dioxide.* Arterial carbon dioxide tension is one of the most potent regulators of CBF. Unlike the response to oxygen, the CBF response to changes in P_aCO_2 is dramatic, such that, within the range of 3.3–10 kPa, for every 0.12 kPa change in P_aCO_2 there is a 1–2 ml/100 g/min change in CBF (doubling P_aCO_2 doubles CBF and halving P_aCO_2 halves CBF). Hypercapnia increases CBF and cerebral blood volume (CBV) and decreases cerebral vascular resistance (CVR) (vasodilation), whereas hypocapnia decreases CBF and CBV and increases CVR (vasoconstriction). These effects represent the most powerful stimulus to the cerebral vascular system and are thought to be the result of changes in extracellular or interstitial H^+ ion concentration. However, after 6–8 hours the CBF returns to baseline values because CSF pH gradually normalizes as a result of the extrusion of bicarbonate.

This cerebrovascular reactivity to an altered P_aO_2 and P_aCO_2 can be reduced or abolished in cases of intracranial hypertension. The loss of reactivity, which is a bad prognostic sign, can be either global or focal.

Neurogenic regulation

It seems likely that specific neuronal centres modify or facilitate autoregulatory responses. Some sympathetic and parasympathetic nerves and several neurotransmitters have been implicated in this mechanism.

Blood haemoglobin concentration

CBF can be influenced by blood viscosity, of which haematocrit is the single most important determinant. Blood viscosity increases logarithmically with increasing haematocrit and the optimal level is probably about 35%.

Blood–brain barrier (BBB)

The BBB is a specialization of the walls of brain capillaries that limits the movement of blood-borne substances into the extracellular fluid of the brain and CSF. Unlike the rest of the body, cerebral endothelial cells are joined to one another by intracellular tight junctions that form a five-layered ring around all cerebral blood vessels preventing any passage of molecules between individual cells. Injury to the brain can cause a breakdown of the BBB allowing normally restricted substances to pass into the brain tissue.

Management of the patient with severe traumatic brain injury (TBI)

Head injuries are the most common cause of death in young adults in the Western world and lead to 9 deaths per 100 000 of the population each year. This represents 1% of all deaths, but 15–20% for those between 5 and 35 years of age, and has a very significant impact on long-term disability. The immediate resuscitation and stabilization of patients with severe TBI and their subsequent intensive care management is aimed at preventing secondary injury to the brain.

Pathophysiology of severe TBI

Injury to the brain following trauma includes both the immediate damage caused at the moment of impact and secondary damage that develops during the first few hours or days after the impact (Table 10.6). Primary brain injury encompasses disruption of brain vessels,

TABLE 10.6	Primary and secondary brain injury
Primary brain injury	Disruption of brain vessels
	Haemorrhagic contusions
	Diffuse axonal injury (DAI)
Secondary brain injury	Extracranial causes: systemic hypotension, hypoxaemia, hypercarbia, disturbances of blood coagulation
	Intracranial causes: haematoma, brain swelling, infection

TYPES OF LESIONS

Extradural haematoma

An extradural haematoma (EDH) is an accumulation of blood in the extradural space between the inner side of the skull and the dura mater. Most (90%) are associated with skull fracture and due to injury of the middle meningeal artery and therefore affect the parietal and parieto-temporal areas. Outcome depends on the level of consciousness at the time of surgery with mortality approaching 20% if unconscious.

Subdural haematoma

A subdural haematoma (SDH) is an accumulation of blood between the inner side of the dura and the arachnoid layer due to tearing of cortical veins. As most patients with acute SDHs have some kind of accompanying brain injury, their prognosis is worse than that of patients with EDHs. They can be classified as acute (ASDH) <3–4 days old, subacute 4–20 days old, and chronic >20 days old. A poor outcome is more likely if SDH is bilateral, accumulates rapidly, or there is >4 hours delay in surgical management of ASDH. Chronic subdural haematoma (CSDH) can occur many weeks after head injury.

Traumatic subarachnoid haemorrhage

Traumatic subarachnoid haemorrhage (SAH) can occur following severe TBI. Traumatic SAH must be quantified on early CT scan since later scans underestimate its incidence and severity. Mortality and poor outcome is twice that seen in patients without the SAH component.

Intracerebral haematoma

Intracerebral haematoma (ICH) usually affects the white matter or basal ganglia and can be the cause of delayed neurological deterioration.

Contusions and lacerations

Haemorrhagic contusions and lacerations are superficial areas of haemorrhage usually affecting the cortex in the frontal and temporal lobes, sustained as the brain hits the bony protruberances of the skull at the site of impact (coup injury) and then the opposite side during deceleration (contrecoup injury).

TYPES OF LESIONS – *continued*

Diffuse axonal injury

Diffuse axonal injury (DAI) is the commonest cause of coma, the vegetative state, and subsequent disability. It is attributed to tearing of nerve fibres at the junction between the grey and white matter because they decelerate at different velocities within the skull and is likely to be a dynamic process at a cellular level that begins soon after trauma and may not be complete for 24 hours. Patients with severe DAI are often in deep coma in contrast to a CT scan that can look quite normal and an initially normal ICP.

Skull fracture

Skull fracture is evidence of major impact to the head and has an associated high incidence of intracranial haematomas. Clinical indicators of a base of skull fracture include periorbital bruising (panda eyes or racoon eyes) and retroauricular bruising (Battle's sign) and may be associated with a cerebrospinal fluid (CSF) leak from the nose (rhinorrhoea) or the ears (otorrhoea). Most leaks close spontaneously.

haemorrhagic contusions, and diffuse axonal injury (DAI) and there is no intervention at present to attenuate such injury. Secondary injury can be divided into intracranial and extracranial causes. Of these, the two main causes, correlating with increased mortality and morbidity, are delay in appropriate surgical management and failure to correct systemic hypoxaemia and hypotension.

Management of the patient with severe TBI in the intensive care unit

Monitoring and assessment

Over and above routine care for general critically ill patients, patients with TBI will require cerebral monitoring to allow measurement of CPP, estimation of CBF, and assessment of the adequacy of oxygen delivery to the brain. This allows therapy to be targeted to specific changes in brain function and to ensure a balance between cerebral metabolic supply and demand:

◆ Intracranial pressure monitoring (Fig. 10.8) provides a physiological variable that is not only useful for diagnosis and prognosis, but also serves as direct feedback to guide the treatment of cerebral perfu-

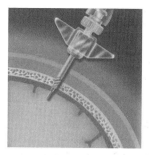 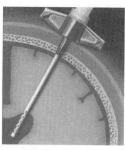

Fig. 10.8 ICP monitoring (a) Intraparechymal (b) Intraventricular. Reprinted with permission from Integra Neurosciences.

sion. ICP can be measured using a subdural, intra-parenchymal, or intraventricular catheter. ICP monitoring is the only way to measure (absolutely) CPP.

♦ Transcranial Doppler ultrasonography (TCD) provides an indicator of CBF and can be used to provide a non-invasive assessment of CPP. TCD can also be used to demonstrate the loss of pressure autoregulation and CO_2 reactivity, which are indicators of poor prognosis after TBI.

♦ Jugular venous bulb oximetry ($S_{jv}O_2$) is used to assess the balance between cerebral oxygen supply and demand after head injury.

Newer techniques for measuring the adequacy of cerebral oxygenation include near infrared spectroscopy, tissue microprobes, and cerebral microdialysis.

Individual monitoring techniques provide information about specific aspects of cerebral function but all have disadvantages and most suffer from significant artefact. Decisions to treat are therefore not usually based on a change in one variable alone. Monitoring of several variables simultaneously (multimodality monitoring) allows cross-validation between monitor, artefact rejection, and greater confidence to make treatment decisions.

When clinical assessment is no longer possible due to sedation or pharmacological paralysis to facilitate ventilation, then there is general agreement that ICP monitoring should be instituted in all patients with severe TBI (GCS ⩽ 8). Uncontrolled intracranial hypertension remains an important cause of mortality and morbidity after severe TBI and in more than one-third of patients ICP exceeds 20 mmHg at some stage While it has never been shown definitively that lowering ICP in patients with intracranial hypertension improves outcome, an ICP > 20 mmHg has been shown to be the fourth most powerful predictor of outcome after age, admission GCS, and pupillary signs, and there is evid-

ence to suggest that treatment to reduce ICP should be initiated if the ICP is 20–25 mmHg. Both ICP and CPP correlate strongly with outcome after TBI with the worse outcomes occurring in patients with an ICP > 20 mmHg and/or a CPP < 60 mmHg.

One of the most controversial areas in the management of severe TBI is the level of CPP required to adequately perfuse the brain. While there is evidence that hypotension following TBI has an adverse effect on outcome there is less evidence to support the concept that induced hypertension, particularly if it is prolonged, is beneficial to the injured brain. A target CPP of 60–70 mmHg is generally advocated.

ICP therapy

ICP therapy is indicated only if raised ICP has been demonstrated by monitoring, if there is CT evidence of increased ICP, or there are clinical signs of developing intracranial herniation.

Sedation

It is common practice for severe TBI patients to be empirically managed with a protocol that includes the routine use of sedatives, analgesics, and neuromuscular blocking agents to facilitate mechanical ventilation and to treat intracranial hypertension.

Intravenous anaesthetic agents cause a dose-dependent reduction in cerebral metabolism, CBF, and ICP whilst maintaining pressure autoregulation and CO_2 reactivity. The use of barbiturates such as thiopental in TBI is controversial and has largely been replaced by propofol, which has similar cerebrovascular effects but a more favourable pharmacological profile. However, there is currently renewed interest in the use of barbiturates for intractable raised ICP.

Potent parenteral narcotics such as fentanyl and morphine are frequently administered to limit pain, facilitate mechanical ventilation, and potentiate the effect of sedation.

Neuromuscular blocking drugs have no direct effect on ICP but may prevent rises produced by coughing and straining on the endotracheal tube. However, such agents are not associated with improved outcome and their use is currently the subject of much debate.

Mannitol

Mannitol is an effective agent to reduce cerebral oedema and ICP in certain settings of intracranial hypertension. However, repetitive administration can potentially increase ICP since mannitol accumulates within brain tissue, reversing osmotic shift and increasing cerebral oedema. This accumulation is most marked when mannitol is in the circulation for long periods as occurs with continuous infusion administration, therefore it should be given in repeat bolus doses. Chronic mannitol therapy is not associated with improvement in neurological outcome and its use should be discontinued when it no longer produces a significant and sustained reduction in ICP.

Hyperventilation

Hyperventilation, which was once the mainstay of treatment to reduce ICP in patients with severe TBI, is now vigorously debated. Its aim is to reduce cerebral blood volume and hence ICP, but it can also cause a significant reduction in CBF. The current guidelines advocate a P_aCO_2 of 4.5–5.0 kPa. Further reductions in P_aCO_2 to 4.0–4.5 kPa should be used only if ICP is >20 mmHg, and levels below 4 kPa considered only when ICP has been shown to be sensitive to P_aCO_2 levels and used only in conjunction with $S_{jv}O_2$ monitoring.

Therapeutic hypothermia

Elevations in temperature worsen outcome after TBI and pyrexia should be avoided. Brain temperature tends to be higher than core temperature and the brain's cerebral metabolic rate for oxygen consumption increases 6–9% for every degree Celsius rise in temperature. Moderate reductions in brain temperature reduce the release of excitatory amino acids and moderate hypothermia to 33–35°C has been shown to be of benefit in animal models. There is some evidence that while hypothermia may not attenuate damage from the primary injury, it may provide a degree of protection against secondary brain injury from hypotension and hypoxia in the early stages following injury. Whether this protection can be sustained over longer periods remains to be determined.

Cooling blankets should only be used in sedated and paralysed patients to avoid a shivering response that may cause a rise in ICP and an increase in oxygen consumption. Persistent hyperpyrexia may be the result of damage to the hypothalamus but microbiological causes should be investigated.

CSF drainage

CSF drainage by insertion of an external ventricular drain is frequently employed to treat intracranial hypertension in severe TBI, and while it is established as a first-line treatment there are no consensual guidelines for its use. Some advocate continuous CSF drainage as long as the ventricle size is normal and intermittent CSF drainage when the ventricle size is small.

Positioning

Head rotation and neck flexion are associated with increased ICP, decreased jugular venous return, and localized changes in cerebral blood flow. It is traditional practice, therefore, to position head injured patients in bed with the head elevated to a maximum of 30° above the heart and in neutral alignment with the trunk in order to reduce ICP, provided that the patient is not hypotensive. Once ICP and CPP monitoring are implemented there is scope for an individualized approach (within these guidelines) to head elevation based on the patient's response.

Neuroprotective drugs

Corticosteroids have been used in the treatment of certain neurological conditions since the 1950s. No one doubts their value in producing rapid improvement in patients with brain tumours associated with oedema and there is evidence of benefit in the early administration of high-dose methylprednisolone in spinal cord injury. However, several prospective randomized clinical trials failed to show that steroid therapy reduces ICP or improves outcome in patients with severe TBI. Currently, the whole issue is being revisited in a large multicentre trial, the CRASH trial (Corticosteroid Randomisation after Significant Head Injury), to determine definitively the effects of high-dose methylprednisolone infusion on death and disability in head injured patients.

Evidence from experimental studies suggests that modification of neurochemical and cellular events with targeted pharmacotherapy can promote functional recovery following TBI. Moreover, it is likely that there is a therapeutic window following injury during which such pharmacological intervention must be initiated in order to be effective. Such drugs (e.g. antioxidants, ion-channel blockers, and membrane stabilizers) aim to protect brain cells from secondary injury by interrupting one or more of the mediating factors that cause tissue damage. However, while animal studies show good effect, there is little clinical evidence to date of brain protection with new drugs.

Respiratory management

A large proportion of patients with severe TBI are hypoxaemic without ventilatory support or added oxygen and many require advanced ventilatory support within a short period of time. Acute lung injury (ALI) (see Chapter 4) is common in patients with isolated head injury, particularly those with a post-resuscitative GCS of 8 or less. It is an additional marker of the severity of brain injury and is associated with an increased risk of morbidity and mortality.

Neurogenic pulmonary oedema (NPE) represents the most severe form of ALI and is seen in cases of fatal or near fatal head injuries and after abrupt elevations in ICP. The exact mechanism responsible for this acute condition is unclear. Primary treatment consists of methods to reduce ICP and appropriate ventilation management, increasing inspired oxygen concentration, controlling carbon dioxide levels, and increasing PEEP to maximize oxygenation with minimal effect on ICP and cardiac output.

The development of non-cardiogenic pulmonary oedema, or adult respiratory distress syndrome (ARDS), complicates the management of severe TBI because many of the therapies used to protect the lungs can raise ICP or decrease CPP. Also the initial catecholamine storm following injury leads to pulmonary changes. The ventilatory strategies used to protect the lungs, such as reduced tidal volume, permissive hypoxemia and hypercarbia, increased levels of PEEP, and prone lying, pose problems for these patients, not only during the acute course of head injury when intracranial pressure may be high, but also in terms of delaying the early rehabilitation therapy which is essential to maximize recovery. The management of fluid balance, BP, and CPP can also be difficult issues. While aggressive CPP management (maintaining CPP > 70 mmHg) decreases the risk of brain ischaemia, it has been shown to increase the incidence of ARDS.

Following head injury, respiratory function may be depressed and a period of apnoea may have occurred at the accident resulting in atelectasis. Aspiration of gastric contents may also occur due to a decreased level of consciousness. Coma, prolonged bed rest, mechanical ventilation and sedation, and a diminished cough reflex make these patients extremely susceptible to pulmonary complications which could further compound their neurological status. Chest physiotherapy is essential in severe TBI patients. However, the care needed to prevent and treat these complications is often associated with significant increases in ICP. Provided that the patient's head and neck are kept in alignment side turning is advocated for chest management, and how long and how often they should remain on their side is determined by intracranial and cardiovascular stability.

Increasing sedation or administering a bolus of sedation may lessen the adverse effects of treatment, but timing is vital if it is to be effective as an adjunct to treatment. During suctioning and chest physiotherapy, the aim is to prevent hypoxaemia (current guidelines recommend a P_aO_2 of >13 kPa in severe TBI) and hypercarbia/hypocarbia and avoid excessive and prolonged increases in ICP. Patients should be pre-oxygenated with 100% O_2 prior to suctioning and, provided that their carbon dioxide levels are not already at the minimum limit, may be mildly hyperventilated. In most cases, the rise in ICP is temporary and returns to baseline in 30–60 s. Suction should be limited to a maximum of two to three passes of catheter in one session to avoid a cumulative effect on ICP.

Cardiovascular management

High levels of sympathetic activity and of circulating catecholamines after severe TBI can have an adverse effect on cardiac function. Cardiac abnormalities after severe TBI include atrial and ventricular arrhythmias, abnormalities of the QRS complex, T wave and ST segment, and QT prolongation, and are most common in patients with diffuse injury, oedema, and contusions. Life-threatening arrhythmias require prompt treatment; however, most cardiac arrhythmias in acute CNS disorders do not require therapeutic intervention.

An inotrope (usually noradrenaline (norepinephrine)) is required in most patients to counteract the hypotensive effects of sedation and facilitate CPP management.

Fluid management

Several factors need to be considered in the fluid management of patients following severe TBI, and these include clinical and laboratory assessment of volume status, the effects of different fluids on CPP and cerebral oedema, osmotic therapy, and water and electrolyte disturbances.

Following TBI the BBB is likely to be disrupted and different fluids can have an effect on cerebral oedema. If the serum osmolarity falls, water moves across the BBB along the altered osmotic gradient, causing cerebral oedema, increased ICP, and decreased CPP. Hypotonic fluids, therefore, should be avoided. Glucose-containing solutions should not be used in the fluid management of patients following severe TBI unless specifically indicated to correct hypoglycaemia (<4 mmol/l) since an increase in glucose levels in ischaemic brain allows anaerobic glycolysis to take place with accumulation of lactic acid. While tight glucose control in the general ICU patient population has shown improved outcome, current guidelines in head injury management advocate glucose levels be kept between 4 and 9 mmol/l. Disturbances of sodium and water balance are common following severe TBI, and accurate diagnosis and treatment is essential (see section on Management of sodium and water balance).

Nutrition

TBI patients have an induced hypermetabolic and hypercatabolic state resulting in increased energy and protein requirements. Early feeding, within hours of injury, is associated with improved clinical outcome and nutritional support should begin within 24 hours following injury, with enteral nutrition the feeding method of choice for nourishing this group of patients.

Several problems can affect the successful delivery of enteral nutrition to TBI patients on intensive care units. In the early stages following injury, delayed gastric emp-

tying/gastroparesis affecting the ability to tolerate feeds is more prolonged than found in patients suffering other types of trauma. In most cases this will improve by 3 weeks post-injury. The exact mechanism for gastroparesis in TBI is unclear but is thought to be related to either the head injury itself, the host of mediators released following cerebral injury, or raised ICP. In many circumstances, the sudden development of intolerance after a period of successful enteral feeding is probably due to a change in clinical status, such as deterioration in neurology or sepsis. In such cases, parenteral feeding may be necessary.

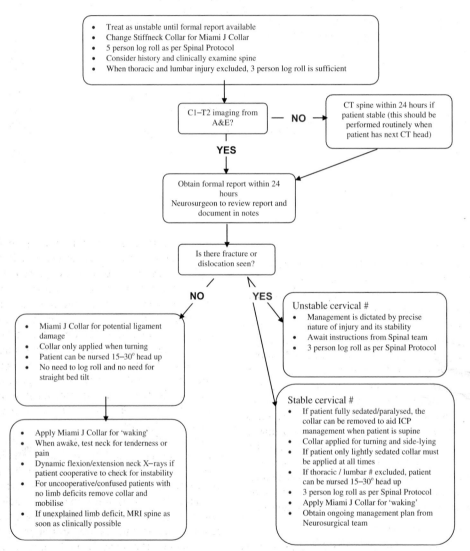

Fig. 10.9 Algorithm for the management of cervical spine in patients with severe TBI

Level of spine involved	Number of people required	Role of each person	Positioning
Multilevel - Cervico-thoracic and Thoraco-lumbar	Unstable – 5 Stable and fixed—moving and handling as for non-spinal patient	1- Head—Team leader 2- Upper body 3- Pelvis, upper thigh 4- Lower leg 5- Skin check, pillow person	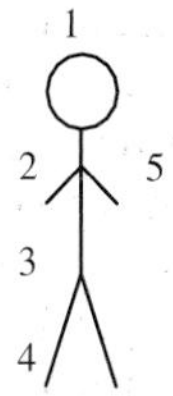
C1 to T4	Unstable – 3 Stable and fixed—moving and handling as for non-spinal patient	1- Head—Team leader 2- Upper body 3- Skin check, pillow person (cross patient's legs for turning)	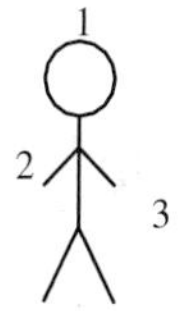
T4 to L5	Unstable – 4 Stable and fixed—moving and handling as for non-spinal patient	1- Upper body—Team leader 2- Pelvis, upper thigh 3- Lower leg 4- Skin check, pillow person	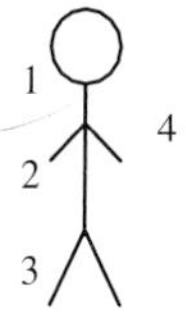

Fig. 10.9 Protocol for turning a spinal patient.

Posture and tone

Patients with neurological dysfunction resulting in abnormal posture and movement are at great risk of developing structural deformity and treatment must be initiated at the onset of neurological damage and continued for as long as the danger of secondary complications exists. The role of the physiotherapist in preventing long-term physical disability in the neurosurgical patient is crucial. Movements are regularly performed on patients who are unconscious in order to maintain muscle and joint range, and passive movements of the limbs may be performed once or twice a day as ICP allows. In addition, splinting of limbs may be required. Different postures and positions and their influence on tone and movement should be considered. For these patients rehabilitation starts from the moment of admission to the intensive care unit and early mobilization is a crucial factor in the rehabilitation process.

Protection of the cervical spine

All severe TBI patients are at risk of having sustained an associated cervical spine injury (Fig. 10.9). In unconscious or sedated patients clinical assessment cannot exclude cervical injury and therefore early diagnostic imaging is essential for patient management. Early imaging also prevents prolonged unnecessary immobilization, with its associated complications. If a fracture or dislocation is diagnosed, management is dictated by the precise nature of the injury and its stability. However, routine radiological examination cannot reliably exclude ligament injury, and in the unconscious patient a cervical collar is often kept in place until such injury can be ruled out. This may mean waiting until the patient has regained consciousness and can describe signs and symptoms.

Cervical collars can cause chin and occipital pressure sores from prolonged tight application and have been shown to occlude skin capillary pressure. They can also cause significant elevation of ICP by obstructing venous drainage. Once bony injury has been excluded, and provided the patient is adequately sedated, the collar can be removed and replaced briefly for turning and repositioning. The collar should be applied when sedation is being weaned and the patient 'woken'.

Management of the patient with subarachnoid haemorrhage (SAH)

Subarachnoid haemorrhage is defined as bleeding into the subarachnoid space (and therefore into the CSF) (Fig. 10.10). Cerebral arteries lie in the subarachnoid space and give off small perforating branches to the brain tissue, and therefore bleeding from these vessels or from an associated aneurysm occurs primarily into this space. Some intracranial aneurysms are embedded within the brain tissue and their rupture causes intracerebral bleeding with or without subarachnoid haemorrhage. Occasionally the arachnoid layer is disrupted and a subdural haematoma results. Following subarachnoid haemorrhage, blood within the CSF can disrupt the reabsorption of CSF and lead to secondary hydrocephalus.

The leading cause of SAH, accounting for about 60% of cases, is rupture of an intracranial saccular aneurysm, which is a dilatation in the wall of an artery, and usually occurs at the junction or bifurcation of arteries. (Other causes include arteriovenous malformation, hypertension, tumours, bleeding diathesis, anticoagulants. and idiopathic.)

The incidence of SAH increases with age, with the peak occurrence between 40 and 60 years and with a female to male ratio of 3:1. The aetiology of cerebral aneurysms remains unclear but several factors are implicated (congenital defects, degenerative change, and hypertension). Hypertension is not only a risk factor of bleeding but is also an unfavourable prognostic factor, increasing poor outcome from 5% to 32%. The cardinal symptom of SAH is the sudden onset of severe headache, present in up to 97% of patients, and this is often accompanied by vomiting.

Despite advances in subarachnoid haemorrhage management, the associated mortality and morbidity remain high with nearly half of the patients dying within 60 days of the initial bleed (ictus). Since management varies depending on the cause, for the purposes of this chapter the management of patients with aneurysmal subarachnoid haemorrhage only will be discussed.

Grading of SAH

The single most important independent predictor of outcome after aneurysmal rupture is the clinical status of the patient on admission after initial resuscitation and stabilisation. A number of clinical grading systems have been proposed and are used to guide treatment or predict morbidity and mortality. The World Federation of Neurological Surgeons (WFNS) Scale, with grading from I to V, uses the GCS to assess the level of consciousness and uses the presence or absence of major focal deficit to distinguish between grades II and III (Table 10.7). Therefore, a grade I SAH with a GCS of 15 is the best and grade V with a GCS of 6–3 is the worst.

Complications of SAH

Rebleeding

The commonest cause of early death after SAH is an immediate rebleed. Rebleeding can occur at any time but most frequently from the third to the eleventh day, with peak incidence around the seventh day after the original bleed. The mortality rate for patients who have a re-bleed from an aneurysm is 80%.

Cerebral vasospasm

Cerebral vasospasm is a leading cause of death and disability and is present in 20–30% of patients with aneurysmal subarachnoid haemorrhage. The presence of blood products around the large arteries at the base of the brain is the most likely cause of vasospasm. It typically occurs about 3–5 days following the initial bleed but onset may be delayed up to 21 days, with the highest risk period between days 3 and 14. The risk of vasospasm is related to the amount of blood on CT, the patient's condition (WFNS Grade I has a 20% risk, WFNS

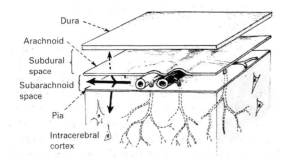

Fig. 10.10 Subarachnoid space. Reprinted from Lindsay, K.W. and Bone, I. (2004) *Neurology and Neurosurgery Illustrated*, with permission from Elsevier.

TABLE 10.7	WFNS Subarachnoid Haemorrhage Grading Scale	
WFNS grade	**GCS score**	**Motor deficit**
I	15	Absent/present
II	14–13	Absent
III	14–13	Present
IV	12–7	Present or absent
V	6–3	Present or absent

Grade V a 75% risk) and the location of the aneurysm (more common with anterior communicating artery aneurysm than with middle cerebral artery aneurysm).

Hydrocephalus

Hydrocephalus occurs when blood impairs either the reabsorption of CSF (communicating) or the intraventricular flow of CSF (non-communicating) and it can develop either acutely (within the first few days) or chronically (in the second week) following SAH. Acute hydrocephalus carries a poor prognosis, and when it causes acute deterioration in conscious level requires urgent CSF drainage with an external ventricular drain.

Seizures

The highest risk of seizures is within the first 24 hours following the SAH but they may occur at any stage, especially if a haematoma has caused cortical damage. Seizures may be generalized or focal. Anti-epileptic medication is not normally prescribed for a first seizure.

Diagnosis of SAH

◆ *Computed tomography* (CT) is the first-line investigation to confirm the diagnosis of SAH. It can also show associated problems such as hydrocephalus and intracerebral haematoma and may help identify the site of an aneurysm.

◆ *Lumbar puncture* is only used when CT imaging is negative but the patient has a history suggestive of SAH. Lumbar puncture commonly reveals an elevated opening pressure with release of blood-stained CSF that does not clear with sequential samples. Xanthochromia (yellow coloration) may take 24 to 46 hours to develop but can be present within 6 hours of the bleed.

◆ *Digital subtraction angiography* (DSA) is the definitive investigation for the identification of aneurysms and for treatment planning. Fifteen to 20% of cases will have a normal angiogram and the aetiology of the haemorrhage in these cases is unclear, but may be due to venous haemorrhage.

◆ *CT angiography* is useful in the unstable patient requiring craniotomy for aneurysmal intracerebral haemorrhage before a cerebral angiogram can be performed.

Cerebral angiography (ideally four-vessel) should be performed within 24 hours of admission and a treatment plan made. The treatment plan would broadly fall into one of three categories: (i) early treatment (clipping/coiling); (ii) late treatment (clipping/coiling) or (iii) no treatment (conservative management).

Treatment

The neurosurgeon, in consultation with the neuroradiologist, will determine which therapeutic option, either surgery (clipping of the aneurysm) or endovascular (coiling of the aneurysm), is most appropriate for each patient. Factors influencing their decision include the site, size, and shape of the aneurysm and the condition of the patient.

Surgical treatment

The ideal goal of surgical treatment is to place a clip across the neck of the aneurysm to exclude it from the circulation. Timing of surgery remains the most controversial aspect of treatment and will depend on the surgeon and the patient. The surgeon has to decide in each case whether to operate early (days 0–3) or to delay surgery until after day 10, both avoiding the highest risk period for vasospasm. Early surgery eliminates the risk of rebleeding and also enables intensive management of vasospasm without danger of aneurysm rupture.

Endovascular treatment

Endovascular coiling (using Gugliemi detachable coils) is being increasingly used as an alternative to surgical clipping. This procedure is minimally invasive and can be carried out at the same time as diagnostic angiography. The approach is via the femoral artery, where a microcatheter is navigated to the aneurysm site and coils are then deposited within the aneurysm sac, sufficient to obliterate it. The coils cause thrombosis by inducing flow stagnation within the aneurysm.

Management of the patient with SAH in the ICU

The main aim in the early management of SAH is stabilization of the patient with optimization for aneurysm obliteration, together with the prevention of secondary cerebral insults. Initial priorities include adequate ventilation and oxygenation, haemodynamic stability, and control of raised intracranial pressure (ICP).

Neurology

Early detection and treatment of a developing neurological deficit may prevent progression from ischaemia to infarction in the SAH patient. The significance of changes, however small, should never be overlooked, e.g. mild weakness, arm drift, dysphasia. Therefore, wherever possible the patient should be clinically assessable. If the patient cannot be assessed clinically (i.e. when sedation is required to facilitate ventilation) then ICP monitoring may be indicated, with a target ICP of 20–25 mmHg and a CPP of 60 mmHg (although the evidence for this is taken from studies in TBI). In most instances if an external ventricular drain is required to treat secondary hydrocephalus there is no need for an ICP bolt to be inserted. However, it may be indicated in some SAH patients with massive intraventricular bleeding where drain function is difficult to assess.

Neurological deterioration, such as a drop in GCS or a focal deficit, in a patient with an untreated aneurysm may be the result of rebleeding, an expanding intracerebral haematoma, vasospasm, or evolving hydrocephalus. Once the aneurysm has been treated such neurological deterioration is likely to be due to either vasospasm or hydrocephalus.

Nimodipine

Nimodipine, a calcium antagonist, has been shown to significantly lower the incidence of deaths caused by delayed cerebral ischaemia and significantly lower the occurrence of cerebral infarcts in patients with aneurysmal subarachnoid haemorrhage and has become standard therapy in the prophylactic treatment of cerebral vasospasm in these patients (Table 10.8).

Respiratory management

Respiratory problems following SAH are a common complication. Neurogenic pulmonary oedema occurs particularly in patients in coma, and in patients with fatal SAH. Cardiogenic pulmonary oedema may be the result of SAH-induced cardiac failure or as a consequence of intensive management.

As in TBI, these patients often need advanced respiratory support in the acute stage. However, there are important differences in their respiratory management. Ventilation should be adjusted to maintain a $P_aO_2 > 13$ kPa and a normal P_aCO_2, not less than 4.5 kPa. Patients with SAH should not be hyperventilated due to the added risk of ischaemia from vasospasm. If sedation is required to facilitate ventilation, any hypotensive side-effects should be avoided with adequate volume expansion and inotropes if necessary. Sedation or neuromuscular blockade should be adequate to prevent an intubated patient with an untreated aneurysm coughing on the ET tube, due to the hypertension and raised ICP that this can induce.

A patient with an untreated aneurysm often needs to be 'woken' and extubated quickly. If extubation is not possible an early tracheostomy may need to be considered to enable sedation to be stopped in order to clinically assess the patient to determine future management.

Cardiovascular management

Cardiac changes in the acute stage following SAH are common and can range from asymptomatic ECG changes to significant life-threatening changes. These changes are attributed to high levels of circulating catecholamines, injury to the posterior hypothalamus, and blood in the CSF affecting brainstem centres and do not necessarily mean poor myocardial function.

ECG abnormalities are common following SAH and are particularly prevalent in the poorer grades. Cardiac changes include SVT, VT, bundle branch block, and sinus arrhythmias. Such arrhythmias usually occur within 48 hours of the onset of SAH but can be delayed for 1 or 2 weeks and can persist for up to 6 weeks post-bleed. In the acute phase pharmacological management should be implemented with care since many of the changes are very brief and aggressive management may lead to a prolonged opposite effect or reduce blood pressure to unwanted levels.

Reactive arterial hypertension for 24 to 48 hours following SAH is common, most probably due to catecholamine release. Extremes of blood pressure should be avoided but account taken of the normal BP for individual patients. High BP in a patient with an untreated aneurysm is more likely to cause a rebleed, and a low BP will exacerbate hypoxic or ischaemic cerebral damage from vasospasm.

Blood pressure management in the patient with an untreated aneurysm

The patient's normal BP should be maintained as far as possible, treating hypotension initially with fluids. Inotropes (usually noradrenaline (norepinephrine)) are

TABLE 10.8	Nimodipine in subarachnoid haemorrhage	
	Oral/nasogastric	**Intravenous (only administered IV if patient not absorbing NG)**
Dose	60 mg	Initial rate of 1mg/hour for first hour. Increased to 2 mg/hour if BP adequate
Timing	4-hourly from diagnosis for 21 days	Continuous infusion
Side-effects	Hypotension can occur in some patients and if so it should be given in divided doses of 30 mg/2-hourly. NB: Nimodipine should never be omitted	Irritant to blood vessels and must be given into a central line and run concurrently with 40 ml/hour normal saline via a dedicated lumen

used only if circulation or urine output cannot be maintained by fluid replacement alone and care should be taken to avoid hypertension and the sudden drop or surge in blood pressure that can occur during pump changes. Gross hypertension should be treated using a short-acting agent, preferably intravenously to allow careful titration (e.g. labetalol) since patients on antihypertensive agents have a significantly higher risk of cerebral infarction.

Blood pressure management once the aneurysm has been treated (clipped or coiled)

Blood pressure management should be guided primarily by the neurological status of the patient aiming for a 'high-normal' BP. Hypertensive therapy including inotropes should be used only as part of a Triple H regime in the presence of clinical vasospasm. Triple H therapy (Hypertensive Hypervolaemic Haemodilution) is a therapeutic approach to prevent delayed ischaemic deficit (DID) by improving CBF using fluids and inotropes to increase MAP, increase circulating volume, and reduce blood viscosity.

Pain management

Headache experienced at the time of SAH is often described as explosive and in the first 48 hours may continue to be intense due to meningeal irritation and raised intracranial pressure. The distress it causes often increases BP to dangerous levels and increases the risk of rebleeding. Effective management of pain and nausea is essential and may calm an otherwise agitated patient. Paracetamol and dihydrocodeine are most commonly used and should be prescribed regularly. Morphine should also be prescribed, ideally by patient-controlled infusion (PCA) in suitable patients. The use of non-steroidal anti-inflammatory drugs (NSAIDs) is not recommended for a patient with an untreated aneurysm as their antiplatelet effects can increase the risk of rebleeding. However, once the aneurysm has been treated NSAIDs may be considered.

Fluid and electrolyte balance

SAH patients are normally maintained on 3 litres of fluid in 24 hours (2 litres normal saline and 1 litre colloid). As in TBI patients, dextrose-containing solutions are avoided and blood glucose is controlled between 4 and 9 mmol/l. Depleted volume states require close monitoring and treatment in view of the risk of cerebral vasospasm following SAH and treatment should aim for a normal/high CVP.

As with TBI patients, disturbances of water and electrolyte balance can occur following SAH. Hyponatraemia (serum sodium < 135 mmol/l) has an associated morbidity and mortality if left untreated. Cerebral salt wasting (CSW) and Syndrome of Inappropriate Antidiuretic Hormone (SIADH) are the two commonest causes and their distinction is important since CSW has an associated depleted circulating volume making spasm a great risk. Diabetes insipidus (DI) is particularly associated with anterior circulation aneurysms. It can also present post-operatively in these patients (see section Management of sodium and water balance).

Nutrition

As in TBI, nutritional support should be commenced as soon as possible.

Positioning

Forced bed rest is a traditional part of SAH management, with patients nursed flat or with head elevation of 15° if there are respiratory complications. Since subcutaneous heparin is not recommended in SAH patients, DVT prophylaxis consists of graduated elastic stockings and mechanical calf compression. Once the aneurysm has been treated, there are no restrictions on mobilizing the patient as their condition allows, except in the case of patients who have been fully anticoagulated following endovascular treatment when some restrictions may apply.

Management of the patient with generalized convulsive status epilepticus

Epilepsy is a condition characterized by periodic disturbances of brain electrical activity that can lead to seizures, loss of consciousness, and sensory disturbances. Any of the classified seizure types can progress to status epilepticus. However, since generalized convulsive status is the form most commonly seen, this section will focus on its management.

Status epilepticus (SE) is a clinical term referring to a series of generalized seizures without recovery of consciousness between attacks lasting for at least 30 min. SE is usually easily diagnosed by observation, with seizures characterized by loss of consciousness, tonic (ongoing) and/or clonic (rhythmic) muscle activity, tongue

---

TRIPLE-H REGIME

- ◆ Hypertensive: MAP 100–110 mmHg
- ◆ Hypervolaemic: CVP 8–15 mmHg
- ◆ Haemodilution: haematocrit 0.3–0.34

biting, and urinary incontinence. However, it is important to note that as the duration of seizures increases convulsive activity may become less obvious as depleted cerebral oxygen supplies are unable to meet demand (electromechanical dissociation), with perhaps only subtle twitching remaining as an outward sign that seizures persist.

Algorithm for treatment of Status Epilepticus

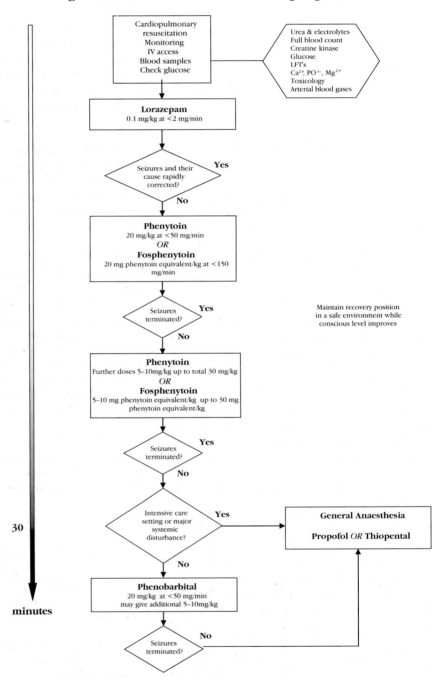

Fig. 10.11 Algorithm for the treatment of status epilepticus. From Chapman, M.G. *et al.* (2001) *Anaesthesia*, **56**, 652, with permission from Blackwell Publishing.

Causes of SE include:

- metabolic abnormalities
- central nervous system infection (e.g. encephalitis, meningitis)
- vascular brain injury
- traumatic brain injury
- drug toxicity (e.g. cocaine, alcohol)
- cerebral anoxic/hypoxic damage
- pre-existing epilepsy
- non-compliance or withdrawal of anticonvulsant drug therapy
- chronic alcoholism
- cerebral tumours/space-occupying lesions.

Management

SE carries a high risk of mortality and morbidity and is therefore a medical emergency, requiring prompt action. Management should be directed at terminating the seizures, preventing recurrence of seizures once status is controlled, investigating and managing the precipitating causes of SE, and managing the potentially serious and cumulative complications of SE.

Many patients will respond to first-line treatment with benzodiazepines; however, it should be noted that all anti-epileptic medication is sedative in nature, therefore these patients will need nursing in a high-dependency environment that has access to resuscitation equipment. In addition, these patients should be nursed in the recovery position, given oxygen therapy, and have continuous ECG, BP, and pulse oximetry monitoring. Steps should be taken to reduce the risk of self-harm/injury occurring during the seizures by removing all unnecessary equipment from the immediate vicinity of the patient.

Figure 10.11 is an algorithm showing the suggested treatment cycle of anti-epileptic drugs that should be considered. If the patient fails to respond to this treatment plan they should be considered to be in refractory status and transferred to the intensive care unit. During prolonged status (60–90 min) the outward signs of motor activity diminish despite the presence of continued electrographic seizures and the patient will require sedation with general anaesthetic agents, thus requiring that the patient be intubated and ventilated. Management is aimed at suppressing this activity by titrating the anaesthetic agents to the neurophysiological monitoring, usually recorded on a portable EEG

monitor, until burst suppression of such activity is achieved. Full supportive treatment of the intubated patient is needed until the seizures stop and they regain consciousness.

Management of the patient with myasthenia gravis

Myasthenia gravis (MG), derived from the Greek for 'severe muscle weakness', is an autoimmune disease of varying severity characterized by relapses and spontaneous remissions. Its incidence is about 1 in 20 000 of the adult population and it is more prominent among women in their second to third decade and among men during their sixth to seventh decade. Without treatment, 20–30% of myasthenics will die from the disease, 39–50% improve spontaneously, and the remainder continue to worsen or remain symptomatic. Its cause is unknown, but the thymus gland may play some role in the autoimmune process since 80% of MG patients have thymic hyperplasia and 15% have thymic tumours.

Pathophysiology

MG affects the neuromuscular junction (Fig. 10.12), specifically the acetylcholine (ACh) receptor sites. Neurotransmission relies on the release of ACh into the neuromuscular junction and its subsequent binding to receptors on the post-synaptic membrane, triggering muscle contraction. The enzyme acetylcholinesterase (AChE) then rapidly breaks down the ACh allowing the muscle to relax. In MG the immune system generates antibodies that bind to these receptor sites, interfering with normal transmission, making it less effective or causing it to fail completely.

Signs and symptoms

The disorder is characterized by weakness and fatigability of voluntary muscles; it typically involves the muscles of the eye, face, and mouth. Skeletal muscles

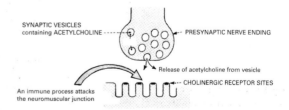

Fig. 10.12 The neuromuscular junction. Reprinted from Lindsay, K.W. and Bone, I. (2004) *Neurology and Neurosurgery Illustrated*, with permission from Elsevier.

can also be affected and in severe cases weakness of the muscles of swallowing and respiration can be life-threatening. The severity of muscle weakness fluctuates, typically worsening with repeated or sustained exertion or towards the end of the day, and is relieved by rest.

Classic signs and symptoms include:

◆ Ocular problems of ptosis and diplopia.

◆ Facial weakness.

◆ Bulbar weakness—difficulty swallowing and managing saliva.

◆ Dysarthria—voice nasal and weak and fades when talking.

◆ Weakness and fatigability of skeletal muscle exacerbated by exercise and worsening as the day goes on.

◆ Loss of strength in limbs—arms more affected than legs and proximal muscles more affected than distal muscles.

◆ Neck muscle weakness with head falling forward.

◆ Respiratory muscle weakness (not usually affected in isolation).

Diagnosis

Diagnosis is based on history, physical examination, electromyography (EMG), which may include diaphragmatic EMG, and confirmatory laboratory testing which should include anticholinesterase drug testing (Tensilon test) and detection of the anti-ACh receptor antibodies. Additionally, MRI/CT scan may be carried out to determine if the thymus gland is enlarged.

The edrophonium chloride (Tensilon) test

Administration of edrophonium chloride is a diagnostic test for MG and produces rapid, but brief, return of muscular power. Edrophonium chloride is a short-acting cholinesterase inhibitor. By decreasing the amount of cholinesterase, edrophonium makes more ACh available to the ACh receptors, thus improving muscle strength. In addition to being used in the diagnosis of MG, it is also used to distinguish between myasthenic crisis, where there is ACh deficiency, and cholinergic crisis, where there is an excess of ACh due to overdose with anticholinesterase drugs.

Edrophonium is administered in incremental doses until clear improvement is seen and is sometimes given as a 'blind' or 'double-blind' test to make the test more objective. Any cholinergic drug can have adverse cardiac effects, such as bradycardia and arrhythmias, and

respiratory effects, such as respiratory muscle weakness, brochospasm, laryngospasm, and increased bronchial secretions. The Tensilon test should, therefore, be carried out by skilled personnel and in an environment that can facilitate emergency respiratory and cardiovascular management. Atropine, the antidote to the muscarinic side-effects of edrophonium, should be available during testing.

Treatment

There is no single therapy that works best for all patients therefore treatment is based on the individual's response to specific therapies:

1. Symptomatic therapy with anticholinesterase agents:
   pyridostigmine (Mestinon)
   neostigmine (rarely used).

2. Disease-modifying approaches:
   immunosuppressant drugs—corticosteroids (e.g. prednisolone), azathioprine
   thymectomy
   plasma exchange (PE)
   intravenous immunoglobulin (IVIg).

Cholinesterase (ChE) inhibitors

Cholinesterase inhibitors delay the breakdown of ACh at cholinergic synapses allowing ACh to accumulate at the neuromuscular junction with prolonged effect. They may also have a direct agonist effect on ACh receptor sites. While they produce dramatic improvement in some patients, treatment with these drugs alone rarely produces normal strength. Pyridostigmine is the drug of choice since it has a long half-life and fewer gastrointestinal side-effects.

Corticosteroids

Prednisolone is given until sustained improvement is seen and this is usually within 3–4 weeks. The drug is then given on alternate days and the dose is gradually reduced over months to the lowest level necessary to maintain improvement. Worsening of symptoms occurs in 50% of patients after commencing prednisolone and this may result in severe bulbar and respiratory muscle weakness sometimes requiring tracheal intubation and ventilation.

Other immunosuppressant drugs

Azathioprine produces improvement in most patients after 4 months but may not show significantly until up to 12 months. Improvement persists for as long as the drug is given, but weakness may return 2 to 3 months after the drug is stopped or the dose is reduced.

Thymectomy

The thymus gland is thought to be responsible for the production of autoantibodies in MG. In 75% of patients the thymus will be hyperplastic and 10% will have a tumour (thymoma). Thymectomy produces best results in young patients with a short history of MG and in the absence of a thymoma. Thymectomy as a treatment for MG should always be an elective procedure with the patient's MG well stabilized prior to surgery. Response to thymectomy may take up to 2 years to show improvement in the patient, with the ultimate aim of maintaining them on lower doses of immunosuppressive medication.

Plasma exchange (PE) and intravenous immunoglobulin (IVIg) therapy

PE and IVIg therapy can be used to produce a rapid but short-term improvement of severe symptoms. Almost all patients will improve after PE. Improvement may begin after the first exchange and is seen within 48 hours

in most patients, continuing for weeks or months after a course of PE.

Management of the myasthenic patient in the ICU

The ICU management will vary depending on whether admission is the result of an acute deterioration in a patient with known MG or new onset in a previously undiagnosed MG patient. In severely ill patients the first priority is to maintain adequate ventilation and protection of the airway.

The development of respiratory insufficiency in MG is due to respiratory muscle weakness as a result of neuromuscular dysfunction and may be complicated by aspiration pneumonia secondary to bulbar weakness. Hypoxaemia, decreased tidal volume, dyspnoea, and abnormal arterial blood gases are all late findings in neuromuscular respiratory failure and are poor indicators of the need for ventilatory support. A more sensitive indicator of progressive respiratory failure is the forced vital capacity (FVC). As the FVC falls, sponta-

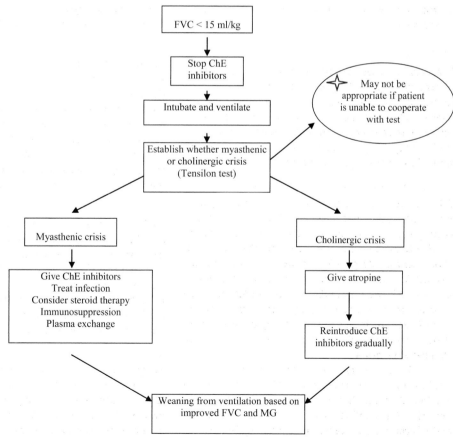

Fig. 10.13 Myasthenic or cholinergic crisis?

neous coughing weakens and there is greater difficulty clearing secretions. Tracheal intubation is generally performed if FVC drops below 15 ml/kg but may be undertaken at a higher FVC if the patient also has bulbar weakness.

When there is an acute deterioration in a known myasthenic, it is vital to distinguish between *myasthenic crisis* and *cholinergic crisis* (Fig. 10.13). The usual cause of myasthenic crisis is infection and the signs and symptoms are those of myasthenia. Cholinergic crisis is caused by over-medication with anticholinesterase drugs and symptoms include abdominal cramping and diarrhoea (muscarinic effects) and profound generalized weakness, excessive pulmonary secretions, and impaired respiratory function (nicotinic effects).

Both are medical emergencies that require prompt tracheal intubation and assisted ventilation. The Tensilon test may reveal whether the patient is over- or underdosed with anticholinesterase drugs, but its use in crisis may not be appropriate since the patient may not be able to cooperate with the test procedure. Delay in intubating the patient while the test is carried out may prove life-threatening. Management should consist of discontinuing all ChE inhibitors and intubating and ventilating the patient as necessary. Any underlying cause of myasthenic crisis, such as infection or electrolyte abnormalities (in particular hypokalaemia, hypocalcaemia, and hypermagnesemia), should be treated. ChE inhibitors should be resumed at a dose lower than before the crisis and gradually increased.

Drug reactions and myasthenia gravis

A number of drugs (including some aminoglycoside antibiotics) exacerbate the blockade at the neuromuscular junction and the use of all drugs must be carefully considered. Some drugs, such as antispasmodics, carry a warning against their use in MG. The decision to extubate a patient with MG after an anaesthetic should be taken with caution.

Management of the patient with Guillain–Barré syndrome

Guillain–Barré syndrome (GBS) is the commonest cause of acute neuromuscular paralysis in the UK with an annual incidence of between 1 and 2 per 100 000 of the population. Despite advances in the treatment and intensive care management of these patients, between 3% and 8% die as a result of potentially avoidable complications, including respiratory failure, respiratory or cardiac arrest, sepsis, pulmonary embolism, or the gen-

eral medical complications of intensive care. A further 10% remain severely disabled up to 1 year later.

Pathophysiology

GBS is an acute inflammatory neuropathy affecting the peripheral nervous system. The underlying pathology is usually demyelination, with secondary axonal degeneration in the most severely affected cases. Two-thirds of patients describe an infectious illness in the 4 weeks prior to the onset of symptoms, suggesting that there is an immune basis for the inflammatory process. Bacterial and viral agents have been implicated and these include *Campylobacter jejuni*, *Mycoplasma pneumoniae*, Epstein–Barr virus, human immunodeficiency virus, and cytomegalovirus.

Signs and symptoms

Neurology

GBS patients usually present with weakness and mild sensory symptoms (usually glove and stocking paraesthesiae). Typically, weakness starts from the feet up and, depending on severity, can gradually involve the rest of the body. Cranial nerves (in particular facial and bulbar) are commonly affected. Areflexia (loss of tendon jerks) is an early sign. In most cases weakness is maximal 3 weeks after the onset of neurological symptoms. Recovery usually begins 2 to 4 weeks after progression of weakness stops, but may, depending on severity, be delayed for months.

Respiratory

Respiratory muscle weakness requiring positive pressure ventilation occurs in 25–30% of patients. Bulbar dysfunction occurs in a similar proportion of GBS patients and may require tracheal intubation for airway protection.

Autonomic dysfunction

Autonomic dysfunction (dysautonomia) is extremely common in GBS patients and occurs in some form in 65% of patients. Sympathetic overactivity resulting in persistent tachycardia and hypertension is the most commonly seen manifestation, although severe parasympathetic manifestations may occur.

Diagnosis

The criteria for diagnosis include history of presenting symptoms (progressive weakness of more than one limb with the duration of progression less than 4 weeks), clinical assessment (areflexia), laboratory studies of CSF (increased protein concentration with normal or only slightly raised white cell count) and blood (viral studies may reveal rising titres to specific viruses), and nerve conduction studies (electromyography (EMG) will show slowed nerve conduction suggesting demyelination).

Treatment

1. *Supportive measures*: good general medical and nursing care; intensive care management; rehabilitation

2. *Specific therapy*: plasma exchange; intravenous immunoglobulin.

Plasma exchange (PE) and intravenous immuno-globulin (IVIg) therapy have been found to be equally effective in promoting recovery from GBS. PE and IVIg are most effective within 1 week of the onset of symptoms or when there has been rapid deterioration in limb power. Due to the ease of administration, IVIg is now the treatment of choice.

Management of the patient with Guillain–Barré syndrome in the ICU

Up to 28% of all GBS cases present with a mild course of the disease, remaining able to walk unaided throughout. Three things will determine whether the remainder will require intensive care management—respiratory failure, bulbar involvement, and autonomic dysfunction.

Respiratory failure

Close monitoring of respiratory function is essential to predict the respiratory needs of this group of patients and is usually done by monitoring the FVC. When the FVC falls to between 15 and 20 ml/kg elective intubation should be considered. Likewise, when the recovering FVC reaches 20 ml/kg weaning is usually commenced. Intubation is often difficult in GBS patients due to autonomic instability. Bulbar dysfunction may require early intubation for airway protection even if the FVC remains adequate. Early tracheostomy should be considered if it is obvious that a prolonged period of artificial ventilation will be required.

Autonomic dysfunction

Autonomic dysfunction is usually benign and does not require any specific therapeutic intervention. However, close monitoring in an intensive care unit is usually required to detect any life-threatening instability. Autonomic instability can cause extreme sensitivity to the effects of drugs, in particular sedatives, analgesics, and inotropes. Postural hypotension and bradycardia induced by vagal stimulation on suctioning are common.

A persistent tachycardia (>120 bpm) is usually treated with short-acting drugs. Severe blood pressure swings should be treated symptomatically with colloid for hypotension and cautious antihypertensive therapy for persistent elevations in blood pressure. Pressor drugs need to be used with great caution and only prolonged hypertensive episodes are treated, using short-acting agents. Delivery of nursing and therapy care should be observed for the effect it may have on the autonomic status of the patient, especially those interventions which may stimulate the autonomic nervous system, such as tracheal suction and chest physiotherapy.

Pain

Pain is a common problem arising from immobility, inflamed nerves, and denervated muscles and it is often refractory to simple analgesics. Pain is often severe, usually neurogenic, and worse with remyelination of the nerves. Types of pain include paraesthesia (tingling, stinging, pins and needles), dysaesthesia (burning), backache and sciatica, meningism (meningeal irritation from swollen nerve roots), joint pain, and occasionally visceral pain (related to autonomic dysfunction). This can be compounded by problems of proprioception in some patients, making symptom relief difficult. Management requires thoughtful use of several types of analgesics. Simple analgesics and NSAIDs may be effective in relieving musculoskeletal symptoms and paracetamol and NSAIDs should be prescribed routinely. Anticonvulsant agents such as gabapentin are effective for paraesthesia and dysaesthesia, while tricyclic antidepressants such as amitriptyline are effective for neurogenic pain. Opioids (e.g. meptazinol) may be required if pain persists.

Sleep

Pain is exacerbated by poor sleep patterns and disorientation caused by the ICU environment. Many patients during the rehabilitation period describe periods of vivid and disturbing dreams, occurring both during the day and at night. Reorientating the patient and giving reassurance can help reduce anxiety and helps promote relaxation prior to sleep. GBS patients often benefit from regular night sedation and access to 'breakthrough' analgesia.

Positioning/rehabilitation

Careful positioning, and passive full-range joint movements can prevent contractures, and physiotherapy input is crucial to address these issues. In addition, intermittent splinting of limbs (wrists, fingers, and ankles) may be needed. A graduated programme, which involves sitting the patient up in bed and on a tilt table to ensure that postural changes can be tolerated, is usually required before the patient can sit out of bed. Positioning can be compromised by the need for head and trunk support and a fully supportive, semi-reclining wheelchair with pressure-relieving cushions is essential.

Communication

The GBS patient presents a challenge in achieving effective communication. Acute GBS, where the patient finds himself paralysed, requiring mechanical ventilation, and totally dependent on others, gives rise to understandable fear and anxiety. Sedation is usually given for the first 24 to 48 hours following intubation but is not appropriate after this period. Early intervention from a speech and language therapist will help identify the most appropriate aids to communication for individual patients. Patients with intact bulbar function can be taught to use a speaking valve with tracheostomy cuff deflation, while patients with impaired bulbar function will need to rely on a blink response to an alphabet board or picture cards in the early stages. If is seems likely that the disease process will be a lengthy one then early tracheostomy will aid lip reading (see Chapter 3).

Management of the patient with acute infection and inflammation of the central nervous system

Any infection of the CNS can have potentially devastating consequences and requires immediate medical attention. Patients often need admission to an intensive care unit for urgent airway protection, mechanical ventilation, and control of raised ICP. They may also require intensive care management for seizure control or because agitation makes them difficult to manage, necessitating sedation and respiratory monitoring.

The infection can be regional (i.e. meningitis), diffuse (i.e. encephalitis), or focal (i.e. brain abscess), and the clinical presentation will vary depending on which part of the CNS is affected. Meningitis is characterized by fever, headache, and neck stiffness, encephalitis is primarily characterized by altered mental status, and brain abscess gives rise to focal deficits. Meningitis is more common than either encephalitis or brain abscess. In meningitis and encephalitis, either syndrome can be accompanied by some features of the other and most cases of meningitis are complicated by some degree of inflammation of the brain tissue (sometimes termed meningoencephalitis).

Meningitis

Meningitis denotes an inflammation of the meninges, usually the arachnoid and pia mater, and the intervening subarachnoid space. There are three main types of meningitis: viral (e.g. herpes simplex virus), bacterial (e.g. *Neisseria meningitides*, *Streptococcus pneumoniae*, *Haemophilus influenzae*), and others (e.g. tuberculous, fungal). The majority of viral causes of meningitis are usually self-limiting, resolve spontaneously with only supportive treatment, and the patient makes a full recovery. Other forms of meningitis, in particular bacterial meningitis, constitute a serious and life-threatening illness. Even with modern treatment, there is significant mortality and of those who survive many will have complications of hydrocephalus, blindness, deafness, cognitive deficits, or epilepsy.

Signs and symptoms

There are certain features common to all types of meningitis, but the speed at which they develop and their intensity will vary depending on the causative organism. Meningitis is not always obvious and some cases may not show the preceding 'typical' signs (this is particularly so with babies). Bacterial meningitis may strike suddenly with the patient lapsing into coma within hours before other symptoms are established. If infection is confined to the spinal meninges the CSF may be purulent without either disturbance of consciousness or even headache. Tuberculous meningitis and cryptococcal meningitis are insidious in onset and the presenting symptoms may not arouse suspicion of meningitis.

More typically the illness is preceded by a respiratory infection, otitis media, or pneumonia, or by a few days of pyrexia and a vague influenza-like state. This is followed by severe frontal/occipital headache, photophobia, drowsiness, and, on examination, non-blanching rash and neck stiffness which is the vital sign of meningeal irritation. This is demonstrated by attempting to bend the head forward so that the chin rests on the chest—neck rigidity will prevent this. In addition, attempting to straighten the knee when the hip is flexed will be painful and restricted (positive Kernig's sign) (Fig. 10.14).

Diagnosis

Diagnosis includes patient history and examination, blood culture, and CSF analysis. Immediate treatment is crucial and lumbar puncture is essential to establish the diagnosis. Patients in coma, with focal neurological signs, or with papilloedema must first undergo CT scanning to exclude a mass lesion prior to lumbar puncture. If CT scanning is not immediately available it is essential to commence antibiotics after taking blood samples for culture rather than risk a significant, and perhaps

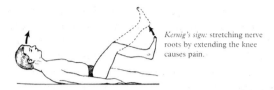

Kernig's sign: stretching nerve roots by extending the knee causes pain.

Fig. 10.14 Signs of meningism. Reprinted from Lindsay, K.W. and Bone, I. (2004) *Neurology and Neurosurgery Illustrated*, with permission from Elsevier.

fatal, delay in initiating treatment. CSF results from lumbar puncture may show a moderate increase in pressure, raised white cell count, raised protein, and a normal or low glucose level.

Viral meningitis

Viral meningitis is caused by a number of different viruses, the commonest being the enteroviruses, spread by the faecal-oral route (common in summer/autumn) and arboviruses (arthropod-borne viruses), transmitted by mosquito bite or tick bite (common in summer/autumn), but often the organism responsible remains unknown. With international travel, tropical viral diseases cannot be excluded and a good history of the patient will establish if this is relevant or not. The onset and symptoms of viral meningitis are similar to the bacterial forms but are usually less severe.

Treatment

Aciclovir is active against herpes simplex virus and should be started immediately. Following this, management is purely supportive and antibiotics are not appropriate. The course of the illness is self-limiting and recovery usually begins within 7–14 days.

Tuberculous meningitis

Tuberculous meningitis is caused by the tubercle bacillus. It may be a primary meningitis but often it is a secondary manifestation of tuberculosis elsewhere in the body, most commonly the lungs The primary lesion may have gone unrecognized and the patient may have been unwell for weeks with gradually increasing headache and listlessness. Untreated tuberculous meningitis may progress over a period of 3 weeks from the non-specific symptoms of fever and lethargy to coma and death.

Treatment

Tuberculous meningitis is treated with the anti-tuberculous drugs rifampicin, isoniazid, and pyrazinamide, the latter two drugs being able to penetrate the meninges. Treatment is normally for 6 months or longer.

Bacterial meningitis

Bacterial meningitis results from invasion of pus-forming bacteria, the commonest being meningococci, pneumococci, and *Haemophilus* (in infants the commonest causes are group B streptococcus and *Escherichia coli*). The onset is acute with bacteria invading the subarachnoid space either directly from adjoining structures such as sinuses or indirectly from the bloodstream. Bacterial meningitis can be fatal or leave the patient with a severe handicap such as deafness or brain injury.

In the UK there are two main types of bacterial meningitis which cause most of the reported bacterial cases, and they are meningococcal and pneumococcal meningitis. *Haemophilus influenzae* type B meningitis (Hib) has been almost eliminated by vaccination of infants.

Meningococcal meningitis (caused by the bacterium *Neisseria meningitidis*) is the most common bacterial form in the UK, accounting for more than half the cases. It is spread by droplet infection and the organism lodges and multiplies in the nasopharynx. It enters the bloodstream giving rise to a generalized septicaemia, pyrexia, and malaise. Invasion of the meninges causes rapidly worsening headache, neck stiffness, and deepening drowsiness. There may be signs of cerebral irritability, photophobia, increased tendon reflexes, vomiting, and generalized or focal seizures may occur. Additionally, a non-blanching haemorrhagic rash may be seen. Meningococcal meningitis is primarily an epidemic disorder, appearing when young people are crowded together. Septicaemia is particularly associated with meningococcal meningitis with about 55% of patients having both meningitis and septicaemia.

Pneumococcal meningitis (caused by the bacterium *Streptococcus pneumoniae*) is indicative of a secondary invasion of the meninges from an adjacent infected site or the result of a bacteraemia. Recent pneumonia, sepsis in the middle ear or sinuses, and a fractured base of skull are frequent causes. It accounts for about one-tenth of meningitis cases, has a high fatality rate, and is associated with a higher risk of permanent neurological damage.

The bacteria which cause both meningococcal and pneumococcal meningitis are very common. They live naturally in the back of the nose and throat or upper respiratory tract and 10–25 per cent of the population are carriers. Only rarely do they overcome the body's natural defences and spread via the bloodstream to the subarachnoid space to cause meningitis (and the incubation period is between 2 and 10 days).

Treatment

Treatment of bacterial meningitis includes the urgent administration of antibiotics, at first empirical and then adapted to the pathogen recovered from the CSF, suppression or removal of the initial infectious focus, steroids, and symptomatic and adjunctive therapy. For meningococcal and pneumococcal meningitis national guidelines suggest treatment with cefotaxime or ceftriaxone. If the patient has a history of anaphylaxis to penicillin or cephalosporins then chloramphenicol should be given.

If a diagnosis of *meningococcal meningitis* is subsequently made then treatment should be benzylpenicillin or ceftriaxone, again substituted by chloramphenicol if the patient has a history of anaphylaxis to penicillin or cephalosporins. With meningococcal meningitis, close contacts of the patient (family, room-mates, nursery school contacts) are at increased risk of cross-infection. All such contacts should be offered antibiotics (rifampicin for 2 days) to eliminate the organism from the nasopharynx.

For meningitis caused by *pneumococci*, ceftriaxone should be given for 10–14 days. If the organism is shown to be penicillin-sensitive then ceftriaxone should be substituted by benzylpenicillin. If the organism is highly penicillin/cephalosporin resistant then vancomycin or rifampicin should be added.

For *Haemophilus influenzae meningitis* ceftriaxone is the drug of choice and this should be prescribed for at least 10 days. Again, if there is a history of anaphylaxis to penicillin or cephalosporins, or if the organism is resistant to ceftriaxone, then chloramphenicol should be prescribed. Rifampicin should be given for 4 days before discharge from hospital.

Encephalitis

Encephalitis is an acute inflammatory process that affects brain tissue and in some cases it will be accompanied by inflammation of the meninges (meningoencephalitis). The majority of cases are caused by viral infection and can manifest either as primary encephalitis, when the virus directly infects the brain, or secondary (post-infectious) encephalitis, where an often innocuous infection is thought to precipitate autoimmune attack of the brain leading to inflammation. Some rare types of encephalitis are caused by amoebae. Like meningitis, the seriousness of the disease depends upon the organism responsible. Bacterial encephalitis will lead to death unless treated, and while some types of viral encephalitis are self-limiting and patients recover fully, others constitute a severe and life-threatening illness.

Signs and symptoms

Onset of encephalitis is usually acute but signs and symptoms of CNS involvement are often preceded or accompanied by a non-specific, acute febrile illness. The classic triad of features of encephalitis are confusion/reduced level of consciousness, fever, and seizures. Seizures may be frequent and spread to involve increasing areas of the body as the cerebral inflammation extends. In secondary encephalitis symptoms usually appear within 1 or 2 weeks of the original infection and typically include fever, headache, behavioural changes, and impaired conscious level but seizures are less common than in primary encephalitis. Unless the meninges are also infected, there is relatively little neck stiffness and Kernig's sign is negative.

Diagnosis

History taking and physical examination can provide clues to the cause, but the diagnosis is usually established on the basis of CSF analysis including viral polymerase chain reaction (PCR), neurodiagnostic studies (CT scan, MRI scan, EEG, and brain biopsy if indicated). Serum and CSF antibody studies are useful in some instances such as in arboviral encephalitis. When recording the history particular attention should be paid to recent illnesses, recent vaccinations, travel, contacts with pets or wild animals, or tick exposure, long-term immunosuppression or possible exposure to HIV, and a recent acquired immunodeficiency syndrome (AIDS) illness.

As in meningitis, lumbar puncture should be performed only after CT scan has excluded a space-occupying lesion in patients in coma or with focal neurological deficits. In viral encephalitis CSF analysis will typically show a normal or moderately elevated opening pressure, a moderate increase in white cell count, normal or elevated protein level, and normal glucose level. Confirmation of diagnosis depends on identification of the virus within the CSF or within brain tissue by means of brain biopsy. Electroencephalography (EEG) is important in patients with encephalitis to exclude non-convulsive status epilepticus.

Bacterial encephalitis

Bacterial pathogens invariably involve inflammation of the meninges out of proportion to their encephalitic components. The exception to this is *Listeria monocytogenes*. Unlike the more common forms of bacterial meningitis, which are mostly restricted to the meninges, *Listeria* also has a propensity to infect the brain tissue itself, and in particular the brainstem. *Listeria* encephalitis is treated with amoxicillin and gentamicin or co-trimaxazole in the penicillin-allergic patient.

Viral encephalitis

More than 100 different viruses are known to cause acute viral encephalitis but the most frequently reported are seasonal enteroviruses and arboviruses and herpes simplex virus.

How and where the virus enters the CNS is virus specific. Some viruses are spread through person-to-person contact (herpes simplex virus (HSV), varicella zoster virus (VZV) associated with chickenpox, measles, mumps, and rubella virus). Important animal carriers are mosquitoes and ticks (arbovirus) and warm-blooded mammals (rabies virus). Some viruses will target specific areas of the CNS, for example HSV selectively affects the inferior frontal and medial temporal lobes. Immunologically compromised patients are particularly susceptible to VZV and cytomegalovirus (CMV).

Treatment

With few exceptions, notably aciclovir for herpes simplex encephalitis (HSE), no specific therapy is available for most forms of viral encephalitis and treatment consists of symptomatic and supportive care. However, since the early administration of antiviral therapy for HSE has been shown to reduce mortality and morbidity (note evidence is only for HSV but VZV is also sensitive), empirical therapy with intravenous aciclovir should be given in all cases of suspected HSE and in addition varicella zoster encephalitis (VZE) until a definitive diagnosis is made. Similarly, until a bacterial cause can be excluded parenteral antibiotics (a cephalosporin) should be commenced. Therefore, all patients with suspected CNS infection should be treated with broad spectrum antibiotics and acyclovir. Treatment should continue until such time as a causative organism is identified or until medically directed otherwise. Secondary or post-infectious encephalitis is treated by immunosuppression, usually with steroids.

The time course for recovery from viral encephalitis can be protracted. However, supportive care should be given for as long as necessary since, even when recovery takes a long time, outcome can still be very good. Behavioural changes can be dramatic and may continue for many months into the recovery stage.

Cerebral malaria

Malaria should always be suspected as the cause of any neurological symptoms in a patient who has returned from an endemic area within the past 2 months. Cerebral malaria frequently presents with non-specific influenza-type symptoms but it can progress to coma and death and therefore requires urgent treatment. Cerebral malaria is treated with intravenous quinine.

Intracranial abscess

Intracranial abscess may develop due to direct spread from adjacent infections in the ear or sinuses, following trauma, either penetrating head injury or closed head injury with base of skull fracture, or alternatively infection can spread through the bloodstream from a distant source. It can also occur as a complication of craniocerebral surgery or in immunologically compromised patients. Two main types of cerebral abscess are intracerebral abscess and subdural abscess (empyema). Chronic otitis media should be suspected in temporal lobe and cerebellar abscess, while frontal lobe abscess should raise suspicions of local sinus infection. While any organism is capable of producing a cerebral abscess, common organisms are *Streptococcus milleri*, anaerobic bacteriodes species, *Proteus* and *E. coli*.

The brain usually goes through a stage of cerebritis before the abscess forms. A capsule, which eventually becomes quite tough and thick, then begins to form around the infected area, a defence mechanism that prevents the infection from spreading through the brain. The abscess then acts as a space-occupying lesion, resulting in raised ICP and focal neurological deficits.

Signs and symptoms

Headaches are a common feature, becoming increasingly severe and leading to confusion and drowsiness, and focal signs and symptoms will usually reflect the site involved. With subdural empyema the spread of infection within the subdural space gives rise to more acute signs of increased ICP. Seizures are also a common feature of intracranial abscess.

Diagnosis

Plain X-rays of the skull may show abnormalities in the frontal sinuses or mastoid air cells indicating a possible source of infection, but CT scan with contrast is the definitive investigation. Blood should be taken for a full count, erythrocyte sedimentation rate (ESR) and blood cultures.

Treatment

Treatment will consist of surgical drainage either via craniotomy or burrhole aspiration of the abscess, identifying the organism responsible and treating with antibiotic therapy, and therapeutic and supportive measures to reduce ICP in severe cases. In addition, the primary source of infection should be investigated and treated.

The algorithm in Fig. 10.15 summarizes the treatment of a patient with a presumed CNS infection.

Management of the patient for brainstem death tests

Determining death by neurological criteria is accepted practice in many countries throughout the world and all the major Western and Eastern religions accept the concept of brain death. There are, however, some dif-

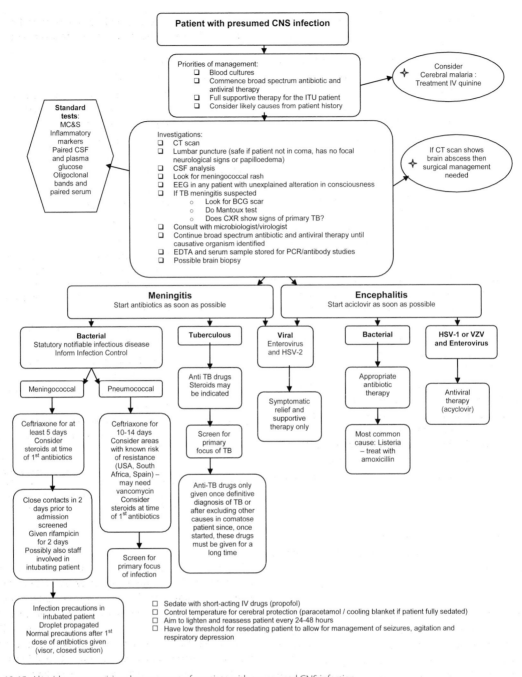

Fig. 10.15 Algorithm summarizing the treatment of a patient with a presumed CNS infection.

ferences in practice between countries regarding the number of physicians required, the additional confirmatory tests recommended, and the time period for testing. Although the same principles apply in adults and children, testing in neonates and infants is more difficult due to size and developmental stage. The time course for maintaining the brain dead patient is limited and prolonged intervention cannot prevent cardiac arrest from haemodynamic instability (despite increasing levels of inotropic support) for more than a few

TABLE 10.9 Stages in the diagnosis of brainstem death

Preconditions	Diagnosis compatible with brainstem death and evidence of irreversible structural brain damage
	Apnoeic coma dependent on mechanical ventilation
Exclusions	Causes of reversible coma and factors causing central depression excluded
	Absence of effects of sedative, hypnotic, analgesic, and muscle relaxant drugs confirmed
	Primary hypothermia excluded
	Metabolic disorders considered with particular emphasis on the correction of abnormal sodium, glucose, and pH levels
Clinical tests	Tests to confirm the absence of brainstem reflexes and the presence of persistent apnoea

TABLE 10.10 Observation and management of the patient prior to and during testing for brainstem death

Neurology	No cranial nerve function
Respiratory	No spontaneous respiration
	Absence of gag reflex on oral suction and absence of cough on tracheal suction
	Normal pH and acid–base balance
	Normalize CO_2 prior to testing
Cardiovascular* and metabolic	MABP ≥60 mmHg (use vasopressors if required)
	Temperature >35°C
	Na^+ 135–155 mmol/l
	K^+ 3.5–4.5 mmol/l
	Glucose 4–9 mmol/l
Sedation	Sedatives, analgesics and muscle relaxant drugs discontinued for >6 hours prior to testing (reversing drugs (e.g. naloxone, flumazenil) and a peripheral nerve stimulator can be used)
Hydration	Intravenous fluids to maintain BP/CVP
	Continue nasogastric feeding
	Insulin infusion if required to keep blood glucose at 4–9 mmol/l
	5% dextrose if required to keep Na^+ below 155 mmol/l
Elimination	DDAVP 0.4 μg if evidence of diabetes insipidus to control electrolyte balance and volume status

* It is recognized that circulatory, metabolic and endocrine disturbances are a likely accompaniment of brainstem death (e.g. hypernatraemia, diabetes insipidus) but these are the effect rather than the cause and, provided that potentially reversible causes of unconsciousness have been excluded, these do not preclude the diagnosis of brainstem death.

days in most cases. Accounts of the preservation of brain dead patients for longer periods have been documented but such cases are very rare and in some cases the evidence is unclear.

The United Kingdom Code of Practice for the Diagnosis of Brain Stem Death (1995) recommends that the definition of death should be regarded as 'irreversible loss of the capacity for consciousness, combined with irreversible loss of the capacity to breathe'. It states that brainstem death, irrespective of its cause, produces irreversible cessation of brainstem function and therefore brainstem death equates with death of the brain and of the individual. In the UK there are three stages in the diagnosis of brain death—preconditions, exclusions, and clinical tests (see Table 10.9).

Timing of brainstem death tests

The time before testing should equal the time taken to meet the essential preconditions and the necessary exclusions (see Table 10.10).

Test procedure

The United Kingdom Code of Practice requires two doctors with expertise in the field to make the diagnosis of brain death (Table 10.11). These will usually be senior clinicians (registered for more than 5 years) with an interest in intensive care medicine and anaesthesia. One should be a consultant and the other a consultant or senior registrar. The preconditions and exclusions must have been satisfied before the tests are carried out and the two doctors must carry out the tests independently of each other. In adults, there is no formal requirement in the UK for a specified time interval between the two sets of tests. It is, however, practice to

allow an interval of 2–4 hours between the first and second tests to allow time for relatives to come to terms with the diagnosis. It is during this period that the subject of organ donation may be broached. If hypoxic injury has occurred (e.g. following cardiac arrest) it is usual to allow at least 24 hours to elapse before brainstem tests are carried out. Although not specifically mentioned in the UK Code of Practice, the 'dolls eyes' response should be tested initially in every case. If present, the patient is clearly not brainstem dead.

Limb and trunk movements

Reflex movements of the limbs and trunk may occur in brainstem dead patients due to spinal reflexes. Their significance should be explained to relatives and staff

TABLE 10.11   Tests for the absence of brainstem function and apnoea

Diagnostic tests	Cranial nerve	Area of brainstem tested
Fixed diameter pupil, unreactive either directly or consensually to sharp changes in light intensity	Optic (II), oculomotor (III)	Midbrain
Absent corneal reflex—no blink occurs when cornea is brushed with gauze	Trigeminal (V), facial (VII)	Midbrain
Absent vestibulo-ocular reflex—no eye movement occurs during or following slow injection of at least 50 ml of ice-cold water into each external auditory meatus (clear access to the tympanic membrane must be established by direct inspection and the head should be flexed at 30°)	Acoustic (VIII), abducens (VI)	Pons
No motor response within the cranial nerve distribution in response to stimuli and no limb response to supraorbital nerve pressure. Absent grimacing to pain. No head movement	Facial (VII), accessory (XI)	Midbrain, medulla
No gag reflex in response to suction catheter passed down the trachea, no slowing of heart rate	Glossopharyngeal (IX), vagus (X)	Medulla
No respiratory movements occur when disconnection from ventilator allows P_aCO_2 to rise above the threshold for respiratory stimulation (6.65 kPa)		Respiratory centre in medulla

Testing for apnoea	Reduce SIMV rate to allow P_aCO_2 to rise to 5.0 kPa prior to testing
	Pre-oxygenate with 100% oxygen for 10 min
	Disconnect from ventilator
	Insufflate oxygen at 6 l/min via suction catheter placed in endotracheal tube to maintain adequate oxygenation during testing
	Allow P_aCO_2 to rise to 6.65 kPa
	Confirm no spontaneous respiration
	Reconnect ventilator

to enable them to understand that they do not involve conscious voluntary movements (i.e. they do not originate in the cerebral cortex).

Documentation

Documented time of death is the time of the first set of brainstem tests when the diagnosis of brain death is confirmed, and not when mechanical ventilation is discontinued. Legally time of death is recognized when the first set of tests indicates brainstem death but death cannot be pronounced and certified until after completion of the second set of tests.

Turning off the ventilator

If the patient is not to be an organ donor, when appropriate time has been given to relatives, the ventilator should be switched off and all infusions discontinued (there should be no 'weaning' process since the patient has been certified dead).

Care of the family

It is well documented that caring for the relatives of a critically ill patient can be extremely stressful. When the patient has had a catastrophic brain injury and is awaiting brainstem tests the stressors can be even greater. These patients are often young, previously fit individuals and the circumstances leading to their admission sudden and tragic. Initial intensive nursing and medical management suddenly changes to supportive care for the patient whose diagnosis is irreversible and often difficult to comprehend. There may be little time for the intensive care team to build up a rapport with the family and for the family to come to terms with imminent loss. These factors alone can make the task of explaining the already complex concept of brainstem death difficult for all those involved.

The nurse's role in preparing the family for the diagnosis of brainstem death and supporting them through the process is crucial. Some relatives may request to be at the bedside when the tests are carried out and will need the support of an experienced and knowledgeable nurse. Despite confirmation of the diagnosis of brainstem death, the patient remains warm to touch and continues to display physiological signs of life (heart rate and blood pressure) until the ventilator is switched off. This can make acceptance of the diagnosis difficult. Relatives should be given appropriate time at the bedside and given the choice to be there when ventilation is discontinued. If they do choose to be at the bedside when the ventilator is switched off, some explanation should be given of possible reflex movements that the patient may make. Some families may want the patient be an organ donor and, once brainstem death has been confirmed, the focus of care will be to fulfil the family's wish.

Approaching the family of a potential organ donor

Broaching the subject of organ donation with a bereaved family is often seen as one of the most difficult stages in the organ donation process and many factors have been identified as potential obstacles to organ donation: dislike of adding to relatives' distress, lack of training in how to approach families, adverse media publicity, fear of being blamed, and fear of saying or doing the wrong thing.

Who can ask?

There are no set rules about who should ask; however, the person asking should be comfortable with the concept of brainstem death and the idea of organ donation. This should be a collaborative approach. The intensive care team who have been involved in the care of the patient and family since admission can provide support and guidance. Involving the transplant coordinator in the initial stages ensures expert advice from someone who can answer all questions regarding the donor process.

When to ask

Some families may spontaneously raise the issue of organ donation prior to brainstem testing and information should be provided as required. The transplant coordinator might be contacted at this point to answer questions about the donor process. However, if the option of donation needs to be broached by the intensive care team, then this should ideally be done in the interval between the two sets of brainstem tests. It is important within this process that the family is given sufficient time to accept the diagnosis of brainstem death.

Management of the patient for organ donation

Once a family has decided that their relative should be an organ donor, the aim of management is to support the patient's organs for transplantation (Table 10.12). Brain death affects nearly every organ system and there are many complications that can make donor management difficult. These complications include hypotension, diabetes insipidus, hypothermia, electrolyte abnormalities, coagulopathy, hypoxia, and cardiac arrhythmias.

At the present time, the only contraindications to organ donation are human immunodeficiency virus (HIV), current malignancy (except malignancy arising from the central nervous system), and Creutzfeldt–Jakob disease (CJD) or a family history of CJD.

Non-heart-beating donors

Non-heart-beating donation is not a new technique but has been practically abandoned in the UK since the

TABLE 10.12	Maintenance of the organ donor	
Respiratory support	PaO2 > 10 mmHg with the lowest possible FiO2 (<0.6)
	Normal pH (7.35–7.45)
	PEEP < 7.5 cm
Cardiovascular support	Maintain intravascular volume (CVP 10 mmHg)
	Treat CVP < 6 mmHg with fluid bolus
	Systolic BP 90–100 mmHg (mean 65 mmHg)
	Vasopressors if required
	HR 100 bpm
	SVR < 1000 dyn/s^5
	Urine output 100 ml/hour (DDAVP for diabetes insipidus)
Endocrine support	Hormone replacement therapy for severe cardiovascular instability or high inotrope requirement (T3, Pitressin, methylprednisolone)
	Glucose 6–11 mmol/l
Haematological support	Fresh frozen plasma (FFP)
	Platelets
Temperature support	Core temperature >35°C
	Warming blankets
	Warmed IV fluids
	Heated and humidified inspired gases

introduction of the brainstem death criteria in 1976. Now, as a result of improvements in surgical techniques, immunosuppression and organ preservation, it is being reconsidered as a valuable option to bereaved families.

Unlike a brainstem dead patient who will be transferred to theatre ventilated with a heartbeat, non-heart-beating donation takes place after a patient has become asystolic. At present, retrievable organs include liver, kidneys, and pancreas; with some centres now looking at the possibility of transplanting lungs from non-heart-beating donors. As good organ function is necessary, most potential non-heart-beating donors will have suffered a neurological insult but will not fulfil brainstem death criteria. Non-heart-beating donation can also be offered to those families who would otherwise refuse donation because they wish to remain with their relative until their heart stops beating.

Management of sodium and water balance

Disturbances of sodium and water balance are common following brain injury and accurate diagnosis and treatment is essential.

Hyponatraemia

Hyponatraemia is defined as a plasma sodium concentration less than 130 mmol/l. Patients with no primary cerebral diseases develop symptoms of hyponatraemia (nausea, anorexia, emesis, confusion, seizures, and impairment of consciousness) with sodium levels below 120–125 mmol/l. In contrast, patients with CNS lesions may demonstrate symptoms at a much higher sodium level. Accurate diagnosis and treatment is essential because of the high risk of seizures if the plasma sodium falls below 120 mmol/l.

Two syndromes leading to hyponatraemia, the syndrome of inappropriate antidiuretic hormone secretion (SIADH) and cerebral salt wasting syndrome (CSW), are most commonly seen in patients with severe TBI and poor grade SAH. Although the serum electrolyte profile of the two syndromes is similar, it is important to distinguish between the two since they require markedly different treatment. SIADH is characterized by increased intravascular volume, water retention, and dilutional hyponatraemia and is treated with volume restriction, while CSW is a state of decreased intravascular volume, increased urine output, and hyponatraemia and is treated by re-establishing normovolaemia.

Syndrome of inappropriate antidiuretic hormone secretion (SIADH)

Antidiuretic hormone (ADH) is passed from the supraoptic and paraventricular nuclei in the hypothalamus and secreted by the posterior lobe of the pituitary gland into the blood. The major function of this hormone is to regulate body fluid tonicity, and plasma osmolality serves as a powerful stimulus for its release. Without the action of ADH, the kidney would generate 20–30 litres of free water per day. SIADH may develop due to persistent release of ADH resulting in increased intravascular H_2O volume, H_2O retention, and dilutional hyponatraemia. SIADH is usually self-limiting and resolves as brain tissue recovers and hypertonic saline is rarely required.

Cerebral salt wasting syndrome (CSW)

Cerebral salt wasting is thought to be due to increased release of atrial natriuretic factor (ANF) from the brain and is characterized by water loss with a low CVP. Hyponatraemia may be associated with not only a progressive naturesis but also a tendency to diuresis, leading to a significant contraction of circulating and extracellular volumes. In CSW, fluid restriction will not correct the hyponatraemia and indeed may be harmful as it will reduce intravascular volume further. This may lead to hypotension and an increased risk of cerebral infarction.

Hypernatraemia

Hypernatraemia may be secondary to dehydration from fluid restriction and the use of osmotic agents for ICP control and this can easily be corrected by the administration of isotonic fluids. Hypernatraemia secondary to dehydration is associated with low urine output and high specific gravity (>1.020). Hypernatraemia can also be iatrogenically induced through excessive use of sodium-containing fluids.

Diabetes insipidus (DI)

Diabetes insipidus may develop after brain injury when there has been damage to the hypothalamus or pituitary gland. It occurs when over 80% of neurons synthesizing vasopressin are destroyed or become temporarily non-functional. It is characterized by a high urine output (> 200 ml/hr) and low urine specific gravity (<1.005).

Diagnosis and treatment

Diagnosis and treatment of disturbances of sodium and water balance are outlined in Tables 10.13 and 10.14.

TABLE 10.13 Diagnosis of disorders of sodium and water balance

Disorder	CVP	Urine output	Specific gravity	Serum Na+ (mmol/l)	Urinary Na+ (mmol/l)	Serum osmolality (mOsmol/kg)	Urine osmolality (mOsmol/kg)
SIADH	High	Low (no evidence of volume depletion)	Normal	Low (<135)	Normal	Low	(High) (compare with serum osmolality)
CSW	Low	High	Normal	Low (<135)	High	High/normal	Variable
DI	Low	High (>1000 ml/4 hour)	Low(≤1.005)	High(>148)	Normal	High	Low

TABLE 10.14 Treatment of disorders of sodium and water balance

SIADH	Restrict water intake to 500–1000 ml per day
	Check urine and serum sodium and osmolality
CSW	Re-establish normovolaemia with the administration of sodium-containing isotonic solutions
	Check urine and serum sodium and osmolality
	In severe cases hypertonic saline should be given over 24–48 hours at a rate to increase sodium concentration by <12 mmol/l/24 hours
DI	If urine output >1000 ml in 4 hours and specific gravity <1.005 give 0.4 μg DDAVP IV
	If urine output remains high after 30 min give further dose of 0.4 μg DDAVP IV
	Accurate fluid balance, aiming for even balance, is essential (urine output should not be chased)
	If sodium >148 mmol/l give glucose 5%, with insulin infusion if needed to keep blood glucose 4–9 mmol/l
	In addition, water can be given via the nasogastric or orogastric tube

Test yourself

Questions

1. Name the three membranes that protect the brain.

2. Which areas of the brain do you associate with the following functions?
   (a) Executive functioning
   (b) Speech
   (c) balance

3. Which cranial nerves are tested in the pupillary response to light?

4. Name the arteries that form the circle of Willis.

5. Name the two components of consciousness and their corresponding brain structures.

6. Give definitions for
   (a) Intracranial pressure
   (b) Cerebral perfusion pressure
   (c) Pressure autoregulation

7. Which of the following is the most sensitive indicator of increasing ICP?
   (a) Blood pressure
   (b) Level of consciousness
   (c) Hemiparesis
   (d) Cushing's reflex

8 Give a brief definition of primary and secondary brain injury.

9. State briefly why it is important to avoid the following after severe TBI.
   (a) Hypotension
   (b) Hypoxia
   (c) Hypercarbia

10. In the WFNS Subarachnoid Haemorrhage Grading Scale what clinical signs are used to grade patients following SAH?

11. What are the main complications of SAH?

12. What three modes of behaviour are used to determine the GCS?

13. What is the highest score you can obtain in the GCS and what is the maximum score in each category?

14. In myasthenia gravis (MG)
    (a) Which part of the CNS is affected?
    (b) What characterizes MG?

15. What is status epilepticus and what is the first line treatment?

16. What is Guillain–Barré syndrome and what are the most typical signs and symptoms?

17. In neuromuscular disorders what is the most sensitive indicator of respiratory failure?

18. Name the intracranial structures that are affected in
    (a) Meningitis
    (b) Encephalitis

19. Give the definition of brainstem death.

20. List possible causes of hyponatraemia and hypernatraemia following brain injury.

Answers

1. Dura mater, arachnoid mater, pia mater

2. (a) Frontal lobe
   (b) Frontal and temporal lobe in dominant hemisphere
   (c) Cerebellum

3. Optic nerve (cranial nerve II) and Oculomotor nerve (cranial nerve III)

4. Anterior communicating artery, middle cerebral arteries, posterior communicating arteries.

5. Arousal: reticular activating system.
   Awareness: cerebral cortex

6. (a) ICP is the CSF pressure within the lateral ventricles
   (b) CPP represents the blood pressure gradient across the brain
   (c) The intrinsic ability of cerebrovascular smooth muscle to maintain a relatively constant CBF over a wide range of perfusion pressures

7. (b) Level of consciousness

8. Primary injury is the damage caused at the moment of impact and secondary injury is the damage that occurs in the hours or days after the injury.

9. After severe TBI
   (a) Autoregulatory mechanisms may be disrupted and therefore CPP is dependent on systemic BP. Hypotension following severe TBI has the highest correlation with morbidity and mortality.
   (b) Hypoxia is associated with increased CBF and is the second most influential cause of secondary brain injury.
   (c) Carbon dioxide is a potent cerebral vasodilator and increases CBF and therefore ICP.

10. GCS and motor deficit

11. Rebleeding, vasospasm, and hydrocephalus

12. Eye opening (E), verbal response (V), motor response (M).

13. Highest score is 15 and in each category the highest score is E4 V5 M6.

14. In myasthenia gravis
    (a) The neuromuscular junction is affected, specifically the acetylcholine receptor sites.

(b) MG is characterized by weakness and fatigability of voluntary muscles, typically involving the muscles of the eye, face, and mouth.

15. Status epilepticus (SE) is a clinical term referring to a series of generalized seizures without recovery of consciousness between attacks lasting for at least 30 min and the first-line treatment is benzodiazepines.

16. GBS is an acute inflammatory neuropathy affecting the peripheral nervous system and patients most typically present with weakness and mild sensory symptoms starting from the feet up.

17. Forced vital capacity (FVC).

18. The intracranial structures involved are
    (a) The meninges, usually the arachnoid and pia mater, and the intervening subarachnoid space
    (b) Brain tissue

19. The irreversible loss of the capacity for consciousness, combined with irreversible loss of the capacity to breathe.

20. Hyponatraemia—SIADH, CSW; hypernatraemia—dehydration, osmotic diuretics, DI.

Bibliography

Alderson, P., Roberts, I. (1997). Corticosteroids in acute traumatic brain injury: systematic review of randomised controlled trials. *British Medical Journal* **314**, 1855–9.

Barker, R.A., Barasi, S., Neal, M.J. (1999). *Neuroscience at a Glance.* Blackwell Science, Oxford.

Bear, M.F., Connors, B.W., Paradiso, M.A. (1996). *Neuroscience: Exploring the Brain.* Williams and Wilkins, Baltimore, MD.

Bouma, G.J., Muizelaar, J.P. (1992). Cerebral blood flow, cerebral blood volume and cerebrovascular reactivity after severe head injury. *Journal of Neurotrauma* Suppl 9, 333–48.

Bratton, S.L., Davis, R.L. (1997). Acute lung injury in isolated traumatic brain injury. *Neurosurgery* **40**(4), 707–12.

Bullock, R., Povlishock, J.T. (1996). Guidelines for the management of severe head injury. *Journal of Neurotrauma* **264**, 1085–8.

Carter, P., Edwards, S. (1997). General principles of treatment. In: *Neurological Physiotherapy: A Problem Solving Approach* (ed. S. Edwards), pp. 87–113. Churchill Livingstone, London.

Chalela, J.A. (2001). Pearls and pitfalls in the intensive care management of Guillaine-Barre syndrome. *Seminars in Neurology* **21**(4), 399–405.

Chapman, M.G., Smith, M., Hirsch, N.P. (2001). Status epilepticus. *Anaesthesia* **56**, 648–59.

Chesnut, R.M. (1995). Secondary brain insults after injury: clinical perspectives. *New Horizons* **3**, 366–75.

Clifton, G.L., Robertson, C.S., Kyper, K. *et al.* (1983). Cardiovascular response to severe head injury. *Journal of Neurosurgery* **3**, 447–54.

Contant, C.F., Valadka, A.B., Shankar, M.D. *et al.* (2001). Adult respiratory distress syndrome: a complication of induced hypertension after severe head injury. *Journal of Neurosurgery* **95**, 560–8.

Crossman, A.R., Neary, D. (1995). *Neuroanatomy: an Illustrated Colour Text.* Churchill Livingstone, Edinburgh.

Cunning, S., Haudek, D.L. (1999). Preventing secondary brain injuries. *Dimensions of Critical Care Nursing* **18**(5), 20–2.

Dearden, N.M. (1998). Mechanisms and prevention of secondary brain damage during intensive care. *Clinical Neuropathology* **17**(47), 221–8.

Drake, G.C. (1988). Report of the World Federation of Neurological Surgeons Committee on a universal subarachnoid haemorrhage rading scale. *Journal of Neurosurgery* **68**, 985–6.

Feldman, Z., Kanter, M.J., Robertson, C.S. *et al.* (1992). Effect of head elevation on intracranial pressure, cerebral perfusion pressure and cerebral blood flow in head injured patients. *Journal of Neurosurgery* **76**, 201–11.

George, M.R. (1988). Neuromuscular respiratory failure: what the nurse knows may make the difference. *Journal of Neuroscience Nursing* **20**(2), 110–17.

Graham, D.I., Hume Adams, J., Nicoll, J.A.R. *et al.* (1995). The nature, distribution and causes of traumatic brain injury. *Brain Pathology* **5**, 397–406.

Greenberg, M.S. (1994). Subarachnoid haemorrhage and aneurysms. In: *Handbook of Neurosurgery* (ed. M.S. Greenberg), 3rd edn, pp. 711–52. Greenberg Graphics, Lakeland, FL.

Gupta, A.K., Summors, A. (eds) (2001). *Notes in Neuronaaesthesia and Critical Care.* Greenwich Medical Media, London.

Hartung, H.P., Willison, H.J, Kieseier, B.C. (2002). Acute immunoinflammatory neuropathy: update on Guillaine-Barre syndrome. *Current Opinion in Neurology* **15**(5), 571–7.

Holly, L.T., Kelly, D.F., Counelis, G.J., *et al.* (2002). Cervical spine trauma associated with moderate and severe head injury: incidence, risk factors and injury characteristics. *Journal of Neurosurgery Spine* **96**(3), 285–91.

Jennett, B. (1991) Diagnosis and management of head trauma. *Journal of Neurotrauma* **8**(Suppl. 1), S15–S18.

Jennett, B., Lindsay, K.W. (1994). *An Introduction to Neurosurgery*, 5th edn. Butterworth-Heinemann, Oxford.

Lawn, N.D., Wijdicks, E.F.M. (2002). Status epilepticus: a critical review of management options. *Canadian Journal of Neurological Science* **29**, 206–15.

Lindsay, K.W., Bone, I. (2004). *Neurology and Neurosurgery Illustrated*, 4th edn. Churchill Livingstone, Edinburgh.

McLeod, A.A., Neil-Dwyer, G., Meyer, C.H.A. *et al.* (1982). Cardiac sequelae of acute head injury. *British Heart Journal* **47**, 221–6.

Maas, A.I.R., Dearden, M., Teasdale, G.M. *et al.* (1997). EBIC guidelines for management of severe head injury in adults. *Acta Neurochirurgica (Wien)* **139**, 286–94.

Martin, N.A., Patwardhan, R.V., Alexander, M.J. *et al.* (1997). Characterisation of cerebral haemodynamic phases following severe head trauma: hypoperfusion, hyperaemia and vasospasm. *Journal of Neurosurgery* **87**, 9–19.

Miller, J.D., Becker, D.P. (1982). Secondary insults to the injured brain. *Journal of the Royal College of Surgeons of Edinburgh* **27**, 292–8.

Morris, C.G.T., McCoy, E. (2004). Clearing the cervical spine in unconscious polytrauma victims, balancing risks and effective screening. *Anaesthesia* **59**, 464–82.

Ng, K.K.P., Howard, R.S., Fish, D.R. *et al.* (1995). Management and outcome of severe Guillain-Barre syndrome. *Quarterly Journal of Medicine* **88**, 243–50.

Oppenheimer, S.M., Cochetto, D.F., Hachinski, V.C. (1990). Cerebrogenic cardiac arrhythmias. *Acta Neurologica* **47** 513–19.

O'Riordan, J.I., Miller, D.H., Mottorshead, J.P. *et al.* (1998). The management and outcome of patients with myasthenia gravis treated acutely in a neurological intensive care unit. *European Journal of Neurology* **5**(2), 137–42.

Palace, J., Vincent, A., Beeson, D. (2001). Myasthenia gravis: diagnostic and management dilemmas. *Current Opinion in Neurology* **14**(5), 583–9.

Palmer, J.D. (ed.) (1996). *Manual of Neurosurgery*. Churchill Livingstone, London.

Parsons, I.C., Wilson, M.M. (1984). Cerebrovascular status of severe closed head injured patients following passive position changes. *Nursing Research* **33**, 68–75.

Piek, J., Chesnut, R.M., Marshall, L.F. *et al.* (1992). Extracranial complications of severe head injury. *Journal of Neurosurgery* **77**, 901–7.

Poulter, A. (1998). The patient with Guillaine-Barre syndrome: implications for critical care nursing practice. *Nursing in Critical Care* **3**(4), 182–9.

Rabinstein, A.A., Wijdicks, E.F.M. (2003). Hyponatraemia in critically ill neurological patients. *Neurologist* **9**(6), 290–300.

Rappaport, Z.V., Vajda, J. (2002). Intracranial abscess: current concepts in management. *Neurosurgery Quarterly* **12**(3), 238–50.

Rees, G., Shah, S., Hanley, C., *et al.* (2002). Subarachnoid haemorrhage: a clinical overview. *Nursing Standard* **16**(42), 47–56.

Robertson, C.S. (2001). Management of cerebral perfusion pressure after traumatic brain injury. *Anaesthesiology* **95**(6), 1513–17.

Robertson, C.S., Valadka, A.B., Hannay, H.J. *et al.* (1999). Prevention of secondary insults after severe head injury. *Critical Care Medicine* **27**, 2086–95.

Ropper, A.H. (ed.) (1993). *Neurological and Neurosurgical Intensive Care*, 3rd edn. Raven Press, New York.

Rosner, M.J., Rosner, S.D., Johnson, A.H. (1995). Cerebral perfusion pressure—management protocol and clinical results. *Journal of Neurosurgery* **83**, 949–62.

Scherer, P. (1986). Coma assessment. *Journal of Nursing* May, 542–55.

Seelig, J.M., Becker, D.P., Miller, J.D. *et al.* (1981). Traumatic acute subdural haematoma: major mortality reduction in comatose patients treated within four hours. *New England Journal of Medicine* **304**(25), 1511–18.

Shafer, P.O. (1999). New therapies in the management of acute cluster seizures and seizure emergencies. *Journal of Neuroscience Nursing* **31**(4), 224–9.

Shorvon, S. (1994). *Status Epilepticus: its Clinical Features and Treatment in Children and Adults*. Cambridge University Press, Cambridge.

Slade, J., Kerr, M.E., Marion, D. (1999). The effect of therapeutic hypothermia on the incidence and treatment of intracranial hypertension. *Journal of Neuroscience Nursing* **31**(5), 264–9.

Smith, M. (1998). Management of the multiple organ donor. *Surgery* 180–4. The Medicine Publishing Company Ltd.

Stone, J.D. Sperry, R.J. *et al.* (eds) (1996). *The Neuroanaesthesia Handbook*. Mosby, St Louis, MO.

Sullivan, J. (2000). Positioning of patients with severe traumatic brain injury: research based practice. *Journal of Neuroscience Nursing* **32**(4), 204–9.

Sutcliffe, A. (2001). Hypothermia (or not) for the management of head injury. *Care of the Critically Ill* **17**(5): 162–5.

Teasdale, G., Jennett, B. (1974). Assessment of coma and impaired consciousness: a practical scale. *Lancet* July 13, 81–4.

Teasdale, G., Jennett, B. (1976). Assessment and prognosis of coma after head injury. *Acta Neurochirurgica* **34**, 45–55.

Twyman, D. (1997). Nutritional management of the critically ill neurologic patient. *Critical Care Clinics* **13**, 39.

Walker, M. (1998). Protection of the cervical spine in the unconscious patient. *Care of the Critically Ill* **14**(1), 4–7.

Watkins, L.D. (2000). Head injuries: general principles and management. *Surgery* 219–24. The Medicine Publishing Company Ltd.

Wijdicks, E.F.M. (2001). *Brain Death*. Lippincott, Philadelphia, PA.

Wijdicks, E.F.M. (2003). *The Clinical Practice of Critical Care Neurology*, 2nd edn. Oxford University Press, New York.

Gastrointestinal problems and nutrition

Introduction

The gastrointestinal (GI) tract has not always been considered an area of vital importance in the care of the critically ill. However, its effectiveness as a defence system and an essential resource for other organs has been increasingly recognized and support of these functions is now considered an essential part of optimal care of the critically ill. The proportion of patients with malnutrition in intensive care has been reported to be as high as 43% (Giner *et al.* 1996) and this group have an increased incidence of complications ($P = 0.01$). In order to improve outcomes as far as possible it is apparent that nutrition forms a vital part of comprehensive and proactive care of the patient. A significant responsibility for the delivery of nutrition falls to the nurse caring for the patient, not only in ensuring that what is prescribed gets delivered but also in monitoring and evaluating the patient's ability to tolerate and assimilate the mode of nutritional delivery. Although the lack of nutrition is not immediately life-threatening, it has been shown to be associated with patient outcome in specific groups within the ICU (Rapp *et al.* 1983, Kudsk 1996).

Anatomy and physiology

The anatomy and physiology of the GI tract will be described briefly, with particular reference to those aspects which have relevance to the critically ill. The GI tract acts as both a point of access and a protective barrier to the external environment.

The major functions of the GI tract include:

♦ Breakdown of complex nutrients.

♦ Absorption of predigested molecules.

♦ Movement of foodstuffs through the digestive tract.

♦ Elimination of waste matter.

♦ Recycling of materials used in digestion.

♦ Protection of vulnerable internal organs from ingested organisms.

The GI tract is mostly under the control of the autonomic nervous system. The oropharyngeal cavity, upper oesophagus, and external anal sphincter are under voluntary control via somatic motor fibres. Most of the GI tract is supplied by both sympathetic and parasympathetic nerves. Parasympathetic innervation is mainly via the vagus and pelvic nerves and sympathetic innervation via the nerves from the spinal cord and pre-vertebral ganglia and from these ganglia to the organs of the gut.

Sympathetic stimulation will decrease gut motility, increase sphincter tone, and decrease exocrine secretions (i.e. discharged via a duct). Parasympathetic stimulation will increase motility, decrease sphincter tone, and increase exocrine secretions. Sympathetic and parasympathetic response can be altered by psycho-emotional stimuli mediated by higher neuronal centres. Thus, fear may increase the viscosity of saliva and decrease the amount secreted producing the characteristic dry mouth, while any strong emotion may increase gut motility.

Gut function

The gut functions of secretion, absorption, and motility are controlled by the interaction of the autonomic nervous system and the endocrine and paracrine systems.

Function is highly organized and integrated within the GI tract allowing movement, digestion, and absorption of food to take place.

Oropharyngeal cavity

Functions of the oropharyngeal cavity are:

♦ mechanical breakdown of food,

♦ swallowing of food bolus (voluntary),

♦ saliva production.

Saliva is a complex substance consisting of:

♦ mucus

♦ salivary amylase, a starch-digesting enzyme,

♦ lingual lipase, a hydrolysing enzyme for lipids,

♦ lysozyme, an enzyme which attacks bacterial cell walls,

♦ lactoferrin, an iron-chelating agent preventing the multiplication of organisms that require iron for growth, and

♦ secretory IgA, an immunoglobulin active against viruses and bacteria (Johnson 1997).

The mucus lubricates and binds food and the enzymes break down carbohydrate and lipids and the other agents protect both the mouth and the upper GI tract from ingestion of pathological organisms. The amount of saliva produced is increased by parasympathetic stimulation and decreased by sympathetic stimulation.

Oesophagus

The oesophagus secretes mucus (for lubrication and protection) and propels food (by peristalsis).

Lower oesophageal sphincter

The lower oesophageal sphincter is the last centimetre of the oesophagus. It prevents reflux of gastric contents by continuous smooth muscle contraction (the muscle relaxes in response to peristalsis to allow food to pass through).

Stomach

The stomach has a primary digestive function but its highly acidic environment also acts as an effective barrier to foreign organisms. Specialized cells within the gastric mucosa secrete the constituents of gastric juice: pepsin, intrinsic factor, hydrogen ions, and mucus. The functions of the stomach are:

- Breakdown of food by pepsin and gastric acid (hydrochloric acid; HCl).

- Production of intrinsic factor (facilitates absorption of vitamin B_{12} by the small intestine).

- Production of gastrin (promotes growth and repair of gastric mucosa and stimulates secretion of pepsinogen and HCl).

Gastric acid secretion is regulated by gastrin and the parasympathetic mediator acetylcholine (ACh); their effect is potentiated by histamine via the H_2-histamine receptors in the gastric mucosa. The basal rate of acid secretion has a diurnal rhythm which is higher in the evening and lower in the morning (Johnson 1997). Other factors which affect secretion include:

- conditioned reflexes such as smell, taste, chewing, swallowing,

- alcohol and caffeine via the gastric chemoreceptors and intramural nerve plexuses in the stomach wall,

- hypoglycaemia via the brainstem and vagal fibres.

Distension of the stomach itself and the presence of digested protein in the intestine will also stimulate further gastric acid release.

The human stomach secretes between 1 and 2 litres of gastric juice per day. Protection of the gastric epithelium from gastric acid is vital as the gastric luminal pH is maintained at a potentially damaging value of 2–3. This protection is achieved by:

1. The luminal surface membranes of gastric mucosal cells fit tightly together forming a barrier against HCl damage. The barrier is impermeable to hydrogen ions maintaining a concentration gradient between epithelium and lumen. This barrier can be disrupted by, among other things, bile salts, alcohol, aspirin, and steroids. Mucosal blood flow and thus oxygenation is an important factor in maintaining mucosal integrity (see later).

2. Secretion of mucus/bicarbonate gel by mucosal cells to cover the mucosal epithelium. The gel is capable of maintaining a pH gradient from approximately 2 on the gastric lumen side to approximately 7.3 on the epithelial side.

Endogenous prostaglandins play a role in maintaining gastric mucosal integrity by influencing mucosal blood flow, stabilizing the mucosal barrier, and stimulating mucus/bicarbonate secretion. Inhibition of the prostaglandins by non-steroidal anti-inflammatory drugs (NSAIDs) may result in gastric erosions or deeper ulceration.

FACTORS AFFECTING MOVEMENT OF NUTRIENTS THROUGH THE GUT

1. Gastric to duodenal delivery of nutrients: antral peristalsis and fundal tone are reduced by the arrival of nutrients and hyperosmolar solutions in the duodenum, maintaining a constant delivery of 1–2 kcal/min.

2. Malabsorbed nutrients (particularly fat) are detected by sensors in the ileum which exert a further inhibitory effect on gastric emptying and small intestinal motility.

3. Additional fibre may reduce glucose absorption thus inhibiting total transit time.

Scott *et al.* (1998)

Enteral nutrition or the presence of any food in the stomach may also be important in maintaining mucosal integrity (see later).

Pancreas

The pancreas secretes both exocrine and endocrine substances. The principal stimulant of enzyme secretion by the pancreatic cells is cholecystokinin (CCK), although secretin also stimulates the water and bicarbonate component. CCK is released in response to amino acids, peptides, and fatty acids in the small intestine and secretin is released in response to a drop in pH in the proximal duodenum below 4.5.

Exocrine function:

- Secretion of water to dilute chyme (a mixture of semi-digested food and gastric enzymes) and increase nutrient absorption.

- Secretion of bicarbonate to neutralize post-gastric chyme.

- Secretion of inactive forms of enzymes including: (i) protein-digesting trypsin, chymotrypsin, elastase, and carboxypeptidase; (ii) fat-digesting lipase and esterase; (iii) starch-digesting amylase; (iv) nucleic acid-digesting nuclease.

In the duodenum, trypsin is activated by the intestinal mucosal enzyme, enterokinase, and trypsin then activates other pancreatic enzymes.

Endocrine secretions, such as insulin and glucagon, are discussed fully in Chapter 16.

Gallbladder

The gallbladder holds and concentrates bile which is a complex mixture of organic components such as bile acids, phospholipids, cholesterol, and bile pigments and inorganic ions such as sodium, potassium and calcium, chloride and bicarbonate (Johnson 1997):

- Bile emulsifies fat into small droplets for degradation by lipase and esterase into micelles (particles with a fatty core and water-soluble coat). Micelles are then transported across the intestinal lumen leaving the bile behind.

- Bile ionizes fat-soluble vitamins into absorbable forms.

- Bile acts to suspend cholesterol, triglycerides, and medium-density lipoproteins in the blood, preventing precipitation and deposition.

Duodenum and jejunum

The duodenum and jejunum constitute the small intestine where absorption of food primarily takes place. A number of other highly complex mechanisms are associated with this part of the gut:

- Secretion of water to further dilute chyme.

- Secretion of bicarbonate to neutralize post-gastric acidic chyme (water and bicarbonate are secreted by Brunner's glands in the mucosa).

- Mucus secretion to protect the duodenal lumen.

- Secretion of enterokinase to convert trypsinogen (inactive form) to trypsin (active form).

- Secretion of secretin and CCK in response to acidity and proteins. These act to stimulate pancreatic secretion and release of the contents of the gallbladder.

- Secretion of maltase, lactase, and sucrase to convert carbohydrates to simple sugars.

- Mixing of chyme to allow exposure of all molecules to the absorptive surface.

- Peristalsis to propel chyme along the small intestine.

- Absorption of carbohydrates by active and passive transport across the intestinal lumen into the bloodstream.

- Absorption of protein as amino acids and protein fragments by active (assisted movement across a concentration gradient) and passive (movement from high to low concentration) diffusion.

- Absorption of fats in the form of fatty acids and monoglycerides by passive transport in the duodenum and the first half of the jejunum.

- Reabsorption of water and electrolytes as well as iron.

Colon

Between 7 and 10 litres of water enter the small intestine over a 24-hour period but only about 600 ml reach the colon where up to 500 ml are then reabsorbed along with sodium, potassium, chloride, and bicarbonate. Other functions within the colon include:

- Secretion of mucus to lubricate faecal material and protect mucosa.

- Mixing of contents to allow exposure to absorptive surface and peristalsis to propel contents.

- Mass movement to propel faecal matter rapidly into the rectum from the sigmoid and descending colon.

- Absorption of water, potassium, and chloride.

- Absorption of folic acid.

- Absorption of ammonia.

Rectum

The rectum is usually almost or completely empty. It fills intermittently and when distended with faecal material the internal sphincter relaxes unless voluntarily overridden. If defaecation is appropriate rectal propulsion moves contents into the anal canal and both internal and external rectal sphincters relax to allow passage of the faecal bolus.

Effect of tonicity of gastrointestinal contents

Tonicity is defined as the effective osmotic pressure of a fluid in relation to plasma. Further details about osmosis and osmotic pressure can be found in Chapter 9.

The GI tract is highly permeable in both directions to water. Water is absorbed passively throughout the stomach and small and large intestines and also secreted into chyme. If the gastrointestinal contents are hypertonic, then osmosis (the movement of water from an area of low solute concentration to an area of high solute concentration across a semi-permeable membrane) into the lumen will occur. If the contents are hypotonic then there will be movement of water from the gastrointestinal contents into the bloodstream. This can obviously affect the fluid and to a certain extent electrolyte balance of the body but it will also affect the amount of fluid in the gut contents. Thus, a hypertonic enteral feed may well produce diarrhoea due to the movement of water into the gut lumen via osmosis.

The immune function of the gut

The dual functions of (1) connection with and (2) protection from the external environment require both accessibility (for absorption of required substances) and complex defences against external harmful organisms.

Protection is achieved by the following mechanisms:

1. The gut mucosa acts as a physical barrier against systemic invasion by bacteria which colonize the gut.

2. The gut epithelial cells prevent migration of organisms.

3. The intestinal walls contain high numbers of lymphocytes and macrophages.

4. The mesentery is filled with regional lymph nodes.

5. Secretory immunoglobulin A (IgA) is produced intraluminally by specialized cells (Peyer's patches). This prevents adherence of bacteria to mucosal cells and is the principal component of the gut mucosal defence system.

6. Kupffer cells (fixed organ-specific macrophages) in the liver and macrophages in the spleen trap and phagocytose bacteria and toxic products if penetration does occur.

In the healthy person this protection is highly organized and effective, but when the patient becomes critically ill a number of factors may compromise the system and allow migration of invading organisms into the circulation (bacterial translocation). These factors are:

1. Altered permeability or loss of integrity of the intestinal mucosa as a result of hypovolaemic ischaemia, sepsis, or endotoxaemia (the presence in the blood of endotoxin, part of the outer membrane of Gram-negative bacteria; see Chapter 12).

2. Decreased host defence mechanisms such as immunosuppression.

3. Increased bacterial numbers within the intestine caused either by overgrowth or intestinal stasis. The normal gut maintains a balance of commensal bacteria which restricts the numbers of any one type. This balance can be disturbed by antibiotics preventing the growth of one organism and thus allowing overgrowth of another.

All of these factors are found frequently in the critically ill patient who is therefore highly vulnerable to overwhelming bacterial invasion.

Protein malnutrition may also affect the integrity of gut mucosa or the immunocompetence of the gut and contribute to an increased risk of bacterial translocation, although this has not been definitely established (Pingleton 1991). Early enteral feeding may protect against loss of mucosal integrity (Moore *et al.* 1989, Kudsk *et al.* 1992).

Absorption and storage of digested food

Absorption primarily takes place in the villi and microvilli which are prominent on the enterocytes or columnar epithelial cells and some goblet cells. These regions are known as the brush border of the intestine.

Carbohydrate

Digestion reduces carbohydrate polymers to monosaccharides (mainly glucose). The intestinal epithelial cells (brush border) contain enzymes, e.g. glucoamylase and sucrase, which split polysaccharides into monosaccharides. Monosaccharides are absorbed in the small intestine by combining with a carrier substance which also binds with sodium. Sodium is then moved into the cell by its own active transport mechanism and the monosaccharide is pulled with it. This active transport allows absorption to occur against a concentration gradient.

Glucose is carried in the bloodstream to the individual cells where it is transported through the cell membrane by a process known as facilitated diffusion (see Fig. 11.1). Glucose is stored as glycogen either in the liver or in muscle cells. This is usually sufficient to maintain blood glucose levels for about 24 hours under normal fasting conditions.

Fat

Digestion of fat is by hydrolysis catalysed by the enzyme lipase. The end products are fatty acids, glycerol, and glycerides. These molecules are highly soluble in the brush border of the epithelial cells and diffuse readily from the intestinal lumen. The molecules are resynthesized and expelled into the lymph system via the

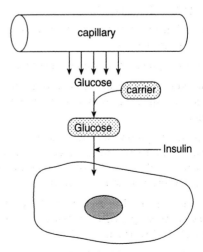

Fig. 11.1 The mechanism of facilitated diffusion of glucose through the cell membrane.

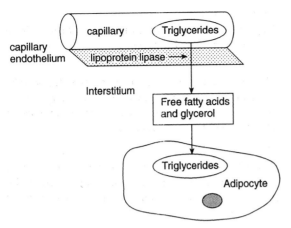

Fig. 11.2 The mechanism of triglyceride (fat) storage in adipocytes.

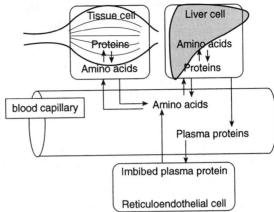

Fig. 11.3 The mechanism of the storage and breakdown of amino acids (proteins).

central lacteals of the villi as small globules of fat called chylomicrons. Lymph is milked from the central lacteals into the abdominal lymphatics by rhythmic contraction of the villi. The chylomicrons are then transported via the thoracic lymph duct to empty into the bloodstream at the junction of the left internal jugular and subclavian vein.

Fat is stored in modified connective tissue cells as triglycerides (see Fig. 11.2). Triglycerides are broken down and resynthesized continuously under the influence of the enzyme lipase. Net breakdown or synthesis is controlled by blood levels of glucose, insulin, catecholamines, and glucagon. High levels of glucose and insulin will increase synthesis and high levels of catecholamines or glucagon will increase breakdown.

Protein

Protein starts to be digested in the stomach by pepsin to form small protein molecules (proteoses, polypeptides, peptones). Pepsin activity is neutralized when the pH changes to alkaline levels. The small protein molecules are further split by trypsin and other enzymes into amino acids and dipeptides and absorbed by active transport into the brush border cells and then taken via the bloodstream to be taken up by cells using the sodium co-transport system utilized by monosaccharides.

The liver and many other cells of the body have the ability to store amino acids and to release them into the bloodstream when levels fall. As a result amino acids are in a state of continual flux from one part of the body to another (Fig. 11.3).

The liver

The liver is one of the most important organs of the body and a wide variety of metabolic functions are per-

formed by the hepatocytes (liver cells). As one of the most essential organs in the body the liver has the ability to regenerate itself. It has both an arterial and venous blood supply with approximately three-quarters of the blood flowing through the liver coming from the portal vein which supplies venous blood. The arterial blood is supplied via the hepatic artery.

The portal vein drains blood from the alimentary canal, spleen, pancreas, and gallbladder containing nutrients for storage and synthesis and debris, including bacteria, for filtration and phagocytosis.

Function of hepatocytes
Carbohydrate metabolism

Glucose homeostasis is maintained by the liver using the following mechanisms:

♦ glycogen storage

♦ gluconeogenesis

♦ release of glucose into plasma.

GLUCONEOGENESIS

Formation of glucose from lactate, pyruvate, amino acids, and glycerol through a series of chemical reactions in the liver cells.

GLYCOGENOLYSIS

The breakdown of glycogen stored in the muscle and liver cells to glucose by enzymes in the liver cells.

When exogenous carbohydrate is not available the blood glucose concentration is maintained by endogenous glucose production, 90% of which is derived from the liver by glycogenolysis or gluconeogenesis. This response is affected by levels of circulating insulin, cortisol, glucagon, adrenaline, and thyroxine.

Degradation of many drugs (including alcohol, benzodiazepines, tranquillizers, phenobarbital, phenytoin, warfarin)

Most drugs metabolized are fat soluble and their conversion by the liver into water-soluble substances facilitates excretion in bile or urine.

Drugs are principally metabolized by hepatic enzymes in a specialized part of the hepatic cell. Two main kinds of chemical change occur:

- non-synthetic—the molecule is changed by oxidation, reduction, hydrolysis,

- synthetic—the molecule is conjugated with other substances such as glucuronic acid, acetic acid, and sulphate.

The pharmacological consequences of drug metabolism vary according to the drug and the reaction it undergoes. Conjugation almost always causes loss of activity (salicylates, paracetamol, and morphine). Acetylation of sulphonamides makes drugs less soluble and therefore potentially more harmful. When two drugs are metabolized by the same microsomal enzymes there may be prolongation of drug action.

Drug metabolism may be impaired in liver disease. The extent to which individual drugs are metabolized in an altered manner is highly variable and care must be taken to avoid overdosage, particularly with sedative drugs.

Elimination of bilirubin

Eighty per cent of bilirubin is derived from haem following the breakdown of haemoglobin in the liver, spleen, and bone marrow. It is not water soluble and is carried in the plasma bound to albumin. In the liver it is transported into the hepatocytes, conjugated with glucuronic acid, and excreted by active transport into the bile. In the terminal ileum and colon, bacteria reduce bilirubin to stercobilinogen which is excreted in the stool. A small amount is reabsorbed and excreted in the urine as urobilinogen.

Fat metabolism

1. Synthesis of lipoprotein from cholesterol, phospholipid, and triglyceride combined with apoproteins.

2. Synthesis of cholesterol and other lipid molecules.

3. Conversion of protein and carbohydrate to fat.

Mineral storage

Hepatocytes store minerals (up to 60% of excess iron) and vitamins, including vitamins A, D, K, B_{12}, and folate.

Production of bile

The primary bile acids (cholic and chenodeoxycholic acid) are produced from cholesterol. They are secreted into bile and then reabsorbed into the portal blood at specific sites in the terminal ileum.

Protein metabolism

1. Synthesis of plasma proteins including albumin, globulins (other than gamma-globulins), transferrin, caeruloplasmin, and components of the complement system.

2. Deamination (breakdown) of proteins and conversion of ammonia to urea.

3. Transamination (movement of amino acids from one molecule to another).

Steroid catabolism

Catabolism of hormones, including insulin, glucagons, cortisol, oestrogens, and contraceptive drugs.

Synthesis of coagulation factors

The following coagulation factors are synthesized by hepatocytes: Factor I, fibrinogen; Factor II, prothrombin; Factor V, proaccelerin; Factor VII, proconvertin; Factor IX, plasma thromoplastin component; Factor X, Stuart factor.

Mononuclear phagocytic function

The mononuclear phagocytic process for clearing the body's own debris and killing and digesting bacteria is carried out by the Kupffer cells in the liver.

Kupffer cells are fixed tissue macrophages sitting in the walls of blood sinuses which can filter particles and foreign bodies/antibody-coated cells etc. The two main functions of the Kupffer cells are:

1. Phagocytosis of bacteria, debris, and other foreign matter in the hepatic sinus blood.

2. Back-up defence mechanism against bacterial translocation into the portal vein.

Assessment of the patient

This should be performed with two goals in mind. The first is to assess the patient's nutritional status and the second is to assess potential GI dysfunction.

History

Useful information can be obtained from the patient if they are able, or relatives if they are not, concerning nutritional status immediately prior to admission. In particular recent weight loss, change in eating habits, and appetite. Other areas which should be explored are bowel function, dental hygiene, and previous GI problems. A history of drug and/or alcohol abuse will also have an impact on the patients nutritional status and should be considered when taking a history.

Physical examination

The patient's general appearance can give a limited evaluation of nutritional state. Obvious signs of obesity and emaciation are easily discernible but muscle wasting (suggesting protein deficiency) may be obscured in the obese patient. Generalized oedema may also mask recognition of muscle wasting and it may only be in the resolution stage of the illness that the degree of loss is apparent. Features of individual vitamin and trace element deficiency, such as dryness, reddening, and petechial haemorrhage of the skin in vitamin C, K, or A deficiencies, may be attributed to other causes such as coagulation disorders.

Jaundice and the almost green tinge associated with bile duct obstruction may be indicators of hepatic dysfunction, although there may be few overt signs until hepatic dysfunction is quite severe.

Examination of the oral cavity

This should be done as part of a general assessment of the patient and includes assessing the condition of the mucosa, teeth (or dentures), and the lips. Signs of inflammation, fungal infection, such as *Candida albicans*, aphthous ulcers, and herpetic lesions should be noted and swabs taken for culture if necessary. Medical staff should be informed.

Teeth need to be examined for blackening, dental caries, wobbling, or loose sockets, and plaque or debris. The gums can be assessed at the same time for signs of inflammation, recession, bleeding, and overgrowth. Bleeding may be related to poor dental hygiene or to coagulation disorders and should be considered in context with the patient's underlying condition. Medical staff should be informed of loose teeth, bleeding gums, and very severe tooth decay, as a dental referral may be necessary.

The patient's breath should also be assessed and any unusual odour such as hepatic foetor (a sweet, musty odour) or ketones (a sweet smell of acetone) should be noted and reported.

Abdominal assessment

The abdomen should be examined for symmetry, size, evidence of distension (taut, swollen skin often with an everted umbilicus), and signs of pulsation (usually visible epigastrically). Dilated veins may be visible and any rashes, scars, or lumps should be noted.

Auscultation of the abdomen to assess bowel sounds should be carried out with the diaphragm of the stethoscope. The absence of bowel sounds cannot be confirmed unless auscultation continues for at least 3 min.

Palpation can be carried out to assess tenderness, muscle resistance, masses, and a fluid thrill (present in ascites). (For details of abdominal palpation see Hudak *et al.* (1990, p. 652).)

Rectal examination may be necessary if the patient complains of constipation or has diarrhoea that may constitute faecal overflow.

Specific problems associated with the gastrointestinal tract

Acute gastrointestinal bleeding

Clinically important gastrointestinal bleeding occurs in 2.8% of mechanically ventilated patients. The risk of bleeding is increased with renal failure and reduced by enteral nutrition(Cook *et al.* 1999).

Acute GI bleeding may be manifested by either:

1. haematemesis—this is usually related to a bleeding point above the duodenojejunal junction, or

2. melaena—altered blood appearing black and tarry from passage through the upper GI tract. If bleeding is copious and current, the patient may pass virtually unaltered blood per rectum.

Assessment of the bleeding patient

Initial assessment of the patient should include the following areas:

1. Physical:
   ◆ Skin—colour, evidence of perspiration, temperature of peripheries.
   ◆ Mucosa—evidence of anaemia.
   ◆ Degree of weakness or obtundation.
   ◆ Level of anxiety, mental state.

2. Haemodynamic:
   ◆ Heart rate, blood pressure, temperature.

3. Fluid status:
   ◆ If there is a central venous catheter, assess CVP.
   ◆ If there is a urinary catheter, assess urine output.
   ◆ If there is a pulmonary artery catheter, assess PA pressures, cardiac output, stroke volume.

4. Respiratory state:

- Respiratory rate, oxygen saturation, arterial blood gases, degree of metabolic acidosis, evidence of respiratory compensation.

If the patient is able to give a history, details should be determined of the frequency and volume of haematemesis or melaena. See Table 11.1 for causes of GI bleeding.

Priorities of management

1. Resuscitation. This refers primarily to replacing and stabilizing blood loss but may also necessitate intubation and ventilation if the patient is unable to sustain adequate blood gases or protect the airway. Supplemental oxygen should always be given. It includes placing large-bore IV access, preferably so that CVP or pulmonary artery occlusion pressure can be monitored, although large peripheral vein access can be used. Fluid is replaced as rapidly as necessary to maintain an adequate circulation. In the first instance, colloid is given urgently while blood is being cross-matched. If the haemoglobin is very low (<5 g/dl) and the patient is compromised then group-specific or at the extreme O-negative blood is necessitated.

2. Monitoring and assessment of the patient's vital signs should be carried out and bloods taken to allow evaluation of arterial blood gases, haemoglobin, clotting, platelets, calcium, and urea and electrolytes.

3. If the patient is aware he/she will require frequent and repeated reassurance and explanation as to what is going on.

Further management

1. If the patient remains hypotensive, in spite of continued fluid resuscitation, investigation of uncontrolled bleeding should be instigated as soon as possible. Otherwise this may be left until the patient's condition has stabilized. Investigation of bleeding may require endoscopy for upper GI bleeding, sigmoidoscopy/colonoscopy for lower GI bleeding, angiography, or even laparotomy.

2. Even if oesophageal varices are suspected, a large-bore nasogastric tube should be inserted to allow drainage and assessment of upper GI bleeding, prevent gastric dilatation, and allow administration of medication. The patient should remain nil by mouth initially in case surgery is required.

3. Treatment can be either surgical, conservative, or using endoscopic or angiographic methods of haemostasis.

Conservative treatment

H_2-receptor antagonists (e.g. ranitidine) or proton pump inhibitors (e.g. omeprazole) are administered to reduce gastric acidity and the accompanying irritation of ulcers. Therapeutic results are best achieved if the gastric pH is kept above 4 and this should be checked 4-hourly. Antacids may have to be administered as well in order to achieve this.

Endoscopic treatment

Sclerosis (fibrosis) of the bleeding point(s) can be performed via the endoscope using either sclerosing agents (adrenaline or alcohol) or, where this is available, electrocoagulation or laser therapy. Preparation of

TABLE 11.1 Causes of gastrointestinal bleeding

Problem	Area affected by problem			
	Upper GI bleeding		Lower GI bleeding	
	Oesophagus	Stomach	Small Intestine	Large Bowel and rectum
Varices	✓	✓ (less common)	✓ (less common)	
Inflammation	✓	✓ (gastritis)		✓ (ulcerative colitis)
Ulcers	✓	✓	✓	
Tumors	✓	✓		✓
Mallory–Weiss tear	✓			
Angiodysplasia		✓ (less common)	✓	✓ (less common)
Crohn's disease			✓	✓
Diverticula			✓ (Meckel's)	
Haemorrhoids				✓
Rectal fissures				✓

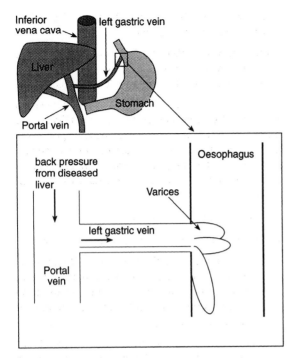

Fig. 11.4 Diagrammatic representation of oesophageal varices.

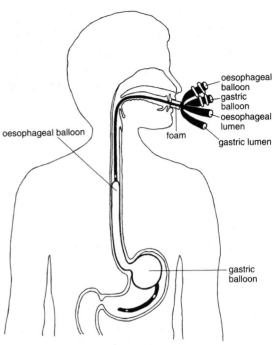

Fig. 11.5 The Sengstaken (modified) tube.

the patient may require iced-water lavage to minimize and clear any active bleeding so that points may be clearly identified and treated.

Oesophageal varices

Aetiology

Oesophageal varices occur when obstruction to the portal vein produces portal hypertension. This may be due to destruction of the hepatic vasculature as in cirrhosis or to obstruction of the portal vein itself. The back pressure produced is transmitted throughout the portal system and has the effect of producing dilatation of the surface blood vessels in the lower oesophagus and, occasionally, the fundus of the stomach and the duodenum (Fig. 11.4). The protruding veins can then become eroded and bleed. Varices should be suspected in patients with acute GI bleeding, particularly with a history/physical examination suggestive of chronic liver damage.

Priorities of management

1. As before, resuscitation of the patient with colloid and blood is of paramount importance.

2. An infusion of vasopressin (antidiuretic hormone) temporarily controls variceal bleeding in 60% of cases. It works by constricting the splanchnic arterioles and increasing their resistance to flow which reduces the amount of blood entering the portal venous system. Its side-effects are systemic hypertension and intestinal colic and it may cause severe ischaemia in the intestine, skin, and heart. Simultaneous infusion of glyceryl trinitrate reduces the coronary and splanchnic vasoconstriction side-effects. Somatostatin or octreotide (a somatostatin analogue) is also commonly used as a first-line splanchnic vasoconstrictor. It is much more expensive, although probably no more effective, than vasopressin.

3. If bleeding is severe a Sengstaken–Blakemore or modified Sengstaken (four-lumen Minnesota) tube should be inserted (Fig. 11.5). This tube is inserted through the nose or mouth and fed into the stomach. It has two balloons which when positioned correctly can apply local pressure to the cardia and the oesophagus. The Sengstaken tube has a lumen for gastric aspiration and the Minnesota tube has an extra lumen in the oesophagus for oesophageal aspiration.

Insertion and care of the Sengstaken tube

This is a difficult manoeuvre which is usually complicated by the agitation of the patient and persistent haematemesis. Particular care should be taken to prevent contamination by blood splashes and all staff involved in the procedure should wear full-face visors, gloves, and plastic aprons.

- Sengstaken or equivalent tube (red rubber or latex tubes should be firmed by placing in a freezing compartment for at least 15 min prior to the procedure)
- Laryngoscope
- Tongue depressor
- Magill's forceps
- Anaesthetic spray
- Lubricating jelly
- Tape to fix the tube
- Piece of sponge, weight, or splint to apply traction
- 50 ml syringe

- The patient requires explanation and preparation for the procedure (see below). They are likely to be considerably distressed and may also be experiencing a degree of hepatic encephalopathy with alterations of perception and behaviour.

- Prior to insertion the balloons should be checked for leaks and patency.

- The tube is inserted with the patient sitting at an angle of about 30° or alternatively in the left lateral position. The choice of position will depend on the patient's conscious level and ability to cooperate.

- When the tube is in position the gastric balloon is inflated with 150–200 ml of air and drawn back until it sits firmly against the cardia of the stomach.

- The tube should be secured with tape and splints or foam applied at the exit point from the nose or mouth in order to maintain traction. Alternatively, firm traction can be maintained using a weight.

- The oesophageal balloon is not usually inflated unless bleeding continues in spite of the gastric tamponade. If it has to be inflated a manometer should be used to ensure that pressures are not greater than 30–40 mmHg (4.5–5.4 kPa). It should not be left inflated for longer than 24 hours as the risk of oesophageal wall ischaemia is high. Some centres do not recommend inflation of the oesophageal balloon at all.

- If the tube has an oesophageal aspiration lumen this should be aspirated frequently or placed on continuous suction in order to prevent build-up of secretions and the danger of aspiration.

- The patient is unable to swallow and saliva will require removal by suction if the patient is unable to spit. Mouth care is essential although difficult to achieve.

Once bleeding is controlled the patient will usually be referred for sclerotherapy, variceal band ligation, or surgery such as transjugular intrahepatic portal systemic shunt (TIPS). TIPS is associated with a reduced incidence of rebleeding from varices although survival is similar to band ligation (Pomier-Layrargues *et al.* 2001) .

Removal of the Sengstaken tube

- The procedure should be explained to the patient.

- The patient should be sitting upright. If there is any concern over the patient's ability to protect his/her airway anaesthetic staff should be consulted to ensure adequate back-up is present to prevent aspiration of any gastric contents.

- If the oesophageal balloon has been inflated this should always be deflated first. Frequently, a period of time is allowed between deflating the oesophageal balloon and removing the tube to ensure that bleeding does not recur.

- Immediately prior to removing the tube the gastric (and oesophageal if this is present) lumen(s) should be aspirated to clear any gastric contents.

- The gastric balloon is then deflated and the tube removed by smooth firm traction.

Stress ulceration

The incidence of histological stress ulceration in ICU patients is high, although the clinical significance of these lesions is much lower. Clinically significant upper

- Where the tube is going.
- How it is going to work.
- The sensations that the patient will experience (e.g. fullness in the stomach, a tube in the mouth and back of the throat, not being able to swallow saliva).
- Likelihood of success: 90% if the tube is used properly.

RISK FACTORS ASSOCIATED WITH STRESS ULCERATION

- Hypoperfusion ischaemia
- Sepsis
- Head injury
- Renal failure
- Multiple trauma
- Respiratory failure and prolonged mechanical ventilation
- Severe burn injuries
- Major surgical procedures
- Fulminant hepatic failure or severe hepatic dysfunction
- Drugs (e.g. non-steroidal anti-inflammatories)

GI bleeding is defined as overt haemorrhage causing haemodynamic instability or requiring transfusion (Cook *et al.* 1999). The number of ulcers that actually cause life-threatening GI bleeding has declined since the late 1980s (Cook *et al.* 1999).

Pathogenesis

A number of factors have been implicated in the development of stress ulcers.

1. Decreased mucosal blood flow

Mucosal blood flow is vital in the maintenance of the gastric mucosal barrier but even a short period of ischaemia may be enough to disrupt the protective function of the mucosa. The mechanism is thought to be a decrease in intramural pH associated with a decreased blood flow limiting removal of hydrogen (H^+) ions, ischaemia, and development of anaerobic metabolism leading to intramural acidosis (Vallet and Lebuffe 1999).

2. Breakdown of the mucosal barrier

Disruption of the mucus-producing cells and reduction in mucus and bicarbonate production and secretion allows back-diffusion of H^+ ions into the mucosa. Factors affecting mucosal breakdown are:

- Bile salts and urea damage the epithelial cells.
- Salicylates and local prostaglandin production inhibit active ion transport and bicarbonate secretion thus reducing the pH gradient between mucosa and gastric lumen.
- Ethanol decreases the thickness of mucus and stimulates histamine release which increases acid secretion.

- Corticosteroids alter the composition and decrease the production of mucus and cause an increase in acid secretion.

3. Increased intraluminal acidity

The level of intraluminal pH is not necessarily a causative factor in itself. Stress ulceration seems to be related to other factors such as the integrity of the mucosal defence mechanisms.

4. Decreased epithelial regeneration

Decreased cellular proliferation and deoxyribonucleic acid (DNA) synthesis in the gastric mucosa have been shown to occur during stress. Thus, regeneration of the mucosal barrier for protection against intraluminal acid is compromised and may lead to ulceration.

5. Lowered intramural pH

It is suggested that the intramural (intramucosal) pH which reflects local ischaemia is a better indicator of the development of stress ulceration than intraluminal pH (Fiddian-Green 1988). The decrease in intramucosal pH can be related to a number of mechanisms which result from poor mucosal blood flow and ischaemia:

- As luminal ions accumulate, they leak back into the mucosa causing a decrease in pH.
- Decreased blood flow causes anaerobic metabolism with a further reduction in pH.
- Vascular permeability is affected by the decrease in mucosal pH causing oedema. This is accentuated by release of histamine and serotonin which cause permeability changes and increased acid secretion.
- Pepsinogen is activated by increased back-diffusion of H^+ ions leading to autodigestion of the mucosa.

While the pathogenesis of stress ulceration remains complex and, as yet, incompletely explained, there are some interventions which have helped to prevent bleeding from stress ulcers. The first and most important is the maintenance of adequate blood flow to the gastric mucosa by early resuscitation of patients with hypovolaemia and concentration on optimal circulatory flow rather than blood pressure. The presence of an acidic intraluminal environment and the loss of the protective mucosal barrier are also thought to be important contributory features.

Neutralizing the acidic intraluminal environment
Antacids

Antacids are suspensions of magnesium and aluminium hydroxides. They act as a base (a substance able to combine with H^+ ions) to neutralize gastric acid. They are effective in reducing the incidence of bleeding provided that the pH is kept above 4. Side-effects include diarrhoea, hypermagnesaemia, increased plasma aluminium levels, and alkalosis. An increased incidence of aspiration pneumonia has been associated with their use, possibly as a result of bacterial overgrowth (Tryba 1991). The requirement of 1- to 4-hourly monitoring of gastric pH and administration of antacid is time-consuming (Konopad and Noseworthy 1988) and there may be difficulty aspirating a representative sample of gastric contents if a fine-bore feeding tube is used.

Histamine (H₂)-receptor antagonists (e.g. ranitidine)

Histamine release is thought to be the method by which increased gastric acid secretion is stimulated. The acid-secreting cells within the stomach respond to the presence of histamine via the H_2 receptor and acid is produced. Ranitidine is the most commonly used H_2 antagonist and has been shown to decrease the incidence of bleeding in selected groups of patients. However, there is no evidence that its use improves the overall survival of critical care patients or that it is effective in clinically important bleeding (Messori *et al.* 2000).

Side-effects of H_2-receptor antagonists include drug interactions, suppression of ADH release, and reports of mental confusion. In addition, cimetidine has caused dysrhythmias, hypotension, and bradycardia, reversible bone marrow depression, and inhibition of cytochrome P-450 in the liver, resulting in altered drug metabolism of diazepam, phenytoin, and propanolol and for these reasons is rarely used.

The increase in intraluminal pH associated with H_2-receptor antagonist use may also result in bacterial overgrowth and an increased incidence of aspiration pneumonia (Messori *et al.* 2000).

Proton-pump inhibitors

Omeprazole binds to and inhibits the potassium-dependent ATPase proton pump of the gastric parietal cell. It does not appear to cause tolerance. However, it requires continuous administration by infusion to maintain gastric pH at >4–6 for more than 12 hours in the critically ill patient (Laterre and Horsmans, 2001).

Improving the protective mucosal barrier

Sucralfate (the basic aluminium salt of sucrose octasulphate) forms a protective barrier over the gastric mucosa and facilitates healing of ulcers while gastric pH is maintained. It has been shown to be effective in the treatment of duodenal ulcers and in the prevention of gastric ulcers (Tryba 1991); however, evidence is conflicting with regard to stress ulceration. There may be less risk of nosocomial pneumonia associated with sucralfate, probably due to the maintenance of gastric pH (Messori *et al.* 2000). It has few side-effects as it is not absorbed from the GI tract.

Enteral feeding has also been suggested as a method of protection from stress ulceration. However, until further studies comparing this with accepted methods have been carried out it is probably advisable to add an alternative form of stress ulcer prophylaxis for high-risk patients such as those with coagulopathies and previous history of gastric or duodenal ulcers.

The incidence of acute GI bleeding from ulcers in the critically ill patient has been dramatically reduced. However, it is likely that this is due as much to general improvements in support of the intensive care patient as to the use of any specific pharmacological agent.

The liver

In the general population, chronic liver disease is much more common than acute liver failure but most patients requiring intensive care are likely to have either acute or acute on chronic liver failure.

Acute liver failure

Incidence and aetiology vary by country and custom with paracetamol (acetaminophen)-induced liver failure more common in the UK, although recent changes restricting dispensed packs to a maximum of 32 tablets may have reduced this (Robinson *et al.* 2000), and *Amanita phalloides* (mushroom) poisoning related liver failure particularly prevalent in France and parts of North America.

Defining types of acute liver failure has been complex and dependent on the interval between onset of jaundice and onset of encephalopathy. Two classifications are currently referred to, those of O'Grady *et al.* (1993) and Bernau *et al.* (1986).

DEFINITIONS OF ACUTE LIVER FAILURE

1. O'Grady *et al.* (1993):

   ◆ hyperacute liver failure (0–7 days)

   ◆ acute liver failure (8–28 days)

   ◆ subacute liver failure (29–72 days)

2. Bernau *et al.* (1986)

   ◆ fulminant hepatic failure (0–14 days)

   ◆ subfulminant hepatic failure (8–12 weeks)

Hyperacute (fulminant) hepatic failure

This is defined as severe impairment of hepatocellular function with concomitant hepatic encephalopathy (see below) in an individual with no evidence of previous liver disease (Levy *et al.* 1991). It can be further subdivided into acute and subacute depending on the length of time from onset to full symptoms. Common causes include viral hepatitis (A, B, C) and paracetamol (acetaminophen) overdose. Other causes include idiosyncratic drug reactions, ingestion of other toxins, e.g. *Amanita phalloides*, acute fatty liver of pregnancy, inhalation of carbon tetrachloride or halothane, and Wilson's disease. Prognosis is poor and mortality remains between 40 and 80% without liver transplantation (Gill and Sterling 2001).

Acute and subacute (subfulminant) hepatic failure

The onset of encephalopathy is delayed and can occur several months after the initial insult. The most frequent causes are viral infections and idiosyncratic drug reactions. Prognosis is very poor and mortality without liver transplantation is more than 80% (Gill and Sterling 2001).

Acute on chronic hepatic failure

This is defined as an acute exacerbation of existing liver disease precipitated by a specific cause. Precipitating causes include: infection, GI haemorrhage (varices, peptic ulcer), administration of sedatives, surgery, high protein load, or any other cause of decompensation of the liver. Short-term survival is better than in fulminant hepatic failure.

Problems associated with acute hepatic failure

Disturbance in conscious level (hepatic encephalopathy)

Encephalopathy (see box for grades of encephalopathy) is the essential clinical feature associated with acute hepatic failure. It is uncertain exactly what causes it but many factors have been implicated. Free fatty acids, mercaptans, phenols, bilirubin, and bile acids have been shown to be toxic. Gamma-aminobutyric acid (GABA), middle molecular weight compounds, and aromatic amino acids have also been associated with encephalopathy. EEG findings typically show diffuse slowing of cortical activity and a high-amplitude waveform of five to seven cycles per second. Subclinical seizure activity can be seen on EEG in grades III and IV which responds to phenytoin and may reduce cerebral oedema.

Cerebral oedema is common in grade III–IV encephalopathy, (>80% of patients with grade IV coma have cerebral oedema) and this is the major cause of death

---

GRADES OF ENCEPHALOPATHY

0: Normal awareness.

I: Mood change, slow mentation, disturbed sleep, usually alert and lucid.

II: Drowsiness, inappropriate behaviour, arousable, and conversant.

III: Marked confusion and disorientation, agitation, stuporose but rousable.

IV: Unrousable to minimal stimuli or no response to noxious stimuli; decerebrate or decorticate posturing.

(Hawker 1990). It is related to disruption of the blood–brain barrier and loss of autoregulation of blood flow. Prognosis is worse as the grade of encephalopathy increases. Diagnosis and management is facilitated by intracranial pressure (ICP) monitoring (see Chapter 10) allowing prompt treatment of increasing ICP.

Coagulopathy

This can cause bleeding at any site including the brain, lungs, and GI tract, as well as retroperitoneal haematoma. Liver synthesis of fibrinogen and factors V, VII, IX, and X is impaired. This is evidenced by prolongation of the prothrombin time which is used as a prognostic index (the greater the prolongation the worse the likely outcome).

Comparison of Factor V levels with Factor XIII (which is synthesized in vascular endothelium) gives a ratio which if greater than 30 has poor prognostic significance.

Alterations in platelet count and function have also been associated with fulminant hepatic failure.

Renal failure

This occurs in approximately 50% of patients and up to 75% of those with grade IV coma. Hepatorenal syndrome refers to a functional renal failure probably due in the majority of cases to generalized intense renal vasoconstriction, the exact mechanism of which is unknown. The blood urea is often low and does not reflect renal function. This is because urea is produced by the liver and production is affected by hepatic failure.

Hypoglycaemia

This is probably related to failure of hepatic gluconeogenesis and can develop rapidly in the early stages. Up to 45% of patients with acute liver failure have hypoglycaemia (Gill and Sterling 2001)

Acid–base and electrolyte imbalance

Hypokalaemia due to inadequate potassium intake, vomiting, and secondary hyperaldosteronism occurs in the early stages of failure. It may later be replaced by hyperkalaemia if renal failure occurs. Hypomagnesaemia, hyponatraemia, hypophosphataemia, and hypocalcaemia can all develop and may exacerbate neurological complications.

Metabolic alkalosis may occur as a response to hypokalaemia and gastric acid loss through vomiting or aspiration. It can also be due to an inability to deal with amino acids in the urea cycle, i.e. removal of the amino radical ($-NH_2$) by conversion into ammonia which combines with carbon dioxide to form urea which is excreted renally.

Metabolic acidosis can occur with paracetamol (acetaminophen) overdose and is also possible as a result of lactic acidosis due to tissue hypoxia.

Respiratory problems

The patient's airway may be compromised due to a decreased conscious level and the ventilatory response to hypoxia is decreased. Patients can develop pulmonary oedema which is thought to be related to alterations in membrane permeability and is associated with cerebral oedema (Levy *et al.* 1991). Furthermore, they develop intrapulmonary shunting leading to ventilation/perfusion mismatch and hypoxaemia. This is due to diffuse dilatation of the pulmonary vascular bed probably as a systemic inflammatory response syndrome (SIRS)-related response.

Cardiovascular problems

Hypotension due to vasodilatation and relative hypovolaemia with high cardiac output and low systemic vascular resistance can occur probably due to circulating inflammatory mediators such as tumour necrosis factor -alpha (TNFα). Arrhythmias related to electrolyte disturbances are common, necessitating continuous monitoring.

Sepsis

The patient is immunocompromised and bacteraemia and fungaemia are common. This is related to reduced reticuloendothelial clearance, impaired leucocyte function, and deficient complement activity. Between 10 and 80% of patients develop bacterial infections (Gill and Sterling 2001).

Management

Due to the high-risk nature of some of the causes of fulminant hepatic failure, source isolation barrier nursing precautions should be followed when caring for these patients.

Encephalopathy

The aims of management are to limit the production of ammonia and avoid precipitating factors such as benzodiazepines. Most ammonia comes from ammonia-forming intestinal bacteria and the breakdown of dietary proteins (Riordan and Williams 1997).

◆ In acute liver failure the absorption of nitrogen should be minimized by low protein intake of less than 40 g/day (Krige and Beckingham 2001). A high-carbohydrate diet to prevent endogenous protein breakdown may also help.

◆ Magnesium sulphate enemas and oral lactulose (a non-absorbable disaccharide) should be given regularly to empty the bowel and therefore reduce re-absorption of protein. The aim is to produce two to four soft stools daily.

◆ Sedation should be avoided unless absolutely essential (if necessary use chlormethiazole, lorazepam, barbiturates, or short-acting anaesthetic agents).

◆ Monitoring of ICP is necessary to effectively manage cerebral oedema (Gill and Sterling 2001). Reduce ICP (aim for <20 mmHg) and maintain cerebral perfusion pressure (aim for > 50 mmHg) using hyperventilation and mannitol. The importance of nursing measures such as maintaining head elevation at >30° and avoiding prolonged coughing or suctioning must be emphasized (full details of these are given in Chapter 10). If these measures prove ineffective, thiopental may be administered (see Chapter 10). Hypotension, hypoxaemia, and hypercapnia should be avoided as these all cause cerebral vasodilatation and thereby increase ICP.

◆ Continuous assessment of the patient's mental state is important so that alterations in conscious level are quickly detected. Patients in the early stages of encephalopathy may be confused and difficult to manage. Considerable nursing time and expertise may be needed to avoid using sedation unless absolutely necessary and to prevent the patient coming to harm.

◆ Reduce sensory load by ensuring a quiet environment with minimal handling and providing reassuring and calming speech and touch (see Chapter 10).

Coagulopathy

◆ Avoid procedures likely to cause bleeding (e.g. prolonged or excessive suction, vigorous mouth care, IM injections).

♦ Bear in mind the potential likelihood of bleeding and observe the patient closely for early indications of covert bleeding.

♦ Administer H_2-antagonists, with or without antacids, to maintain gastric pH >4.

♦ Administer fresh frozen plasma (FFP), whole blood, and platelets as prescribed. This is generally only necessary if spontaneous bleeding occurs or prior to an invasive procedure. The aim is to keep the haemoglobin between 8 and 12 g/dl and to treat bleeding problems.

♦ Vitamin K (10 mg IV) is usually prescribed on a daily basis for 2–3 days.

Renal failure

Many patients with acute liver failure develop anuric renal failure, this is usually due to acute tubular necrosis (Phillips *et al.* 2000). Prevention is the most important aspect of management by:

♦ correction of precipitating causes (especially hypovolaemia),

♦ use of mannitol to promote diuresis,

♦ avoidance of nephrotoxic drugs and high-dose furosemide (frusemide).

Early commencement of continuous renal replacement therapy is preferred to intermittent dialysis due to the reduced fluid shifts involved and their effect on cerebral perfusion (Gill and Sterling 2000).

Hypoglycaemia and nutrition

♦ Monitor blood glucose levels hourly. If blood glucose is <3.5 mmol/l, 10–20% glucose should be infused to maintain normoglycaemic blood levels.

♦ Nutrition should consist of low-protein, high-carbohydrate feed.

♦ Some authorities suggest higher than normal levels of vitamins.

♦ Enteral feeding is possible provided that the patient has not recently bled and the GI tract is functioning.

♦ There is little evidence at present that use of high-branched-chain, low-aromatic amino acid feed formulae improves the level of encephalopathy.

Acid–base and electrolyte management

These are a common problem and should be monitored/managed carefully. Hyponatraemia, hypokalaemia, alkalosis, and acidosis may all occur.

♦ Monitor potassium levels frequently and correct as necessary.

♦ Consider correction of metabolic alkalosis by correction of potassium deficiency.

♦ Respiratory alkalosis associated with hyperventilation and metabolic acidosis does not usually require treatment

Respiratory problems

The patient may need to be intubated in order to protect the airway. If grade III or IV encephalopathy is present elective ventilation is recommended (Riordan and Williams 1997). If severe hypoxaemia, hypoventilation, or fitting occurs the patient should be ventilated. Airway pressures should be kept as low as possible and use of PEEP minimized, IPPV may be used to hyperventilate to reduce ICP in severe cerebral oedema.

Cardiovascular problems

♦ Optimal intravascular volumes should be maintained using either CVP, PA pressure measurements, or other methods of monitoring cardiac output and blood volume such as the oesophageal Doppler.

♦ Treat any causes of hypotension such as hypovolaemia, arrhythmias, and, if necessary, maintain the circulation with inotropes and/or vasopressors.

Risk of infection

♦ Scrupulous attention should be paid to infection control measures. Infective complications occur in 20–36% of patients probably due to impaired neutrophil function, low serum complement concentrations, and decreased humoral response (Vargo and Rudy 1988).

♦ Regular cultures should be taken and appropriate antibiotics prescribed if organisms are found.

♦ Note that there is a high incidence of fungal infections which need to be recognized and treated early.

Chronic hepatic failure

Chronic hepatic failure is characterized by jaundice, ascites, and encephalopathy. The two main causes of chronic hepatic failure are persistent hepatitis and cirrhosis. It is most likely that patients admitted to the critical care unit with chronic hepatic failure will either have suffered an acute decompensation, most commonly due to GI bleeding, or infected ascites. There may be an alternative cause for admission and the chronic liver failure is a secondary pathology.

CAUSES OF CIRRHOSIS OF THE LIVER

- Alcohol
- Infection
- Metabolic disorders (fibrocystic disease, Wilson's disease, glycogen storage disease)
- Drugs (methotrexate, methyldopa)
- Cholestasis
- Immunological factors
- Congestion (hepatic venous outflow obstruction)

Problems associated with chronic hepatic failure

Encephalopathy

The mechanism for development of encephalopathy is presumed to be similar to that of acute hepatic failure but development is slower and cerebral oedema is rare. It is usually known as portal-systemic encephalopathy in chronic failure due to the development of a portal–systemic collateral circulation (caused by portal hypertension). This allows bypassing of the liver by the blood supply of the GI tract and direct entry of toxins to the systemic circulation. The problem is often precipitated by an increased protein load in the gut, particularly following GI haemorrhage.

Ascites

This is not solely due to portal hypertension in cirrhosis. Sodium and water retention are increased by a decreased renal blood flow, and increased release of renin leading to secondary aldosteronism. The secondary aldosteronism is intensified by failure of the liver to metabolize aldosterone and vasopressin. Hypoalbuminaemia due to liver failure will lower colloid osmotic pressure and encourage the formation of oedema.

Oesophageal varices

The pathogenesis of oesophageal varices and their management were discussed earlier in this chapter.

Management

Treatment of the precipitating factor is the most important aspect of management. Blood cultures and diagnostic paracentesis should be taken to rule out infected ascites and active measures should be carried out to prevent further GI bleeding.

Encephalopathy

Management is as for acute hepatic failure (see earlier) except that cerebral oedema is less likely to be a problem.

Ascites

- Sodium restriction of <40 mmol/24 hours.
- Fluid restriction of 1500 ml/24 hours.
- Diuretic therapy.
- Paracentesis (drainage of ascites via an indwelling catheter) with or without infusion of salt-poor albumin.

Oesophageal varices

Management of oesophageal varices was described earlier on this chapter.

Jaundice

This word 'jaundice' refers to the yellow appearance of the skin and mucous membranes seen with an increased bilirubin concentration in the body fluids. It is detectable when the serum bilirubin concentration exceeds 50 µmol/l.

Causes of jaundice are either haemolysis, obstruction, or hepatocellular.

Haemolytic jaundice

An increased rate of destruction of red blood cells produces an increased amount of bilirubin which is excreted by the liver until its capacity is overwhelmed. The jaundice is usually mild, as the healthy liver can excrete up to six times the normal bilirubin load. Causes of haemolytic jaundice include drugs, erythrocyte abnormalities (e.g. sickle-cell disease), and malaria.

Obstructive jaundice

Jaundice occurs due to obstruction of the excretion of bilirubin anywhere between the biliary canaliculi and the ampulla of Vater. Causes of large duct obstruction include gallstones in the common bile duct, biliary duct strictures, sclerosing cholangitis, carcinoma of the head of the pancreas, and other tumours. Causes of small duct obstruction include drugs and alcohol, which damage liver cells and bile ducts, primary diseases of the hepatocytes, such as viral hepatitis, severe bacterial infections, Hodgkin's disease, primary biliary cirrhosis, and pericho1angitis associated with ulcerative colitis.

Jaundice can be prolonged and severe and the patient will pass pale or clay-coloured stools due to the lack of bilirubin entering the gut. Urine will be dark due to renal excretion of conjugated bilirubin.

Hepatocellular jaundice

Jaundice results from the inability of the liver to transport bilirubin into the bile as a result of liver cell damage. Common causes are alcohol, drugs, and hepatitis

B. Drugs, such as salicylates, oral contraceptives, and rifampicin, can interfere with bilirubin metabolism. The mechanisms are:

- displacement of bilirubin from protein binding in the blood (e.g. salicylates),

- impairment of bilirubin uptake and transport (e.g. rifampicin),

- blockage of excretion into the canaliculi (e.g. oral contraceptives).

Liver dysfunction

Critically ill patients may develop liver dysfunction as part of multiple organ failure. This can be either as a result of circulatory disturbance or as a reaction to one or more of the drugs used in treatment. Factors involved are numerous and may produce both hepatocellular damage and intrahepatic cholestasis. Decreased hepatic perfusion and hypoxia are a likely cause although cholestasis due to extrahepatic bile duct obstruction may also occur.

Management depends on the precipitating cause, but is usually dependent on treating the underlying disease. If drugs are suspected as a cause then they are discontinued and an alternative used.

Liver support systems

Liver transplantation is considered the only fully effective treatment for acute liver failure which does not respond to supportive management (Gill and Sterling 2001). However, the growing disparity between donor availability and demand has meant that many patients do not receive a donor organ in time. There has therefore been a concentrated research focus on alternative liver assist devices to allow support until either a donor can be found or until liver function is recovered. These support systems fall into two types:

1. *Extracorporeal blood purification techniques.* This involves use of a double-sided albumin-impregnated hollow-fibre dialysis membrane (which adsorbs molecules onto its surface). Blood travels through one side of the membrane allowing adsorption of protein-bound toxins onto the membrane and albumin is then run through the other side of the membrane and removes the toxins via the concentration gradient (in a similar manner to haemodiafiltration; see Chapter 9). The albumin is then run through a charcoal filter, an ion-exchange resin, and another dialyser run against ordinary dialysate. This clears all the toxins picked up by the albumin which is then returned to the pa-

tient circuit in a closed loop. This is known as the molecular adsorption recycling system (MARS). It is still undergoing extensive trials, but on the basis of early work may be beneficial for both acute and acute on chronic liver failure (Sorkine et al. 2001).

2. *Biological liver support systems.* This technique combines the use of artificially generated hepatocytes in a system based again on a dialyser. The hepatocytes are grown in the dialyser plates themselves or attached to a matrix within the dialyser. There are problems with the short life of the hepatocytes and the lack of replication which requires a new supply of hepatocytes every 6–7 hours. Although research in humans is still in a very early stage, there may be potential if these difficulties can be overcome (Sorkine et al. 2001).

Liver transplantation

This procedure is necessary in patients who have severe acute liver failure or chronic, irreversible, and progressive liver disease which does not respond to alternative medical and surgical interventions. Between 1994 and 1998 in the UK a total of 3102 liver transplants were carried out, of which 87 per cent were first transplants. The mean age at first transplantation was 42 years (range 0–76 years). The most common indications for transplantation were primary biliary cirrhosis, alcoholic cirrhosis, and post-hepatitis C cirrhosis (Hartley et al. 2001)

Major contraindications are extrahepatic malignancy, severe sepsis, and active alcoholism.

Relative contraindications are portal vein thrombosis, severe cardiopulmonary or renal disease, age over 55 years, past multiple abdominal operations, psychological instability, and positive hepatitis B e-antigen.

CONDITIONS IN WHICH LIVER TRANSPLANT MAY BE APPROPRIATE

- Biliary atresia
- Inborn errors of metabolism
- Chronic active cirrhosis
- Primary biliary cirrhosis
- Sclerosing cholangitis
- Primary hepatic malignancy
- Acute liver failure
- Subacute hepatic necrosis

Donors

Live organ donation

Development of techniques in splitting livers to pro-duce firstly reduced-size grafts from adult donors for children and then in producing split liver-transplants where two recipients could be transplanted with one donor liver have resulted in the technique of live organ donation of livers in adults. This is possible because of the segmental structure of the liver (allowing surgical division with vascular and biliary access) and the regenerative capacity of the liver itself (Seaman 2001). Although a success rate of over 87% at year one has been quoted (Seaman 2001) there is a risk to the donor as well as the recipient due to the large volume of liver tissue required (about 65%) in adults. The technique is growing in specific centres Liu *et al.* (2002) have recently published a study of 16 live donor transplant recipients, 14 of the recipients and all the donors survived. However, this should still be considered experimental until further work is published.

Cadaveric organ donation

The same criteria for approach to donation are required as for any other organ (see Chapter 10 and Hawker 1990).

Transplantation

Orthotopic (replacement of the recipient's liver with that of the donor) transplantation is the usual method. Donor livers can be maintained for between 8 and 20 hours using a perfusion solution.

Blood loss can be high and transfusion requirements may range from 10 to 100 units. Fresh frozen plasma (FFP) and platelets are also required in large quantities.

CLINICAL CRITERIA FOR CADAVERIC LIVER DONORS

- Age less than 55 years
- No hepatobiliary disease or severe liver trauma
- Acceptable liver function tests and coagulation profile
- Size and ABO compatibility with available recipient
- No extracerebral malignancy
- No active systemic or hepatic infection
- Negative HIV and hepatitis B serology
- Negative cytomegalovirus (CMV) serology

(Hawker 1990)

Post-operative management

1. *Haemodynamic problems*:

   - Monitoring and management of intravascular volume is vital and patients have pulmonary artery catheters *in situ* to allow assessment of fluid status as well as cardiac output. Suboptimal circulating volumes are corrected using blood, colloid, and crystalloid as appropriate.

   - Hypotension not related to low intravascular volume is corrected using inotropes. The specific inotrope will depend on peripheral vascular resistance and cardiac output (see Chapter 6).

   - Hypertension occasionally occurs and must be controlled to protect the integrity of the vascular anastomoses. Treatment is usually related to the underlying cause, such as inadequate sedation or continuing cerebral oedema, in patients with previous acute hepatic failure. Occasionally, anti-hypertensive agents are required.

   - Hypothermia is common due to the length of operation and the use of bypass. Gradual warming is instituted using foil blankets.

2. *Respiratory problems*: the majority of patients are ventilated post-operatively to allow optimal respiratory support. PEEP at moderate levels is used to minimize basal atelectasis. Active chest physiotherapy is then required to prevent further problems. Pleural effusions are common and the majority resolve spontaneously or with diuretic therapy. Development of ARDS is associated with intraabdominal sepsis, allograft rejection, and hepatic artery thrombosis.

3. *Metabolic disturbances*:

   - Hypokalaemia can be severe due to absorption of potassium into the reperfused hepatocytes. Potassium supplements are given routinely unless serum levels are high.

   - Hyperglycaemia may require insulin to maintain normal blood glucose levels.

   - Metabolic alkalosis is probably related to the large amounts of citrate in transfused blood as well as hypokalaemia.

4. *Bleeding and coagulopathy*: continuous bleeding is usually surgical in origin and may necessitate a return to theatre. Coagulopathy can usually be controlled using FFP and platelet infusions.

5. *Immunosuppression*: the exact programme and timing of immunosuppression varies but the primary agents used are prednisolone, azathioprine, and ciclosporin. Newer agents, such as polyclonal and monoclonal antilymphocyte globulin preparations, are used in some centres as initial immunosuppression which is then followed by ciclosporin long term. Ciclosporin is a highly effective immunosuppressant but its use carries the risk of a number of side-effects (e.g. nephrotoxicity), some of which can be severe.

6. *Infection*:
   - The patient will be susceptible to infection due to his/her state of chronic ill health or acute liver failure pre-operatively. This will then be compounded by the introduction of immunosuppressive drugs.
   - Bacterial infections occur frequently post-operatively and are treated with the appropriate antibiotics. Fungal infections (*Candida albicans* and *Aspergillus* most commonly) are treated with amphotericin B. Viral infections can also occur and require acyclovir.
   - Patients should be nursed in side-rooms with protective isolation. Scrupulous care is required for all clean and aseptic procedures.

7. *Renal dysfunction*: This occurs in up to two-thirds of transplant patients post-operatively. It may result from continued bleeding and poor renal perfusion, sepsis, and poor allograft function. The drugs used for immunosuppression and to treat infection can be highly nephrotoxic. Management consists of maintaining intravascular volume. The aim is to produce 0.5 ml/kg/hour urine.

THE PATIENT EXPERIENCE OF TRANSPLANT

Categories of experience include:

1. Facing the inevitable
2. Recapturing the body
3. Emotional chaos
4. Leaving the experts
5. Family and friends
6. The threat of graft rejection
7. Honouring the donor

Forsberg *et al.* (2000)

---

8. *Neurological dysfunction*: patients who have undergone transplant for acute liver failure will require continual ICP monitoring throughout the postoperative period. Neurological assessment is regularly carried out to monitor status in all liver transplant patients. Complications, such as fitting, can occur which are usually associated with ciclosporin neurotoxicity or hypomagnesaemia. Other neurological problems may occur as a result of intracerebral haemorrhage, hepatic or metabolic encephalopathy, and opportunistic infection.

9. *Pain*: an opiate, such as morphine, is usually given as an infusion or intravenous bolus. Some centres also use a sedative, such as diazepam, to reduce the patient's awareness of discomfort and facilitate ventilation.

10. *Psychological problems*: there are numerous psychological problems associated with adjusting to transplantation. The nearness of death will have caused fear and anxiety and a necessity to confront their own mortality. The adjustment to accepting the presence of another person's organ within their own body may also take considerable support and rationalization. Forsberg *et al.* (2000) have identified a range of profound emotions experienced by transplant recipients in their phenomenological study of the patient experience. Patients require trained counselling and support which must be an important part of any transplant programme.

11. *Nutritional deficit*: patients are often severely malnourished pre-operatively due to prolonged liver disease. Energy expenditure is significantly raised by the stresses associated with transplantation and patients are hypercatabolic in the post-operative phase. Nutrition is therefore urgently required and can be given either enterally or parenterally.

12. *Liver dysfunction*: liver function usually returns to normal soon after transplantation but up to two-thirds of patients suffer some degree of liver dysfunction. In the extreme situation the graft fails to function immediately due to ischaemic injury and there is total hepatic failure. Retransplantation is the only possible course, although prognosis is poor. There may be some lesser degree of failure related to technical complications, such as bleeding, and these may be repaired on return to theatre. Rejection is the commonest cause of graft dysfunction and occurs to some extent in most patients usually 2–3 weeks later. Rejection can occur slowly

and progressively or acutely. Treatment consists of increasing levels of steroids and use of antilympho-cyte globulin or monoclonal antilymphocyte anti-body (OKT3). Survival following liver transplant is now around 80% at 1 year and 60% at 5 years. It is an accepted form of treatment both in end-stage liver disease and acute liver failure.

Acute pancreatitis

This condition occurs in about 1 in 10 000 people and is largely associated with alcohol abuse or gallbladder dis-ease (75% of cases).

The exact aetiology of the disease is unknown but its pathogenesis involves the activation of pancreatic enzymes within the pancreas rather than in the duo-denum (see earlier). This leads to autodigestion and an acute inflammatory response. It is thought that in the case of alcohol this is caused by irritation and protein precipitation which obstructs the acinar ductules and traps enzymes within the pancreas. The irritant factor in gallbladder disease is thought to be bile which due to biliary tract abnormalities may reflux back and irritate the pancreas. Blockage of the pancreatic duct by gall-stones may also precipitate pancreatitis. Many of the multisystem problems associated with pancreatitis (res-piratory complications, cardiac abnormalities, impaired renal function, disseminated intravascular coagulation, etc.) are related to the transfer of enzymes and pro-ducts of pancreatic tissue destruction to the circulation. This is thought to happen via the lymphatic drainage of the pancreas. Overall mortality associated with the disease has steadily reduced over the past 20 years to between 4 and 8% (Bank *et al.* 2002). Outcome is related

---

SIGNS AND SYMPTOMS OF ACUTE PANCREATITIS

- Acute epigastric and peri-umbilical pain
- Nausea and vomiting
- Abdominal distension associated with a small bowel ileus or pseudocyst in severe disease
- Low-grade pyrexia, occasionally hypothermia
- Shock: ↑ pulse, ↓ BP, etc.
- Retroperitoneal haemorrhage showing as either Grey–Turner sign—grey discoloration (bruising) over the flanks—or Cullen's sign—bruising in and round the umbilicus

---

LABORATORY DATA ASSOCIATED WITH ACUTE PANCREATITIS

- Serum amylase is high (usually >1000 IU/l)
- Serum lipase is high in 75% of cases
- Total calcium levels are decreased (this may be due to hypoalbuminaemia or extravascular pre-cipitation)
- Ionized calcium levels may also decrease due to intraperitoneal combination with free fatty acids
- Hyperglycaemia is common (this is related to either hyperglucagonaemia or, more commonly, insulin deficiency)
- Hyperbilirubinaemia
- Raised transaminase and alkaline phosphatase levels
- Hypoalbuminaemia

RANSON SCORE FOR PROGNOSTIC FACTORS IN ACUTE PANCREATITIS

On admission:

- Age >55 years
- White cell count >16,000/mm^3
- Glucose >11mmol/l
- LDH >400 IU/l
- AST >250 IU/l

Within 48 hrs of hospitalization:

- Decrease in Hct >10%
- Increase in blood urea >1.8 mmol/l
- Calcium <2 mmol/l
- P_aO_2 < 8 kPa
- Base deficit >4 mmol/l
- Fluid deficit >6 litres

Mortality rates:

- 0–2 risk factors: mortality rate <1%
- 3–4 risk factors: mortality rate ≈15%
- 5–6 risk factors: mortality rate ≈40%
- >6 risk factors: mortality rate ≈100%

to the severity of the disease and the vast majority of deaths occur in the 25% of patients with most severe form of the disease (Wyncoll 1999). This group should be treated in specialized referral centres.

Diagnosis of pancreatitis is difficult and is usually based on a number of differential diagnoses as well as the interpretation of laboratory data. The use of CT scans is also considered an effective method of assessment of acute pancreatitis and associated complications (Wyncoll 1999).

Strategies for management

Correction of hypovoloemia and fluid volume imbalances

The release of vasoactive substances following auto-digestion of pancreatic tissue causes alterations in permeability of the capillary membrane. This leads to large losses of fluid into the extravascular space and particularly into the peritoneal space. Fluid losses lead to a low circulating blood volume with reactive constriction of the splanchnic (abdominal organ) blood vessels resulting in poor perfusion of the pancreas, further damage to pancreatic tissue, and a continuing downward spiral in the patient's condition.

Further fluid losses related to nasogastric aspiration and vomiting must also be taken into account:

◆ Adequate volume loading is essential in the management of these patients and should be given under CVP or PA pressure monitoring. The fluid of choice will depend on the clinical situation and can be crystalloid or colloid, although blood may be used in haemorrhagic pancreatitis if the haemoglobin is low.

◆ Crystalloid fluid replacement should continue at a rate suitable for the patient's normal fluid requirements. The aim is to preserve organ perfusion and maintain renal function with a urine output >0.5 ml/kg/hour.

Correction of electrolyte imbalances

Imbalances in calcium, magnesium, phosphate, and potassium are also related to alterations in capillary permeability, nasogastric losses, vomiting, and diarrhoea. Calcium levels are reduced as a result of intraperitoneal saponification (combination to form a soap-like compound) with free fatty acids released during fat necrosis. Alcohol abusers may also suffer from diet-related decreases in these levels:

◆ Levels should be monitored and corrected as required.

◆ The patient should also be observed for signs of hypocalcaemia.

◆ Continuous ECG monitoring is useful for signs of, and arrhythmias associated with, hypokalaemia and hypomagnesaemia. Regular measurements of elec-

---

SIGNS OF HYPOCALCAEMIA

◆ *Chvostek's sign*: twitching of the lip and cheek in response to tapping of the side of the face over the facial nerve in the parotid gland.

◆ *Trousseau's sign*: carpopedal spasm with wrist and metacarpophalangeal joints flexed and interphalangeal joints extended when a blood pressure cuff placed on the same arm is inflated to just above systolic pressure. (The response should occur within 2 min.)

---

trolytes from arterial blood samples should be taken to monitor potassium levels.

Haemodynamic disturbances

These are related to the acute inflammatory process as well as hypovolaemia, hypocalcaemia, hypokalaemia, and possible myocardial depressant factors:

◆ There is a need for continuous monitoring of blood pressure, ECG, CVP, or PA, and cardiac output if myocardial depression is suspected.

◆ Ideally, the patient should be catheterized in order to monitor urine output.

◆ Intravascular volume should be optimized and electrolyte levels corrected. If cardiac output remains low, inotropes will be required or vasopressors if in high-output shock.

Compromised respiratory function

Hyperventilation may occur as a response to the acute pain associated with pancreatitis. Pain relief is important in limiting this response. Respiratory complications occur in 30–50% of patients and up to 70% are hypoxaemic. There are a number of possible contributory factors:

◆ Increased likelihood of developing ARDS (see Chapter 4). Non-cardiogenic pulmonary oedema occurs in 10–30% of patients.

◆ Pleural effusions may form from the passage of pancreatic exudate via lymph channels into the chest, or extravasation of exudate through the diaphragm.

◆ Pseudocysts or abscesses may form a fistula into the chest cavity.

◆ Atelectasis may occur as a result of hypoventilation due to pain-related splinting of the abdominal wall.

Management consists of supporting respiratory function with appropriate oxygen therapy and ventilation when necessary. Monitoring should include pulse oximetry and frequent arterial blood gases.

Pain

The epigastric and peri-umbilical pain in acute pancreatitis is caused by extravasation of inflammatory exudate and enzymes into the retroperitoneum. This may lead to digestion of the fat in the pancreatic bed and surrounding tissue. Another cause may be distension of pancreatic ducts and obstruction of the ampulla of Vater or swelling of the head of the pancreas producing duodenal obstruction.

- Analgesia is essential, usually by opiate infusions. Pethidine is the opiate of choice and morphine should be avoided due to its increased ability to cause spasm of the sphincter of Oddi.

- Localized analgesia, such as nerve blocks or ganglion blocks, may be useful, although epidurals should be used with caution.

- Other methods of pain relief, such as warmth, positioning, and relaxation, may have a minimizing effect but are unlikely to take the pain away completely.

- Continuous nasogastric aspiration and nil by mouth should be instituted in order to limit pancreatic stimulus to release enzymes.

Hyperglycaemia

This can occur secondary to hyperglucagonaemia and insulin deficiency. Insulin infusion titrated to blood glucose levels should be used.

Nutrition

The role of enteral nutrition in acute pancreatitis is still under debate. The stimulant effect that food in the stomach may have on the pancreas in severe pancreatitis is thought to be a stressor and many centres continue to recommend parenteral nutrition. However, the jejunal route can be used for feeding without pancreatic stimulation and this has been shown to be beneficial even in severe pancreatitis, with reduced septic complications ($P < 0.01$) and fewer total complications (Windsor *et al.* 1998). Some centres have infused elemental feed intragastrically without apparent harm (Schlichtig and Ayres 1988). The feed should be high in carbohydrate and low in fat to minimize pancreatic secretion. Patients with small bowel obstruction should not receive enteral feed.

In mild, uncomplicated, pancreatitis nutritional support may not be necessary, initially. However, in moderate to severe pancreatitis nutritional support should be instituted early with placement of a jejunal tube or parenteral nutrition if this is unsuccessful (Wyncoll 1999).

Secondary infection

Administration of high-dose IV antibiotics such as imipenem or cefuroxime may be beneficial in reducing infectious complications (Wyncoll 1999).

INDICATIONS FOR ENDOSCOPY

- Acute gastrointestinal haemorrhage (identification of site and haemostasis)
- Biopsy of lesions such as tumours and ulcers
- Placement of duodenal and jejunal feeding tubes
- Sclerosis of oesophageal varices
- Removal of ingested foreign objects
- Studies of biliary and pancreatic ducts

Surgery or drainage of abscesses/necrosis

Surgical debridement or radiologically-guided drainage is occasionally indicated, particularly if the general state of the patient deteriorates.

Endoscopy

Oesophagogastroduodenoscopy (OGD) is the examination of the upper GI tract using a flexible fibreoptic instrument which is passed into the mouth and down the oesophagus to allow direct visualization of the mucosal surface. It is also possible to carry out procedures such as sclerosis of varices, and to take biopsies of lesions such as ulcers, via an instrument channel within the scope.

The critically ill patient is most likely to require endoscopy for investigation of GI haemorrhage, epigastric pain, and possibly to carry out haemostasis of bleeding varices or ulcers.

Preparation of the patient for endoscopy

The patient should be adequately resuscitated from any bleeding prior to endoscopy. In addition, an explanation of the procedure, reasons for it, and likely sensations should be given. Routine gastric lavage prior to the procedure is unnecessary. Increased levels of sedation may be required during the procedure. Endoscopy can cause hypoxaemia in any patient with cardiorespiratory compromise and monitoring of ECG, arterial blood pressure, and oxygen saturation should continue throughout the procedure. If necessary, the inspired oxygen concentration may have to be increased.

Following the procedure, the patient should be observed for signs of further bleeding and/or perforation (see Table 11.2 for haemostasis).

Delivery of nutritional support

Most critically ill patients are unable to meet their own nutritional requirements in the normal way. They must therefore be assessed and the most appropriate type of support decided on the basis of that assessment.

TABLE 11.2	Haemostasis of bleeding points
1. Chemical methods	Injection of sclerosants, such as adrenaline and alcohol, directly into the base of an ulcer
	Use and efficacy: Can control arterial bleeding in over 90% of cases
2. Thermal methods	Electrocoagulation: monopolar and bipolar diathermy. Heater probe. Laser photocoagulation
	Use and efficacy: Haemostasis of most vessels apart from brisk arterial bleeding. Can control arterial bleeding from peptic ulcers. Effective in 80–90% of ulcer bleeds. Can reduce the incidence of arterial rebleeding from ulcers

Assessment of the patient's nutritional status and requirements

This is difficult in the critically ill patient; problems are caused not only by the alteration in metabolic function associated particularly with sepsis and trauma, but also by other stressors (for details see Chapter 3).

Most of the methods for assessing nutritional status and requirement were produced for a relatively well population and may not apply to the critically ill. Suggested methods are described below with details of their application in intensive care.

Anthropometry

Daily weight is not a reliable measure of nutritional status in the critically ill. The fluid balance fluctuations associated with the illness or therapy may produce considerable changes in weight which are unrelated to nutrition. Weight loss itself also gives little indication of the composition of that loss. Thus, a 2 kg weight loss in starvation may have a ratio of fat to protein of 2:1, but in the hypercatabolic patient the ratio may be 1:4 (Berger and Adams 1989) with much graver consequences.

Measurement of skinfold thickness and midarm muscle circumference have also been used to gauge muscle mass (for details of the technique see Goodinson 1987) but this too has problems in the critically ill patient. Oedema may seriously alter the measurement, changes develop slowly, and there can be considerable interoperator variation.

Measurements of hand-grip muscle strength by dynamometry and respiratory muscle strength using maximal inspiratory force have been used but are affected by other variables such as patient cooperation and respiratory muscle fatigue.

CALCULATION OF NITROGEN BALANCE

Nitrogen balance = (intake − loss/24 hours).

Intake (g/24 hours) = protein/6.25 (g/24 hours).

Loss (g/24 h) = urinary urea (mmol/l) × urinary volume/24 hours (litres) × 0.028.

Assessment of nitrogen balance

Loss of protein stores can be profound in acute illness. Finn *et al.* (1996) found up to 17% of body stores were lost in 21 days in multiple trauma patients, two-thirds of which was skeletal muscle mass.

Nitrogen balance, as the end product of amino acid breakdown, can provide an insight into whether protein (and therefore lean body mass) is being gained or lost. Intake of nitrogen (usually in the form of protein) is compared to nitrogen losses as urinary urea in a 24-hour urine collection (about 90–95% of nitrogen is excreted in the urine). The difference between the two is termed the nitrogen balance and may be neutral or negative but is rarely positive in the critically ill (Schlichtig and Ayres 1988).

An estimate of faecal losses of 4 g/day of nitrogen has been suggested. However, in the parenterally fed patient with minimal or absent stools this will overestimate the losses, and vice versa in the patient with diarrhoea. It must therefore be added to the nitrogen balance calculation with caution.

The usefulness of nitrogen balance in assessing the patient's nutritional state is debatable. Assumptions are made that a steady state exists within the body pool of nitrogen, but this may not be the case. For instance, a rising blood urea in acute renal failure will affect the amount of urinary urea lost giving a falsely low level of nitrogen loss. Correct interpretation of nitrogen balance is therefore important and assessment of the patient's overall nutritional status must be made in order to evaluate the results correctly.

Levels of serum proteins as nutritional indicators

Most investigators have concluded that levels of serum proteins do not accurately assess whole-body nutritional status in individual patients (Schlichtig and Ayres 1988). There are a number of other factors involved in the critically ill patient which alter the levels of these proteins without affecting nutritional status. The most commonly used indicator has been albumin; however, albumin levels are frequently low in the critically ill due to:

- fluid shifts producing comparative dilution,
- movement of proteins into extravascular spaces through leaky capillary membranes,

PLASMA PROTEINS USED TO ASSESS NUTRITIONAL STATE

Serum albumin

May fall precipitately in the critically ill without significant nutritional deficit. It rises slowly in repletion.

Serum transferrin

Can also be raised in iron deficiency. It frequently underestimates nutritional status in the critically ill. It rises earlier than albumin in repletion.

♦ dilution by infusion of artificial colloids,

♦ decreased liver production due to liver dysfunction associated with the disease state.

Thus, despite the absence of significant malnutrition, low albumin levels may be found and are considered to be a non-specific indicator of illness.

Indirect calorimetry

This is the only clinical method currently available that can provide a reasonably accurate assessment of the individual patient's energy requirements (McClave *et al.* 2001). It is a technique whereby the patient's energy expenditure is calculated from the inspired and expired gases (i.e. the amount of oxygen consumed and the amount of carbon dioxide produced by the patient). These gases are consumed and produced during the oxidation of food substances and the amount of oxygen and carbon dioxide can be directly related to the amount of food oxidized to produce energy:

$C_6H_{12}O_6$ (carbohydrate) $+ 6O_2 = 6H_2O + 6CO_2 +$ energy (kcal).

It requires a stand-alone metabolic monitor, such as the Datex Deltatrac, or a ventilator that incorporates metabolic monitoring. It is also possible to use the technique of mass spectrometry (different constituents of a gas are detected by passing them through an electron beam which ionizes them, and then a magnetic field which separates the ionized molecules by their mass and electric charge); however, this is a very expensive alternative and is rarely available clinically.

The advantages of indirect calorimetry for assessment of energy expenditure are that:

1. It is accurate for the individual patient (as opposed to formulae and tables which are accurate for a population of patients).

2. If continuous measurements are performed, changes in metabolic rate (for instance, as a result of activity or drugs) are measured (Weissman *et al.* 1989).

3. It gives an immediate answer to the patient's energy requirements rather than waiting for laboratory analysis, etc.

Other information may be gained from the use of indirect calorimetry, such as an indirect measure of the work of breathing. If the patient is being weaned from the ventilator and support is decreased, provided no other changes in the patient's condition are occurring, then the increase in oxygen consumption will reflect the increased work required from the patient to compensate for the decrease in ventilatory support.

The disadvantages of indirect calorimetry for assessment of energy expenditure are that:

1. Its accuracy decreases with increasing inspired oxygen concentrations; an error >5% exists with $F_iO_2 > 0.6$. it is therefore more inaccurate in the critically ill patients who are least able to tolerate the effects of either over- or underfeeding.

2. The assumption that steady-state conditions exist may not always apply. In particular, body carbon dioxide pools are likely to increase and decrease if there are pH imbalances and this may produce an inaccurate reading.

3. If the patient is on haemofiltration, there may be carbon dioxide loss across the filter membrane in solution in the ultrafiltrate and as bicarbonate. This results in potential underestimation of carbon dioxide production by the indirect calorimeter and therefore underestimation of energy expenditure.

4. Hypoventilation and hyperventilation will also affect the measurement of expired gases as carbon dioxide accumulates or is blown off. This results in over- or underestimation of energy expenditure.

5. A major disadvantage of this method is the cost of the equipment which may make its routine use prohibitive.

If used correctly, indirect calorimetry is the most accurate way of assessing the individual critically ill patient's energy needs (Carlsson *et al.* 1984, Weissman *et al.* 1986, Van Lanschot *et al.* 1986).

Markers of gut function

A number of factors are used in assessing the function of the gut, but some are more useful than others and all should be assessed before a decision on function is made (Table 11.3).

TABLE 11.3 Factors involved in deciding the mode of nutritional support

Gut function	Oral/oesophageal route	Mastication and swallowing	Mode of nutritional support
Gut is fully functioning	Oral oesophageal route is patent	Patient is able to masticate and swallow	Patient can eat a normal diet
Gut is functioning, although tolerance of certain foods may be affected	Oral/oesophageal route is patent	Patient may have difficulty with mastication but can swallow	Patient can eat a modified diet
Gut is functioning, although tolerance of certain foods may be affected	Oral/oesophageal route may have some degree of restriction or damage so that whole foods are not tolerated	Patient may have difficulty with mastication but can swallow	Patient can take nourishing fluids only
Gut is functioning, although tolerance of certain foods may be affected or parts of the gut, such as the stomach, may not function	Oral/oesophageal route may be restricted or damaged or gastric function may be absent	Patient has difficulty masticating or swallowing	Patient requires enteral feed via a nasogastric/duodenal tube or gastrostomy/jejunostomy tube
Gut is not functioning or requires rest from stimulation			Patient requires parenteral nutrition

Presence or absence of bowel sounds

These are frequently used as an absolute indicator of gut function but their presence or absence should be interpreted with caution. Bowel sounds are produced by the disruption of the gas–fluid interface of the intestinal and gastric lumen by peristaltic waves. The largest areas of gas–fluid interface are in the stomach and the colon—the two areas of the bowel most sensitive to loss of function. In some circumstances, gastric and colonic function may be affected but small bowel function may continue or return more quickly following an insult. Bowel sounds may thus be absent although only parts of the gut are non-functioning. As the small bowel is the major site for absorption of nutrients it may still be possible to feed the patient enterally using a nasoduodenal tube or

jejunostomy tube placed directly into the small bowel. Bowel sounds should therefore be interpreted in context with other indicators of bowel function such as pain, distension, vomiting, gastric aspirate, and diarrhoea.

High volumes of nasogastric aspirate

There is no definitive level at which the amount of aspirate clearly indicates absence of gut function. Volumes used as a cut-off point reflect the amount of feed being given and the likely amount of gastric secretions. Gastric secretions are approximately 2 litres per day in the healthy person but can be increased by stimulation, such as the presence of a nasogastric tube (Guyton 1985, p. 678). The amount of aspirate used in some ICUs as a cut-off point for continuing or commencing enteral feed is 200 ml after a 4-hour period without aspiration (McClave *et al.* 1992). (Again, this must be considered in context with other factors.)

Vomiting/regurgitation of feed

This is a dangerous situation if the patient is unable to protect his/her airway as the risk of aspiration is considerable. Endotracheal intubation should not be considered totally protective as aspiration of feed is not uncommon in intubated patients despite fully inflated endotracheal tube cuffs. Patients should be nursed in the semi-recumbent position (45° to the horizontal) to reduce the risk of regurgitation . Enteral feeding should always be stopped and the patient assessed for other signs of intolerance such as abdominal distension, pain, and diarrhoea, if vomiting or regurgitation is evident. If there is no evidence of an abdominal disorder then drugs that increase gastric motility and emptying, such as metoclopramide, may be given to improve gas-

---

INDICATIONS FOR PARENTERAL NUTRITION

1. GI tract obstruction (adhesions, hernia, carcinoma of the oesophagus or colon, intussusception, volvulus, and diverticular disease)

2. Prolonged paralytic ileus (post-surgery, peritonitis, post-spinal injury)

3. Enterocutaneous fistulae

4. Malabsorption and short-bowel syndromes (<100 cm)

5. Inflammatory intestinal disease (some patients with Crohn's disease, or ulcerative colitis)

6. Very severe pancreatitis and cholecystitis

SUGGESTED FACTORS ASSOCIATED WITH INCREASED RISK OF REGURGITATION OF FEED AND NOSOCOMIAL PNEUMONIA

- Presence of enteral feeding tube (Kearns *et al.* 2000, Tejada Artigas *et al.* 2001)
- Size of enteral feeding tube—not supported by evidence (Metheny *et al.* 1986, Ferrer *et al.* 1999)
- Placement of enteral feeding tube—not supported by evidence (Strong *et al.* 1992, Kearns *et al.* 2000)
- Position of patient—(Drakulovic *et al.* 1999)
- Increased delay in gastric emptying (Mentec *et al.* 2001)

FACTORS THAT HAVE BEEN IMPLICATED IN DIARRHOEA INCLUDE

- Lactose intolerance (Berger and Adams 1989)
- Antibiotic therapy (Schlichtig and Ayres 1988)
- Other drug therapy such as digoxin (Koruda *et al.* 1987)
- Zinc deficiency (Schlichtig and Ayres 1988)
- Feed osmolality (Keohane *et al.* 1984)
- Low serum albumin levels (Brinson and Pitts 1989)
- Bacterial contamination of feeds
- Infection such as *Clostridium difficile* (Bliss *et al.* 2000)
- Fat malabsorption

tric emptying, and feed restarted cautiously at a low rate.

Assessment of nasogastric aspirate or vomit

The colour, amount, pH, and consistency of nasogastric aspirate or vomit can provide useful information. It should be observed and recorded. Gastric or duodenal bleeding will either appear as a normal red colour if it has spent little time in the stomach itself or will be altered to the so-called 'coffee grounds' (brownish-black particles) if it remains in the stomach for any length of time. Normal biliary and gastric secretions appear green. Bile that has had little time in the stomach, and is therefore unaltered, is yellow.

Diarrhoea

Between 15 and 52% of critically ill patients develop diarrhoea (Adam and Batson 1997, Montejo 1999, McClave *et al.* 1999). Many of the causes are not simply related to intolerance of enteral feed, although this may aggravate the situation. The patient should be investigated and treated for likely causes prior to discontinuing enteral feeding for diarrhoea. For further details see care of the enterally fed patient.

Assessment of bowel movements

There is a considerable variation in the normal frequency of bowel movements between individuals and the patient's history should be referred to before deciding whether there is a problem with constipation or diarrhoea. In spite of a generally held belief to the contrary, patients are as likely to become constipated in critical care as they are to experience diarrhoea due to the use of opioids, low-residue feeds, etc. (Adam and Batson 1997). Montejo (1999) found an incidence of constipation in 15.7% and of diarrhoea in 14.7% of the 400 intensive care patients studied in the Spanish multicentre prospective survey of gastrointestinal complications. Information about gastrointestinal dysfunction can be obtained from a thorough assessment of the patient's stools and an accurate record of frequency, consistency, and texture (see Table 11.4).

Pain

Acute abdominal pain is frequently associated with gut dysfunction and should always be treated seriously. It is

TABLE 11.4 Types of diarrhoea

Frequency	Colour	Texture	Cause
Occasional	Black	Tarry	Old bleeding—upper GI tract: melaena
Frequent depending on the rate of bleeding	Dark red	Viscous but liquid	Fresh bleeding: melaena
Constant	Brighter red	Liquid	Rectal bleeding: haemorrhoids
Frequent	Green/khaki	Soft stool or liquid	Infective: *Clostridium* difficile, Salmonella
Frequent	Pale brown/clay coloured	Loose, bulky, may float or be frothy	Malabsorption, obstruction of the biliary duct
Frequent	Bloody	Loose with obvious blood	Ischaemic or infarcted bowel
Frequent	Flecks of blood and mucus	Loose with mucus	Ulcerative colitis, Crohn's disease

CONDITIONS PRODUCING ABDOMINAL PAIN/TENDERNESS

- (Perforated) peptic ulcer
- Dissecting or ruptured aneurysm
- Pancreatitis
- Ruptured ectopic pregnancy
- Cholecystitis
- Acute renal infections
- Crohn's disease
- Pelvic inflammatory disease
- Ulcerative colitis
- Hepatitis
- Diverticulitis
- Occlusion of mesenteric artery
- Appendicitis
- Ileus
- Bowel obstruction
- Peritonitis

Rare but recognized extra-abdominal causes

- Myocardial disease
- Respiratory disease
- Diabetic or thyroid crisis
- Spinal cord lesion
- Acute intermittent porphyria
- Pneumonia
- Lead poisoning
- Endometriosis
- Sickle-cell disease
- Trauma to spleen and kidney

CAUSES OF ABDOMINAL DISTENSION

- Intestinal obstruction
- Malabsorption
- Peritonitis
- Abdominal haemorrhage (see Chapter 13)
- Ascites
- Gas
- Paralytic ileus
- Gut wall oedema

rhoea it should be taken as a sign of gut dysfunction, any enteral feeding should be discontinued and senior medical staff informed.

Priorities of care

There are two major categories in priorities of care:

1. Prevention of gastrointestinal problems associated with critical illness.

2. Maintenance of nutritional intake.

Prevention of gastrointestinal problems

Aspiration of stomach contents

The incidence of aspiration in critically ill patients has been quoted as high as 38% (Winterbauer *et al.* 1981). It is a potentially lethal complication leading to pneumonia or ARDS, and it is important to avoid any potentiating circumstances. It is should always be borne in mind that even intubated patients or those with tracheostomies can aspirate gastric contents in spite of an inflated cuff.

INCREASED RISK OF ASPIRATION IS ASSOCIATED WITH:

- Reduced level of consciousness
- Diminished or absent cough or gag reflexes
- Incompetent oesophageal sphincters
- Delayed gastric emptying (such as that associated with diabetes or malnutrition)
- Paralytic ileus
- Displacement of enteral feeding tube either into the oesophagus or into the pharynx itself (can be associated with vigorous coughing or retching)
- Presence of an enteral feeding tube

an important sign in ileus, peritonitis, obstruction, etc., and if accompanied by other signs such as abdominal distension and vomiting, feed should be stopped immediately and medical staff informed.

Distension

The abdomen may be distended for a number of reasons and care should be taken in assessing this. However, when associated with pain, vomiting, or diar-

Strategies to avoid aspiration include:

- Monitor gastric residual volumes (the amount of gastric aspirate in the stomach) 4-hourly when feeding is being established and 8-hourly once it is established (note: some individual critical care feeding protocols may differ).

- Check gastric residual volumes prior to any vigorous head-down procedures such as postural drainage and if necessary aspirate gastric contents.

- Nurse the patient in a 30–45° upright position to reduce the risk of reflux, provided cardiovascular status allows.

- Monitor the tube position externally by marking the entry site with tape or ink on the tube and checking that this has not migrated outwards.

- Monitor the tube position internally by performing gastric aspiration and confirming a satisfactory position on chest X-ray.

Nosocomial pneumonia

Bacterial transfer from the stomach to the oropharynx and trachea is recognized as a major factor in the development of nosocomial pneumonia in ventilated patients (Tejada Artigas *et al.* 2001). Increased growth of organisms in the stomach is associated with an increase in gastric pH (Pingleton 1991). A rise in gastric pH can be due to the use of H_2-receptor antagonists, antacids, and enteral feeding. In a review of associated risk factors for ventilator associated pneumonia Tejada Artigas *et al.* (2001), found an incidence of 54% of nosocomial pneumonia in ventilated patients who were continuously enterally fed.

The use of selective decontamination of the digestive tract (SDD) has been successful in reducing the incidence of nosocomial pneumonia in certain critical care populations (Meijer *et al.* 1990), in particular, the multiple trauma patient, patients with stays of more than 5 days in critical care, surgical critical care patients (Van Dalen 1991), and acute necrotizing pancreatitis patients (Wyncoll 1999). However, it has not made any difference to length of stay in critical care nor to mortality in any but a small subgroup of patients (multiple trauma patients) and is only routinely used in a few centres.

Strategies to reduce the incidence of nosocomial pneumonia include:

- Elimination/reduction of the factors contributing to the incidence of aspiration (see above).

- Avoidance of exogenous bacterial contamination (see Chapter 3).

- Avoidance of use of antacids or H_2 antagonists if possible (see earlier).

- In certain groups of patients (see above), use of SDD may be appropriate.

Stress ulceration and acute bleeds

This is discussed in the section on acute Gl bleeding (see earlier).

Maintenance of nutritional intake

Nutritional support does not constitute part of first-line life-saving interventions but has an essential role in the treatment and recovery of the critically ill patient. Progressive weight loss adds to debility, and patient mortality and morbidity correlate closely with loss of body weight. Loss of more than 30% of body weight is usually fatal (Apelgren and Wilmore 1983).

In a study of 129 patients admitted to critical care, Giner *et al.* (1996) identified 43% as malnourished. This group had a significantly higher incidence of complications. It is thus important both to identify patients likely to be at risk and to ensure that nutritional support meets their needs.

The goal of nutritional therapy in the acute phase of critical illness is to provide sufficient calories and protein to maintain body weight and reduce nitrogen loss. It is not usually possible to replenish body stores until the recovery phase of critical illness due to the levels of catabolic hormones associated with the stressed state.

Immunonutrition

A number of nutrients have been associated with specific effects on the immune response in critically ill patients. As nosocomial infection is associated with an increased risk of both morbidity and mortality in the

---

NUTRITIONAL SUPPORT IS INDICATED IN THE FIRST INSTANCE IN:

- Hypercatabolic patients: burns, multiple trauma, sepsis, and major operations

- Patients with greater than 10% body weight loss

Nutritional support may be unnecessary in the first instance in:

- Acute but quick resolving illness, e.g. cardiac surgery on relatively healthy patients, some major surgery requiring short-term critical care intervention, some drug overdoses, etc.

NUTRIENTS ASSOCIATED WITH ALTERING INFLAMMATORY RESPONSE

- *Glutamine*: major fuel source for activated immune cells and enterocytes (cells that line the intestine), may also act as a precursor for glutathione (extracellular antioxidant).

- *Arginine*: a precursor to nitric oxide with immunoregulatory properties, essential for wound healing and lymphocyte response.

- *Omega-3 polyunsaturated fatty acids*: associated with down-regulation of inflammatory response by altering the arachidonic acid pathway (see Chapter 12).

- *Nucleotides*: important for lymphocyte reproduction.

critically ill, it would be extremely advantageous if immune function could be manipulated by the addition of one or more of these nutrients.

There have been over 60 studies of feeds combining various immune-enhancing nutrients (usually three or more in each feed), with a variety of results and recommendations. However, a recent systematic review of the evidence (Heyland *et al.* 2001) found that when these immune-enhanced feeds were directly compared with standard feeds in a randomized controlled trial there was no difference in mortality. There were decreased numbers of infectious complications and length of stay associated with their use but the heterogeneity of the groups studied means that no real conclusions can be drawn.

The addition of individual immunonutrients such as glutamine or arginine may have a more positive effect on mortality, especially in the longer term (Griffiths *et al.* 1997), or in specific patient groups (Houdijk *et al.* 1998).

It remains to be seen whether the use of these nutrients and the specific dose will be formally associated with improved outcome in the critically ill.

Modes of nutrition

Provision of complete nutritional support can be accomplished in either enterally, parenterally, or by a combination of the two. Considerable debate exists as to the advantages and disadvantages of each method, but none can be used exclusively in the critical care unit. The decision as to which method is best for the individual patient must be made on the basis of GI function, metabolic problems, and the knowledge of the potential risks and advantages of each route. One method may have to be substituted for the other as the

patient's condition changes. Nevertheless, there are a number of good reasons for attempting to use enteral nutrition where possible.

The advantages of enteral nutrition are:

- It is more physiological, using the normal route for absorption and subject to the checks and balances associated with the uptake of oral nutrition.

- It is cheaper (an important aspect in view of limited resources).

- It does not require central venous access with the associated risks of insertion, infection, etc.

- It preserves gut mucosal integrity.

- It has a possible role in modifying the immune response to stress if administered in the early stages following trauma (Moore *et al.* 1989).

The disadvantages of enteral nutrition are:

(1) It is associated with diarrhoea (14.7%; Montejo 1999). This can cause dehydration, electrolyte imbalance, skin excoriation, and discomfort as well as increasing nursing workload considerably.

(2) In many cases, patients who are enterally fed do not always receive the amount of feed prescribed; in some cases they may not receive even basic metabolic requirements (Rapp *et al.* 1983, McClave *et al.* 1999, De Jonghe *et al.* 2001). This appears to be related to functional problems (Adam and Batson 1997) associated with the technique including: (i) stopping feeds for an hour each time absorption is checked, (ii) keeping patients nil by mouth for excessive periods prior to procedures, (iii) poor systems for checking that the amount prescribed is actually delivered.

(3) There is a possible increased risk of nosocomial pneumonia associated with continuous enteral feeding. The mechanism is thought to be related to the increase in gastric pH which allows bacterial colonization of the stomach and retrograde migration of the organisms via the oesophagus to the respiratory tract.

(4) Not all patients will be capable of absorbing enteral feed. It is possible to feed a high percentage of critically ill patients enterally but this requires a commitment to the method and a willingness to tackle associated problems.

Differences in metabolism between parenteral and enteral feeding

The assimilation of digested enteral feed occurs via the portal system and the liver. Parenteral feed passes directly into the circulation.

Amino acids, with the exception of branched-chain amino acids, are extracted by the liver from the enteral route. Branched-chain amino acids pass directly into the systemic circulation and are taken up primarily by muscle. However, in parenteral administration, all amino acids enter the systemic circulation although the same pattern of uptake is then followed.

Carbohydrate normally passes directly from the intestine to the liver, but in parenteral feeding it first passes into the circulation, which may have an effect on the levels of insulin-mediated uptake by the liver.

The metabolism of fat may also be affected by parenteral administration as hepatic steatosis (fatty liver) is a complication which is not seen in enterally fed patients. The mechanism is not known but is related to high levels of glucose feeding previously more common prior to the introduction of lipid solutions.

These differences have led to the assumption that enteral nutrition is better controlled by the body as it more closely mimics the normal oral diet. It is subject to the physiological feedback mechanisms which dictate hormone release, and support the balance between anabolism/catabolism and the maintenance of blood levels of nutrients.

Complications associated with enteral feeding
Mechanical
Due to:

♦ Knotting of the tube (Fig. 11.6).

♦ Clogging or blockage of the tube due to (i) fragments of inadequately crushed tablets, (ii) adherence of feed residue, (iii) incompatibilities between feed and medication given (e.g. phenytoin).

♦ Incorrect placement (usually in the bronchial tree).

♦ Nasopharyngeal erosions and discomfort.

♦ Sinusitis and otitis.

♦ Oesophageal reflux and oesophagitis.

♦ Tracheo-oesophageal fistula.

♦ Ruptured oesophageal varices.

♦ Pyloric or intestinal obstruction by gastrostomy or jejunostomy tubes.

Nausea and vomiting
Due to:

♦ high infusion rates

♦ large gastric volumes

♦ fat or lactose intolerance

♦ hyperosmolality

♦ delayed gastric emptying.

Aspiration
See section on priorities of care.

Diarrhoea
(See also section on markers of gut function.) Diarrhoea has been particularly associated with enteral feeding in the critically ill. It does not necessarily indicate that the gut is unable to function and the patient should be assessed for precipitating factors which can be dealt with before feed is discontinued.

Abdominal distension/delayed gastric emptying
Due to:

♦ critical illness

♦ formula (associated with high density, high lipid content)

♦ medication (opiates)

♦ ileus

♦ gastric atony

♦ medical conditions such as pancreatitis, diabetes, malnutrition, or post-vagotomy.

Cramping
Due to:

♦ lactose intolerance

♦ high fat content formulae

♦ malnutrition-related malabsorption.

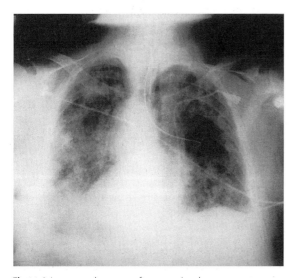

Fig 11.6 Incorrect placement of nasogastric tube.

Constipation

Constipation can be related to:

- opiate infusions
- previous laxative abuse
- long-term feeding regimens (particularly low-fibre formulae).

Hyperglycaemia

Hyperglycaemia is associated with sepsis, age, renal insufficiency, diabetes, steroid therapy, and high-caloric-density formulae.

High rates of infusion, or inadequate endogenous insulin production and inadequate exogenous insulin supplementation can also induce hyperglycaemia. Prolonged hyperglycaemia may develop into hyperosmolar, hyperglycaemic non-ketotic dehydration, and coma (HHNK), although this is unlikely to develop in the critical care area where close monitoring and management will respond to this early.

Hypercapnia

High levels of carbohydrate in feeds can produce large amounts of CO_2 that require increased minute volumes and respiratory rate in order to be excreted. This may precipitate ventilatory failure in the patient with compromised respiratory function or in the weaning patient.

Electrolyte and trace element abnormality

- Hypernatraemia due to high sodium intake and dehydration.
- Hyponatraemia due to overhydration and GI water loss (diarrhoea, drains, etc.) as well as insufficient sodium intake.
- Hyperkalaemia, usually associated with renal insufficiency and metabolic acidosis.
- Hypokalaemia, usually associated with diarrhoea, high-dose insulin, or diuretics, but can also be due to insufficient intake or replacement.
- Hyperphosphataemia, usually caused by renal dysfunction in tube-fed patients.
- Hypophosphataemia occurs in the same way as hypokalaemia but may also be seen in malnourished patients when feeding is restarted (refeeding syndrome) along with low serum levels of zinc, copper, and magnesium.

Complications associated with parenteral feeding

These complications also include the risks associated with central venous catheter placement, as well as the metabolic and infectious complications of parenteral delivery itself.

Insertion of central venous catheter

1. *Pneumothorax.* This is a recognized complication, the frequency of which is usually associated with the expertise of the operator but is quoted at 5%. It is most likely to occur when insertion is on the left as the left pleural dome is higher. There is an increased risk with mechanical ventilation, CPAP, obesity, and chest deformities.

2. *Arterial puncture.* Accidental puncture of the carotid artery often only requires digital pressure. However, significant bleeding can occur if the subclavian artery is punctured especially in patients with coagulation abnormalities, including platelet dysfunction. Accidental injury to the thoracic duct may produce chylothorax and, although rare, can occur with a left-sided approach.

3. *Catheter misplacement.* This is usually misdirection up into the neck from the subclavian approach and is more common with right-sided approaches because of the abrupt descent of the vena cava from the junction point of the right subclavian vein. Occasionally, the catheter may pass down the subclavian vein from a jugular approach. It is also possible to perforate a vessel and place the catheter into the neck tissue, mediastinum, or pericardium. This may result in a large haematoma, upper airway obstruction, hydro- or haemopneumothorax or pericardial tamponade.

The presence of a central venous catheter

Bacterial and fungal infections occur in between 3 and 7% of patients. The infecting organism is commonly *Staphylococcus aureus* (a skin commensal). Most infections are thought to be due to poor insertion technique or failure to observe infection control protocols (see Chapter 3).

Metabolic complications

1. *Hyperglycaemia.* Causes include persistent gluconeogenesis, blunted insulin response, decreased sensitivity to insulin, impaired peripheral utilization of glucose or phosphate, and chromium deficiency. Late development in a stable patient may signal a new infection or complication.

2. *Hypoglycaemia.* A sudden discontinuation of feed may induce hypoglycaemia, particularly if the patient is receiving insulin concurrently. The insulin should usually be discontinued or reduced prior to stopping the feed and, if this is not possible 10–20% glucose may be commenced. Blood glucose should be frequently monitored.

3. *Hyperlipidaemia.* Lipid clearance may be impaired in liver disease. Rapid infusion of lipid may also result in transient hyperlipidaemia.

4. *Hepatic dysfunction.* Abnormal liver function tests (LFTs) and fatty infiltration of the liver can develop in carbohydrate-based parenteral nutrition. It is treated by reducing the number of calories or increasing the proportion of fat.

5. *Acid–base disturbances.* Hyperchloraemia can develop from amino acid metabolism but the resulting acidosis is usually mild and most amino acid preparations contain acetate as a buffer. Metabolic alkalosis can be seen with diuretic use, continuous nasogastric drainage, or corticosteroid therapy if concomitant replacement of sodium, potassium, and/or chloride ions is inadequate.

6. *Electrolyte imbalance.* Generally, sodium, potassium, chloride, and bicarbonate are monitored and corrected before problems occur. However, significant body deficiencies may not be reflected by plasma levels due to the effect of pH and serum albumin levels or hormonal influences, such as aldosterone or ADH, which are often altered in the critically ill. Occasionally, magnesium, calcium, and phosphate may become imbalanced. Hypophosphataemia is often seen when parenteral nutrition is first started following a period of semi-starvation. This is due to poor prior intake of phosphate, increased glucose phosphorylation, and augmented intracellular transport of phosphates once feeding is restarted. Plasma phosphate levels below 0.3–0.5 mmol/l can cause haemolysis, rhabdomyolysis, respiratory failure, and hamper weaning attempts. This may persist for several days after adequate replacement. Other effects include arrhythmias, decreased myocardial contractility, 2,3-DPG deficiency, seizures, diminished tissue sensitivity to insulin, abnormal calcium and magnesium metabolism, decreased sensitivity to vasoactive drugs, generalized tissue hypoxia, and ATP deficiency.

Other complications associated with parenteral feeding

◆ Precipitation of respiratory failure and failure of weaning due to excessive carbohydrate administration (see earlier).

◆ Hyperosmolar states with an excessive osmotic diuresis.

◆ Abnormal platelet function and hypercoagulability states.

◆ Anaemia after prolonged use of IV lipids.

Many of the potentially serious complications associated with parenteral feeding can be avoided or controlled by rigorous monitoring and observation of the patient. A high index of suspicion for complications should also be maintained.

Nutritional requirements (Tables 11.5–11.9)

It is only possible to give an approximate guide to the amount of nutrients required by the individual patient.

TABLE 11.5 Monitoring nutritional support

Variable to be monitored	Enteral nutrition	Parenteral nutrition
Electrolytes	Daily	Daily
Serum magnesium, calcium, phosphate	Twice weekly	Twice weekly
Acid–base status	Daily	Daily
Gastric residuals (aspirate)	4-hourly when starting feeding; 8-hourly when established	As required by pathology
Abdominal function (distension, vomiting, nausea, diarrhoea, constipation)	Continuously	As required
Flow rate and volume infused	Hourly	Hourly
Blood glucose	8-hourly	1–2-hourly at first; when stable 4–6-hourly
Urinalysis for glucose and ketones	Daily	Daily
Urea and creatinine (plasma)	Daily	Daily
Urea and creatinine clearance (urinary)	24-h urine collection weekly	24-h urine collection weekly
Weight (if mobile or on a weigh bed)	For fluid status: daily. For nutritional status: weekly	For fluid status: daily. For nutritional status: weekly
Haematological and coagulation screens	Every 1–2 days	Every 1–2 days
Serum albumin, proteins, LFTs, trace elements (e.g. copper, zinc, etc.)	Weekly	Weekly

TABLE 11.6 Daily nutritional requirement during enteral and parental nutrition

Nutrient	Amount per day	Influencing factors
Protein (nitrogen)	0.7–1.0 g/kg/day (0.15–0.3 g/kg/day)	Hypermetabolism can increase protein requirements to 1.5–2.0 g/kg/day
Carbohydrate	Need will depend on the patient's energy requirements two-thirds of which are usually provided by carbohydrate, and one-third by fat. A useful quick estimate of requirements is: Male: 25–30 kcal/kg/day Female: 20–25 kcal/kg/day	Patients with respiratory insufficiency or those who are weaning after long-term ventilation may not cope with the high carbon dioxide levels associated with high intakes of carbohydrate. Energy requirement can then be supplied as one-half fat and one-half carbohydrate
Fat	The minimum amount of fat necessary to prevent fatty acid deficiency is 1 litre of 10% fat emulsion (e.g. intralipid) weekly. However, usually the amount of fat delivered is aimed at providing energy rather than preventing deficiency and is adjusted to between one-third and one-half of total calories required. A useful quick estimate of requirements is 0.8–1.0 g/kg/day (Scott *et al.* 1998)	Tolerance of intravenous fat can be limited (see parenteral nutrition complications) and the amount delivered may need to be adjusted if this is the case

Note: This table represents only a rough guide, and each patient should be assessed individually.

TABLE 11.7 Electrolyte requirements during enteral or parenteral nutrition

Typical daily requirement	Additional factors
Sodium 70–100 mmol/day	More may be needed with loop diuretic therapy or increased GI losses such as diarrhoea or fistulae etc. Less may be needed in oedema and hypernatraemia
Potassium 70–100 mmol/day	More may be needed during early repletion, post-obstructive diuresis, loop diuretic therapy and increased GI losses. Less may be required in renal failure
Magnesium 7.5–10 mmol/day	As above
Calcium 5–10 mmol/day	
Phosphate 20–30 mmol/day	More may be needed in early nutritional repletion when there may be dramatic falls in serum phosphate (see refeeding syndrome). Less may be required in renal failure

TABLE 11.8 Trace element requirements during enteral and parenteral nutrition (from the Parenteral and Enteral Group of the British Dietetic Association, 1997)

Trace element	Recommended daily dietary allowance		Effects of deficiency
	Enteral nutrition (μmol/l)	Parenteral nutrition (μmol/l)	
Zinc	110–145	145	Impaired cellular immunity, poor wound healing, diarrhoea
Chromium	0.5–1.0	0.2–0.4	Insulin-resistant glucose intolerance, elevated serum lipids
Copper	16–20	20	Hypochromic microcytic anaemia, neutropenia
Iodine	1–1.2	1.0	
Selenium	0.8–0.9	0.25–0.5	Cardiomyopathy
Molybdenum	0.5–4.0	0.2–1.2	
Manganese	30–60	5–10	CNS dysfunction
Fluoride	95–150	50	

Factors, such as age, weight, sex, severity of illness, use of catecholamines, body temperature, and injury, will all affect nutrient and energy needs. Electrolyte and fluid balance are also important factors in deciding the composition of feeds.

The exact requirements for trace elements in the critically ill have not been determined but deficiency can have significant effects on a number of metabolic

TABLE 11.9 Vitamin requirements during enteral or parenteral nutrition (from the Parenteral and Enteral Group of the British Dietetic Association, 1997)

Vitamin	Recommended daily dietary allowance	
	Enteral nutrition	Parenteral nutrition
A (retinol) 5000 (μg)	600–1200	800–2500
B$_1$ (thiamine) (mg)	0.8–1.1	3–20
B$_2$ (riboflavin) (mg)	1.1–1.3	3–8
Niacin (mg)	2–18	40
B$_6$ (pyridoxine) (mg)	1.2–2.0	4.0–6.0
B$_{12}$ (cyanocobalamine) (μg)	1.5–3.0	5–15
C (ascorbic acid) (mg)	40–60	100
D (cholecalciferol) (μg)	5	5
E (δ and α tocopherol) (mg)	10	10
Folic acid (μg)	200–400	200–400
K (phytomenadione) (μg/kg)	1	0.03–1.5
Pantothenic acid (mg)	3–7	10–20
Biotin (μg)	10–200	60

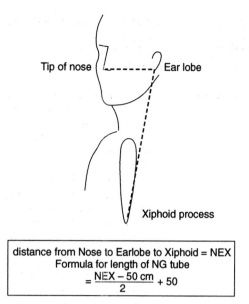

$$\text{distance from Nose to Earlobe to Xiphoid} = \text{NEX}$$
$$\text{Formula for length of NG tube}$$
$$= \frac{\text{NEX} - 50 \text{ cm}}{2} + 50$$

Fig. 11.7 Calculation of the length of the nasogastic tube.

processes. Most enteral feeds contain stated amounts of most essential trace elements. Multiple additives for parenteral feeding may be supplemented as necessary.

Insertion of nasogastric and duodenal feeding tubes

Enteral feeding tubes are normally inserted blind by appropriately experienced nursing staff. However, the presence of an endotracheal tube cuff increases the difficulty of entry to the oesophagus by pressing on its soft walls and decreasing its size. It may therefore be necessary to insert the tube under direct visualization of the pharynx. This is usually carried out by senior medical staff. (Note: The ET tube cuff does not provide complete protection against inadvertent tracheal intubation with the nasogastric tube.)

The technique for insertion will differ slightly according to the type of tube but the principles are the same.

Principles of insertion.

1. Explanation to the patient is required whether they are sedated or awake. This should include: the need for the tube, where the tube will be placed, likely sensations that the patient may feel and how long the tube is likely to be in place.

2. Insertion is treated as a clean rather than aseptic technique with hand-washing prior to commencement and non-sterile gloves worn for protection of the operator.

3. Measurement of the length of tube is required to ensure placement within the stomach or duodenum. This can be fairly accurately measured using the formula shown in Fig. 11.7 (for 91% of tubes placed within the stomach, Hanson 1979). However, in practice the more simple method of measuring nose to ear to xiphisternum is a reasonable approximation of length. Most tubes are marked at 10 cm intervals and the stomach should be reached by the time the 40 cm mark is at the nares.

4. Placement in the duodenum requires insertion of at least 85 cm of feeding tube to allow direct passage or to allow a coil in the stomach which may then be passed into the duodenum (Whatley *et al.* 1984).

5. Lubrication is necessary to promote atraumatic insertion. Some tubes are pre-lubricated and require placing in water to activate the lubricant, others require lubricating jelly.

6. The tube is inserted along the floor of the nose; this avoids the sensitive conchae and will provide a guide through the nasal cavity to the nasopharynx. If the patient is conscious they may assist insertion by swallowing once the tube is felt at the back of the nasopharynx.

7. Once the tube has been inserted, the position should be checked. The following methods are suggested, although the only certain method of checking placement for fine-bore tubes is by X-ray:

◆ Auscultation over the epigastric region during insufflation of 20 ml of air into the tube. Bubbling air should be clearly heard. (Note: It is still possible to hear bubbling air if the tube is in the lung (Metheny *et al.* 1990).)

◆ Aspiration of gastric contents and testing of the pH of fluid withdrawn. A pH of <4 indicates gastric placement. Care must be taken with critically ill patients and those receiving H_2 antagonists or antacids, as the gastric pH may be as high as 5–6. It is also possible to withdraw tracheobronchial secretions in certain conditions with a low pH (Metheny and Clouse 1997), e.g. pH 7.0–7.29 (malignancy), pH 6 (oesophageal rupture), and pH 5.5 (empyema).

8. If the tube has a guidewire it should be removed once the tube is in the correct position. If there is difficulty withdrawing the guidewire, 1–2 ml water inserted into the tube may assist in lubricating its passage.

Care of the enterally fed patient with a nasogastric tube
Checking gastric residual volumes (aspirate)

◆ Residual volumes should be checked 4-hourly when feeding is first commenced and then 8-hourly once the feed has been running without large amounts of residual volumes. This may differ according to unit protocols.

◆ It is unnecessary to stop feeds for an hour in order to check residual volumes. The minimal time necessary to demonstrate reduced absorption has not yet been determined but it is probably less than 30 min even with reduced gastric motility.

◆ If all is well following a check for residual volumes, the rate of feed delivery should be increased to cover delivery of the feed volume missed prior to the check.

◆ It is possible to aspirate fine-bore nasogastric tubes of 1.5–2.0 mm internal diameter. A 50 ml syringe should be used which exerts less pressure and is therefore less likely to cause the tube to collapse.

◆ Gastric residual volumes of less than 200 ml have been found to be an acceptable cut-off limit in practice. There is little published research in this area and recommendations range from 'more than 1.5 times the previous hour's input of feed' (Koruda *et al.* 1987) to '<200 ml' (Armstrong *et al.* 1991, McClave *et al.* 1992).

◆ If residual volumes of 200 ml or more are obtained, the feed is either held at the current level if feeding is just building up, or reduced to a lower rate if the feed has been in progress for some time. Volumes are then checked again 4 hours later and the manoeuvre repeated. If this occurs three times in succession, or is accompanied by vomiting and abdominal pain or distension, the medical staff should be informed and the feed stopped. There is little evidence to support either returning residual volumes to the patient or discarding them. In a very small study, Booker *et al.* (2000) found no significant difference in weight, electrolyte levels, or CO_2 between patients randomized to have either discarded or returned gastric residual aspirates. The only noted, though not significant, difference was that two tubes clogged in the return group and no tubes clogged in the discard group.

◆ Stimulants of intestinal motility may be used including metoclopramide and erythromycin if the patient has no acute signs of feed intolerance but continues to have high volumes of gastric residuals.

◆ Feeding into the duodenum may still be possible and should be tried if there is no evidence of general gut dysfunction (pain, distension, vomiting). Care should be taken when feeding into the duodenum, and may require assessment of gastric contents regularly by aspiration, either using a double-lumen tube with a gastric outlet or by inserting a nasogastric tube.

Prevention of tube obstruction

◆ Avoid giving crushed tablets down the enteral tube. Any drugs given in the nasogastric tube should be either soluble or in the form of linctus. A 20–30 ml flush of water should be given following administration of drugs; more may be required if crushed tablets are given.

◆ Some authorities recommend flushing the tube with at least 30 ml of water every 4 hours during continuous feeding (Kohn and Keithley 1989).

◆ Water is the most appropriate fluid for flushing tubes (Metheny *et al.* 1988).

◆ Use a continuous delivery method of feeding (drying and encrustation between feeds may obstruct the tube).

◆ Use a polyurethane or PVC material tube as these have a larger internal diameter and better flow rates than silastic tubes (Metheny *et al.* 1988).

Prevention of tube displacement

◆ Use a firm but easily removable tape to attach the tube to the nose or face.

◆ The point of entry into the nose should be marked on the tube with fine tape once correct placement has been established. This can then be checked to ensure it remains in the same place. (Note: This does not guarantee the tube has remained in the stomach. It is possible for it to be brought up by vigorous coughing or retching and sit coiled in the mouth or oropharynx, particularly when the patient is unconscious.)

♦ Check tube placement after any vigorous coughing or retching using the methods described above.

Diarrhoea

Causes are frequently multifactorial in the critically ill patient so the whole patient should be reviewed to identify all relevant factors as follows:

1. Drugs:

♦ Drugs that have been particularly associated with diarrhoea are: antibiotics, magnesium-containing antacids, electrolyte elixirs, large amounts of hypertonic sugary elixirs, digoxin, methyldopa, and laxatives.

♦ The patient's drugs should be reviewed and alternatives sought where possible, to those which may be implicated in diarrhoea. Hypertonic elixirs can be diluted prior to administration.

♦ Addition of a *Lactobacillus acidophilus* preparation, such as live yoghurt, may help restore normal gut flora.

♦ It may be appropriate to give antidiarrhoeal drugs, such as loperamide, and codeine phosphate for drug-related diarrhoea, with the exception of antibiotic-related diarrhoea. Cholestyramine has been suggested for diarrhoea caused by *Clostridium difficile* toxin as it binds the toxin to the resin (Koruda *et al.* 1987).

2. Bacterial contamination:

♦ Potential sources of bacterial contamination should be investigated and a stool specimen sent for culture, sensitivity, and *C. difficile* toxin.

♦ Feed should not be hung at room temperature for more than 12 hours and feed bags should not be 'topped up'. Feed-giving sets should be changed every 24 hours.

♦ Ready-made feed should be used wherever possible. If feed has to be reconstituted on the unit, or substances added, great care should be taken to maintain sterility.

2. Feed constituents:

♦ High-osmolality, high-fat-content, and high-lactose-content feeds have all been associated with diar-

rhoea. In fact, most formulae no longer contain lactose and research has shown conflicting evidence of the link between high osmolality and diarrhoea (Keohane *et al.* 1984). Problems with fat tolerance are more likely with special feeds such as Pulmocare (50% of non-protein calorie content from fat, 50% from carbohydrate). If appropriate, an alternative feed with less fat or a lower osmolality may be tried instead.

♦ In same cases a bulking agent such as methylcellulose or psyllium hydrophilic mucilloid has been used to good effect (Heather *et al.* 1991).

4. Albumin levels. Hypoalbuminaemia may cause osmotic diarrhoea if it is associated with a lowering of capillary oncotic pressure (COP). However, artificial colloids may maintain an adequate COP despite a low albumin level. If the COP is reduced, feed within the intestinal lumen creates an osmotic gradient with fluid moving into, rather than out of, the intestine, resulting in a loose watery stool.

5. Intestinal effects of malnutrition and parenteral nutrition:

♦ Malnutrition is associated with a loss in the number and height of intestinal villi and decreased levels of brush border enzymes. The effect of this is a reduction in the absorptive capability of the intestine. Similar effects can be seen following long periods of parenteral feeding (Koruda *et al.* 1987). There is also some evidence to show that intestinal epithelial cells may benefit from direct uptake of glutamine from feed given via the intestinal tract as a source of energy, for maintenance of the intestinal barrier and the gut's immune function.

♦ Commencement of enteral feeding in a malnourished patient may require very slow increase in delivery rates and use of a peptide-based formula which is more easily absorbed.

♦ In same cases, it may be appropriate to feed both enterally and parenterally to encourage return of gut function and to maintain a suitably high level of nutritional intake.

Many critically ill patients with diarrhoea associated with enteral feed can be managed simply by altering the feed formula, reviewing implicated factors, and adjusting treatment accordingly. Frequently, enteral feeding can be continued at a reduced level until the appropriate treatment has been started. Diarrhoea should not prevent enteral feeding unless it is associated with severe absorptive disorders or infection such as *C. difficile*.

Evaluating delivery of feed

There is good evidence to suggest that patients do not always get the amount of feed that is prescribed and some may get only a small proportion of what is prescribed (Adam and Batson 1997, McClave *et al.* 1999). Evaluation of the feed delivery should include a method of comparing feed delivered to feed prescribed on a daily basis. If no mechanism exists for this and no review is carried out then the patient may become malnourished before the deficit is detected.

- Feed should be prescribed in *calories* per 24 hours rather than *millilitres* per hour.

- The total calorie intake over 24 hours should be calculated by the nurse; any large deficit or excess, and the reasons for it, should be reported to the dietitian or medical staff.

- Nursing evaluation should include details of the patient's ability to absorb and tolerate enteral feed.

The most important aspects of feeding are that the patient receives what he/she requires in the form best suited to his/her ability to absorb and utilize it.

Care of the parenterally fed patient

Insertion of the central venous catheter

Details for insertion of a central venous catheter are given in Chapter 5. In some units, a dedicated port of a triple-lumen line is considered adequate for short-term parenteral feeding. However, long-term feeding should be either via a tunnelled feeding line or a Hickman catheter. Debate continues as to whether the risk of inserting a tunnelled feeding line into a critically ill patient outweighs the (slightly increased) incidence of infection in triple lumen lines.

Infection of central venous catheters: mechanisms and management.

1. Infection by migration of organisms down the dermal tunnel, preceded by colonization of the skin surrounding the site of insertion. Colonization may occur from insertion or during redressing.

Management strategy:

- Scrupulous aseptic technique (surgical gowns, sterile gloves, povidone-iodine skin preparation, removal of any blood from insertion site prior to dressing) when inserting or dressing the catheter.

- Use of an occlusive dressing which should be re-dressed according to unit policy.

2. Bacterial colonization of the tip. This is generally as a result of bacteraemia from another source. The problem is then compounded by the formation of a fibrin sheath within 3 days of insertion which acts as a shield to bacteria against systemic antibiotics.

Management strategy:

- Maintenance of a high index of suspicion for catheter infection.

- Removal of the catheter if patient shows evidence of infection (without any other obvious cause) and send tip for culture—appropriate systemic antibiotics can then be prescribed if indicated.

- Change non-tunnelled lines if there is evidence of infection at the site or systemically.

3. Colonization of the hub or intraluminal segment of the catheter. This is generally due to contamination during tubing changes or by the infusion of contaminated solutions.

Management strategy:

- Scrupulous aseptic technique (sterile field, surgical gloves, spray hub, and connections with isopropyl alcohol) during changes of administration set or infusions.

- Change the administration set every 24 hours unless using pre-mixed 48-hour infusion bags when the administration set should be changed with the infusion bag.

4. Infected infusate. This is less likely than in many other IV infusions due to the amino acid content of the feed which decreases the pH. However, if lipid emulsion is present in the bag, bacterial and fungal growth will be supported. Lipid emulsion alone is almost as good a growth medium as that normally used to culture organisms.

Management strategy:

- Pre-mixed bags prepared in sterile conditions should be used wherever possible. If not, scrupulous aseptic precautions should be taken in setting up individual bottles and bags for concurrent infusion.

- Infection rates have been shown to be reduced to between 1 and 2% by employment of specially trained personnel. This is probably due to both an increased understanding of the risks as well as a high level of competence in manipulating lines. The same standards should be expected of the critical care nurse in order to limit the likelihood of infection in the highly vulnerable patient.

Prevention of intolerance of glucose load

Hyperglycaemia associated with stress (see Chapter 3) is often exacerbated by infusing exogenous glucose. Insulin levels may rise in response to the glucose but are either insufficient to maintain normoglycaemia or appear not to function adequately to allow sufficient glucose uptake in the liver and tissues. This may be compounded by the failure of glucose infusions to suppress hepatic gluconeogenesis in the critically ill. The response to a glucose infusion may reflect the patient's degree of illness and reduction in insulin requirements may be an early sign of recovery. Conversely, increasing insulin requirements may indicate a new wave of sepsis. This should be interpreted with caution in patients with accompanying liver disease as gluconeogenetic mechanisms are impaired.

The mangement strategy is:

- Regular monitoring of blood glucose is essential with 15–30 min measurements in the hour following commencement or discontinuation of parenteral nutrition and following any sharp rise or fall (Krzywda et al. 1993).

- Intravenous insulin infusions should be titrated to maintain blood glucose <10 mmol/l. Van den Berghe et al. (2001) have completed a randomized, controlled trial of 1548 patients which showed that maintaining a blood glucose <6.1 mmol/l is associated with a reduction in mortality ($P = 0.04$). However, further study is required before this is general practice.

- Large changes in insulin infusion rates are not recommended because of the dangers of hypo- and hyperglycaemia. Insulin infusions should not be stopped abruptly even when the blood glucose is very low; it is better to infuse more glucose in order to maintain blood levels and reduce insulin as necessary to avoid rebound hyperglycaemia.

- Infusion rates of glucose should be kept within the limits of metabolic requirements and if tolerance limits the amount to below acceptable levels for nutrition, further calories should be given as lipid infusion.

- Infusion should be continuous and via an infusion pump to deliver a constant rate of feed.

- Consideration should be given to discontinuation of insulin infusions prior to stopping parenteral nutrition in order to avoid hypoglycaemia.

Prevention of problems from volumes of fluid infused

Due to its hypertonicity, most parenteral feed requires a considerable amount of fluid volume to deliver the nutritional requirements of the patient. This may cause fluid overload in the patient in renal failure or in critically ill patients who have problems with oedema. Parenteral nutrition may have to be discontinued until either renal replacement therapy is commenced or the patient passes sufficient volumes of urine, and fluid overload is less of a problem.

PSYCHOSOCIAL EFFECTS OF PARENTERAL NUTRITION

- Dependence on catheter and infusion pump
- Loss of potential comfort source
- Loss of taste and pleasure associated with eating
- Anxiety about whether it will ever be possible to eat again
- Anxiety about effects of the feed itself and its ability to provide adequate nutrition
- Loss of social aspects of eating (togetherness, communication, family relationships)

The managment strategy involves accurate calculation of fluid balance and hourly monitoring of intake and output.

Psychological aspects

Many of the psychosocial problems associated with parenteral nutrition (see box) do not apply to the critically ill as they may have little awareness of the need for food or lack of it. It is also unlikely that their parenteral feeding will continue in the long term. However, during the convalescent phase the patient may become more aware and the route for feeding, reason, and length of time it will continue, should be carefully explained.

Test yourself

Questions

1. Review the function of hepatocytes. In the event of major liver dysfunction, how would the patient be affected?

2. What are the main problems associated with enteral feeding in the critically ill?

3. What are the main problems associated with parenteral feeding in the critically ill?

4. What are the priorities in acute gastrointestinal bleeding?

Answers

1. a. Hepatocytes maintain glucose homeostasis, synthesise coagulation factors and plasma proteins, metabolise many drugs, deaminate other proteins, metabolise and synthesise fats, eliminate bilirubin, catabolise steroids and hormones, store minerals and vitamins, form part of the mononuclear phagocytic process.

   b. Primary effects for the critically ill patient are coagulation dysfunction, extended drug effects, poor maintenance of blood glucose levels, altered level of consciouness, increased vulnerability to infection, rising bilirubin levels and jaundice.

2. Poor gastric motility.

Increased risk of aspiration pneumonia.

Intolerance and inability to achieve nutritional goals.

Associated diarrhoea.

Mechanical problems

3. Requirement for a dedicated central venous access lumen.

Poor tolerance of the glucose load.

Increased risk of infection.

High fluid volumes.

Potential loss of intestinal endoluminal integrity.

4. Resuscitation—replacement and stabilization of blood loss (initially using colloid, then blood as available).

Ensuring adequate venous access to allow sufficient replacement fluids.

Investigation of cause (usually by endoscopy).

Treatment of cause.

References and bibliography

Adam, S.K. (1990). An investigation into nutritional delivery, prescription and need in the ventilated, enterally fed ITU patient. *M.Sc. thesis*. King's College, University of London.

Adam, S., Batson, S. (1997). A study of problems associated with the delivery of enteral feed in critically ill patients in five ICUs in the UK. *Intensive Care Medicine* **23**, 261–6.

Apelgren, K.N., Wilmore, D.W. (1983). Nutritional care of the critically ill patient. *Surgical Clinics of North America* **63**, 497–507.

Armstrong, R.F., Bullen, C., Cohen, S.L., *et al.* (1991). *Critical Care Algorithms*. Oxford University Press, Oxford.

Bank, S., Singh, P., Pooran, N., *et al.* (2002). Evaluation of factors that have reduced mortality from acute pancreatitis over the past 20 years. *Journal of Clinical Gastroenterology* **35**, 50–60.

Belknap M.D., Davidson, L.J., Flournoy, D.J., *et al.* (1990). Contamination of enteral feedings and diarrhea in patients in intensive care units. *Heart and Lung* **19**, 362–70.

Berger, R., Adams, L. (1989). Nutritional support in the critical care setting (part I). *Chest* **96**, 139–50.

Berger, R., Adams, L. (1989). Nutritional support in the critical care setting (part 2). *Chest* **96**, 372–80.

Bernau, J., Rueff, B., Benhamou, J.P.(1986). Fulminant and subfulminant hepatic failure: definitions and causes. *Seminars in Liver Disease* **6**, 97–106.

Bliss, D.Z., Johnson, S., Savik, K., *et al.* (2000). Fecal incontinence in hospitalized patients who are acutely ill. *Nursing Research* **49**, 101–8.

Booker, K.J., Niedringhaus, L., Eden, B., *et al.* (2000). Comparison of 2 methods of managing gastric residual volumes from feeding tubes. *American Journal of Critical Care* **9**, 318–24.

Brinson, R.R., Pitts, W.M. (1989). Enteral nutrition in the critically ill patient: role of hypoalbuminemia. *Critical Care Medicine* **17**, 367–70.

Carlsson, M., Nordenstrom, J., Hedenstierna, G. (1984). Clinical implications of continuous measurement of energy expenditure in mechanically ventilated patients. *Clinical Nutrition* **3**, 103–10.

Cook, D., Heyland, D., Griffith, L., *et al.* (1999). Risk factors for clinically important upper gastrointestinal bleeding in patients requiring mechanical ventilation. *Critical Care Medicine* **27**, 2812–17.

De Jonghe, B., Appere-De-Vechi, C., Frounier, M. *et al.* (2001). A prospective survey of nutritional support practices in intensive care unit patients: What is prescribed? What is delivered? *Critical Care Medicine* **29**, 8–12.

Elpern, E.H., Jacobs, E.R., Bone, R.C. (1987). Incidence of aspiration in tracheally intubated adults. *Heart and Lung* **16**, 527–31.

Ferrer, M., Bauer, T.T., Torres, A., *et al.* (1999). Effect of nasogastric tube size on gastroesophageal reflux and microaspiration in intubated patients. *Annals of Internal Medicine* **130**, 991–4.

Fiddian-Green, R.G. (1988). Splanchnic ischaemia and multiple organ failure in the critically ill. *Annals of the Royal College of Surgeons of England* **70**, 128–34.

Forsberg A, Backman L, Moller A. (2000). Experiencing liver transplantation: a phenomenological approach. *Journal of Advanced Nursing* **32**, 327–34.

Fromant, P., Farman, J. (1987). Looking after the liver patient. *Care of the Critically Ill* **3**, 34–7.

Gill, R.Q., Sterling, R.K. (2001). Acute liver failure. *Journal of Clinical Gastroenterology* **33**, 191–8.

Giner, M., Laviano, A., Meguid, M.M., *et al.* (1996). In 1995, a correlation between malnutrition and poor outcome in critically ill patients still exists. *Nutrition* **12**, 23–9.

Goodinson, S.M. (1987). Anthropometric assessment of nutritional status. *Professional Nurse* **2**, 388–93.

Griffiths, R.D., Jones, C., Palmer T.E. (1997). Six-month outcome of critically ill patients given glutamine-supplemented parenteral nutrition. *Nutrition* **13**, 295–302.

Guyton, A.C. (1985). *Anatomy and Physiology*. Holt-Saunders, Philadelphia, PA.

Hanson, R.L. (1979). Criteria for length of nasogastric tube insertion for tube feeding. *Journal of Parenteral and Enteral Nutrition* **3**, 160–3.

Hartley, P., Petruckevitch, A., Reeves, B., *et al.* (2001). The National Liver Transplantation Audit: an overview of patients presenting for liver transplantation from 1994 to 1998. *British Journal of Surgery* **88**, 52–8.

Hawker, F. (1990). Liver transplantation. In: *Intensive Care Manual* (ed. T.E. Oh), 3rd edn, pp. 240–5. Butterworth, Sydney.

Heather, D.J., Howell, L., Montana, M., *et al.* (1991). Effect of a bulk-forming cathartic on diarrhoea in tube-fed patients. *Heart and Lung* **20**, 409–13.

Houdijk, A.P.J., Rijnsburger, E.R., Jansen, J. *et al.* (1998). Randomised trial of glutamine-enriched enteral nutrition on infectious morbidity in patients with multiple trauma. *Lancet* **352**, 772–6.

Hudak, C.M., Gallo, B.M., Benz, J.J. (1990). *Critical care nursing: a holistic approach*, 5th edn. Lippincott, Philadelphia, PA.

Johnson, L.R. (1997). *Gastrointestinal Physiology*, 5th edn. Mosby-Yearbook, St Louis, MO.

Kearns, P.J., Chin, D., Mueller, L., *et al.*. (2000). The incidence of ventilator-associated pneumonia and success in nutrient delivery with gastric versus small intestinal feeding: a randomized clinical trial. *Critical Care Medicine* **28**, 1742–6.

Keohane, P.P., Attrill, H., Love, M., *et al.* (1984). Relation between osmolality of diet and gastrointestinal side effects in enteral nutrition. *British Medical Journal* **288**, 678–80.

Kohn, C.L., Keithley, J.K. (1989). Enteral nutrition: potential complications and patient monitoring. *Nursing Clinics of North America* **24**, 339–51.

Konopad, E., Noseworthy, T. (1988). Stress ulceration: a serious complication in critically ill patients. *Heart and Lung* **17**, 339–48.

Koruda, M.J., Guenter, P., Rombeau, J.L. (1987). Enteral nutrition in the critically ill. *Critical Care Clinics* **3**,133–53.

Krige, J.E.J., Beckingham, I.(2001). Portal hypertension-2. Ascites, encephalopathy and other conditions. *British Medical Journal* **322**, 416–18.

Krzywda, E.A., Andris, D.A., Whipple, J.K. *et al.* (1993). Glucose response to abrupt initiation and discontinuation of total parenteral nutrition. *Journal of Parenteral and Enteral Nutrition* **17**, 64–7.

Kudsk, K.A., Croce, M.A., Fabian, T.C. *et al.* (1992). Enteral versus parenteral feeding: effects on septic morbidity after blunt and penetrating abdominal trauma. *Annals of Surgery* **215**, 503–11.

Laterre, P.F., Horsmans, Y.(2001). Intravenous omeprazole in critically ill patients: a randomized, crossover study comparing 40mg with 80mg plus 8 mg/hour on intragastric pH. *Critical Care Medicine* **29**, 1931–5.

Lee, B. Chang, R.W.S., Jacobs, S. (1990). Intermittent nasogastric feeding: a simple and effective method to reduce pneumonia among ventilated ICU patients. *Clinical Intensive Care* **1**, 100–2.

Levy, G.A., Chung, S.W., Sheiner, P.A. (1991). Approach to the patient with severe liver failure. In: *Update in Intensive Care and Emergency Medicine*, Vol. 14 (ed. J.L. Vincent), pp. 590–7. Springer, Berlin.

Liu, C., Fan, S., Lo, C.M., *et al.* (2002). Right-lobe live donor liver transplantation improves survival of patients with acute liver failure. *British Journal of Surgery* **89**, 317–22.

McClave, S.A., Snider, H.L., Lowen, C.C. *et al.* (1992). Use of residual volume as a marker for enteral feeding intolerance: prospective blinded comparison with physical examination and radiographic findings. *Journal of Parenteral and Enteral Nutrition* **16**, 99–105.

McClave, S.A., Sexton, L.K., Spain, D.A. *et al.* (1999). Enteral tube feeding in the intensive care unit: factors impeding adequate delivery. *Critical Care Medicine* **27**, 1252–6.

McClave, S.A., McClain, C.J., Snider, H.L. (2001). Should indirect calorimetry be used as part of nutritional assessment? *Journal of Clinical Gastroenterology* **33**, 14–19.

Meijer, K., Van Saene, H.K.F., Hill, J.C. (1990). Infection control in patients undergoing mechanical ventilation: traditional approach versus a new development—selective decontamination of the digestive tract. *Heart and Lung* **19**, 11–20.

Mentec, H., Dupont, H., Bocchetti, M., *et al.*. (2001). Upper digestive intolerance during enteral nutrition in critically ill patients: frequency, risk factors, and complications. *Critical Care Medicine* **29**,1955–61.

Messori, A., Trippoli, S., Vaiani, M., *et al.* (2000). Bleeding and pneumonia in intensive care patients given ranitidine and sucralfate for prevention of stress ulcer: meta-analysis of randomized controlled trials. *British Medical Journal* **321**, 1103–6.

Metheny, N.A., Clouse, R. (1997). Bedside methods of detecting aspiration in tube-fed patients. *Chest* **111**, 724–31.

Metheny, N., Eisenberg, P., Spies, M. (1986). Aspiration pneumonia in patients fed through nasoenteral tubes. *Heart and Lung* **15**, 256–61.

Metheny, N., Eisenberg, P., McSweeney, M. (1988). Effect of feeding tube properties and three irrigants on clogging rates. *Nursing Research* **37**, 165–9.

Metheny, N., Dettenmeier, P., Hampton, K., *et al.* (1990). Detection of inadvertent respiratory placement of small-bore feeding tubes: a report of 10 cases. *Heart and Lung* **19**, 631–8.

Miller, T.A. (1987). Mechanisms of stress-related mucosal damage. *American Journal of Medicine* **83**(6A), 8–14.

Montejo, J.C. (1999). Enteral nutrition-related gastrointestinal complications in critically ill patients: a multicentre study. *Critical Care Medicine* **27**, 1447–53.

Moore, F.A., Moore, E.E., Jones, T.N., *et al.* (1989). TEN versus TPN following major abdominal trauma—reduced septic morbidity. *Journal of Trauma* **29**, 916–23.

O'Grady, J.G., Williams, R. (1989). Aspects of intensive care following liver transplantation. *Care of the Critically Ill* **5**, 67–9.

O'Grady, J.G., Schalm, S.W., Williams, R. (1993). Acute liver failure: redefining the syndromes. *Lancet* **342**, 273–5.

Petrosino, B.M., Christian, B.J., Wolf, J., *et al.* (1989). Implications of selected problems with nasoenteral feedings. *Critical Care Nursing Quarterly* **12**, 1–18.

Phillips, M.G., Harry, R., Wendon, J. (2000). The hepatorenal syndrome. In: *Year Book of Intensive Care and Emergency Medicine, 2000* (ed. J.L. Vincent), pp. 390–402. Springer, Berlin.

Pingleton, S.K. (1991). Enteral nutrition and infection: benefits and risks. In: *Update in Intensive Care and Emergency Medicine*, Vol. 14 (ed. J.L. Vincent), pp. 581–9. Springer, Berlin.

Pomier-Layrargues, G., Villeneuve, J-P., Deschênes, M. *et al.* (2001). Transjugular intrahepatic portosystemic shunt (TIPS) versus endoscopic variceal ligation in the prevention of variceal rebleeding in patients with cirrhosis: a randomised trial. *Gut* **48**, 390–6.

Rapp, R.P., Young, B., Twyman, D. *et al.* (1983). The favourable effect of early parenteral feeding on survival in head-injured patients. *Journal of Neurosurgery* **58**, 906–12.

Riordan, S.M., Williams R. (1997). Current concepts: treatment of hepatic encephalopathy. *New England Journal of Medicine* **337**, 473–9.

Robinson, D., Smith A.M.J., Johnston, G.D.(2000). Severity of overdose after restriction of paracetamol availability: retrospective study. *British Medical Journal* **321**, 926–7.

Schlichtig, R., Ayres, S.M. (1988). *Nutritional Support in the Critically Ill*. Year Book Medical Publishers, Chicago, IL.

Scott, A., Skerratt, S., Adam, S. (1998). *Nutrition for the Critically Ill: a Practical Handbook*, p. 67. Arnold, London.

Seaman, D.S. (2001). Adult living donor liver transplantation: current status. *Journal of Clinical Gastroenterology* **33**, 97–106.

Sheiner, P.A., Greig, P.D., Levy, G.A. (1990). Perioperative management of the liver transplant patient. In: *Update in Intensive Care and Emergency Medicine*, Vol. 10 (ed. J.L. Vincent), pp. 706–19. Springer, Berlin.

Sorkine, P., Ben Abraham, R., Szold, O. (2001). Liver support systems. In: *Yearbook of Intensive Care and Emergency Medicine 2001*, (ed. J.L. Vincent), pp. 619–27. Springer, Berlin.

Strong, R.M., Condon, S.C., Solinger, M.R., *et al.* (1992). Equal aspiration rates from postpylorus and intragastric-placed small-bore nasoenteric feeding tubes: a randomized, prospective study. *Journal of Parenteral and Enteral Nutrition* **16**, 59–63.

Tejada Artigas, A., Bello Dronda, S., Chacun Valles, E. *et al.* (2001). Risk factors for nosocomial pneumonia in critically ill trauma patients. *Critical Care Medicine* **29**, 304–9.

Tryba, M. (1991). Sucralfate versus antacids or H$_2$-antagonists for stress ulcer prophylaxis: a meta-analysis on efficacy and pneumonia rate. *Critical Care Medicine* **19**, 942–9.

Van Dalen, R. (1991). Selective decontamination in ICU patients: benefits and doubts. In: *Update in Intensive Care and Emergency Medicine*, Vol. 14 (ed. J.L. Vincent), pp. 379–86. Springer, Berlin.

Van den Berghe, G., Wouters, P., Weekers, F. *et al.* (2001). Intensive insulin therapy in critically ill patients. *New England Journal of Medicine* **345**, 1359–67.

Van Lanschot, S.J.B., Feenstra, B.W.A., Vermeij, C.G., *et al.* (1986). Calculation versus measurement of total energy expenditure. *Critical Care Medicine* **14**, 981–5.

Vargo, R.L., Rudy, E.B. (1988). Infection as a complication of liver transplant. *Critical Care Nurse* **9**, 52–62.

Weissman, C., Kemper, M., Damask, M.C., *et al.*. (1984). Effect of routine intensive care interactions on metabolic rate. *Chest* **86**, 815–18.

Weissman, C., Kemper, M., Askanazi, J., *et al.*. (1986). Resting metabolic rate of the critically ill patient: measured versus predicted. *Journal of Anaesthesiology* **64**, 673–9.

Weissman, C., Kemper, M., Elwyn, D.H., *et al.* (1989). The energy expenditure of the mechanically ventilated critically ill patient: an analysis. *Chest* **89**, 254–9.

Whatley, K., Turner, W.W., Dey, M., *et al.* (1984). When does metaclopromide facilitate transpyloric intubation? *Journal of Parenteral and Enteral Nutrition* **8**, 679–81.

Windsor, A.C., Kanwar, S., Li, A.G. *et al.* (1998). Compared with parenteral nutrition, enteral feeding attenuates the acute phase response and improves disease severity in acute pancreatitis. *Gut* **42**, 431–5.

Winterbauer, R.H., Durning, R.B., Barron, E., *et al.* (1981). Aspirated nasogastric feeding solution detected by glucose strips. *Annals of Internal Medicine* **95**, 67–8.

Wyncoll, D.L. (1999). The management of severe acute necrotising pancreatitis: an evidence-based review of the literature. *Intensive Care Medicine* **25**, 146–56.

CHAPTER 12

The systemic inflammatory response, sepsis, and multiple organ dysfunction

Introduction

One of the greatest challenges currently facing those who work in critical care is the patient suffering from multiple organ dysfunction and the systemic inflammatory response syndrome. These patients are acutely ill with many wide-ranging problems requiring an array of the most complex forms of organ support and intervention. At present, there is no definitive form of treatment and a variety of therapies may be tried.

A major factor in the problem is that any organ or system in the body may be affected (although some, such as the lungs, kidneys, and clotting system, are more vulnerable) and each individual will have differing degrees of organ dysfunction producing different requirements for support.

The number of patients admitted to critical care units in the US with sepsis and septic shock was estimated by Angus *et al.* (2001), from a study of 847 hospitals in seven states, to be 383,000 per year.

In spite of considerable improvements in the management of sepsis, mortality rates remain very high with 30–50% of patients still dying from severe sepsis (Friedman *et al.* 1998, Bernard *et al.* 2001).

The lack of clinically specific definitions of the condition, the varying causes, and the numerous co-morbidities (e.g. cancer, immunosuppression, COPD) has made early identification and management difficult, resulting, in some cases, in delays in treatment (Lyseng-Williamson and Perry 2002). This varied case mix complicates comparisons of treatment and research into the condition.

A recent consensus conference (Levy *et al.* 2003) has attempted to develop a staging system for describing sepsis itself. It consists of predisposition, infection, response, and organ dysfunction (PIRO) and will allow discrimination between morbidity resulting from infection and morbidity resulting from response to infection (Table 12.1).

Definitions

Systemic inflammatory response syndrome (SIRS) and multiple organ dysfunction syndrome (MODS) have been known previously under a variety of different names. The use of these terms was considered misleading and an alternative definition suggesting an inflammatory component was put forward (ACCP/SCCM 1992). The 'Bone criteria' for defining sepsis and inflammatory responses evolved from this (see boxes and Table 12.2).

SIRS describes the non-specific generalized inflammatory response of the body to an extrinsic insult, of which infection is only one cause. *Sepsis* is the term used when the cause of SIRS is infection, and severe sepsis refers to sepsis plus organ dysfunction. *Septic shock* is severe sepsis and hypotension which is not responsive to adequate fluid resuscitation.

MODS was previously known as multiple organ failure, progressive/sequential organ failure, or multisystem organ failure. This was felt to denote a situation that was either present or absent rather than a progressive development along a continuum of physiological

TABLE 12.1 Possible signs of systemic inflammation in response to infection (Levy et al. 2003)	
Infection[a], documented or suspected, and some of the following[b,c]	
General variables	Fever (core temperature >38.3°C)
	Hypothermia (core temperature <36°C
	Heart rate >90 bpm or >2 S.D. above the normal value for age
	Tachypnoea
	Altered mental status
	Significant oedema or positive fluid balance (>20 ml/kg over 24 hours)
	Hyperglycemia (plasma glucose >120 mg/dl or 7.7 mmol/l in the absence of diabetes
Inflammatory variables	Leucocytosis (WBC count >12 000 μl^{-1})
	Leucopenia (WBC count <4000 μl^{-1})
	Normal WBC count with >10% immature forms
	Plasma C-reactive protein >280 above tht normal value
	Plasma procalcitonin >2 S.D. above the normal value
	Haemodynamic variables
	Arterial hypotension[b] (SBP < 90 mmHg, MAP < 70, or an SBP decrease >40 mm Hg in adults or <2 S.D. below normal for age)
	$S_V O_2$ > 70%[b]
	Cardiac index (CI) >3.5 litres/min m²
Organ dysfunction variables	Arterial hypoxemia ($P_a O_2$:$F_i O_2$ < 300)
	Acute oliguria (urine output <0.5 ml kg^{-1} hour^{-1} or 45 mmol/l for at least 2 hours)
	Creatinine increase >0.5 mg/dl
	Coagulation abnormalities (INR > 1.5 or APTT > 60 s)
	Ileus (absent bowel sounds)
	Thrombocytopenia (platelet count <100 000 μl^{-1})
	Hyperbilirubinaemia (plasma total bilirubin >4 mg/dl or 70 mmol/l)
Tissue perfusion variables	Hyperlactataemia (>1 mmol/l)
	Decreased capillary refill or mottling

WBC, white blood cell; SBP, systolic blood pressure; MAP, mean arterial blood pressure; $S_V O_2$, mixed venous oxygen saturation; INR, international normalized ratio; APTT, activated partial thromboplastin time.
[a]Infection defined as a pathological process induced by a microorganism.
[b]$S_V O_2$ > 70% is normal in children (normally 75–80%) and CI 3.5–5.5 is normal in children; therefore *neither* should be used as signs of sepsis in newborns or children.
[c]Diagnostic criteria for sepsis in the paediatric population are signs and symptoms of inflammation plus infection with hyper- or hypothermia (rectal temperature >38.5 or <35°C), tachycardia (may be absent in hypothermic patients) and at least one of the following indications of altered organ function: altered mental status, hypoxemia, increased serum lactate level, or bounding pulses.

TABLE 12.2 Table of definitions

Term	Definition
Bacteraemia	The presence of viable bacteria in the blood
Septicaemia	An imprecise term used in a number of different ways to describe: (1) the presence of microorganisms or their toxins in the blood, (2) sepsis syndrome (see box). Its use is no longer recommended
Sepsis	Systemic inflammatory response with an infective cause
Septic shock	Sepsis-induced hypotension (BP < 90 mmHg or reduced by 40 mmHg from baseline without another cause), which is unresponsive to fluid resuscitation with manifestations of hypoperfusion, such as oliguria, altered mental state etc.
Severe sepsis	Sepsis complicated by organ dysfunction
Apoptosis	Genetically programmed cell death
Anergy	A general loss of immune responsiveness indicating deficient T-cell function

SYSTEMIC INFLAMMATORY RESPONSE SYNDROME (SIRS)

The systemic inflammatory response to a variety of severe clinical insults, manifested by two or more of the following conditions:

- Temperature >38°C
- Heart rate >90 bpm
- Respiratory rate >20 breaths/min or hyperventilation with a P_aCO_2 < 4.3 kPa (32 mmHg)
- WBC >12 000 or <4000 cells/mm³, or 10% immature neutrophils

MULTIPLE ORGAN DYSFUNCTION SYNDROME (MODS)

Presence of altered organ function in an acutely ill patient such that homeostasis cannot be maintained without intervention. This can either occur directly as the result of a well-defined insult or as a secondary result of the host response induced in SIRS.

SEPSIS SYNDROME (after Bone et al. 1989a)

- Hypo- or hyperthermia (<35.6°C/96°F or >38.3°C/101°F)
- Heart rate >90 bpm
- Respiratory rate >20 breaths/min
- Evidence of inadequate organ perfusion/function:

    alteration in mental status

    arterial hypoxaemia (P_aO_2 < 9.6 kPa/72 mmHg)

    an elevated plasma lactate level

    urine output below 0.5 ml/kg/hour for at least 1 hour

Sepsis syndrome does not require the presence of a positive blood culture nor hypotension.

TRIGGERS OF SIRS

- Trauma
- Pancreatitis
- Major burns
- Major surgical procedures
- Infection
- Haemorrhage/major blood transfusion
- Ischaemic tissue
- Periods of inadequate perfusion followed by reperfusion

the underlying pathophysiology, and the biochemical or immunological mechanisms. In addition they do not consider microbiological classifications, even though responses to anti-inflammatory therapies may differ in Gram-positive and Gram-negative infections and the therapies themselves appear to be more effective in patients with documented infections.

Bacterial sepsis

Traditionally, Gram-negative organisms (e.g. *Escherichia coli*, *Pseudomonas aeruginosa*, *Klebsiella* and *Enterobacter* species) were the commonest cause of severe sepsis and septic shock (Bochud and Calandra 2003). These infections are mostly in the lung, abdomen, blood, or urinary tract. However, they have now been overtaken by Gram-positive sepsis due to staphylococci (e.g. *Staphylococcus*

derangement and the term 'multiple organ dysfunction syndrome' was introduced (ACCP/SCCM 1992).

More recently (Abraham *et al.* 2000), these definitions have been criticized because they make no reference to

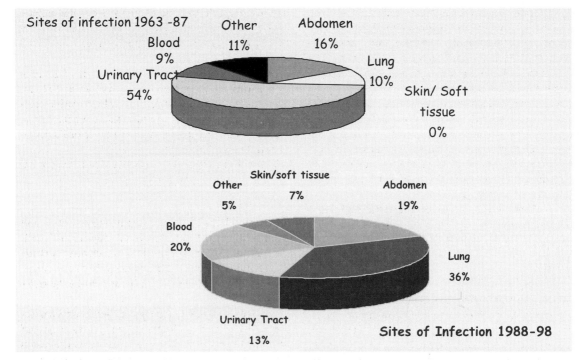

Fig. 12.1 Sites of infection associated with sepsis. (Based on data taken from Bochud *et al.* 2001.)

aureus, coagulase-negative staphylococci), streptococci (e.g. *Streptococcus pneumoniae*), and enterococci. These infections are commonly respiratory, blood, and skin/soft tissue based or catheter-related (Fig. 12.1).

The inflammatory response in bacterial sepsis is due as much to release of components of the bacterial cell wall and enzymes as to the bacteria itself.

Toxins and degradative substances associated with bacteria

Exotoxins

These are proteins released into the environment following their synthesis in the cytoplasm of the cell. They often react with a single target tissue to cause specific damage (e.g. nerves, cardiac muscle). They are produced by both Gram-negative and -positive bacteria.

Endotoxin

This is a structural component of bacterial cells, an integral part of the cell wall, and is released as the cell lyses. They are large lipopolysaccharides, and toxicity is associated with the lipid A portion of the molecule.

Enzymes

Gram-negative bacteria contain a periplasmic space in the cell wall which produces hydrolytic enzymes including lipases, phosphatases, and proteases.

Gram-positive bacteria produce hydrolytic exoenzymes as they do not have a periplasmic space.

Examples of specific degradative substances include:

♦ Streptokinase (streptococci): dissolves fibrin clots thus preventing isolation of infection.

♦ Hyaluronidase (pneumococci, streptococci, staphylococci): digests hyaluronic acid in the basement membrane permitting tissue penetration.

♦ Leucocidin (staphylococci, streptococci): disintegrates phagocytes.

♦ Haemolysin (clostridia, staphylococci): dissolves red blood cells, inducing anaemia and limiting oxygen delivery.

Pathophysiology of SIRS and MODS

The prevailing theory of development of SIRS is that it occurs as the result of an insult that triggers the exaggerated, generalized inflammatory response and leads to the clinical and pathological sequelae of organ dysfunction and failure. However, it is now recognized that there is an anti-inflammatory response as well (Munford and Pugin 2001, Hotchkiss and Karl 2003), as a result of early findings of immunosuppression at the onset of sepsis in some patients (Heidecke 1999). This may overtake the pro-inflammatory response leading to immuno-suppression, anergy (loss of immune responsiveness), and increased susceptibility to further infections. Additional depression of the immune response may arise from increased apoptosis (programmed cell death) of lymphocytes (Hotchkiss *et al.* 1999).

Sepsis (the infective trigger) remains the most common single cause of development of MODS but 40–50% of patients do not have positive blood cultures or an identifiable septic focus (Huddleston 1992). In this case, a treatment dilemma arises as it is possible that an undiagnosed bacterial infection is actually present meriting antibiotic therapy.

The effect of the increased production of these inflammatory factors is to initiate a highly complex common series of pathways of response, as follows.

Inflammatory/immune response

A series of complex interactive mechanisms are activated via humoral (non-cellular) and cellular mediators. These involve both innate (non-specific) first-line defence and adaptive (specific) immune mechanisms (see Chapter 15). In normal circumstances these are subject to extensive inhibitory regulators such as feedback loops and redun-dant pathways. In the case of an overwhelming inflammatory response, these inhibitory systems can fail to control activation and a cycle of continuous reactivation can occur.

Activation of the inflammatory response often leads to concomitant activation of coagulation and alterations in haemostatic balance. Several circulating components play a role in both processes: tissue factor, the kallikrein/kinin cascade, complement, Factor XII (Hageman factor), and platelets.

The mechanism of tissue damage due to inflammatory response is represented in Fig. 12.2.

Endothelial damage

The endothelium is highly susceptible to activation and damage, particularly by white blood cell/endothelial cell interactions. Other inflammatory mediators, such as tumour necrosis factor (TNF), released from monocyte/macrophages and other cells, will also damage the endothelium.

The endothelium has a major function in anticoagulation. When damaged, it loses many properties integral to anticoagulation and can become the source of pro-coagulant substances such as tissue thromboplastin and tissue factor.

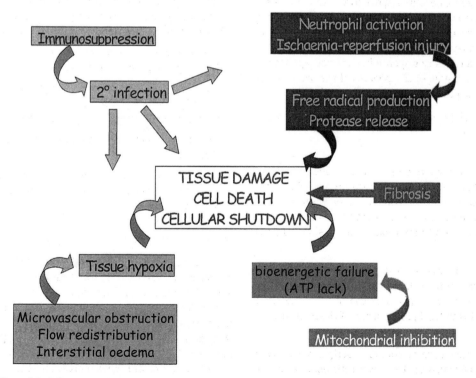

Fig. 12.2 Effects of the inflammatory response.

The three major effects of endothelial damage are:

- release of further mediators and potent vasoactive substances, e.g. prostaglandins, thromboxanes, nitric oxide, endothelins,
- potentiation of coagulation,
- increased capillary permeability.

If activation is widespread then coagulation abnormalities are likely and altered capillary permeability will produce diffuse interstitial oedema and alterations in intravascular fluid volume as fluid passes into the interstitial space.

Neuroendocrine activation

There is an acute phase endocrine response with release of adrenocorticotrophic hormone (ACTH), glucocorticoids, catecholamines (epinephrine (adrenaline) and norepinephrine (noradrenaline)), growth hormone, endorphins, and prolactin. There is increased cardiac output and blood flow to vital organs, with redistribution of blood flow away from secondary organs, increased capillary permeability, and increased blood glucose (for full details see Chapters 3 and 16).

Inflammatory pathways (see Fig. 12.3)
Humoral (plasma enzyme cascades)

Complement   Classically, this is activated by antigen/antibody complexes or alternatively by specific microorganisms. It is a complex cascade through a series of

approximately 20 circulating proteins. Their major function is to initiate and enhance the inflammatory response and help destroy pathogens. The roles of the complement cascade are:

- Induction of inflammation.
- Opsonization (coating with opsonin to enhance binding to phagocytic cells) of foreign particles.
- Cellular activation of phagocytic cells (e.g. neutrophils, macrophages/monocytes).
- Direct target cell lysis (rupture of the cell membrane).

The effect is protective if complement activation is regulated and localized to the site of injury. If large amounts of complement activation occur and appear systemically, then actions become detrimental. This effect is manifested by overwhelming vasodilatation, increased capillary permeability, and phagocytic activation with concomitant release of toxic by-products.

Coagulation and fibrinolysis   The mechanisms of coagulation and fibrinolysis work interdependently, producing a fine balance of haemostasis which, once disrupted, can be difficult to control (Fig. 12.4). Activation of coagulation occurs in response to injury, localized inflammation, and damage to the endothelium. The localized response provides an excellent protective mechanism which, in unregulated circumstances leading to systemic involvement, will rapidly produce coagulopathy and severe dis-

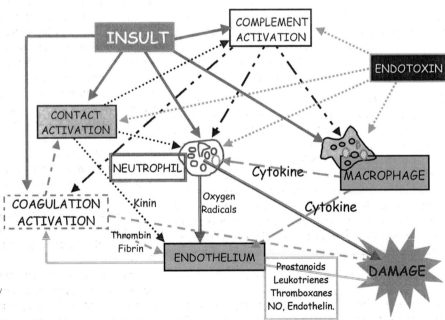

Fig. 12.3 The inflammatory pathways (mechanisms of inflammation).

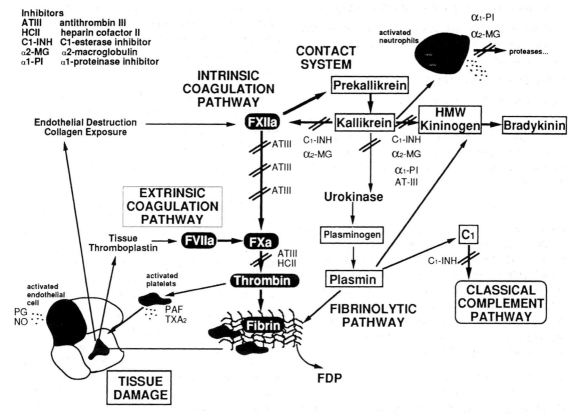

Fig. 12.4 The coagulation, contact, and fibrinolysis pathways.

seminated intravascular coagulation (DIC). The effects are seen as an increased incidence of vascular obstruction, with the potential to cause tissue ischaemia and organ damage. In DIC, there are the combined problems of intravascular coagulation and haemorrhage due to the depletion of clotting factors and platelets.

Kallikrein/kinin The contact system is activated at the same time as the coagulation cascade through Factor XII (Hageman factor). Although the role of this system is not clearly defined, it includes enhancement of the inflammatory response and the fibrinolytic cascade and a possible role in renal blood flow and blood pressure regulation. Bradykinin is the major metabolite produced by the cascade. It has a potent vasodilator effect and has also been shown to increase capillary permeability in some tissues. The kinins also indirectly activate complement, further propagating the inflammatory response.

Cellular (white blood cells, platelets, endothelium, mast cells, and fibroblasts)
White blood cells These include neutrophils, monocytes (circulating macrophages), and lymphocytes. The

primary function of neutrophils is surveillance and phagocytosis of foreign pathogens. They are drawn to the site of injury by chemotactic attraction to chemical products of cell destruction or foreign organisms. The neutrophil phagocytoses the pathogen by releasing proteases (cytotoxic enzymes such as elastase and catalase), and highly reactive oxygen-related molecules collectively referred to as oxygen-derived free radicals. These radicals attack the pathogen in combination with the proteases secreted from the neutrophil causing cell death and phagocytosis.

There is often some release of these highly toxic substances into the extracellular environment and this can result in local tissue damage and organ dysfunction.

The effects of mediators and enzymes synthesized and released by activated neutrophils include vascular endothelial damage and parenchymal damage (Table 12.3).

Proteases, such as elastase, can damage the extracellular matrix. The normal function of proteases is to digest bacteria and other foreign protein matter but they will also act as enzymatic catalysts for the enzyme cascades:

TABLE 12.3 Table of mediators released by white cells as an inflammatory response

Mediator	Lymphocytes	Macrophages	Neutrophils
Oxygen-derived free radicals		✓	✓
Proteases (collagenase, elastase)		✓	✓
Interleukins	✓	✓	✓
Platelet-activating factor		✓	✓
Prostaglandins			✓
Leucotrienes		✓	✓
Nitric oxide (NO)		✓	✓
Tissue factor (thromboplastin)			✓
Tumour necrosis factor	✓	✓	
Interferons	✓ (gamma)	✓	
Antibodies	✓		
Colony-stimulating factors	✓		

complement, coagulation, kallikrein/kinin, fibrinolysis. Their action is potentiated by the presence of oxygen radicals which damage enzymes normally responsible for breaking down and eliminating proteases.

The primary functions of macrophages (mature tissue-based monocytes such as the Kupffer cells in the liver) and monocytes (immature mobile cells circulating in the blood) are: (a) to engulf and phagocytose foreign pathogens or antigens and process them for presentation to lymphocytes, thus stimulating specific lymphocytic proliferation and (b) to produce inflammatory mediators known as monokines (cytokines).

Lymphocytes form sensitized cells and antibodies which are highly specific to a particular foreign pathogen.

In cell-mediated immunity, the T lymphocytes proliferate in response to presentation of the antigen surface of a macrophage to T-cell lymphoid tissue. This is stimulated to produce numerous antigen-specific cells by macrophage release of the cytokine interleukin-1 (IL-1). In humoral immunity, the B lymphocytes recognize the antigen and differentiate into antibody-producing cells. The antibodies bind with the antigen producing an antigen/antibody immune complex which is removed by phagocytic cells in the mononuclear phagocyte system. Lymphocytes also produce mediators which are known as lymphokines.

Platelets These react to disruption of the endothelium and exposure of the underlying collagen basement membrane. The shape of the platelet alters from the normal disc to a swollen sphere and it develops numerous projections known as pseudopods. These two manoeuvres expand the surface area available for adhesion and increase the likelihood of aggregation. During the shape change, adenosine diphosphate (ADP) is released which initiates platelet aggregation. Thromboxane A_2 (TXA_2) is also extruded and causes vasoconstriction and further stimulation of platelet aggregation. This effectively activates platelet surface stickiness but the von Willebrand factor must be present for adhesion to the exposed collagen and fibrinogen must be present for formation of the platelet plug. In addition, release of platelet surface pro-coagulant from the platelet initiates formation of a fibrin plug. The liberated ADP and TXA_2 activate more platelets until the aggregate is large enough to plug the vessel effectively.

Uncontrolled and excessive platelet activation triggered by a major insult will result in disruption of the normal coagulation mechanisms and development of DIC.

Mast cells These are found in almost all tissues. The mast cell mediates the inflammatory response to injury by releasing mediators (see below) following stimulation either from direct injury or the presence of endotoxin, complement, or bradykinin. The effects include vasodilation (histamine and prostaglandins), increased capillary permeability (histamine and leucotrienes), chemokinesis—increased white blood cell movement (histamine)—and bronchoconstriction (histamine and leucotrienes).

Effects of mediators produced by the inflammatory response

There are numerous mediators produced by the inflammatory response and it is beyond the scope of this chapter to describe the function and actions of all of them. However, some of the more important mediators will be briefly described. Mediators are produced primarily by immune cells although they are also generated in the endothelium and other cells.

Arachidonic acid metabolites

Arachidonic acid (AA) is a normal constituent of cell membranes that is released as a result of the contact of the enzyme phospholipase A_2 with injured cell walls. Arachidonic acid metabolism produces mediators known as eicosanoids which are essential for activation of macrophages. The two pathways of AA metabolism are the cyclooxygenase and lipooxygenase pathways. Their action is summarized in Fig. 12.5.

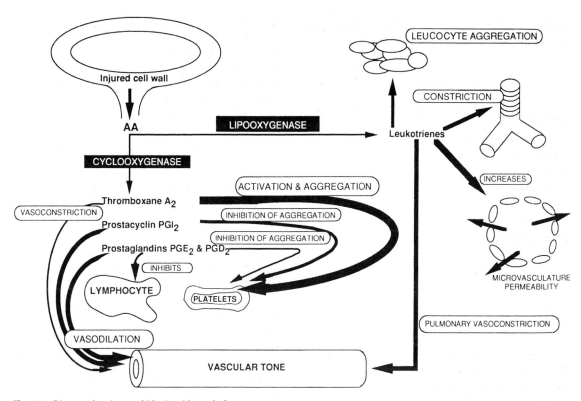

Fig. 12.5 Diagram showing arachidonic acid metabolism.

Tumour necrosis factor

Tumour necrosis factor (TNF) is a polypeptide cyto-kine produced primarily by activated macrophages. TNF release is stimulated by lipopolysaccharide (LPS), microorganisms, ischaemic tissue, and tissue debris. It may well have a central role in the pathogenesis of multiple organ dysfunction and its actions include:

1. Neutrophil activation to produce oxygen-derived free radicals and proteases.

2. Platelet–neutrophil–endothelial interactions.

3. Endothelial activation leading to increased vascular permeability, expression of adhesion molecules to cause leucocytes to adhere to the endothelial surface, and release of endothelial-derived inflammatory mediators (Abbas *et al.* 1997)

4. In high quantities TNF is a pyrogen (induces fever), stimulates secretion of other cytokines (e.g. IL-1 and -6), acts on hepatocytes to stimulate the acute phase response, activates the coagulation system, and sup-presses bone marrow stem cell division (Abbas *et al.* 1997).

TNF also has valuable functions in the normal inflammatory/ immune response.

Interleukins (including IL-1, -6, -8, -10)

Interleukins are released in a number of inflammatory conditions, such as rheumatoid arthritis, haemodialysis, and transplant rejection, as well as sepsis and trauma.

They are also released by activated macrophages and other cells and are associated with inducing pro-coagulant activity in the endothelium and mediating leucocyte adhesion, decreased vascular responsiveness to catecholamines, increased muscle proteolysis, and negative nitrogen balance. IL-1 also produces leuco-cytosis, fever, enhanced T-cell, B-cell, natural killer cell, macrophage, and polymorphonuclear (PMN) cell acti-vity and proliferation, enhanced antibody production, and stimulation of production of acute phase proteins.

IL-1 has a naturally occurring inhibitor IL-1 receptor antagonist (IL-1ra), which is produced by mononuclear phagocytes, and may be responsible for regulating the inflammatory response.

IL-6 is probably a second-stage messenger released by macrophages, endothelial, and other cells in response to TNF or IL-1. Its most important actions are: (a) the stimulation of acute phase protein production in the liver, (b) antibody production, (c) as a growth factor for B cells and malignant plasma cells, and (d) the maintenance of the metabolic response to surgical stress.

Platelet activating factor

Platelet-activating factor (PAF) is a lipid mediator produced from the cell membranes of many different inflammatory response cells and damaged endothelium.

Once in the circulation, PAF initiates platelet activation and the morphological changes associated with the ability to aggregate. Other actions include:

◆ promotion of neutrophil adhesion,

◆ bronchoconstriction,

◆ relaxation of vascular smooth muscle (Abbas *et al.* 1997),

◆ stimulation of oxidative burst (i.e. production of oxygen-derived radicals),

◆ neutrophil degranulation (release of oxygen-derived radicals and digestive enzymes).

Once PAF enters the systemic circulation, excessive platelet activation leads to clot formation and platelet plugs, as well as vasoconstriction. This results in abnormalities of the microcirculation as well as exacerbation of any pre-existing coagulopathies.

Nitric oxide

Nitric oxide, formerly known as endothelium-derived relaxant factor, is a potent vasodilating mediator which is released from many different cell types as well as the endothelium. It has other properties including cytotoxicity, decreased platelet aggregation, mitochondrial dysfunction and neural transmission. Sepsis is associated with very high levels of NO caused by increased expression of the inducible form of NO synthase. NO is currently thought to be the major mediator involved in producing sepsis-related hypotension.

These numerous mediators and inflammatory responses provoke pathophysiological changes in the following three major areas of body function (Table 12.4).

Maldistribution of circulating volume

The factors involved in maldistribution of circulating volume are numerous. Many of the released mediators cause vasodilatation while others vasoconstrict. Some affect capillary vascular permeability, causing intravascular fluid to move both into peripheral venous vessels where it pools, or to pass through the capillary membrane into the interstitial space (known as the 'third'

PHYSIOLOGICAL FUNCTIONS OF TNF

◆ Enhancement of phagocytic activity of neutrophils and macrophages

◆ Initiation of hepatocyte resistance to invasion (particularly parasitic)

◆ Enhancement of lymphocyte activity

◆ Stimulation of interleukin-l, platelet-activating factor, and gamma-interferon release

◆ Induction of fever

◆ Stimulation of collagenase production leading to tissue remodelling

---

TABLE 12.4 Pathophysiological derangements associated with mediators and the neuroendocrine response

1. Maldistribution of circulating blood volume	Systemic vasodilatation
	Increased microvascular permeability
	Vascular obstruction related to cellular aggregation, microthrombi, and tissue oedema
	Selective vasoconstriction
	Endothelial damage
	Coagulation/microvascular thrombi
	Loss of autoregulation
2. Imbalance of oxygen supply and demand	Maldistribution of circulating volume
	Microvascular abnormalities
	Increased oxygen demand due to pain, fever, tachycardia, restlessness, etc.
	Oxygen extraction defects
	V/Q mismatch
	Intrapulmonary shunt
	Excessive cellular activity
	Myocardial depression
3. Alterations in metabolism	Hypermetabolism
	Hyperglycaemia
	Protein catabolism and gluconeogenesis
	Resistance to insulin
	Excessive cellular activity
	Fatty acid mobilization and increased oxidation
	Hepatic dysfunction and lactate production

fluid space). Another factor in maldistribution is the obstruction to blood flow within the microvasculature caused by clumping of white cells in response to the initial injury and development of microthrombi stimulated by kallikrein, PAF, and thromboxanes. Normal peripheral vascular autoregulatory mechanisms are also dysfunctional during the hyperdynamic phase of SIRS resulting in vasodilatation and localized vasoconstriction with inappropriate closure of pre-capillary sphincters.

Imbalance of oxygen supply and demand

In healthy tissue, decreases in oxygen delivery do not initially lower oxygen consumption because tissue oxygen extraction is increased proportionately (see Chapter 6).

When available oxygen to the tissues falls below a critical level, tissue extraction can no longer increase to compensate and oxygen consumption will fall when there is a further fall in oxygen delivery. This is known as supply-dependent oxygen consumption.

It is postulated that in SIRS an impairment of tissue oxygen extraction capacity occurs which may lead to oxygen supply dependency at normal or increased levels of overall oxygen delivery (Schumacker and Cain 1987). Pathological supply dependency in SIRS may be due to:

1. Maldistribution of blood flow (see above).

2. Cellular defects. An impairment of oxidative metabolism has been demonstrated in sepsis in some human studies (Brealey 2002). This suggests an inability to utilize oxygen by the cells and is related to mitochondrial inhibition by nitric oxide. Paradoxically, in sepsis, the tissue PO_2 is elevated, supporting this cellular hypothesis that oxygen is available but utilization is decreased.

3. Impaired oxygen diffusion. This is hypothesized to be due to:

   ◆ an increase in interstitial fluid widening the distance between capillaries and cells,

   ◆ shorter capillary transit time (due to low SVR and high cardiac output) preventing unloading of oxygen from haemoglobin (Dantzker 1989),

   ◆ 'shunting' of blood away from the nutrient capillaries.

Catabolic alterations in metabolism

Principal alterations seen in the early phase of sepsis are hypermetabolism, hyperglycaemia, protein catabolism, resistance to utilization of exogenous substrates, and inadequate reserves of substrates. However, in subsequent phases of sepsis there may be decreased metab-

olism. The majority of these alterations are associated with the response of the hypothalamus and sympathetic nervous system to a major stress (for details see Chapters 3 and 16).

Specific organ dysfunctions associated with SIRS and sepsis

Central nervous system involvement in MODS

CNS failure in multiple organ dysfunction is defined as a decreased level of consciousness ranging from confusion to coma that cannot be explained by physical, drug, or metabolic abnormalities. In a review of medical critical care patients, the highest incidence of neurological complications was seen in sepsis patients (38.8%) (Barlas et al. 2001).

Sepsis, circulatory, and microcirculatory perfusion deficits and reperfusion injury are all significant factors in the process of development of CNS failure. The exact mechanisms are still unclear; suggested factors include:

1. Disordered amino acid transport and metabolism. Increased plasma levels of aromatic and sulphur-containing amino acids (specifically phenylalanine and glutamine) are found in the brain and CSF of patients with sepsis. Accumulation of these substances could play a role in vasodilatation and altered cerebral function.

2. Altered neurotransmitter concentration. Increased levels of serotonin (5-HT) and 5-hydroxyindoleacetic acid (5-HIAA) have been found in animal studies. Their effects are compatible with the encephalopathic changes associated with MODS.

3. Brain microabscesses. These are produced by blood-borne contaminants which may block cerebral arterioles causing ischaemia. They may also initiate hyperaemia, oedema, and petechial haemorrhages.

Actions of cytokines and mediators such as nitric oxide.

Circulatory and microcirculatory perfusion deficits

Cerebral cellular metabolism relies on adequate supplies of oxygen and glucose. If the supply of both oxygen and glucose is inadequate due to perfusion deficits, anaerobic metabolism takes place producing accumulation of lactic acid and eventual intracellular acidosis. When intracellular pH falls below 5.5, or ATP is exhausted, irreversible cell damage occurs.

Cellular acidosis decreases the uptake of calcium ions (Ca^{2+}) by the mitochondria and sarcoplasmic reticulum thus increasing intracellular levels of Ca^{2+} This activates enzymes, such as phospholipases and proteases, which are capable of destroying cell membranes and intra-cellular organelles. Cellular acidosis will also inhibit mitochondrial respiration, further blocking ATP synthesis.

ATP depletion occurs and calcium shifts, prostaglandin synthesis, release of oxygen-derived radicals, and membrane damage result.

The excitatory neurotransmitters glutamine and aspartate may also have a role in the ischaemic process. The result is a major loss of functioning cerebral tissue which is probably reversible if the patient survives.

Cerebral reperfusion injury

Reperfusion injury refers to damage occurring after circulation has been restored. The phenomenon is due to the generation of toxic oxygen-derived radicals or reactive oxygen species (ROS) as a by-product of oxygen-supported conversion of hypoxanthine to xanthine and uric acid, both from mitochondria and white cells. Hypoxanthine is produced when ATP degrades during ischaemia. When oxygen is reintroduced the excess hypoxanthine which has built up is converted to xanthine and ROS (Collard and Gelman 2001). Cell damage also results from the accumulation of free fatty acids and prostaglandins (see Fig. 12.6).

Two processes have been associated with reperfusion injury: post-ischaemic hypoperfusion and the no-reflow phenomenon.

1. *Post-ischaemic hypoperfusion.* This occurs after periods of complete global ischaemia and is seen as a 15–20 min period of hyperaemia (high blood flow) followed by vasospasm-induced hypoperfusion. The hyperaemia occurs as a result of loss of autoregulation and from the difference in blood viscosity of stagnant blood and circulating blood reperfusing the microcirculation. Vasospasm lasts for 6–34 hours and is thought to be a response to calcium activation and increased production of thromboxane A_2.

2. *The no-reflow phenomenon.* This is less common and occurs for 1–3 days after ischaemia. There is a continued decrease in cerebral blood flow despite normal mean arterial and cerebral perfusion pressures. Processes contributing to the no-reflow phenomenon are:

  ◆ oedema

  ◆ vasospasm

  ◆ increased blood viscosity with red blood cell sludging

  ◆ hypermetabolism

  ◆ membrane damage

  ◆ intracellular or mitochondrial calcium shifts

  ◆ release of oxygen-derived free radicals.

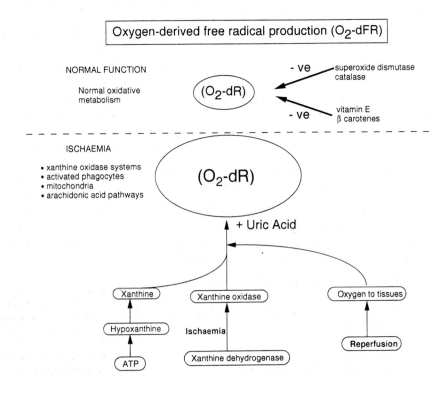

Fig. 12.6 The generation of oxygen-derived radicals.

CNS dysfunction associated with MODS

CNS involvement in MODS is not always associated with a period of hypoxia and metabolic causes are still unknown. It is generally an indicator of poor prognosis (Sprung *et al.* 1990).

Three distinct types of dysfunction are seen:

* septic encephalopathy,
* critical illness polyneuropathy and myopathy,
* neuroendocrine exhaustion or failure.

Septic encephalopathy

In septic encephalopathy neurological alterations are diffuse ranging from altered concentration and intermittent confusion to seizures and coma. EEG changes are also variable but the degree of abnormality correlates with the degree of encephalopathy. An increased mortality is associated with increasing severity of encephalopathy (Eidelman *et al.* 1996). A mortality rate of between 33 and 49% has been associated with severe encephalopathy in sepsis (Sprung *et al.* 1990, Eidelman et al 1996).

Critical illness polyneuropathy

Critical illness polyneuropathy (CIP) increases patient mortality and can significantly prolong recovery time. It is associated with primary axonal degeneration of motor and sensory fibres and denervation atrophy of limb and skeletal muscles (Witt *et al.* 1991). This usually presents clinically as profound limb and chest wall weakness, although sensory deficits can occur alone or in combination. A primary critical illness myopathy (CIM) with muscle degeneration that is not secondary to muscle denervation is also recognized, either alone or in combination with a polyneuropathy when it is termed critical illness myopathy and neuropathy (CRIMYNE) (Latronico 2003).

Neuroendocrine exhaustion

Neuroendocrine exhaustion or failure occurs as part of a biphasic neuroendocrine response seen in prolonged critical illness. In this case, reduced hypothalamic stimulation results in impaired pulsatile release of a number of anterior pituitary hormones and poor stimulation of their target tissues (Van den Berghe *et al.* 2001) and is associated with the following problems:

* altered release of hypothalamic products such as vasopressin, thyrotropin-releasing hormone, growth hormone-releasing hormone, and corticotrophin releasing-factor,
* glucose intolerance,
* failure to mount a febrile response,

* neurogenic pulmonary oedema,
* sick euthyroid syndrome,
* hypoadrenal response, producing a relative adrenocortical insufficiency which is associated with poor outcome (Rothwell *et al.* 1991).

The presence of these problems suggests that the body is no longer able to mount an effective response to the neuroendocrine triggers associated with SIRS. However, this has yet to be established, with a number of conflicting results from studies on adrenal response (Schroeder *et al.* 2001).

Patient assessment for neurological and muscular involvement

Assessment should include the following:

1. *Conscious level* (although this can be impossible to assess due to the levels of sedation required to maintain ventilation). A high index of suspicion should be maintained if the patient appears unresponsive when sedation is reduced. Sedation should be reduced when the patient appears totally unresponsive, even during unpleasant procedures such as suction or turning (for further details see Chapter 10). Glasgow coma scores are associated with the grade of encephalopathy and mortality (Eidelman *et al.* 1996).

2. *Mental agitation and confusion.* This is often apparent when the patient is first admitted and other causes must be excluded (e.g. hypoxaemia). It can herald a further septic episode in a patient who has previously been recovering with no evidence of mental confusion.

3. *Profound weakness and muscle wasting* may only become apparent as the patient is recovering from MODS. It can be distinguished from simple weakness related to normal catabolic muscle wasting by electrophysiological studies which will show evidence of primary axonal degeneration of both sensory and motor fibres or myopathic changes (Bednarik *et al.* 2003).

4. EEGs may exhibit evidence of changes consistent with *metabolic or anoxic encephalopathy* and a few will show evidence of profound abnormalities.

Respiratory system involvement in MODS

Respiratory system involvement in MODS occupies a range of dysfunction from acute lung injury (ALI) to acute respiratory distress syndrome (ARDS).

ALI is defined by the following clinical findings:

1. Diffuse acute pulmonary infiltrates seen on CXR associated with decreased pulmonary compliance.

DEFINITION OF RESPIRATORY FAILURE

Blood gases:

◆ PO_2 < 8.0 kPa, patient breathing air and at rest

◆ ± PCO_2 > 6.5 kPa in the absence of primary metabolic alkalosis

◆ ± pH < 7.25 in the absence of primary metabolic acidosis

Patient:

◆ respiratory rate >40 or <6–8 breaths min

◆ deteriorating vital capacity (<15 ml/kg)

2. A P_aO_2:F_iO_2 ratio <300 mmHg (40 kPa).

3. Pulmonary artery wedge pressure of <18 mmHg (i.e. non-cardiogenic origin).

4. A precipitating factor.

ARDS includes all the above but the P_aO_2:F_iO_2 ratio is <200 mmHg (26.7 kPa).

There is usually evidence of respiratory failure (dyspnoea, tachypnoea, tachycardia, agitation).

Pathogenesis of ARDS

The underlying pathophysiology traditionally consists of three overlapping phases: an inflammatory or exudative phase, a proliferative phase, and, finally, a fibrotic phase (Bellingan 2002). It is now apparent that these phases are not distinct (for instance markers of fibrosis can be found on day 1 of ARDS) and the disease process is also complicated by other variables such as episodes of nosocomial pneumonia and possible ventilator-induced lung injury.

Inflammatory or exudative phase

Initial disruption of the alveolar epithelium and endothelial damage occurs releasing mediators that cause increased capillary permeability, neutrophil and platelet aggregation, and pulmonary vasoconstriction. This results in alterations to microcirculatory flow and V/Q mismatch. Capillary membrane disruption also allows movement of fluid and protein into the interstitium. Atelectasis occurs as a result of interstitial oedema compressing alveoli. This compounds the decreased lung compliance caused by decreased surfactant production.

Proliferative phase

Direct parenchymal damage occurs as a result of mediator and macrophage action and necrosis from hypoxia. This damage ultimately causes fibrosis in alveolar tissue, further decreasing lung compliance. The net result is progressive alveolar collapse, intrapulmonary shunting, and hypoxaemia.

Fibrotic phase

Increasing scarring and fibrosis occur with replacement of alveolar epithelial tissue and derangement of vasculature. This reduces lung compliance thereby increasing the work of breathing, decreasing the tidal volume, and resulting in CO_2 retention. Also, because of the alveolar obliteration and interstitial thickening, gas exchange is reduced which contributes to hypoxia and ventilator dependence (Bellingan 2002).

The pulmonary fibrosis in ARDS may take some time to resolve and can lead to persistent pulmonary problems both during weaning and after patients leave the critical care unit. Recovery of lung function can be slow, with some patients taking up to 12 months to return to baseline while others have persisting abnormalities (McHugh et al. 1994).

Patient assessment for ARDS

General appearance

Patient colour, respiratory function and pattern, level of fatigue, mental state, signs of sweating and distress (see Chapter 4 for details).

Lung fields

Auscultation in ARDS may sound clear or may detect isolated or generalized crackles or wheezes (see Chapter 4 for details).

Chest X-ray

This is commonly anteroposterior in critical care, as a portable X-ray is usually necessary for sick patients. The typical early ARDS picture is non-specific with clear lung fields or scant infiltrates. There may also be unilateral lobar consolidation or diffuse lung involvement related to precipitating factors. Later interstitial oedema may be evident and the picture becomes one of diffuse alveolar infiltrates, sometimes termed 'white-out' (Hobbs and Mahajan 2000).

Pulse oximetry

Patients are usually hypoxaemic from the early stages of ARDS and S_aO_2 will be <90% on air. Additional inspired oxygen will improve S_aO_2 initially, but requirements will continue to rise making CPAP or mechanical ventilation necessary.

Pulmonary secretions

Volume, colour, and texture should be assessed. There are usually minimal, loose white secretions present in the early stages of ARDS. As the disease progresses secretions become thicker and more profuse, often due to secondary infection. Specimens should be sent for microbiological culture.

Arterial blood gases

In the early stages of ARDS, the patient's P_aO_2 will be low and the P_aCO_2 will be either normal or low if the patient is hyperventilating in response to hypoxaemia. The pH will be normal or slightly alkalotic if the P_aCO_2 is low.

In the later stages, as the patient tires and respiratory failure ensues, the P_aCO_2 will rise with a decrease in pH due to a mixed respiratory and metabolic acidosis. The P_aO_2 will remain low in spite of increased inspired oxygen concentrations of up to $F_iO_2 = 1.0$.

Ventilator observations

Compliance will be decreased usually to a static compliance of less than 20–30 ml/cmH$_2$O. The decreased compliance will result in high airway pressures during positive pressure ventilation, increasing the risk of barotrauma and alveolar damage if the pressure is not limited to less than 30 cmH$_2$O plateau pressure.

The limitation of tidal volumes to between 6–8 ml/kg (ideal body weight) has been associated with a reduction in risk of mortality of 22% (ARDS Network 2000). The overall goal of intervention is to reopen and stabilize collapsed, but potentially functional, alveolar units while minimizing barotrauma and variations in expansion of different areas of the lung caused by the disease process (see Chapter 4 for details).

Inspired oxygen requirements are often increased to greater than F_iO_2 of 0.6 in order to achieve oxygen saturations of >90%. There are potential concerns about oxygen toxicity at higher concentrations, although the impact on patients is still far from clear.

The use of inhaled nitric oxide and prone positioning (see Chapter 4 for details) to improve ventilation/ perfusion matching have been included in the management of patients with severe ARDS, though neither strategy has been associated with outcome improvement (Dellinger et al. 1998, Gattinoni et al. 2001).

Heart rate

The patient will be tachycardic due to hypoxaemia as well as a number of other factors (mediator and catecholamine release, pyrexia, low systemic blood pressure).

Pulmonary hypertension

Pulmonary artery pressures show increased pulmonary systolic and diastolic pressures with normal pulmonary artery wedge pressures. Pulmonary artery wedge pressures may rise if there is associated cardiac dysfunction.

ARDS is a feature in between 25 and 42% of sepsis patients and despite recent developments mortality remains high at around 30–40% (Herridge et al. 2003). Many of those who survive will have persistent functional impairment up to a year after discharge from hospital. Successful patient management requires respiratory support, identification and treatment of precipitating causes, and expert monitoring and prevention of further morbidity.

Cardiovascular involvement in MODS

A major part of the cardiovascular dysfunction seen in SIRS and sepsis is related to the loss of peripheral vasoautoregulatory mechanisms and the need to maintain tissue oxygenation in spite of increasing hypoxaemia. A confounding factor in the ability of the myocardium to respond is a depressant effect on function often associated with SIRS.

The loss of peripheral autoregulation and excess NO production leads to inappropriate vasodilatation, maldistribution of flow, and decreased oxygen extraction. The appropriate circulatory response to this tissue hypoxia is to increase cardiac function by increasing heart rate and contractility in an attempt to meet tissue demands. Preload and afterload are reduced by the fall in arterial and venous tone. The decreased preload leads to a decreased contractility (Starling effect) which is compensated by the reduction in peripheral vessel resistance to flow. If adequate intravascular volume is maintained then cardiac output rises to meet tissue oxygen demands and a hyperdynamic response is evident. The hyperdynamic response consists of:

- increased cardiac output
- increased heart rate
- decreased systemic vascular resistance

Myocardial dysfunction

This may be evident early in the course of sepsis. However, myocardial depression can persist even after correction of hypoxia, acidosis, and electrolyte disturbance, suggesting that the inflammatory response itself has suppressed myocardial function. Once the sepsis has resolved, the depression reverses, usually within 7–10 days (Pathan et al. 2002).

Several factors and mediators have been implicated in its development:

1. Loss of autoregulation of coronary blood flow resulting in excessive vasodilatation, high coronary blood flow, and reduced oxygen extraction.

2. Maldistribution of coronary blood flow: microcirculatory disturbances and scattered necrosis have been reported.

3. Alterations in myocardial substrate extraction: reliance on lactate and endogenous cardiac reserves as a major fuel source rather than the normal substrate (free fatty acids).

4. Myocardial oedema and altered calcium metabolism.

5. Altered response to sympathetic nervous system stimuli: decreased sensitivity to circulating catecholamines due to down-regulation of α-adrenergic receptors.

6. Myocardial depressant factors. There is strong evidence supporting the presence of myocardial depressant factors. These factors appear to reduce ventricular contractility by one-third or more and are probably linked to TNFα and IL-1β and mediated by mechanisms that include nitric oxide and cyclic GMP generation (Krishnagopalan *et al.* 2002).

7. Endotoxin may play a direct role in depressing myocardial function but the mechanism has not as yet been fully established.

8. Interleukin-2 has been shown to induce heart failure and haemodynamic changes when used as immunotherapy in cancer patients.

Many other mediators are thought to be implicated in myocardial dysfunction but their roles have yet to be clarified.

The net result is that while cardiac output may remain normal or even increased there is a decrease in ventricular ejection fraction with accompanying biventricular dilatation (Parker and Fink 1992). In addition, there is an abnormal response to fluid volume loading showing a smaller increase in left ventricular end diastolic volume and stroke work index for an increase in pulmonary artery wedge pressure (Ognibene *et al.* 1988). This is reversible as the patient recovers.

Patient assessment of cardiovascular dysfunction
Heart rate and rhythm
Tachycardia is a feature of the patient with SIRS. Atrial and occasionally ventricular arrhythmias can occur which may diminish cardiac output and exacerbate hypotension.

Mean arterial pressure (MAP)
MAP is not a good indicator of flow. However, a MAP of at least 60 mmHg is usually necessary to maintain the perfusion pressure of vital organs.

Urine output
Urine output in a catheterized patient allows continuous assessment of renal perfusion as a marker of general organ perfusion. The aim is to maintain a urine output of >0.5 ml/kg/hour. However, the quality of the urine produced may be poor and daily measurement of plasma urea and creatinine levels are required for assessment of renal function.

Stroke volume (SV), cardiac output (CO) and pulmonary artery wedge pressure (PAWP)
Ideally, monitoring of the effect of fluid challenges on SV and CO should be carried out. There are now several ways of achieving this (see Chapter 5). Fluid resuscitation should then be carried out as a series of fluid challenges against serial measures of SV, CO and if using a pulmonary artery catheter, PAWP.

CO in the patient with sepsis or SIRS can either be normal or, more usually, raised if the patient has been adequately fluid resuscitated. In most critical care units, the thermodilution technique remains the established method of determining CO. It will also allow calculation of oxygen delivery and consumption. However, it is also possible to use Doppler ultrasonography, PiCCO®, lithium dilution CO measurement with pulse contour analysis, or transthoracic bioimpedence techniques, all of which offer a less invasive method of determining CO (although not oxygen delivery and consumption).

Gut tonometry
This is a method of monitoring regional (gut) blood flow and perfusion (see Chapter 5). A thin silicone balloon wrapped around the end of a fine-bore tube is placed in the stomach. The balloon contains air and acts as a semi-permeable membrane allowing equilibration with the CO_2 released from the gut mucosa over a period of about 30 min. The air in the balloon is aspirated periodically to measure the partial pressure of the CO_2. A value of the pH of the gut mucosa (pHi) can then be determined from calculations using the partial pressure of CO_2 obtained. Recent work suggests that the PCO_2 gap (the difference between gastric mucosal PCO_2 and arterial PCO_2) at 24 hours after admission to critical care may be a useful predictor of prognosis (Levy *et al.* 2003), although, in the same study, the arterial lactate level was similarly effective.

Sublingual capnometry, a less invasive method of monitoring proximal mucosal PCO_2 under the tongue, has recently been developed extending from this concept (Weil *et al.* 1999). There is a direct correlation between $P_{sl}CO_2$ and gastric CO_2 (Marik and Bankov 2003). The technique takes less than 5 min and may prove to be a useful marker of adequate resuscitation/ tissue perfusion in the critically ill patient (Boswell and Scalea 2003).

Arterial base deficit
A rapidly developing arterial base deficit, measured doing routine blood gas analysis, is highly suggestive of

tissue ischaemia or infarction. Correction of the metabolic acidosis is achieved by treating the underlying cause rather than by giving bicarbonate.

Lactate

Blood lactate levels may be a good indication of global ischaemia. Levels >2 mmol/l reflect increased lactate production and this is often associated with tissue hypoxia. Blood lactate is an end product of anaerobic respiration which occurs when pyruvate entry into the tricarboxylic acid (Krebs) cycle is blocked by a lack of oxygen. It is now recognized that hyperlactataemia may also be due to a variety of other causes including accelerated glycolysis, ATP hydrolysis, and inactivation of pyruvate dehydrogenase (which blocks pyruvate entry into the mitochondrial Krebs cycle). However, a normal blood lactate level does not necessarily indicate that all organs are adequately perfused.

Temperature

The septic patient may exhibit either pyrexia or, occasionally, a hypothermic response. Pyrexia may be accompanied by tachycardia and hypotension associated with vasodilatation and efforts may be necessary to cool the patient in order to reduce metabolic demands if the patient's ability to meet oxygen demand is compromised.

Gastrointestinal involvement in MODS

Splanchnic hypoperfusion occurs as part of the compensatory mechanisms associated with a decrease in cardiac output. Perfusion is reduced as a result of the vasoconstrictive response and blood flow diversion which produce supply-dependent oxygen consumption and an oxygen deficit. Non-specific complications include hypokinetic gastric function with large gastric aspirates.

Effects on gastrointestinal organs can be severe, particularly at mucosal level where rapidly proliferating cells have a high oxygen and substrate requirement:

◆ *Stomach*. Disruption of the mucosal barrier occurs with development of mucosal and submucosal ischaemia. This leads to an increased risk of ulceration and stress ulcer bleeding. Gastric motility is also reduced.

◆ *Small intestine*. Disruption of the mucosal barrier occurs and there is a loss of gut mucosal integrity which may lead to translocation of luminal organisms (see Chapter 11 for further information).

◆ *Pancreas*. Pancreatitis (an inflammatory response resulting from premature activation of pancreatic enzymes) can occur (see Chapter 11 for further information). Pancreatitis is itself a trigger for a further systemic inflammatory response.

◆ *Gallbladder*. Acalculous cholecystitis (inflammation unrelated to gallstones) can develop.

◆ *Colon*. Disruption of the mucosal barrier and an increased translocation of luminal organisms may result. Colitis may also develop.

Patient assessment for gastrointestinal involvement
Abdomen

Observation, palpation, and ausculation should be carried out for evidence of distension, discomfort and pain, and presence of bowel sounds (see Chapter 11 for further information).

Faeces

Note the presence of diarrhoea—colour, consistency, frequency. Note the presence of blood.

Gastric intolerance

The following can occur: nausea, vomiting, and large aspirates (>200 ml) from the nasogastric tube.

Pancreatic enzymes

Test for serum amylase (see Chapter 11 for further information) to indicate pancreatic dysfunction.

Gut tonometry and sublingual capnometry

Monitoring the partial pressure of gut luminal carbon dioxide (P_gCO_2) may be a useful indicator of both the efficacy of fluid resuscitation and prognosis, but this has yet to be established in routine clinical practice.

Ultrasound can be used to diagnose acalculous cholecystitis as well as identify fluid collections within the abdomen.

Liver involvement in MODS

Liver dysfunction is not usually seen until several days after the development of other organ dysfunction. The serum bilirubin exceeds 20–30 μmol/l and is associated with other markers of hepatic dysfunction such as increased hepatic enzymes (see box), increased prothrombin time or hepatic encephalopathy.

At present, there is no clearly identified mechanism of liver dysfunction in MODS, although a number of theories have been put forward. It is likely that the

---

CLINICAL MARKERS OF HEPATIC DYSFUNCTION

◆ Raised serum bilirubin (>20–30 μmol/l) (jaundice)

◆ Raised AST and LDH (at least twice normal levels)

◆ Abnormal prothrombin time or INR

◆ Hepatic encephalopathy (see Chapter 11)

effects of various mediators released by neutrophils and damaged tissue may cause shunting, altered vascular permeability, and further platelet activation within the liver itself, thus producing localized areas of ischaemia.

An alternative theory suggests Kupffer cells (tissue-based macrophages within the liver) are the source of hepatic dysfunction. They are stimulated by endotoxin or other inflammatory mediators circulating from either the trigger or secondary dysfunction sites, to release toxic mediators. These mediators act on the closely situated hepatocytes altering their function but not causing cell death. The presence of any pre-existing liver disease is likely to precipitate liver dysfunction.

Effects of liver dysfunction

Demands placed on the liver's metabolic functions (see Chapter 11) during the hypermetabolic phase are enor-

TABLE 12.5 Effect of SIRS/sepsis on liver function

Liver function	Effect of SIRS/sepsis
Protein metabolism	Increased rate of gluconeogenesis
	Concomitant rises in protein catabolism and urea production
	Increased urinary nitrogen excretion
	Decreased clearance of amino acids resulting in high levels of phenylalanine and tyrosine
Lipid metabolism	Lipolysis and lipogenesis may occur, resulting in (a) high levels of serum lipids and (b) decreased peripheral lipid clearance
	Reduced hepatocyte utilization of ketones produced from lipid conversion
Hepatic protein synthesis	Increased synthesis of acute-phase reactant proteins
	Decreased synthesis of albumin and transferrin
	Depletion of fibronectin (enhances phagocytosis) levels
Detoxification of drugs, toxins, and hormones	Increased levels of hormones normally detoxified by the liver such as ADH and aldosterone
	Higher serum levels, prolonged duration of action, and increased toxicity may occur of drugs normally metabolized by the liver
Clotting factors	Bleeding and DIC may be accentuated by limited removal of activated clotting factors
	Reduced clotting factor synthesis

mous. In conjunction with this, the combined effect of circulating mediators and possible hypoperfusion on hepatic cell function is potentially highly damaging. The result is deranged carbohydrate, protein, and lipid metabolism as well as a dysfunctional immune response, reduced protein synthesis, and impaired detoxification processes (Table 12.5).

Patient assessment for liver dysfunction

Conscious level and neurological status

This should take other factors such as sedation and neurotrauma into consideration but any features of encephalopathy (see Chapter 10) should be assessed.

Conjunctival and skin colour

These should be observed for a yellow tinge indicating jaundice (see Chapter 11 for details).

Skin, mucous membranes, and invasive line sites

These should be inspected daily for evidence of coagulation abnormalities which give rise to bleeding from gums, purpura, bleeding from line sites, etc.

Urinalysis

Daily urinalysis should be done to check bilirubin levels.

Liver function tests

These should be carried out at least every 2–3 days in the acute phase (see Chapter 11 for details).

Clotting tests

These should be carried out on a daily basis.

Renal involvement in MODS

Either pre-renal failure or a direct renal effect by toxins or inflammatory mediators can result in renal dysfunction. Pre-renal failure occurs as a result of decreased renal perfusion. This can be reversed if perfusion is restored. Recent theories on cell hibernation as a response to ischaemia are based on the finding that kidney histology (cell structure) is essentially normal in spite of severe biochemical and physiological dysfunction (Hotchkiss and Karl 2003) and that following an episode of sepsis and renal failure baseline renal function is usually recovered. This suggests that there is a 'programmed shutdown' of the kidney in response to a prolonged insult which allows subsequent recovery of function. Previous theories were based on the development of acute tubular necrosis as a result of ischaemia, toxins such as endotoxin and mediators, or as a drug-related response. Full details of the pathogenesis of acute renal failure and acute tubular necrosis (ATN) are given in Chapter 9.

The clinical course of renal dysfunction has four phases:

1. Onset. A potentially reversible stage, which may correspond with pre-renal failure. It may last hours to days depending on the cause. The disease course following ischaemic causes is generally shorter than for toxic causes.

2. Oliguric–anuric phase. Lasts 1–6 weeks. The glomerular filtration rate is significantly reduced with total body fluid overload, high blood urea and plasma creatinine levels, electrolyte abnormalities, and resulting metabolic acidosis. Evidence of uraemic symptoms may also be present.

3. Diuretic phase. An increased urine output is accompanied by a gradual increase in renal function. Urine output may be more than 2–3 litres per day with little or no evidence of concentration or excretion. Gradually, the urinary urea increases and sodium falls. Acidosis and electrolyte imbalance begin to improve.

4. Recovery phase. Glomerular filtration usually returns to at least 70–80% of normal within 1–2 years. Mild to moderate residual renal dysfunction may remain, though the need for long-term dialysis is very rare if the kidneys were previously healthy.

Patient assessment for renal involvement

The patient should be assessed for:

* oedema (peripheral and pulmonary), nausea, vomiting, pruritis, and other symptoms of uraemia (see Chapter 9),

* urine output (the aim is > 0.5 ml/kg/hour),

* urinalysis for specific gravity, protein, glucose, and blood ± urinary sodium and urea, ± urine: plasma osmolality,

* blood urea,

* plasma creatinine,

* blood potassium,

* blood pH,

* intravascular fluid volume status (see also cardiac assessment).

Haematological involvement in MODS

The manifestations of coagulopathy most commonly seen in MODS are:

1. Bleeding from line sites and wounds due to depletion of clotting factors.

2. Bleeding into the skin, ranging from petechiae to gross echymosis as well as from mucosa and gums.

3. Stress ulcer, peptic ulcer, and other causes of gastrointestinal bleeding are more common.

DIC is a pathological over-stimulation of normal coagulation which paradoxically causes both microvascular thrombi (which deplete normal stores of clotting factors and activate the fibrinolytic system) and bleeding due to the resultant lack of clotting factors and overactive fibrinolysis (full details are given in Chapter 14). Although DIC occurs as a result of almost any severe disease process, there are a number of particular factors which pre-dispose to its development. These are:

* arterial hypotension,

* inadequate tissue perfusion,

* stasis of capillary blood flow (Hudak *et al.* 1990).

DIC represents the severe end of a continuum of dysfunction of the haematological system and can often occur as a response to SIRS. (A list of trigger factors for DIC can be found in Chapter 14.)

Patient assessment for haematological involvement

The following should he assessed/observed.

* skin for evidence of petechiae, purpura, bruising, and haematomas,

* gums and mucous membranes for bleeding,

* sclera and conjunctiva for haemorrhage,

* intravenous cannulae sites, arterial cannulae sites, chest drain sites, wounds, tracheostomy sites for bleeding,

* sputum during endotracheal suctioning for bleeding,

* urinalysis for evidence of haematuria,

* stools for evidence of melaena and nasogastric aspirate for evidence of gastric bleeding,

* measurement of haemoglobin, platelet count, thrombin time, prothrombin time, D-dimer levels (the fibrin-specific degradation fragment D is measured using monoclonal antibodies and is a marker of DIC), fibrinogen level, partial thromboplastin time (PTT).

Table 12.6 gives a summary of manifestations of organ failure associated with SIRS and MODS.

Priorities and principles of management in SIRS and MODS

Priorities

As with any critical illness the initial resuscitation response is to assess and support the airway, breathing, and circulation (ABC):

TABLE 12.6 Summary of manifestations of organ failure associated with SIRS and MODS

System	Manifestation
Neuromuscular	Encephalopathy
	Peripheral neuropathy
	Peripheral myopathy
Respiratory system	Acute respiratory distress syndrome (ARDS)
Renal system	Acute renal failure
Gastrointestinal	Pancreatitis
	Gastric and intestinal stasis or hypokinesis
	Acalculous cholecystitis
	Stress ulceration and gastrointestinal bleeding
Hepatobiliary	Elevation in liver function enzymes to more than twice normal levels
	Serum bilirubin >20–30 times
	Prolonged INR or PT
Cardiovascular	Decreased response to catecholamines
	Loss of microvascular regulatory tone and peripheral vasodilatation
	Central myocardial depression
Coagulation	Thrombocytopenia
	Clinical evidence of bleeding
	Disseminated intravascular coagulation (DIC)
Neuroendocrine	Altered growth hormone release in prolonged critical illness
	Altered anterior pituitary function

1. *Airway.* A patent airway is likely to be threatened in the patient who is comatose and aspiration is a high risk in the obtunded patient. Intubation should be considered early rather than following a catastrophic event.

2. *Breathing.* Oxygen therapy and, if necessary, ventilatory support should be instituted to maintain oxygen saturations of 90–95%. If ventilation is required, the aim is to limit the risk of barotrauma using alternative modes and low tidal volumes (6–8 ml/kg) and, in some circumstances, allowing carbon dioxide levels to rise (permissive hypercapni).

3. *Circulation.* The main aim is the rapid restoration of organ perfusion and perfusion pressure. Initially, fluid volume status should be optimized using colloid challenges (aliquots of 200 ml) followed by measurement of CVP or PAWP, and SV. If this is unsuccessful in restoring perfusion pressure, vasoactive drugs are required.

Early interventions

Once the patient is stabilized, any injuries should be actively treated with particular reference to the removal of any necrotic tissue, debriding burn eschar, and stabilizing fractures. Drainage of any collections or abscesses should also be carried out urgently. If these are not dealt with they will form a focus for further stimulation of the inflammatory/ immune response.

Further soft tissue damage and inflammation should be minimized.

Blood, urine, and other cultures, such as CSF, pleural fluid, or pus, should be sent to microbiology to attempt identification of any source of sepsis.

Appropriate antibiotics should be prescribed and administered, either as a broad-spectrum cover prior to microbiological results or according to culture sensitivities if these are available.

Further interventions

These are aimed at supporting failing organs or preventing further dysfunction.

Metabolic

Any metabolic derangement should be corrected promptly, although an acceptable degree of abnormality may be tolerated. Body temperature should be maintained within the normothermic range of 36.0–37.5°C.

Strict control of blood glucose levels (4.4–6.1 mmol/l) in the surgical critical care population (Van den Berghe *et al.* 2001) has been shown to improve mortality.

Infection

Any focus of infection, such as abscesses, should be located and drained. Prevention of secondary infection is essential and strict asepsis, care of intravenous cannulae, and all aspects of infection control should be observed.

Renal

Furosemide (frusemide) or dopamine have no effect on improving renal function but they may potentially convert oliguria to a more normal urine output. Continuous haemofiltration and diafiltration can be used to support renal dysfunction and, if metabolic acidosis is severe, to normalize the pH.

Nephrotoxic and hepatotoxic drugs should be avoided where possible or levels monitored (for example, gentamicin).

Gastrointestinal tract

Prophylaxis against GI bleeding including proton pump inhibitors, H_2 antagonists, sucralfate, and enteral feeding may be considered. Restoration of adequate organ perfusion is paramount.

Provision of appropriate nutrition based on individual requirements and monitoring and maintenance of electrolyte and trace element levels should be carried out.

Haematological

Haemoglobin levels of 7–9 g/dl should be maintained (Hebert *et al.* 1999). Blood transfusions are probably not necessary in most patients unless Hb is <7 g/dl. Exceptions are patients with coexisting acute myocardial infarcts or unstable angina (Hebert 2001). Any clotting abnormalities should be corrected to acceptably abnormal levels using clotting factors, platelet transfusions, etc.

Musculoskeletal

Pressure areas should be protected from damage by position change where possible or special support beds used where necessary. Early passive movements and mobilization will assist in preventing contractures and avoid decreased range of movement. Frequent changes in position will be beneficial for V/Q matching as well. Further details can be found in Chapter 3.

Further insults capable of triggering the immune/inflammatory response should be avoided; particularly hypoxaemia and organ hypoperfusion.

Circulation

A major objective in management of the patient with SIRS is the maintenance of tissue perfusion. As discussed previously in this chapter, the inflammatory response is associated with three distinct pathophysiological problems:

- maldistribution of circulating volume,
- imbalance of oxygen supply and demand,
- alterations in metabolism.

All of these affect the ability of the cardiovascular system to respond to tissue oxygen requirements. In addition, the myocardial depressant factors associated with SIRS may reduce the myocardial response still further.

Monitoring circulatory disturbance (see also Chapter 5)

It is necessary at the outset to use comprehensive haemodynamic monitoring to establish the extent of cardiovascular derangement. Ideally, the patient should have a pulmonary artery thermodilution catheter (or other form of blood flow monitoring) placed to allow monitoring of cardiac output, and other variables. If a fibre-optic thermodilution catheter with continuous S_vO_2 monitoring is available this can be useful to provide an assessment of therapeutic interventions when cardiac output is decreased.

Evidence of global tissue hypoxia can be monitored by measuring blood lactate or base deficit. The aim is to reduce blood lactate to <2.0 mmol/l (Armstrong *et al.* 1991). The degree of ischaemia in the gut can be measured by the gastric mucosal CO_2 which may be a marker of gut hypoperfusion and hypoxia (Gutierrez *et al.* 1992).

Supporting the circulation

Optimizing intravascular fluid volume

A recent study of early optimization of tissue oxygen delivery (Rivers *et al.* 2001) showed that patients who were given additional fluid resuscitation, erythrocyte transfusion, inotropic therapy, and ventilatory support to achieve normal central venous oxygen saturation of greater than 70% had a significant absolute reduction in hospital mortality of 16%. They also required less fluid, vasopressors, mechanical ventilation, and pulmonary artery catheterization once admitted to critical care. Of the patients who survived, the goal-directed therapy group had a significantly shorter duration of mechanical ventilation and length of hospital stay. It is therefore likely that early and aggressive intervention in this way can influence the development of the disease.

Serial measurements of SV, CO, and PAWP can be used to assess the response to fluid resuscitation (see Chapter 6 for details). The aim is to continue volume loading until the CO and SV show no further improvement. Occasionally, in cases of severe ARDS, the intravascular volume may be kept purposefully lower to reduce the extracapillary fluid shift.

The MAP should usually be maintained at >60–70 mmHg, though lower levels may be tolerated by younger patients. The aim is to maintain a pressure compatible with continued renal and cerebral perfusion. Markers of renal perfusion are a continued urine output of >0.5 ml/ kg/hour and measures of blood urea and creatinine. Markers of cerebral perfusion are more difficult to obtain but conscious level and alertness are useful indicators if the patient is not fully sedated and/or paralysed.

If fluid administration does not improve the SV further but the MAP remains below 60 mmHg (higher in previously hypertensive patients) then vasopressors or inotropes should be considered. Vasopressors (e.g. norepinephrine (noradrenaline)) are used in high-output states with low SVR and inotropes (e.g. dobutamine) in low-output states. Epinephrine (adrenaline) is both an inotrope and a vasopressor and can be used for either effect. The choice of drug will depend on the individual critical care unit and the patient.

Circulatory optimization and the use of 'supranormal' levels of CO and oxygen delivery

Shoemaker et al. (1988) showed that high-risk surgical patients who were maintained at high levels of CO and oxygen delivery using fluid and inotropes peri-operatively had a greatly improved outcome compared with those who were managed conservatively. It was theorized that higher (so-called 'supranormal') levels of CO and oxygen delivery were required in order to cope with the stress of surgery. This concept was then adopted for patients in septic shock (Edwards et al. 1989) with the goals of:

- an increased oxygen delivery of >600 ml/min/m²,
- a cardiac index of >4.5l/min/m²
- an oxygen consumption >170 ml/min/m².

However, randomized controlled studies have failed to show any improvement in outcome through the use of 'supranormal goals' in critically ill as opposed to high-risk patients.

A recent meta-analysis of optimization by Kern and Shoemaker (2002) of 21 clinical studies looked at the effect of this intervention over the time-course of high-risk surgical, septic, and trauma patients and found that improvement was only evident when optimization occurred early (i.e. 8–12 hours post-operatively or prior to onset of organ failure). This is echoed by the results from the randomized controlled study by Rivers et al. (2001) where early identification and optimization of sepsis patients resulted in a significant ($P = 0.009$) reduction in mortality from 46.5% in the control group to 30.5% in the treatment group.

Clearly, there is growing evidence for early detection of sepsis with prompt target-directed intervention before organ failure occurs.

Supporting respiration

Physical measures supporting gas exchange and alternative modes of ventilation are employed to achieve the aims of:

- maintaining saturations (usually) >90 %,
- minimizing the incidence of barotrauma by keeping airway plateau pressures below 30 cmH₂O.

The overall goal of intervention is to reopen and stabilize closed, but potentially functional, alveolar units while minimizing barotrauma and variations in expansion of different areas of the lung caused by the disease process. Secondary goals are to: (1) reduce F_iO_2 to the minimum acceptable level, (2) allow adequate carbon dioxide excretion, (3) avoid haemodynamic compromise, and (4) maintain adequate oxygen transport.

The conventional approach to ventilatory support in the patient with ARDS was volume-cycled ventilation with tidal volumes of 10–15 ml/kg and flow rates that maintained an inspiratory–expiratory ratio of 1:2 to 1:4. Increments of PEEP were added to both improve recruitment of non-aerated alveoli and to prevent airway closure and alveolar collapse.

Newer strategies now involve the use of lower tidal volumes (6–8 ml/kg), higher levels of PEEP (up to 20 cmH₂O) and other unproven support options for oxygenation such as prone positioning and inhaled nitric oxide or prostacyclin (see Chapter 4 for more details).

Specific therapies

There are currently a wide range of possible therapies being studied for their effect on sepsis, SIRS, and the development of MODS.

Activated protein C (drotrecogin alpha)

Recombinant human activated protein C has anti-inflammatory, anticoagulant, and antifibrinolytic properties. It inactivates factors Va and VIIIa preventing the generation of thrombin which is strongly pro-inflammatory. It also has direct anti-inflammatory effects including blocking of monocyte production of cytokines and cell adhesion.

In a large trial of 1690 patients, Bernard et al. (2001) showed a significant reduction ($P = 0.005$) of 6% in mortality when used on patients with severe sepsis. However, it is associated with an increased risk of bleeding and thus should be used with caution in patients with coagulopathies, increased bleeding risk, or a need for surgery. It is only approved for use in patients with the most severe forms of sepsis (two or more organ failures (Europe) or an APACHE II score of over 25 (USA)) and is extremely expensive, even by current drug standards, at over approx £5000 to £6000 per 96-hour course.

Steroids

The use of high-dose corticosteroids in septic shock was discontinued as a result of two large randomized controlled multicentre trials (Veterans Administration Systemic Sepsis Cooperative Study Group 1987, Bone et al. 1989b). The results showed no improvement in overall outcome; moreover there was increased mortality due to secondary infection in the group treated with steroids.

However, a recent study by Annane et al. (2002) showed improved survival in patients with septic shock treated within 6 hours of presentation with low-dose hydrocortisone (50 mg q.d.s.) and fludrocortisone (50 μg/day). The benefit was only apparent in those who did not respond to ACTH stimulation suggesting they had relative adrenal insufficiency.

There is also some limited evidence of improvement when steroids are given to patients in the fibroproliferative phase of ARDS (Meduri *et al.* 1991). The role of steroids in the treatment of sepsis requires more work before their full therapeutic capability is established.

Plasmapheresis

The exchange of plasma, resulting in the removal of circulating mediators and replacement of depleted levels of protease inhibitors, may have a beneficial effect on patients with septic shock and multiple organ failure. Studies to date are small or anecdotal but there is some evidence to suggest a reduction in mortality in septic shock patients (Barzilay *et al.* 1989).

Strict glycaemic control

Tight control of blood glucose levels using insulin therapy had a major effect on surgical critical care patient mortality (4.5% compared with 8% in the control group), especially those patients with a septic focus (Van den Berghe *et al.* 2001). In this study, the treatment group had their blood glucose level maintained at 4.4–6.1 mmol/l while the control group level was kept below 11.1 mmol/l. The frequency of episodes of sepsis was reduced in the treatment group by 46%.

ANTI-INFLAMMATORY AGENTS NOT SHOWN TO IMPROVE OUTCOME IN SEPSIS

- Anti-endotoxin (HA-1A) monoclonal antibody (endotoxin-specific antibody)

- Bactericidal permeability-increasing protein (BPI) and endotoxin receptor antagonists

- Anti-TNF (tumour necrosis factor) antibody

- Interleukin-1 receptor antagonist (naturally occurring interleukin-1 inhibitor)

- Nitric oxide synthase inhibition

- Antithrombin III—protection from excess protease (enzyme catalyst) action

- Soluble TNF receptors

- Platelet activating factor (PAF) antagonist

- Tissue factor pathway inhibitor

Mechanisms are still unknown but include the reduced oxidant production and potential anti-apoptotic effect of insulin and the protection from impaired phagocytosis seen with hyperglycaemia.

Immunomodulatory agents

Many anti-inflammatory agents have shown disappointing results in large randomized controlled trials, although there may be greater effect in patients who are severely ill (Eichacker *et al.* 2002). This is, in part, related to poor trial design. The newer concept of a later hypoimmune state has provided a new focus for research in immune-enhancing therapies for septic patients. Possible contenders are interferon-γ, a potent macrophage activator, and IL-12, an immune stimulant.

Antioxidants

Free radical scavengers, xanthine oxidase inhibitors, antioxidants, and iron-chelating agents have all been studied for possible beneficial effects in SIRS, though few large randomized controlled trials have been performed. Procysteine (an analogue of *N*-acetylcysteine) showed no benefit in the biggest of the antioxidant trials (Bernard *et al.* 1997). Oxygen-derived free radicals incite lipid peroxidation of cell membranes, which means that the radical reacts with the polyunsaturated fatty acid in the cell membrane. This alters membrane fluidity, secretary function, and ionic gradients causing increased permeability and oedema. A more potent radical (the hydroxyl ion) is generated by combination of free iron with other free radicals such as hydrogen peroxide.

It seems from the complexity of the pathways involved in the systemic inflammatory response that a single therapeutic answer is unlikely. What is certain is that considerable further work is required to understand the mechanisms involved and to catalogue the effect of each therapy. Until this is carried out and effective interventions are identified the mainstay of patient care will remain the support of failing organs and the prevention of further damage and infection.

Test yourself

Questions

1. List all the organs affected by SIRS and sepsis.

2. What are the main pathophysiological derangements associated with sepsis?

3. What are the priorities of management?

4. In relation to the priorities of management, how does the nursing care affect the management aims of sepsis?

Answers

1. Central nervous system
   Neuroendocrine system
   Respiratory system
   Cardiovascular system
   Gastrointestinal system
   Liver
   Renal system
   Haematological system

2. Maldistribution of circulating volume.
   Imbalance of oxygen supply and demand.
   Catabolic alterations in metabolism.

3. Resuscitation to ensure airway, breathing, and circulation are supported.
   Identifiable foci such as trauma or ischaemic tissue are treated.
   Blood, urine, and other cultures are sent to identify sepsis sources.
   Broad-spectrum antibiotics are prescribed if sensitivities are not available.
   Organ support such as renal therapy is initiated.
   Metabolic derangements are corrected.
   Prevention of further complications such as secondary infection, gastrointestinal bleeding, hypoxia

4. Early recognition of, and immediate response to, difficulties with airway, breathing, circulation.
   Alert and responsive monitoring of the patient's condition to detect early changes.
   Scrupulous hygiene and infection control measures.
   Careful and thorough examination of the patient to locate potential causes of sepsis.
   Preventive care such as ensuring head up >45°, regular position changes, good humidification and suction to prevent secondary pneumonia.

References and bibliography

Abbas, A., Lichtman, A.H., Pober, J.S. (1997). *Cellular and molecular immunology.* W.B.Saunders, Philadelphia.

Abraham, E., Matthay, M.A., Dinarello, C.A., *et al.* (2000). Consensus conference definitions for sepsis, septic shock, acute lung injury, and acute respiratory distress syndrome: time for a reevaluation. *Critical Care Medicine* **28**, 232–5.

ACCP/SCCM (American College of Chest Physicians/Society of Critical Care Medicine) Consensus Panel (1990). Ethical and moral guidelines for the initiation, continuation and withdrawal of intensive care. *Chest* **97**, 949–58.

ACCP/SCCM (American College of Chest Physicians/Society of Critical Care Medicine) (1992). Consensus conference: definitions for sepsis and organ failure and guidelines for the use of innovative therapies in sepsis. *Critical Care Medicine* **20**, 864–74.

The Acute Respiratory Distress Syndrome Network (2000). Ventilation with Lower Tidal Volumes as Compared with Traditional Tidal Volumes for Acute Lung Injury and the Acute Respiratory Distress Syndrome. *New England Journal of Medicine* **342**, 1301–8.

Angus, D.C., Linde-Zwirble, W.T., Lidicker, J., *et al.* Epidemiology of severe sepsis in the United States: analysis of incidence, outcome, and associated costs of care. *Critical Care Medicine* **29**, 1303–10.

Annane, D., Sebille, V., Charpentier, C., *et al.* (2002). Effect of treatment with low doses of hydrocortisone and fludrocortisone on mortality in patients with septic shock. *Journal of the American Medical Association* **288**, 862–71.

Armstrong, R.F., Bullen, C., Cohen, S., *et al.* (1991). *Critical Care Algorithms,* pp. 80–2. Oxford University Press, Oxford.

Barlas, I., Oropello, J.M., Benjamin, E. (2001) Neurologic complications in intensive care. *Current Opinion in Critical Care* **7**, 68–73.

Barzilay, E., Kessler, D., Berlot, G., *et al.* (1989). Use of extracorporeal supportive techniques as additional treatment for septic-induced multiple organ failure patients. *Critical Care Medicine* **17**, 634–7.

Bednarik, J., Lukas, Z., Vondracek, P. (2003). Critical illness polyneuromyopathy: the electrophysiological components of a complex entity. *Intensive Care Medicine* **29**, 1504–14.

Bellingan, G.J. (2002). The pulmonary physician in critical care; the pathogenesis of ALI/ARDS. *Thorax* **57**, 540–6.

Bennett, E.D. (1991). New agents—pentoxifylline and dopexamine. *Clinical Intensive Care* **2**(suppl.), 72–82.

Bernard, G.R., Reines, H.D., Halushka, P.V., *et al.* (1991). Prostacyclin and thromboxane A_2: formation is increased in human sepsis syndrome. *American Review of Respiratory Disease* **144**, 1095–101.

Bernard, G.R., Artigas, A., Brigham, K.L. *et al.* (1994). The American–European Consensus Conference on ARDS: definitions, mechanisms, relevant outcomes, and clinical trial coordination. *American Journal of Respiratory and Critical Care Medicine* **149**, 818–24.

Bernard, G., Wheeler, A.P., Arons, M.M., *et al.* (1997). A trial of antioxidants N-acetylcysteine and procysteine in ARDS. The Antioxidant in ARDS Study Group. *Chest* **112**, 164–72.

Bernard, G.R., Vincent, J.L., Laterre, P.F., *et al.* (2001). Efficacy and safety of recombinant human activated protein C for severe sepsis. *New England Journal of Medicine* **344**, 699–709.

Bochud, P.Y., Glauser, M.P., Calandra, T., International Sepsis Forum (2001). Antibiotics in sepsis. *Intensive Care Medicine* **27**, S33–S48.Bone, R.C. (1992). Phosoholipids and their inhibitors: a critical evaluation of their role in the treatment of sepsis. *Critical Care Medicine* **20**, 884–90.

Bochud, P.Y., Glauser, M.P., Calandra, T. (2001). Antibiotics in sepsis. *Intensive Care Medicine* **27**, S33–S48.

Bochud, P.Y., Calandra, T. (2003). Pathogenesis of sepsis: new concepts and implications for future treatment. *British Medical Journal* **326**, 262–6.

Bone R.C.(1996). Immunologic dissonance: a continuing evolution in our understanding of the systemic inflammatory response syndrome(SIRS) and the multiple organ dysfunction syndrome (MODS). *Annals of Internal Medicine* **125**, 680–7.

Bone, R.C., Fisher, C.J., Clemmer, T.P., *et al.* (1989*a*). Sepsis syndrome: a valid clinical entity. *Critical Care Medicine* **17**, 389–93.

Bone, R.C., Slotman, G., Maunder, R. and the Prostaglandin E$_1$ Study Group (1989*b*). Randomized double-blind, multicenter study of prostaglandin E$_1$ in patients with the adult respiratory distress syndrome. *Chest* **96**, 114–19.

Boswell, S., Scalea, T.M. (2003). Sublingual capnometry: an alternative to gastric tonometry for the management of shock resuscitation. *AACN Clinical Issues: Advanced Practice in Acute and Critical Care* **14**, 176–84.

Brealey, D., Brand, M. Hargreaves, I., Heales, S., *et al.* (2002). Association between mitochondrial dysfunction and severity and outcome of septic shock. *Lancet* **360**, 219–23.

Collard, C.D., Gelman, S. (2001) Pathophysiology, clinical manifestations and prevention of ischemia-reperfusion injury. *Anesthesiology* **94**, 1133–8.

Dantzker, D. (1989). Oxygen delivery and utilisation in sepsis. *Critical Care Clinics* **5**, 81–98.

Dellinger, R.P., Zimmerman, J.L., Taylor, R.W., *et al.* (1998). Effects of inhaled nitric oxide in patients with acute respiratory distress syndrome: results of a randomized phase II trial. *Critical Care Medicine* **26**, 15–23.

Edwards, J.D., Brown, C.S., Nightingale, P., *et al.* (1989). Use of survivors' cardiorespiratory values as therapeutic goals in septic shock. *Critical Care Medicine* **17**, 1098–103.

Eichacker, P.Q., Parent, C., Kalil, A., *et al.* (2002). Risk and the efficacy of antiinflammatory agents. *American Journal of Respiratory and Critical Care Medicine* **166**, 1197–205.

Eidelman, L.A., Putterman, D., Putterman, C. *et al.* (1996). The spectrum of septic encephalopathy: definitions, etiologies, and mortalities. *Journal of the American Medical Association* **275**, 470–3.

Fisher, C.J., Opal, S.M., Dhainaut, J.F. *et al.* (1993). Influence of an anti-tumour necrosis factor monoclonal antibody on cytokine levels in patients with sepsis. *Critical Care Medicine* **21**, 318–27.

Friedman, G., Silva, E., Vincent, J.L. (1998). Has the mortality of septic shock changed with time. *Critical Care Medicine* **26**, 2078.

Gattinoni, L, Tognoni, G., Pesenti, A., *et al.* (2001). Effect of Prone Positioning on the Survival of Patients with Acute Respiratory Failure. *New England Journal of Medicine* **345**, 568–73.

Gutierrez, G., Bismar, H., Dantzker, D., *et al.* (1992). Comparison of gastric intramucosal pH with measures of oxygen transport and consumption in critically ill patients. *Critical Care Medicine* **20**, 451–7.

Heidecke, C.-D., Hensler, T., Weighardt, H. *et al.* (1999). Selective defects of T lymphocyte function in patients with lethal intraabdominal infection. *American Journal of Surgery* **178**, 288–92.

Hebert, P.C., Wells, G., Blajchman, M.A., *et al.* (1999). A multicenter, randomized, controlled clinical trial of transfusion requirements in critical care. Transfusion Requirements in Critical Care Investigators, Canadian Critical Care Trials Group. *The New England Journal of Medicine* **340**, 409–17.

Hébert, P., Yetisir, E., Martin, C., *et al.* (2001). Is a low transfusion threshold safe in critically ill patients with cardiovascular diseases? *Critical Care Medicine* **29**, 227–34.

Herridge, M.S., Cheung, A.M., Tansey, C.M., *et al.* (2003). One-year outcomes in survivors of the acute respiratory distress syndrome. *New England Journal of Medicine* **348**, 683–93.

Hobbs, G., Mahajan, R. (2000). *Imaging in anaesthesia and critical care* p. 42 Churchill Livingstone, Edinburgh.

Hotchkiss, R.S., Karl, I.E. (2003). Medical progress: the pathophysiology and treatment of sepsis. *New England Journal of Medicine* **348**,138–50.

Hotchkiss, R.S., Swanson, P.E., Freeman, B.D., *et al.* (1999). Apoptotic cell death in patients with sepsis, shock and multiple organ dysfunction. *Critical Care Medicine* **27**, 1230–59.

Hudak, C.M., Gallo, B.M., Benz, J.J. (1990). *Critical Care Nursing: a Holistic Approach*, p. 818. Lippincott, Philadelphia, PA.

Huddleston, V.B. (1992). *Multisystem Organ Failure: Pathophysiology and Clinical Implications*, p. 308. Mosby Year Book, St Louis, MO.

Kern, J.W., Shoemaker, W. (2002). Meta-analysis of hemodynamic optimization in high-risk patients. *Critical Care Medicine* **30**, 1686–92.

Krishnagopalan, S., Kumar, A., Parrillo, J., *et al.* (2002). Myocardial dysfunction in the patient with sepsis. *Current Opinion in Critical Care* **8**, 376–88.

Latronico, N. (2003). Neuromuscular alterations in the critically ill patient: critical illness myopathy, critical illness neuropathy or both? *Intensive Care Medicine* **29**, 1411–13.

Levy, B., Gawalkiewicz, P., Vallet, B., *et al.* (2003). Gastric capnometry with air-automated tonometry predicts outcome in critically ill patients. *Critical Care Medicine* **31**, 474–80.

Levy, M., Fink, M., Marshall, J., *et al.*, for the International Sepsis Definitions Conference (2003). 2001 SCCM/ESICM/ACCP/ATS/SIS International Sepsis Definitions Conference. *Critical Care Medicine* **31**, 1250–6.

Lyseng-Williamson, K.A., Perry, C.M. (2002). Drotrecogin alfa (activated). *Drugs* **62**, 617–30.

Malcolm, D.S., Zaloga, G.P. (1990). Adjunctive pharmacotherapy in sepsis. *Infections in Medicine* **10**, 41–8.

Marcy, T.W., Marini, J.J. (1991). Inverse ratio ventilation in ARDS: rationale and implementation. *Chest* **100**, 494–504.

Marik, P.E., Bankov, A. (2003). Sublingual capnometry versus traditional markers of tissue oxygenation in critically ill patients. *Critical Care Medicine* **31**, 818–22.

Matthay, M.A. (1989). New modes of mechanical ventilation for ARDS: how should they be evaluated. *Chest* **95**, 1175–6.

Meduri, G.U., Belenchia, J.M., Estes, R.J., *et al.* (1991). Fibroproliferative phase of ARDS: clinical findings and effects of corticosteroids. *Chest* **100**, 943–52.

McHugh, L.G., Milberg, J.A., Whitcomb, M.E. *et al.* (1994). Recovery of function in survivors of the acute respiratory distress syndrome. *American Journal of Respiratory and Critical Care Medicine* **150**, 90–4.

Munford, R.S., Pugin, J. (2001). Normal responses to injury prevent systemic inflammation and can be immunosuppressive. *American Journal of Respiratory and Critical Care Medicine* **163**, 316–21.

Ognibene, F., Parker, M., Natanson, C., *et al.* (1988). Depressed left ventricular performance: response to volume infusion in patients with sepsis and septic shock. *Shock* **93**, 903–11.

Parker, M.M., Fink, M.P. (1992). Septic shock. *Journal of Intensive Care Medicine* **7**, 90–100.

Pathan, N., Sandiford, C., Harding, S., *et al.* (2002). Characterization of a myocardial depressant factor in meningococcal septicaemia. *Critical Care Medicine* **30**, 2191–8.

Rivers, E., Nguyen, B., Havstad, S., *et al.* (2001). Early goal-directed therapy in the treatment of severe sepsis and septic shock. *New England Journal of Medicine* **345**, 1368–77.

Rossaint, F., Falke, K.J., López, F., *et al.* (1993). Inhaled nitric oxide for the adult respiratory distress syndrome. *New England Journal of Medicine* **328**, 399–405.

Rothwell, P.M., Udwadia, Z.F., Lawler, P.G. (1991). Cortisol response to corticotropin and survival in septic shock. *Lancet* **337**, 582–3.

Schroeder, S., Wichers, M., Klingmüller, D., *et al.* (2001). The hypothalamic-pituitary-adrenal axis of patients with severe sepsis: altered response to corticotropin-releasing hormone. *Critical Care Medicine* **29**, 310–16.

Schumacker, P.T., Cain, S.M. (1987). The concept of a critical oxygen delivery. *Intensive Care Medicine* **13**, 223–9.

Shoemaker, W.C., Appel, P.L., Kram, H.B., *et al.* (1988). Prospective trial of supranormal values of survivors as therapeutic goals in high-risk surgical patients. *Chest* **94**, 1176–86.

Sinclair, S., Singer, M. (1993). Reviews in medicine: intensive care. *Postgraduate Medical Journal* **69**, 340–58.

Sprung, C.L., Peduzzi, P.N., Shatney, C.H., *et al.* (1990). Impact of encephalopathy on mortality in the sepsis syndrome. *Critical Care Medicine* **18**, 801–6.

Tuchschmidt J., Fried, J., Swinney, R., *et al.* (1989). Early hemodynamic correlates of survival in patients with septic shock. *Critical Care Medicine* **17**, 719–23.

Van den Berghe, G. (2001). Neuroendocrine axis in critical illness. *Current Opinion in Endocrinology and Diabetes* **8**, 47–54.

Van den Berghe, G., Wouters, P., Weekers, F., *et al.* (2001). Intensive insulin therapy in critically ill patients. *New England Journal of Medicine* **345**, 1359–67.

Veterans' Administration Systemic Sepsis Co-operative Study Group (1987). Effect of high-dose glucocorticoid therapy on mortality in patients with clinical signs of systemic sepsis. *New England Journal of Medicine* **317**, 659–65.

Weighardt, H., Heidecke, C.-D., Emmanuilidis, K. *et al.* (2000). Sepsis after major visceral surgery is associated with sustained and interferon-(gamma)-resistant defects of monocyte cytokine production. *Surgery* **127**, 309–15.

Weil, M.H., Nakagawa, Y., Tang, W. *et al.* (1999). Sublingual capnometry: a new noninvasive measurement for diagnosis and quantitation of severity of circulatory shock. *Critical Care Medicine* **27**, 1225–9.

Witt, N.J., Zochodne, D.W., Bolton, C.F., *et al.* (1991). Peripheral nerve function in sepsis and multiple organ failure. *Chest* **99**, 176–84.

Trauma

Chapter contents

Introduction

The management of the trauma patient demands considerable skill from the many disciplines involved in patient care. Injuries may range from simple, single organ damage to severe multiple injuries, and initial management is centred on the immediate identification of life-threatening injuries and the maintenance of the airway, breathing, and circulation. Continuous reassessment of the patient's clinical state and adequate monitoring of vital signs are essential from the moment the patient arrives in the emergency department.

The aim of continuous reassessment and intensive monitoring is the early detection of deterioration and the prevention of secondary complications.

The initial management of the trauma patient can be considered as four distinct phases (ACS 1984). These strategies begin at the scene of the trauma and continue until the patient is stabilized prior to transfer to the ICU.

Initial management

There are four stages in the initial management of the trauma patient:

1. Primary survey.

2. Resuscitation phase.

3. Secondary survey.

4. Definitive care phase.

Primary survey

This takes place at the scene of the trauma by pre-hospital staff and continues on arrival in the emergency department. The primary survey is concerned with the identification and management of life-threatening injuries and the following areas must be *simultaneously* assessed:

+ Airway maintenance and cervical spine control.

+ Breathing and ventilation.

+ Circulation and haemorrhage control.

+ Dysfunction of the central nervous system—neurological status.

+ Exposure—the patient is completely undressed for rapid assessment of injuries.

The patient's vital functions must be assessed quickly and treatment priorities established.

Airway

A patent airway must be established by chin-lift or jaw-thrust manoeuvres. Debris, blood clots, and loose-fitting false teeth should be removed from the mouth. High-concentration oxygen therapy ($F_iO_2 = 0.60$) should be immediately instituted by facemask. There is no place for low-concentration oxygen administration in the trauma patient as urgent correction of hypoxaemia is imperative. Endotracheal intubation, cricothyroidotomy, or tracheostomy may be required to maintain a patent airway. The possibility of cervical spine injuries should always be suspected, particularly in patients with multiple trauma or blunt trauma above the clavicle (including whiplash injuries). The patient's head should not, therefore, be hyper-extended to maintain the airway if a neck injury is possible.

Breathing

The chest must be exposed to assess respiratory movement as ventilation may be impaired even though the patient has a patent airway.

The following are the most common traumatic conditions that compromise ventilation and must be considered if ventilation is inadequate:

+ tension pneumothorax,

+ open pneumothorax,

+ flail chest with pulmonary contusions,

+ severe head injuries.

Circulation

A rapid assessment of the patient's haemodynamic status is essential. Initial observations include heart rate, blood pressure, skin colour, and capillary return. Hypotension following trauma is presumed to be due to hypovolaemia until proven otherwise. External haemorrhage should be controlled by direct pressure on the wound or by the use of pneumatic splints. Pneumatic antishock garments (e.g. a military antishock trouser (MAST) suit) may be useful in controlling haemorrhage from injuries to the abdomen and lower extremities.

Haemorrhage into the thoracic and abdominal cavities, and around fracture sites, may account for major blood loss.

Dysfunction of central nervous system

A rapid neurological assessment must be made in order to evaluate the patient's level of consciousness, pupillary size, and reaction. A more detailed neurological examination is performed in the secondary survey (see later).

Exposure and examination

The patient should be undressed and a rapid assessment made of injuries to the trunk and limbs.

Resuscitation phase

The management of shock must be initiated, patient oxygenation reassessed, and haemorrhage control re-evaluated. Hypovolaemic shock is corrected by replacement of lost intravascular volume by blood, colloids, or crystalloids. If not contraindicated, a urinary catheter should be inserted to monitor output. Life-threatening conditions identified in the primary survey should be constantly reassessed as management continues.

Secondary survey

This begins after the life-threatening conditions have been identified and treated and shock therapy has begun. The secondary survey involves a thorough head-to-toe examination and assessment of the patient where each region of the body is examined in detail. In this phase, laboratory studies, X-rays, scans, and special investigations such as peritoneal lavage are carried out.

Definitive care phase

In this phase, all of the patient's injuries are managed comprehensively: fractures are stabilized, the patient is transferred to the operating theatre if immediate operative measures are necessary, or the patient is stabilized in preparation for transfer to the ICU or other specialist area.

Arrival at the critical care unit

The critical care staff should be informed in advance of the impending arrival of the patient. The time prior to receiving the patient must be spent preparing the bed area and assembling the necessary equipment. The nurse must anticipate all eventualities.

- If the patient is to remain spontaneously breathing, prepare equipment for administering humidified oxygen.

- If mechanical ventilation is required, ensure the ventilator is functioning correctly and is set appropriately for delivery of oxygen, minute or tidal volume, and respiratory rate. The patient may then be connected on arrival. If possible, prepare appropriate infusions of sedative and/or analgesic drugs.

- Suction equipment must be tested and ready for use. A manual rebreathing bag should be connected to the oxygen supply.

- Other basic supplies and apparatus should be available as per unit protocol.

- Depending on the patient's injuries, an appropriate bed or pressure-relieving mattress may be required

(e.g. Stryker frame for spinal injuries).

- If required, prepare traction in advance and ensure this can be affixed to the particular bed used.

- Prepare a range of volumetric pumps for the immediate administration of drugs and fluids.

- Pressure bags for rapid volume transfusions may be needed. If continuous pressure monitoring is required, these too should be prepared in advance.

- Such patients are often hypothermic on arrival due to exposure and infusion of cold fluid. Blood warmers and body warming devices (e.g. Bair Hugger) may be needed.

- Continuous ECG monitoring is essential. Ensure the monitor is working correctly, set the alarm limits, and have skin electrodes ready to attach.

- Ensure that a sphygmomanometer and stethoscope, or a semi-automatic sphygmomanometer, are at the bedside. Pulse oximetry is extremely useful as an immediate guide to patient oxygenation, especially prior to the insertion of an intra-arterial cannula for blood gas analysis. A variety of temperature probes may be required. An oral thermometer may be ade-

---

CHECKLIST FOR EQUIPMENT PREPARATION

- Humidified oxygen/ ventilator
- Suction
- Rebreathing bag
- Special bed or pressure-relieving mattress
- Traction
- Volumetric pumps
- Pressure bags
- Skin electrodes for ECG monitoring
- Sphygmomanometer, stethoscope
- Pulse oximeter
- Temperature probes (skin/rectal), thermometer
- Primed transducers for invasive monitoring
- Trolley for central venous/arterial cannulation
- Nasogastric tube
- Blood/body warming devices
- Chest drain sets

quate but consider the need for recording core temperature if the patient is hypothermic. Skin probes may be required if there is vascular injury to the limbs.

♦ Anticipate the need for central vein cannulation or recannulation as emergency insertion may not have been sterile. Prepare a trolley with the necessary catheters (e.g. triple-lumen central venous, pulmonary artery).

♦ Anticipate the need for nasogastric tube insertion.

When the patient arrives in the critical care unit, his/her clinical state may vary from conscious, alert, breathing spontaneously, and haemodynamically stable, to unconscious, endotracheally intubated, mechanically ventilated, hypoxaemic, and shocked. The subsequent nursing and medical management will therefore depend entirely on the extent of the patient's injuries and alterations in clinical state. Constant reassessment of the patient's condition is essential. Continual monitoring of vital signs is important for the early detection of deterioration and the institution of appropriate treatment quickly and effectively.

The extent of use of invasive and non-invasive monitoring devices will depend on the degree of the patient's injuries and the facilities available on the critical care unit. For a full description of patient monitoring refer to Chapters 5 and 6.

> When the patient arrives the immediate nursing priorities are to the Airway, Breathing, and Circulation, all of which should have been stabilized prior to transfer but may have deteriorated during transfer.

If the patient is breathing spontaneously and requires oxygen therapy, connect them to the prepared humidified oxygen system at the prescribed concentration and flow. If the patient is being mechanically ventilated, confirm that the ventilatory settings are correct then connect to the ventilator. Ensure that the alarm limits are set appropriately, and chest expansion is adequate and symmetrical.

Connect the patient to the ECG monitor and note the heart rate and rhythm. If a central venous catheter is *in situ*, attach to the prepared transducer or manometer. Ensure that infusions in progress are running correctly and that any wound or chest drains and the bladder catheter are correctly positioned. Check that chest drains are not clamped and ascertain if suction is required. Check chest drain patency and volume of drainage.

RECORD IMMEDIATE BASELINE OBSERVATIONS OF:

♦ Heart rate and rhythm

♦ Blood pressure

♦ Central venous pressure

♦ Respirations or ventilator recordings

♦ Temperature

♦ Neurological status

♦ Chest/abdominal drainage volumes

The correct positioning of the patient will depend on the injuries sustained. For instance, a spontaneously breathing patient with a flail chest should sit erect if his/her cardiovascular status and other injuries allow. Patients with actual or suspected fractures of the neck or spine will need extreme care in positioning and must remain flat with the appropriate area immobilized. Fractured limbs must be carefully positioned and supported. Any traction must be correctly fitted and the end of the bed elevated if appropriate and not contraindicated (e.g. spinal injury).

If the patient is stable at this point and no immediate treatment is necessary, a full nursing assessment should now be carried out. If the patient is haemodynamically unstable, ventilatory support inadequate, or the patient is in pain, then these aspects must be corrected first.

General nursing assessment

This involves a thorough head-to-toe examination of the patient by the nurse and will provide the starting point from which any change can be determined. The nurse must continually observe and reassess, document and report changes, and be aware of the significance of deviations from the baseline measures.

Respiratory injuries

For a full description of respiratory assessment refer to Chapter 4. The following are essential observations in the trauma patient.

Respiratory rate and depth

Record the respiratory rate if the patient is breathing spontaneously. Note the depth of respirations. Is the patient using accessory muscles to aid breathing? Is there stridor? (a sign of upper airway obstruction). A respiratory rate greater than 20 breaths/min should alert the nurse to the possibility of respiratory compromise. Pulse oximetry and blood gas analysis should be used as an adjunct to observation and examination.

Chest movements and air entry

Is the chest moving symmetrically with each respiration? Is there air entry in all regions? If chest movement is unilateral, or air entry poor in any region, consider intraluminal bronchial obstruction (e.g. blood, clot, tooth), malposition of the endotracheal tube (if intubated), pneumothorax, haemothorax, rupture of a bronchus, or pulmonary contusions. Bear in mind that the patient may have underlying respiratory disease such as asthma or chronic obstructive airways disease.

If the patient has multiple rib fractures and/or a flail segment this may impair movement of the chest wall. If the patient is breathing spontaneously, paradoxical chest wall movement may be evident over the flail segment (see section on chest injuries).

Respiratory pattern

Note the pattern of respiration. Is it regular? Particular patterns of respiration are characteristic of particular head injuries in spontaneously breathing patients. For example, Cheyne–Stokes respirations (periodic rapid and slow breathing) is seen in bilateral cerebral hemisphere damage, hyperventilation in midbrain injuries, apneustic (prolonged inspiration) in pontine injuries, and ataxic (random) in medullary injuries. For further details see Chapter 10.

Skin

Examine the skin of the chest for bruising, lacerations, and abrasions which may indicate underlying injuries (e.g. seat-belt marks). Feel for subcutaneous emphysema which is due to air leaking into the subcutaneous tissues either from external (e.g. stab wound) or from internal (e.g. fractured ribs lacerating underlying lung) injuries. Observe for cyanosis, which can occur if there is rapid deterioration, e.g. due to a tension pneumothorax.

Pain

Does the patient complain of pain or tenderness over any particular area of the chest? Does he/she have pain on inspiration that limits chest movement? If chest drains are *in situ*, note the contents (e.g. blood, haemoserous), and the presence of bubbling and swinging of the fluid level with respiration.

Cardiovascular injuries

A 12-lead ECG should be performed. Continuous ECG monitoring should be in progress to immediately detect any change in rate or rhythm. Feel the pulse from time to time. Is it rapid, thready, irregular, or full and bounding? Are all central pulses present? Bear in mind that the patient may have underlying cardiovascular disease that is being treated (e.g. beta-blockers, a permanent pacemaker). Limb injuries (e.g. fractures, compartment syndrome) may compromise peripheral perfusion. Peripheral pulses, swelling, and temperature should be frequently monitored.

The frequency of blood pressure recordings will depend on the extent of the patient's injuries. Continuous monitoring by means of a transduced intra-arterial cannula allows changes in blood pressure to be detected immediately. This is essential in multiply injured or shocked patients if rapid treatment is to be effected. Changes in blood pressure should not be taken in isolation but always related to changes in other variables, such as heart rate, central venous pressure, pulmonary artery pressures, and stroke volume. Consider the effects of drug therapy as a cause of the change in blood pressure (e.g. analgesia or sedation); a fall may be accentuated in a hypovolaemic patient.

Note if there is bleeding over wound sites and drains and measure these losses frequently.

Neurological injuries

A full neurological assessment must be undertaken as soon as possible. This will indicate the severity of the

---

SUMMARY OF RESPIRATORY ASSESSMENT

- Respiratory rate and depth
- Chest movements and air entry
- Respiratory pattern
- Skin (bruising, lacerations, emphysema, colour)
- Pain

SUMMARY OF CARDIOVASCULAR ASSESSMENT

- Heart rate and rhythm
- Blood pressure
- Central venous pressure, pulmonary artery pressure
- 12-lead ECG
- Central and peripheral pulses
- Bleeding (drains, wounds, etc.)
- Limb swelling and temperature differences

injury and provide the baseline for sequential appraisal and the detection of deterioration. The Glasgow Coma Scale provides a quantitative measure of the level of consciousness and is the sum of the scores of three areas of assessment: eye opening, best motor response, and best verbal response, each being graded separately. For a full description refer to Chapter 10.

Pupil size and their response to light must also be evaluated. A difference in pupil diameter of more than 1 mm is abnormal. A sluggish response, or lack of response, to light may indicate intracranial injury; however, the effect of medications (e.g. atropine, opiates) must be considered.

The nurse should observe any spontaneous limb movements for equality, though limb fractures or injuries may inhibit movement. The muscle tone should be assessed for flaccidity and asymmetry. Spasticity (e.g. following spinal cord transection) is a late sign. If spontaneous movements are minimal the response to painful stimuli must be determined. A decrease in the amount of movement or the need for more stimulus on one side is significant and may suggest an intracranial, spinal, or nerve injury.

The frequency of recording of neurological observations will depend on the patient's neurological status and the presence of actual or potential head injury. The nurse should also examine the scalp for lacerations, bruising, and obvious deformity. Bruising behind the ears may indicate bleeding into the mastoid spaces—a late sign of a basal skull fracture. The presence of otorrhoea or rhinorrhoea is also suggestive of a basal skull fracture. Leakage of cerebrospinal fluid is also suggested by measurement of the glucose level which is at least half that of the blood glucose level.

Renal injuries

Unless the patient is fully conscious and haemodynamically stable, urine output will usually be monitored hourly by means of a urinary catheter and collecting system. However, certain conditions contraindicate the use of a urethral catheter, these include trauma, or sus-

> **SUMMARY OF NEUROLOGICAL ASSESSMENT**
>
> ◆ Conscious level: Glasgow Coma Scale
> ◆ Pupillary response
> ◆ Limb movement and response to stimuli
> ◆ Examine scalp (lacerations, cerebrospinal fluid leakage, bruising)

> **SUMMARY OF RENAL ASSESSMENT**
>
> ◆ Urine output
> ◆ Urinalysis
> ◆ Urine colour (haematuria, myoglobinuria)
> ◆ Examine genitalia

pected trauma, to the urethra. Observe for urethral bleeding. In these cases, a suprapubic catheter is usually inserted.

Routine urinalysis should be carried out on all patients and the urine observed for frank haematuria, clots, debris, and colour change. Haematuria is an important sign of potential genitourinary trauma. Note the urine colour—black urine suggests myoglobinuria, which follows muscle damage and breakdown (rhabdomyolysis). A 'positive' dipstick to haemoglobin may indicate either haemoglobin or myoglobinuria. Examine the genitalia and note any bruising, lacerations, or oedema, which may indicate underlying injury. Urine output should be maintained at a minimum of 0.5 ml/kg/hour in adult patients

Gastrointestinal injuries

All mechanically ventilated patients should have a nasogastric tube inserted unless this is contraindicated (e.g. nasal or basal skull fractures), in which case an orogastric tube should be inserted. Gastric dilatation is common after major trauma as well as in ventilated patients. The gastric aspirate should be left to drain freely and should be aspirated regularly. Observe aspirate and test for blood.

Examine the abdomen for bruising, grazes, and lacerations, particularly in the regions of the liver, spleen, and kidneys, which may indicate underlying organ damage. Is the abdomen painful in any particular region? Does the abdomen look distended? Is it rigid on palpation? Is there any evidence of bleeding per rectum (or per vagina)?

Assess the patient's nutritional state and consider the need for early feeding (see Chapter 11).

> **SUMMARY OF GASTROINTESTINAL ASSESSMENT**
>
> ◆ Oro- or nasogastric tube (if not contraindicated)
> ◆ Measure gastric aspirate and test for blood
> ◆ Examine abdomen (bruising, pain, rigidity)
> ◆ Note bleeding per rectum (or per vagina)

SUMMARY OF SKIN AND LIMB ASSESSMENT

- Note bruising, lacerations, and swelling
- Skin temperature and colour
- Peripheral perfusion and pulses
- Check plaster casts, splints, traction

Skin and limb injuries

Note any bruising, lacerations or swelling. Feel the skin temperature and note the colour. The hypovolaemic patient may appear ashen-faced with cool, pale extremities. Look for cyanosis—peripherally in the nail beds and centrally in the lips and tongue. Pressing the tip of a digit on the skin to blanch it and observing the return of colour can test the efficiency of capillary refill in each limb. This is immediate in the well-perfused patient. Note if any limb is particularly cool. Check that distal pulses are present, and that pressure dressings, splints, plaster casts, or traction on limbs are not impeding the circulation. Ensure that pressure is not exerted on healthy skin by plaster casts or traction devices (observe for tissue swelling and breaks in the skin).

The patient and relatives

A concise medical and social history will need to be taken from the patient or relatives to aid the planning of your nursing care. Do not ask relatives to repeat information if this is already contained within the medical notes, although it is vital that correct addresses and telephone numbers of next-of-kin are confirmed.

Establish a short-term plan of action from the medical staff and relay this information to the patient and relatives. Encourage them to ask questions, explain the use of any equipment attached to the patient, and ensure that they are regularly informed of progress and developments. Document any information that the patient or family have been told by medical staff concerning the injuries and outcome. A greater understanding of the patient's injuries and a good rapport with nursing and medical staff will help relatives cope with the frightening environment of the critical care unit.

Trauma is always sudden and unexpected and, unlike the routine post-operative patient who has a planned admission to the unit, there can be no preparation time to allow the patient or relatives to adjust mentally. The patient's injuries may have a profound effect on normal daily living and family life. Financial and work problems may ensue. Emotional and perhaps professional support will be needed to help the family cope with these. Social workers, ministers of religion, and external organizations (such as those for head- and spine-injured patients) can offer great comfort, support, and advice. Never forget that amidst the abundance of wires and tubes is a person who will need your constant care and reassurance and who is probably frightened about his/her injuries and worried about their effects on his/her future.

Head injuries

Head injuries are a common consequence when trauma results from vehicular or sports accidents, or falls in the home or work place. In the UK around one million people suffer from some form of head injury each year.

Many patients with head injuries are managed in general CCUs that have no facilities for monitoring intracranial or cerebral perfusion pressure. Severe head injuries still have a high morbidity and mortality and the management of such patients must be directed at preventing secondary brain damage and providing the best conditions for recovery from any brain damage already sustained (see Table 13.1 for types of head injury).

Pathophysiology

The detailed anatomy and physiology of the brain is described in Chapter 10.

The brain, cerebrospinal fluid, blood, and extracellular fluid are contained within the rigid structure of the skull. The brain is poorly anchored within the skull and its soft consistency renders it liable to move in response to acceleration or deceleration. Bruising (contusions) can occur when there is contact between the interior skull and the surface of the brain; internal shearing forces can cause axonal tracts within the white matter to stretch and tear. Mild stretch injury, with reversible loss of function, is responsible for the transient disturbance of consciousness known as 'concussion'.

Skull fractures alone do not cause neurological disability and severe brain injuries can occur without skull fractures. A patient with a skull fracture is, however, at risk of having, or developing, intracranial damage. Close observation is necessary to detect early signs of neurological deterioration.

Since the volume within the cranial vault is constant, increasing the volume (by oedema, haemorrhage, or haematoma) will directly increase the intracranial pressure (ICP). Increases in ICP are initially compensated by movement of cerebral venous blood into the systemic circulation. As the pressure rises further, there is com-

TABLE 13.1 Types of head injury

Scalp	Abrasions, contusions, lacerations, avulsions	The rich blood supply to the scalp may cause wounds to bleed profusely. Always suspect underlying fractures and potential intracranial damage. Is there any foreign body (e.g. glass) remaining?
Fractures	Simple, linear	Impact causes a simple crack in the bone with no break in the skin
	Simple, depressed	A portion of bone is pushed inwards
	Compound, depressed	A violent blow causes pieces of bone fragment to be driven into the intracranial cavity
	Open	A direct pathway or opening through the scalp laceration into the cerebral substance. The dura is torn; CSF may leak from the wound or the brain tissue may be visible. This type of fracture is an important potential source of intracranial infection
	Basal	Characterized by CSF leakage from the ear (otorrhoea) or nose (rhinorrhoea) which may be mixed with blood. Ecchymosis (bruising) in the mastoid area behind the ear ('Battle sign') is a late sign appearing several hours after the injury. Periorbital ecchymosis ('raccoon eyes') is a sign of a cribriform plate fracture
Diffuse	Concussion	Caused by stretching of axonal shafts in white matter with reversible loss of function. Results in temporary confusion or loss of consciousness
	Diffuse axonal	Microscopic damage throughout brain caused by tearing or stretching of axonal tracts. Not amenable to surgery. Characterized by prolonged and deep coma, often decerebrate/decorticate posturing and autonomic dysfunction causing high fever, sweating, hypertension. Mortality is high
Focal	Contusion	Macroscopic damage occurring in a relatively local area, often beneath an area of impact (coup contusions) or areas remote from impact (contrecoup contusion). Often prolonged periods of coma, mental confusion, or obtundation. May cause herniation and brainstem compression if large or associated with pericontusional oedema. Alcoholic patients are prone to delayed bleeding into contusions
	Intracranial haemorrhage (i): acute epidural	Bleeding from a tear in a dural artery or in the dural sinus. Rare but may be rapidly fatal. Causes loss of consciousness followed by a lucid period, then a secondary depression of conscious level. A hemiparesis develops with a fixed dilated pupil on the side opposite the haematoma
	Intracranial haemorrhage (ii): acute subdural haematoma	Bleeding commonly from rupturing of bridging veins between cerebral cortex and dura. Also seen with lacerations of the brain or cortical arteries. Often seen as underlying brain injury. Causes decreased level of consciousness and possible epileptic seizures if the clot irritates the cerebral cortex
Lacerations	Impalements and bullet wounds	Impaled objects must be removed at operation. Outcome depends on location, size of injury, and the patient's condition. Patients in coma following bullet wounds have a high mortality. The larger the calibre and the higher the velocity of the bullet the more likely death will occur. A bullet that does not penetrate the skull may still result in an intracranial injury

pression of brain tissue and decreased cerebral arterial blood flow. If this continues, the ICP rises at the expense of cerebral blood flow and results in brain ischaemia. Brain tissue dies when its blood supply is interrupted for only a few minutes. The brain also has no metabolic reserves and is thus wholly dependent on arterial blood flow to meet its metabolic needs. The cerebral perfusion pressure (CPP) is measured by subtracting ICP from mean arterial pressure. CPP is thus decreased by a raised ICP and it may fall below the perfusion pressure necessary to maintain cerebral blood flow. Ischaemic injury resulting from a decreased CPP may involve all cerebral tissue or any focal areas. When compartmental pressure gradients develop from local areas of injury, brain shifts can occur within the cranial cavity, the most important being uncal or tentorial herniation (coning) which causes brainstem compression and catastrophic neurological injury.

CONSEQUENCES OF RAISED INTRACRANIAL PRESSURE

- Alterations in the level of consciousness
- Headaches, photophobia, nausea, vomiting
- Bradycardia and hypertension
- Coma
- Brain death

CARDIOVASCULAR SIGNS OF RAISED INTRACRANIAL PRESSURE

- Decreased heart rate
- Decreased respiratory rate
- Raised blood pressure
- Raised temperature
- Widened pulse pressure

Changes in vital signs in patients with raised intracranial pressure

As ICP increases, the heart rate and respiratory rate decrease and blood pressure and temperature rise. There may be irregular patterns of respiration with Cheyne–Stokes or Kussmaul breathing (see Chapter 4). If brain compression causes the circulation to fail, the pulse and respiration become rapid and temperature usually rises but does not follow a consistent pattern. The pulse pressure (the difference between systemic systolic and diastolic pressure) widens. Immediately preceding this, there may be a period of rapid fluctuations in pulse varying from a slow rate to a rapid one. Death will ensue unless effective interventions are achieved. These changes in vital signs must be assessed in relation to the patient's responsiveness (for more details of recognition and management of raised intracranial pressure see Chapter 10).

Secondary brain damage

The brain requires continuous perfusion with well-oxygenated blood. A reduction in mean arterial blood pressure below 60–80 mmHg, particularly when the intracranial pressure is raised, may cause ischaemic neuronal damage if sustained for more than a few minutes. The brain is normally able to regulate its own blood supply to maintain a constant perfusion pressure despite wide variations in systemic blood pressure. However, when injured, the brain loses this capacity. The brain is thus particularly vulnerable to ischaemic dam-

TABLE 13.2 Causes of secondary brain damage

	Cause	Secondary to
Extracranial	Hypoxia	Brainstem damage causing decreased respiratory drive
		Haemo/pneumothorax
		Pulmonary contusions
		Rib fractures
		Aspiration pneumonitis/infection
		Fat emboli /pulmonary emboli
		ARDS
	Hypotension	Hypovolaemic shock
Intracranial	Compression from haematomas	Subdural
		Extradural
		Intradural (intracerebral/subarachnoid)
	Venous engorgement leading to cerebral oedema	
	Secondary infection	Meningitis, brain abscess

age in the presence of hypotension, hypoxaemia, or hypovolaemia. Secondary brain damage can often be caused by extracranial or intracranial insults and may be prevented by rapid treatment (see Table 13.2).

Treatment

Basic requirements

The first priority in dealing with any patient with a head injury is to stabilize the airway, breathing, and circulation and thus prevent further secondary cerebral damage resulting from hypotension and hypoxia. Management thereafter will depend on the patient's condition and the presence of other injuries. Cervical spine injuries should always be suspected in all patients. Particular care must be taken to stabilize the cervical spine until neck injury has been excluded by X-rays and a specialist opinion sought.

Not all unconscious patients will require intubation; a Guedel or nasopharyngeal airway may be adequate to maintain a patent airway as long as a gag reflex is present. However, adequate blood gas tensions must be maintained and so the patient should be intubated and mechanically ventilated to prevent hypoxaemia. Obviously, other causes such as a pneumothorax should first be excluded. Most severe head injuries will require intubation, particularly if the GCS is less than 8. In order to reduce detrimental changes in cerebral and systemic blood pressure rapid sequence intubation should be performed with adequate sedation and neuromuscular blockade.

Hyperventilation

This may be required if a patient's condition is rapidly deteriorating because of raised ICP. The question of hyperventilation in head injury is a subject of some controversy and some studies have suggested that therapeutic hyperventilation does not improve outcome. The objective of hyperventilation is to induce hypocapnia since the arterial P_aCO_2 level profoundly affects cerebral blood flow. When the P_aCO_2 is abnormally elevated, cerebral vasodilatation occurs, increasing intracranial blood volume and thus ICP. A reduction in P_aCO_2 hence reduces intracranial blood volume and ICP. Studies now suggest that the P_aCO_2 should be maintained at the lower end of the normal range (4.5 kPa) while maintaining a normal pH (Wright 1999, Wong 2000). This usually requires endotracheal intubation, mechanical ventilation, and, often, neuromuscular blockade. Excessive hypocapnia can reduce cerebral circulation to the point where cerebral ischaemia occurs. Blood gases must therefore be carefully monitored and, if available, the patient's end tidal CO_2 should be continuously monitored so that prompt changes in ventilation can be made. Sudden potentially life-threatening increases in ICP can be treated with aggressive short-term hyperventilation.

The cerebral vasoconstrictor response to hypocapnia does not last for more than 24–48 hours and therefore prolonged hyperventilation, if used, must be reviewed regularly. The cerebral vascular resistance appears to normalize within 4–6 hours of hyperventilation. The P_aCO_2 should therefore be elevated slowly when discontinuing hyperventilation in order to prevent rebound cerebral vasodilatation and increased ICP.

Nursing procedures

See Chapter 10 for details of ICP monitoring.

The patient with a raised ICP should not be stimulated unnecessarily and should be nursed in a quiet environment. The ICP is raised by agitation, coughing, and pain and nursing procedures should therefore be aimed at minimizing these. In the intubated patient with a raised ICP, endotracheal suction should be carried out only as often as is necessary for clearance of secretions. If secretions are minimal the frequency of suctioning should be reduced. Chest percussion and physiotherapy will also increase ICP. Blocking the ICP response to these procedures can be achieved by careful positioning of the patient with head-up tilt at 30° and with the neck in a neutral position. Tapes securing the endotracheal tube should not be tied too tightly as venous return may be impeded thus increasing ICP. Ventilate with 100% oxygen immediately prior to, and after, suctioning. In the unconscious patient, passive limb movements and regular turning must be instituted and a pressure-relieving mattress may be required. Bladder catheterization will also be necessary.

Always anticipate complications arising from the head injury. Nursing management should be directed towards identification and prevention of these potential problems. Should complications develop, immediate medical or surgical intervention may be necessary.

Assessment

Frequent neurological assessment of the head-injured patient is vital to detect changes early and to effect rapid treatment. These may initially be performed at 15–30 min intervals (see Chapter 10 for assessment procedures). Any deterioration must be reported and documented immediately.

Sedation and analgesia

Narcotics and non-depolarizing muscle relaxants do not alter cerebrovascular resistance and will not raise ICP provided that blood gas tensions remain unaltered. Ideally, short-acting agents should be used which can be stopped to allow a fairly rapid assessment of underlying neurological function. Antagonist agents, such as flumazenil and naloxone, should be used with caution after head injury as they may induce epileptic seizures and increase cerebral metabolism. Sedation and analgesia is often a problem, as both opiates and benzodiazepines may cause respiratory depression in spontaneously breathing patients and thus enhance the possibility of secondary brain damage. Paracetamol, dihydrocodeine, or codeine phosphate are usually safe and effective. In the mechanically ventilated patient, analgesia should not be withheld, especially if other injuries such as limb fractures have been sustained. Adequate sedation will help reduce the effects of any potential stimuli that may increase ICP. Propofol is extremely useful as the drug has a short half-life and does not alter pupillary response; however, it can reduce systemic blood pressure which will have a deleterious effect on cerebral perfusion. Propofol is also potentially epileptogenic but this does not appear to be of major clinical concern. In the case of a raised ICP which does not respond to hyperventilation and dehydration therapy (see later) the use of intravenous barbiturates, such as thiopental, should be considered as these reduce cerebral metabolism and oxygen consumption.

Dehydration therapy

The ICP can often be reduced by dehydration therapy using the osmotic diuretic mannitol with or without furosemide (frusemide). Following an infusion of 100 ml of 20% mannitol (or 200 ml of 10% solution), a reduction in ICP is seen within 10–20 min as brain water follows the osmotic gradient into the vasculature with a consequent diuresis. The duration of reduction in ICP following mannitol may last from 2 to 6 hours and repeated boluses may be required to maintain the ICP below 20 mmHg. Mannitol does cross the blood–brain barrier and will therefore lose some of its efficacy with repeated use. A serum osmolality of 310–320 mOsmol/kg should not be exceeded. Maintenance fluids are reduced to approximately half the daily requirement. Careful monitoring of heart rate, blood pressure, CVP, and blood electrolytes is essential during such therapy in order to avoid excessive hypovolaemia and electrolyte disturbances. This is especially important if the patient has sustained other injuries causing haemodynamic instability.

Positive end expiratory pressure (PEEP)

PEEP may be necessary in the hypoxaemic mechanically ventilated patient. However, PEEP will raise intrathoracic pressure, which may impede cerebral venous return and thus elevate ICP. Without ICP monitoring it is difficult to assess the magnitude of this effect, though PEEP levels of up to 10 cmH$_2$O are usually well tolerated.

Seizures

Epileptic seizures may occur with any head injury, either from direct irritation of the cortex, space-occupying lesions (e.g. haematoma), or from secondary causes such as hypoxia, hypotension, and hypoglycaemia. Prolonged or repetitive seizures may be associated with intracranial haemorrhage. Seizures are usually treated aggressively since they may cause cerebral hypoxia, brain swelling, and raised ICP. Respiratory function, length of time, and a description of the seizures must be carefully documented on a 'seizure chart'. Appropriate medication should be instituted (usually intravenous phenytoin). Ensure the safety of the patient at all times; side-rails should be used on the bed and padded with pillows to prevent injury.

Metabolic

Stress-induced diabetes mellitus may be a complication of head injury. Blood and urine should be regularly tested for glucose and insulin therapy prescribed as necessary. Blood glucose levels must be kept within the normal range. Hyperglycaemia may lead to secondary brain damage by increasing the osmotic pressure resulting in cerebral ischaemia (Woodrow 2000). Diabetes insipidus is caused by damage to the hypothalamus or posterior pituitary gland. It occurs quite commonly in severe bead injuries, and particularly brain death, but may follow fairly minor trauma. This results in failure of appropriate antidiuretic hormone (ADH) secretion resulting in the passage of large volumes of dilute urine. Intravenous fluid replacement will usually be necessary to prevent hypovolaemia and vasopressin therapy is usually required (see Chapter 9). Vital signs and blood electrolytes should be carefully monitored and the urine specific gravity should be regularly ascertained. Fluid balance must be carefully documented. Conversely, inappropriate ADH secretion may occur with head injury resulting in oliguria and fluid retention.

Infection

Infection may be a complication of head injury, either directly from an open head wound or skull fracture, especially if CSF leakage is present, or from cannulae and drain sites. These may give rise to meningitis or brain abscesses. Careful monitoring of temperature and bacteriological culture of potential sites of infection is necessary. Prophylactic antibiotic therapy, such as benzyl penicillin, is now considered only for those with basal skull fractures or compound vault fractures. Tetanus prophylaxis should not be overlooked when lacerations or penetrating injuries occur.

Miscellaneous

Gastric dilatation is common after any trauma and the risk of aspiration cannot be overemphasized. Vomiting and retching will increase ICP and should be avoided by the use of anti-emetics (e.g. metoclopramide). All semiconscious or unconscious patients should have gastric aspiration performed regularly by placement of an oro- or nasogastric tube. A nasogastric tube is never inserted in patients with frontal basal skull fractures because of the risk of passage of the tube into the cranium. Feeding should be commenced as early as possible; this should ideally be enterally unless contraindicated (see Chapter 11). Glucose is a vital metabolic requirement of the brain and although the injured brain has a lowered cerebral metabolism it is more susceptible to lack of this substrate. Prolonged deprivation may cause secondary brain damage. Regular blood glucose measurements are therefore essential and supplemental intravenous glucose may be required. Early institution of feeding will also prevent the development of stress ulceration. Prophylactic ulcer medication is not generally indicated unless there is a coagulopathy or a relevant past history (e.g. known peptic ulceration, indigestion, alcohol abuse).

Myocardial ischaemia and injury are common in head-injured patients, either due to associated chest trauma and cardiac contusions, or to an association with elevated plasma catecholamines causing tachycardia, hypertension, and increased cardiac output, thus imposing excess work on the heart. A 12-lead ECG must be taken and continuous ECG monitoring should be in progress.

Hyperthermia is harmful to the head-injured patient since elevations in body temperature increase the metabolic rate of the brain and will elevate carbon dioxide levels. The higher the temperature, the greater the risk to the patient. Methods of cooling should be instituted immediately (e.g. antipyretics, fanning, tepid sponging, cooling mattress).

Agitation and restlessness may be a sign that the unconscious patient is getting better or, more ominously, that the patient is deteriorating. Restless patients must not be sedated without excluding hypoxia, hypo-

tension, metabolic derangement, a full bladder, or pain from other injuries. The patient must be assessed for the development of any focal change (e.g. unequal pupils, non-use of one or more limbs). The patient should be prevented from harming him- or herself (e.g. by using padded side-rails) or from dislodging cannulae and tubes.

Figure 13.1 shows a schema for the entire process of head injury management.

Maxillofacial and upper airway trauma

Maxillofacial and upper airway injuries are common, and the majority result from vehicular accidents, physical violence, or sporting injuries. Many patients with severe maxillofacial injuries will have other associated injuries; cervical spine trauma must always be suspected. Consequently, extreme care must be taken to stabilize the neck when the airway is being secured. Sharp trauma, such as knife and gunshot wounds, causes lacerations and penetrating injuries that may damage the

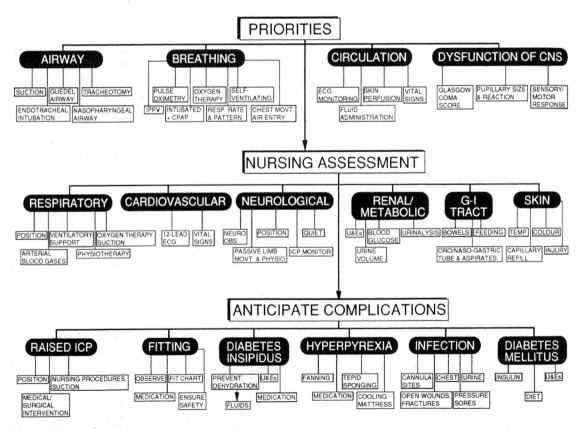

Fig. 13.1 Schema of head injury management.

air passages, blood vessels, nerves, and oesophagus. Blunt trauma may cause bone fractures and damage to the larynx and trachea leading to severe airway problems.

Injuries to the face and neck can be life-threatening because they may severely compromise the airway and cause major haemorrhage. The management priorities are to therefore secure and maintain a patent airway and to prevent hypovolaemic shock due to massive bleeding from the facial skeleton and soft tissues. Airway management poses particular problems in these patients because the very nature of the trauma means that access may be obstructed. Once the airway has been secured and haemorrhage controlled, further definitive management should be deferred until other potential life-threatening injuries have been dealt with.

Airway management

Initial management will include assessment of the injury, the patient's conscious level, colour, and ability to maintain a patent airway. Suction can be applied but, depending on the site and extent of the trauma, particular problems may be encountered.

Oral intubation or emergency tracheotomy may be required if a patent airway cannot be maintained. This may be particularly necessary in the following circumstances in order to maintain effective gas exchange:

- Bilateral anterior mandibular fracture or symphyseal fracture may cause the tongue to lose its anterior insertion. In the supine patient the tongue may then drop back and occlude the oropharynx. To open the airway a suture is placed through the tongue and secured with tape to the side of the face.

- The oral cavity or airway may be blocked by teeth, dentures. vomitus, bone fragments, blood, or foreign bodies. These can also block the larynx, trachea, or main bronchi. Attempts should be made to scoop out debris with a gloved finger and suction applied with a large-bore Yankauer suction catheter.

- A maxillary fracture may be displaced and block the nasal airway. To open the airway the maxilla must be disimpacted by pulling it forwards.

- Haemorrhage may obstruct the airway, and results from bleeding vessels in open wounds or from the nose if the maxillary artery or ethmoidal vessels are damaged. Direct pressure to wounds and suction will be required to open the airway.

- Soft tissue swelling and oedema may obstruct the airway. Although not usually an immediate phenomenon, early intubation may prevent airway obstruction.

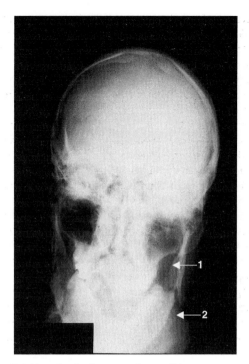

Fig. 13.2 X-ray showing fracture to the mandible.

Trauma to the larynx or trachea may cause obstruction of the airway by swelling or displacement of structures (e.g. vocal cords or epiglottis). If the airway is threatened and anatomical disruption makes intubation difficult or impossible, an emergency cricothyroidotomy or a tracheostomy must be performed. Nasal intubation is never attempted when mid-facial injuries are present or a basal skull fracture is suspected.

Specific maxillofacial fractures

Mandible

This is easily fractured because of its prominent position (Fig. 13.2). It may cause airway obstruction if fractured bilaterally at the angle or body of the mandible and often causes haematoma and swelling of the neck and floor of mouth. Definitive treatment consists of internal wiring or plating.

Maxilla

Airway obstruction and fracture of nasal bones, orbit, zygoma, soft tissue injury, and ocular damage often accompany this injury. Le Fort classified these fractures into three types, but there may be a combination:

- *Le Fort I.* The least severe. A dento-alveolar fracture which separates the palate from the remainder of the facial skeleton.

♦ *Le Fort II*. The fracture extends from the lower nasal bridge through the medial wall of the orbit and crosses the zygomatic-maxillary process.

♦ *Le Fort III*. The most severe. The fracture completely separates the midfacial skeleton from the base of the upper nasal bridge, most of the orbit, and across the zygomatic arch. The fracture involves the ethmoid bone and may affect the cribriform plate at the base of the skull.

Le Fort II and III fractures are often associated with basal skull fractures and may lead to CSF leakage, meningitis, and pneumocranium. Nasal intubation (nasotracheal or nasogastric) must never be carried out due to the risk of passing the tube through the cribriform plate into the cranial cavity. Definitive surgery involves internal fixation with wiring and plating and intermaxillary fixation. External fixation is often required.

Zygoma and orbit

Fracture and displacement of the zygoma can disrupt the lateral wall and floor of the orbit. Subconjunctival ecchymosis and periorbital swelling may be present. Unstable fractures require internal or external fixation, stable fractures can be reduced by operation and no other active management is usually required. Fractures of the orbital walls may tear or compress the optic nerve and blindness is usually immediate and permanent.

Nasal

This injury is very common. Haemorrhage may be severe and nasal packing may be required. Closed reduction and external splinting may be required.

Larynx

Fractures of the larynx are usually caused by blunt trauma. These may severely compromise the airway and necessitate immediate tracheostomy. Surgical exploration and repair is then necessary.

Specific nursing management

Airway and breathing

Constant and careful observation of the airway is essential in any patient with maxillofacial injuries. Soft tissue swelling and oedema rarely present as an immediate problem but swelling can increase insidiously. Always remember that a patient who does not have an endotracheal tube or tracheostomy *in situ* is at risk of developing airway problems at a later stage.

Depending on the patient's injuries, the airway may be maintained by the patient him/herself, by a Guedel or nasopharyngeal airway, an endotracheal tube, or a tracheostomy. Humidified oxygen therapy will usually be required, but the patient may not necessarily require mechanical ventilation unless his/her injuries are severe or there are other injuries that necessitate this.

Ensure that oxygen masks are not tight fitting if there are facial fractures or wounds. Nasal prongs may be more comfortable in some patients but oxygen cannot be humidified by this method. Never use nasal prongs if there is evidence of rhinorrhoea.

Specific respiratory assessment will include observation for any difficulty in breathing and evidence of stridor or increasing oedema of the neck, face, and mouth. Pulse oximetry is a useful guide to patient oxygenation but an intra-arterial cannula may be required for monitoring blood gases.

A patient who is tachypnoeic, tachycardiac, and in respiratory distress may have a foreign body lodged in a main bronchus. A chest X-ray and bronchoscopy will be required if no other cause is apparent, such as pneumothorax or pulmonary embolus.

In general, patients are best nursed in an upright position if other injuries and the haemodynamic status allow. This encourages drainage of blood, saliva, and CSF away from the airway, reduces venous pressure and encourages fluid reabsorption.

Circulation

Significant haemorrhage can occur in patients with closed injuries to the bony structures of the middle third of the face (maxilla, nose, and ethmoids). Steady bleeding from the nose and oral cavity into the soft tissues of the face can cause profound swelling of the cheeks and a tense skin. Careful monitoring of blood pressure and pulse are essential. Even a small puncture wound that is continually trickling arterial blood can cause significant blood loss and may be overlooked. It is important to be aware of the potential for raised intracranial pressure if there are associated head injuries.

Wounds

Clear guidelines must be obtained from the medical staff regarding specific wound management. Check the scalp for lacerations, bruising, and foreign bodies, such as glass fragments. All wounds should be observed for signs of haemorrhage, haematoma formation, and infection. Monitor temperature regularly and swab and culture any suspected sites of infection. If external fixation has been used to stabilize fractures ensure that pin sites are kept clean and dry.

Mouth

The mouth must be kept clean, moist, and free of infection. This may be difficult in the patient who has his/her jaws wired together or is unable to take oral fluids. Patients who have had major oral surgery and have sutures or skin grafts within the oral cavity may require very frequent mouth care (hourly) and this must be carried out with great care in the immediate post-operative period.

If the jaws are wired together a pair of wire cutters must be available at the bedside and the nurse must be aware as to which wires should be cut if the airway is compromised. Anti-emetics should be given regularly if the patient is nauseated as vomiting must be prevented. A Yankauer suction catheter should be at hand.

Eyes

Observe for peri-orbital swelling (associated with fractures of the zygoma or maxilla) and subconjunctival ecchymosis (haemorrhage) which may be due to direct trauma to the globe or a fracture of the zygoma. A 'blow out' fracture is caused by a direct blow on the eyeball which causes such a rise in intraorbital pressure that the orbital contents are forced through the orbital floor and herniate into the antrum. As well as bruising and endophthalmus, this causes a tethering of the eyeball where the muscles become trapped in the hemia limiting elevation of the eye and causing diplopia.

Pooling of tears in the eye may indicate damage to the lacrimal apparatus. If present, proptosis or exophthalmus suggests haemorrhage within the orbital walls. Ask the patient if he/she can see clearly. Does he/she have diplopia? Ascertain the normal visual acuity (does he/she wear spectacles normally?). Is there a contact lens or foreign body in the eye? Small particles that have sufficient force to penetrate the tough wall of the eyeball are generally metallic. Retained iron particles in the eye will gradually dissolve and the brown pigment is then dispersed through the ocular tissues but the sight is destroyed. Glass may remain inert for years. Pyrogenic infection of the eyeball often follows penetrating injuries.

Nose

Observe for bleeding or rhinorrhoea. If present, rhinorrhoea suggests a cribriform plate fracture. Never pass a nasogastric or nasotracheal tube in such a patient as the cranial cavity maybe intubated. Ask the patient if he has any difficulty breathing through his/her nose. Does the nose look deformed in any way?

Ears

Observe for bleeding or otorrhoea. Look behind the ears for bruising over the mastoid process (Battle sign) which may indicate a basal skull fracture.

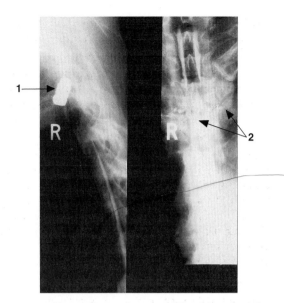

Fig. 13.3 Myelogram showing thoracic spinal cord disruption by a bullet injury. The track of the bullet is visible by the debris (arrowed).

Spinal injuries

The most common causes of spinal injuries are vehicular accidents (including motorcycles), diving accidents, and falls. Less commonly they occur as a result of gunshot wounds and sporting activities (Fig. 13.3).

They are often associated with other injuries, particularly to the head and chest. Any unconscious, multiply injured patient must be assumed to have spinal damage until this is excluded by an expert opinion. The first aid management is extremely important, as considerable damage to the spinal cord can be caused by inexpert care at the scene of the trauma and in the transfer of the patient to hospital. This section will not discuss the first aid management of spinal injuries but will be concerned with the acute management of the patient on the ICU.

The spinal cord is most often damaged in the cervical region but the thoracolumbar region is also at risk. In this region the spinal canal is narrower relative to the width of the spinal cord and any vertebral displacement is more likely to cause damage to the cord. Injury to the cord leads to bruising or mechanical destruction of the nerves, haemorrhage, and oedema. Some of the cord damage may be reversible, but up to 4 weeks will be required to assess the degree of final damage.

The management of the airway, breathing, and circulation must take priority. However, spinal injury must be considered when establishing these priorities and precautions should be taken to prevent exacerbation of any neurological damage.

Nursing priorities

Airway with cervical spine control

In high cervical spine injuries intubation may be required in order to protect the airway and/or provide a means of ventilatory support. Vertebral fractures above C5 lead to loss of diaphragmatic function and those above C8 to loss of intercostal function. There may also be other injuries to the head or chest that necessitate intubation in order to maintain effective oxygenation or to secure the airway. The intubation procedure must be carried out by an experienced anaesthetist with an assistant responsible for controlling the head and neck and minimizing spinal movement. A difficult intubation should be anticipated and the necessary accessories such as a fibre-optic laryngoscope or bronchoscope should be at hand. In patients with acute cervical cord injury, pharyngeal stimulation by a Guedel airway, endotracheal tube, or suction may provoke a vagal reflex causing severe bradycardia or asystole. This should be anticipated and can be prevented by the administration of atropine prior to the procedure. In patients with actual or suspected cervical spine injuries the neck must be stabilized at all times using a rigid collar of an appropriate size that grips the chin. However, collars alone are inadequate and lateral support must be given by the use of a sandbag each side of the head (with the head in a neutral position) or by manual stabilization during movement of the patient or during specific procedures. In the ICU, stabilization of the neck and spine must be continued throughout any procedures (e.g. X-rays, insertion of CVP lines). If X-rays confirm spinal damage, more definitive stabilization may be considered such as the use of skull tongs, halopelvic traction, or spinal fusion.

Breathing

The patient with a cervical spine injury who is breathing spontaneously requires very careful observation of his/her respiratory function. Ascending oedema of the traumatized cervical cord may result in deterioration of respiratory status shortly after admission and equipment for manual ventilation must be at the bedside.

Blood gas analysis and/or pulse oximetry should be used to identify hypoxaemia as early as possible.

> Hypoxaemia can lead to neurological deterioration and must be avoided.

It may be necessary to monitor vital capacity if there is any doubt that respiratory function is inadequate or could possibly deteriorate. This is particularly so in patients with fractures above C8. A forced vital capacity of less than 10–15 ml/kg body weight may indicate the need for ventilatory support.

Patients with spinal injuries should be nursed on a specific type of bed capable of lateral tilting and longitudinal elevation whilst keeping the spine straight (e.g. Stoke Mandeville, Parragon, or Stryker frame). This will ensure that the spine is always in a neutral position and the patient can be tilted head up and feet down to an angle of approximately 45°. This will increase functional residual capacity and is particularly important in patients who have other chest trauma but are breathing spontaneously. Atelectasis is common, and the ability to expectorate may be impaired. Regular physiotherapy is therefore essential and the use of narcotic drugs, which further suppress respiration, should be avoided.

Circulation

All patients with an acute spinal injury should have continuous ECG monitoring. Patients with injury to the cervical or high thoracic cord may have reduced sympathetic outflow between the T1 and L2 segments. This will cause hypotension and bradycardia and is known as neurogenic or 'spinal' shock. Atropine may be needed if the heart rate falls below 50 bpm with associated hypotension (systolic BP < 80 mmHg). This type of shock is purely neurogenic in origin and must be distinguished from hypovolaemic shock, which may also be present in the multiply injured patient (characterized by hypotension and tachycardia). Aggressive fluid replacement is detrimental in patients with purely neurogenic hypotension as it precipitates pulmonary oedema. Patients with bradycardia and hypotension may be subjected to a fluid challenge with close monitoring of central venous (and/or pulmonary artery wedge) pressure. The response should be observed and measurements made before more fluid replacement is given. Hypotensive patients unresponsive to fluid replacement may need vasopressor support.

> Hypotension and inadequate tissue perfusion may lead to irreversible neurological damage, careful monitoring of vital signs is therefore essential.

Abdominal or other occult trauma may not be easily recognized in the tetraplegic patient since the abdominal wall is anaesthetized and flaccid. The classical signs of a rigid, painful abdomen following visceral perforation or haemorrhage may not therefore be apparent. Close monitoring of vital signs and an awareness of potential injury is important. Peritoneal lavage, ultrasound, and X-ray procedures may be performed if there is a suspicion of abdominal trauma. Some patients may feel shoulder tip pain if abdominal injury is present.

Specific nursing management

Paralytic ileus and gastric dilatation are common after spinal cord trauma. A nasogastric tube should be passed (unless contraindicated) and aspirated regularly. Enteral feeding may take time to become established because of this.

Acute urinary retention will develop in tetraplegic and paraplegic patients unless the sacral segments have been spared. A urethral catheter should be inserted (unless contraindicated) and urine output monitored closely. Infection of the urinary tract can become a major problem and catheterization should be carried out under strict aseptic conditions. Regular urinalysis, testing for the presence of white cells, and microbiological culture should be performed. Body temperature should be monitored.

Constipation is often a problem and bowel care should be given according to specific unit protocols. This will include the regular administration of laxatives and enemas.

The prevention of pressure sores is vital and meticulous attention must be paid to regular changes of position. Proper positioning is important to prevent pressure on heels and bony prominences, with padding (such as a pillow) placed between the inner surfaces of the knees and between the medial malleoli of the ankles. The skin should be kept clean and dry and hypoalbuminaemia avoided by adequate nutrition.

The patient will develop atrophy of the extremities owing to disuse and, if their condition allows, passive exercises should be carried out with a range of movements that preserve joint motion and stimulate circulation. The positioning of joints and limbs is important in order to prevent deformities such as footdrop. The patient must be maintained in proper alignment at all times; however, there may be limitations to positioning and limb movements in the multiply injured patient.

Chest injuries

The majority of chest injuries are caused by blunt trauma. Such injuries may result from a high-velocity impact (e.g. a rapid deceleration as seen in road traffic accidents), a low-velocity impact (e.g. a direct blow to the chest), or from crushing trauma to the chest. Less commonly (in the UK), penetrating injuries, such as knife and gunshot wounds, are also seen. Many patients with severe intrathoracic injuries, such as laceration of the heart, aorta, or major airways, do not survive to reach hospital. Patients with chest trauma also often have other injuries such as head, spinal, abdominal, and maxillofacial damage. Some will be multiply injured. The priorities of management are, as always, maintenance of airway, breathing, and circulation, with identification and correction of life-threatening injuries.

Nursing priorities

Airway and breathing

A patent airway must be secured; intubation or tracheostomy may be required, depending on the patient's injuries. Chest injury often leads to tissue hypoxia. This may be caused by diminished blood volume, failure to ventilate the lungs adequately, ventilation/perfusion mismatch, or changes in intrapleural pressures, which lead to lung collapse with displacement of mediastinal structures. Hypoxia must be corrected and interventions are aimed at ensuring that adequate amounts of oxygen are delivered to the parts of the lung that are capable of normal ventilation and perfusion. CPAP or BiPAP may be useful tools to avoid atelectasis in spontaneously breathing patients and to assist breathing in those with a flail chest injury. If intubation is necessary to secure the airway, mechanical ventilation will normally be required. IPPV will be necessary in patients who are unconscious, have severe respiratory distress, or associated head injuries, where hypoxia must be avoided. A chest X-ray will have been taken as a matter of priority in the casualty department of any patient with suspected chest injuries. Many serious injuries including fractures, haemo- or pneumothorax, cardiac tamponade, ruptured diaphragm, dissecting aorta, and major airway disruptions can be diagnosed. Pneumothoraces should ideally be identified and drained before mechanical ventilation is instituted, although this may not always be possible. Close monitoring of arterial blood gases is essential and appropriate levels of oxygen must be administered to correct hypoxaemia.

In the self-ventilating patient careful and continuous monitoring of respiratory function must be made. Signs of respiratory distress may indicate the need for further interventions (see Chapter 4). Note that central cyanosis may be a late or absent sign of hypoxaemia in patients with a decreased haemoglobin as a result of haemorrhage.

Circulation

Patients with major cardiac or vascular lacerations may have had haemorrhage arrested by a tamponade effect. Rapid transfusion and the subsequent increase in arterial and intracardiac pressures may result in uncontrollable and fatal bleeding. Such injuries must be identified before resuscitation elevates the systolic blood pressure to >100 mmHg.

Continuous ECG and monitoring of vital signs is essential. Myocardial contusions are common in chest injuries and may give rise to tachyarrhythmias and conduction abnormalities. Large blood losses may result from haemothoraces and tearing of thoracic vessels. Observe for signs of hypovolaemia (see Chapter 6). Is the patient peripherally cool and poorly perfused? Look at the patient's colour. Is he/she pale? Are there signs of obvious bleeding (e.g. from chest or wound drains)?

Specific chest injuries

Pulmonary contusions

These occur when shearing or crushing forces are applied to the thoracic cage and cause disruption of the microcirculation. Extravasation of red cells and plasma occurs and these fluids fill the alveoli. This results in interstitial haemorrhage and alveolar collapse in the contused area. Gas exchange is impaired as perfusion is maintained in the unventilated lung segments causing intrapulmonary shunting and subsequent hypoxaemia. The infiltrates are usually absorbed after 3–5 days but may progress in complicated cases. A chest X-ray will reveal localized areas of contusion and haemorrhage.

Management is aimed at ensuring adequate ventilation and treating hypoxaemia. If severe, intubation and mechanical ventilation may be required. Pain control is important. Intercostal nerve blocks or epidural analgesia are extremely useful. A patient with adequate pain relief will breathe more deeply, be cooperative with physiotherapy, and clear secretions more effectively. Supplemental oxygen therapy with or without non-invasive ventilation should be given and blood gases monitored. If the patient is mechanically ventilated, manoeuvres to improve oxygenation are aimed at reducing the shunt (e.g. postural changes), increasing the F_iO_2, increasing the functional residual capacity by the use of PEEP, and improving tracheobronchial toilet by effective suctioning and physiotherapy.

Rib fractures

Blood loss and disruption of the underlying lung tissue are associated with rib fractures. The sharp edges of the fractured rib may lacerate the underlying lung causing haemorrhage. Any number of ribs may be fractured, and if several ribs are fractured in more than one place, or the broken ribs are combined with fracture dislocations of the costochondral junctions or sternum, this is known as a flail segment and moves independently of the rib cage. The negative intrapleural pressures generated on inspiration will pull this segment inwards creating a paradoxical movement and thus compromise ventilation by reducing tidal volume. A flail segment itself is not an indication for mechanical ventilation but the functional consequences must determine the necessity for ventilatory support. Recent studies have shown a decreased mortality in patients with extensive rib fractures using a conservative approach to pain relief, as opposed to routine mechanical ventilation, provided that the P_aO_2 remains above 6.6 kPa on an F_iO_2 of 0.5, the vital capacity remains above 10 ml/ kg and the respiratory rate below 40 breaths/min. Non-invasive ventilation may be a useful adjunct.

Adequate analgesia is absolutely essential in patients with rib fractures. Pain will inhibit inspiration and lead to atelectasis in the basal segments, prevent adequate coughing and clearance of secretions, and limit effective physiotherapy. If there are few unilateral rib fractures, oral analgesia, intercostal nerve blocks, or thoracic epidural analgesia may be sufficient, but in multiple fractures intravenous analgesia may be needed in addition. A minitracheotomy may prevent intubation if there is difficulty in clearing secretions. Chest strapping is not recommended as this will only serve to inhibit effective ventilation.

Close monitoring of blood gases will be required and pulse oximetry will be useful. Careful observation of respiratory function is vital. Assist with physiotherapy and encourage the patient to breathe deeply and cough to clear secretions. Position the patient in an upright and comfortable position if his/her condition allows. Assess the effect of any analgesia given and review this if pain persists.

Pneumothorax (simple, open, tension) and haemothorax

Chest injuries are often accompanied by either the collection of blood in the chest cavity (haemothorax) from torn intercostal vessels or haemorrhage from lacerated lung tissue, or the escape of air from injured lung into the pleural cavity (pneumothorax). Often both blood and air are found in the pleural cavity (haemopneumothorax). The lung on that side of the chest is compressed and ventilation is impaired. A small pneumothorax (<5% haemothorax volume) can be allowed to resolve spontaneously provided it is not compromising ven-

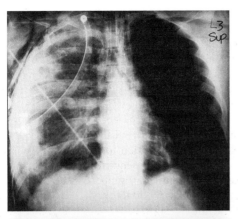

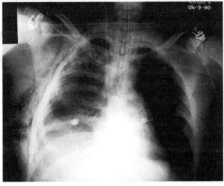

Fig. 13.4 X-ray showing fractured ribs, pulmonary contusions, and pneumothorax. Before (a) and after (b) insertion of chest drain on left side.

tilation and is not enlarging. A chest drain (or needle aspiration) will, however, usually need to be inserted particularly if the patient requires mechanical ventilation (Fig. 13.4).

A tension pneumothorax is a medical emergency and requires immediate decompression. In this situation, air is drawn into the pleural space from a lacerated lung or through a hole in the chest wall. Air that enters with each inspiration is trapped and cannot be expelled, therefore tension builds up. The lung is compressed and collapses, pushing the mediastinal structures (heart, trachea, and great vessels) towards the unaffected side of the chest (mediastinal shift), impairing ventilation in the other lung and decreasing venous return. Thus, tension pneumothorax results in impairment of cardiovascular as well as respiratory function. Collapse and electromechanical dissociation may rapidly result. The diagnosis of tension pneumothorax is made clinically; there is usually no time to take a chest X-ray before treatment is instituted. The patient will become progressively more hypoxaemic and may be tachy-cardiac and hypotensive. Air entry will be absent over the affected area and chest movement reduced. The trachea will be deviated away from the affected side, the neck veins are distended, and the patient will become progressively cyanosed. Immediate decompression is obtained by inserting a needle into the second intercostal space in the mid-clavicular line of the affected hemi-thorax. The ability to aspirate air into the syringe attached to the needle will confirm the diagnosis and converts the injury to a simple pneumothorax. A chest drain should now be inserted. If there is failure to aspirate air from the needle, the needle and syringe should be withdrawn but the possibility of a pneumothorax now exists as a result of the needle insertion.

Massive blood loss may result from haemothoraces that are usually caused by penetrating injuries lacerating systemic or pulmonary vessels. Such injuries may be accompanied by hypovolaemic shock and insertion of a chest drain may reveal a considerable amount of blood in the chest cavity. Concurrent drainage of the haemothorax and volume resuscitation is required. Some patients will require surgical intervention and this is usually dependent on the continuing rate and volume of blood loss. Very careful measurement of blood in the chest drain is required (every 15–30 min) with continuous monitoring of vital signs as fluid replacement is given.

An open pneumothorax is caused by a penetrating injury to the chest, which leaves an open hole between the atmosphere and the chest cavity. Equilibrium between intrathoracic pressure and atmospheric pressure is immediate and if the opening in the chest wall is more than two-thirds the diameter of the trachea air will pass preferentially into the chest through the hole (causing a 'sucking' chest wound). Ventilation is impaired and the patient will become hypoxaemic. The hole must be sealed immediately with an occlusive dressing and taped securely on three sides only. Leaving one side of the dressing open will allow air to escape as the patient exhales, but as the patient breathes in the dressing is occlusively sucked over the wound preventing air from entering. If the hole is sealed completely, air will accumulate in the thoracic cavity resulting in a tension pneumothorax. This is a temporary measure; a chest drain should be inserted remote from the open wound. Surgical closure of the wound is often required.

Low-pressure suction (up to 10 kPa) may be applied to chest drains in order to aid evacuation of air and blood from the pleural cavity. Pressure levels must be checked regularly and chest drain tubing observed to identify blood clots blocking the tubing and impairing drainage (for comprehensive care of chest drains refer to Chapter 4). If the patient is making any spontaneous inspiratory effort, two chest drain clamps must always be available at the bedside in case of accidental disconnection of the tubing. A tension pneumothorax or a pneumothorax drain that is bubbling (i.e. a bronchopleural fistula) must not be clamped or air will build up in the chest cavity.

Pericardial tamponade

This results from penetrating or blunt trauma which cause the pericardium to fill with blood from the heart or great vessels. The pericardium is a fibrous structure, and even relatively small amounts of fluid in the pericardial sac will restrict cardiac filling. Cardiac tamponade is characterized by an increase in heart rate and central venous pressure, and a decrease in blood pressure and cardiac output. Peripheral perfusion will be poor and the neck veins may become distended due to the increase in central venous pressure. Pulsus paradoxus (disappearance or weakening of the radial pulse on spontaneous inspiration) may be palpated. Large, cyclical, beat-to-beat variations may also be seen in the monitored systemic blood pressure trace that is related to the phases of the respiratory cycle.

Treatment is by pericardiocentesis where blood is aspirated by needle and syringe from the pericardium. If the blood in the pericardium is clotted, aspiration may prove impossible. If the patient is moribund open thoracotomy may be required with creation of a pericardial window. Cardiac tamponade caused by penetrating trauma will need surgical exploration and repair.

Myocardial contusion

This is caused by blunt trauma to the chest or by deceleration trauma. It is comparable in diagnosis and treatment to a myocardial infarction. ECG changes will be apparent: usually non-specific ST segment and T wave changes. Dysrhythmias are common and may be fatal. Tachyarrhythmias, multiple premature ventricular ectopics, and conduction disturbances (heart block and bundle branch block) often occur. Serial cardiac enzymes will be elevated. Continuous ECG monitoring is essential as the onset of dysrhythmias may be sudden. Cardiogenic shock may result from myocardial contusions; if so, inotropic support and intra-aortic balloon counterpulsation may be required to maintain systemic arterial pressure.

Diaphragmatic rupture

This usually follows penetrating or blunt trauma to the abdomen and may result in the abdominal contents being forced into the chest through a laceration in the diaphragm. The liver usually prevents herniation through the right hemidiaphragm and it is therefore most commonly seen on the left side. Herniation of the stomach into the chest may become evident when a nasogastric tube is seen in the chest cavity on X-ray. Early IPPV may mask the signs of respiratory distress that would be evident in the self-ventilating patient. Penetrating injuries into the abdomen may lacerate the diaphragm and cause a haemothorax. Most patients with a diaphragmatic rupture will require surgical exploration and repair.

Major airway injuries

Blunt or penetrating trauma may cause rupture of the trachea or bronchus, or tears and punctures of the lung tissue. The presence of surgical emphysema is a sign of airway injury; with transection of the trachea or bronchus this may be extensive in the mediastinum and subcutaneous tissues. Pneumothorax and haemothorax are commonly associated and usually require drainage. Rupture of a large bronchus may cause haemoptysis and atelectasis of the affected lung. Patients with complete transection of the trachea often die rapidly of asphyxia but an adequate airway may exist and treatment is usually by surgical repair. Patients with tracheal rupture may have stridor, aphonia, and respiratory distress. Considerable problems may be encountered in endotracheal intubation. Blind intubation may prove fatal and fibre-optic intubation may be required.

Penetrating injuries are often accompanied by injuries to the oesophagus, carotid artery, and jugular vein; missile injuries may cause extensive tissue destruction.

Aortic rupture

This usually occurs as a result of deceleration trauma but occasionally from penetrating trauma. Tears of the aorta and pulmonary arteries are frequently fatal: 90% of patients will die at the scene of the injury. Most survivors will have had the blood loss contained by a haematoma, and an intact adventitia (outer wall) may prevent immediate death. Initial severe hypotension will occur with the loss of up to 1000 ml of blood and the patient will usually respond to rapid fluid resuscitation. However, hypotension may be recurrent or persistent and blood transfusion will be necessary to maintain an adequate oxygen carrying capacity and arterial pressure. A chest X-ray may show a widened mediastinum, tracheal shift to the right, and blurring of the aortic outline. Early angiography would be indicated if the patient's condition permits but urgent surgical repair may be required.

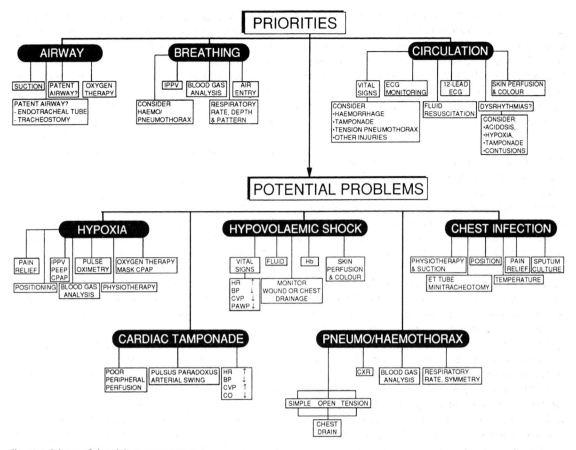

Fig. 13.5 Schema of chest injury management.

Fig. 13.5 Shows a schema summarizing the management of chest injuries.

Abdominal and pelvic injuries

Penetrating injuries, particularly stab and gunshot wounds, are common causes of abdominal trauma in young men. Blunt trauma most often results from road traffic accidents and falls; many of these patients will have associated injuries to the head, spine, chest, and genitourinary system. These injuries will complicate management, and it must be remembered that patients with abdominal injuries have the potential for severe haemorrhage and an increased risk of post-traumatic sepsis. Injuries resulting from blunt trauma to the abdomen are the most difficult to diagnose; in the multiply injured patient, the signs of intra-abdominal injury (pain, guarding) may be difficult to assess or may be masked by other injuries.

Immediate management is aimed at identifying the presence of abdominal injury rather than making an accurate diagnosis of a specific injury. The liver, spleen, and kidneys are the major organs involved in blunt trauma. Visceral disruption can occur as a result of rapid deceleration, a direct blow, or shearing forces. The compulsory use of seat belts in vehicles has reduced mortality from head and maxillofacial injuries but has significantly increased the incidence of damage to the thoracic cage, liver, spleen, and mesentery.

Diagnosis can be aided by various procedures such as peritoneal lavage, computed tomography, ultrasonography, X-rays, and selective angiography. Peritoneal lavage is performed by installation of a litre of normal saline into the peritoneal cavity through a percutaneous catheter; this fluid is then drained out through the same catheter and examined for blood. The technique is accurate in 95% of cases in detecting intra-abdominal haemorrhage (including bleeding from pelvic fractures) and is helpful in evaluating the need for laparotomy.

Injuries sustained from penetrating trauma will depend upon the type of weapon or object, its path or trajectory and, in the case of gunshot wounds, the velocity and calibre of bullet. Stab wounds will penetrate adjacent structures but bullets may have a circuitous or tumbling action causing extensive tissue damage involving multiple organs.

Abdominal injuries

Initial resuscitation priorities of the patient with abdominal trauma are maintenance of airway, breathing, and circulation. Specific treatment of abdominal injuries should not delay correction of hypoxaemia and tissue perfusion. Urgent laparotomy may be indicated if hypovolaemia persists after adequate fluid replacement and the cause cannot be attributed to other injuries. In the ICU the patient must be carefully observed for increasing abdominal pain, rigidity, or tenderness. Continuous monitoring of vital signs is essential. It is important to be alert for haemodynamic changes that indicate haemorrhage (tachycardia, hypotension, low CVP, poor peripheral perfusion, pale colour) or the need for excessive fluid replacement that does not improve the cardiovascular status. The abdominal cavity is a potential reservoir for major occult blood loss and injury must always be suspected if there is bruising or superficial lacerations (e.g. from seat belts) which may indicate damage to underlying organs.

Unless contraindicated, a urethral catheter should be inserted in patients with severe abdominal trauma in order to monitor urine output. The presence of haematuria is an important sign of potential genitourinary damage, although such damage can occur without any subsequent haematuria. Similarly, a naso- or orogastric tube should be inserted (unless contraindicated) in order to decompress the stomach, reduce the risk of pneumonic aspiration of stomach contents, and detect the presence of upper gastrointestinal injury (if blood is aspirated). Remember that patients whose prime insult is not to the abdomen may still have the potential for abdominal injury. Trauma to the lower chest (e.g. rib fractures or stab wounds) may damage the underlying abdominal viscera. This is because the diaphragm rises to the level of the fourth intercostal space at full expiration. Up to 60% of gunshot wounds and 25% of stab wounds in this region of the chest will cause abdominal injury.

Pelvic fractures

Pelvic fractures may cause massive and sometimes uncontrollable haemorrhage (4 litres or more of blood

SIGNS OF HAEMORRHAGIC SHOCK

- ◆ Tachycardia
- ◆ Hypotension
- ◆ Low CVP
- ◆ Low PAWP
- ◆ Poor peripheral perfusion

may be lost). However, 75% of patients will become haemodynamically stable after initial fluid resuscitation. The associated muscles are also very vascular, and major veins and arteries in the pelvis can easily be disrupted by trauma. The mortality of patients with open pelvic fractures exceeds 50% and associated rectal and genitourinary injuries are common. Approximately 30% of patients with pelvic fractures also have a ruptured bladder and torn urethra.

Severe haemorrhage may be difficult to control and pneumatic antishock garments (e.g. a MAST suit) may be useful in initial resuscitation. Immobilization and internal external fixation may help control bleeding but surgical repair of torn vessels or angiography and embolization may be required.

Genitourinary injuries

Upper genitourinary injuries (kidneys, upper ureters, and renal vessels)

Injuries to the kidneys are most often caused by blunt trauma (sporting injuries, falls, vehicular accidents, and assaults): 40% of patients will have associated or multiple injuries that may obscure the signs and symptoms of renal trauma. Penetrating trauma directly to the kidney from stab or gunshot wounds are easy to diagnose but may cause injury to other organs, such as the spleen, liver, pancreas, bowel, and duodenum, or perforate the diaphragm. Damage from penetrating trauma can be severe and extensive, particularly from gunshot wounds causing laceration of the renal vessels, kidney, and ureters.

Direct blows to the back resulting in bruising and abrasions may indicate underlying renal damage and in any patient sustaining deceleration trauma there is potential for genitourinary injury. Rapid deceleration (as in falls) may cause tearing of the renal vessels, intimal tearing, or rupture of the ureters at the pelvi-ureteric junction. Direct blows to the abdomen can crush the kidney between the anterior end of the 12th rib and the lumbar spine. Fractures to the lower ribs or spinal processes should therefore raise suspicion of renal injury. Vehicular accidents may cause renal injury if a seat belt, steering wheel, or other external mechanical forces crush the kidney anteriorly between the abdominal wall and the paravertebral muscles.

Renal trauma can be categorized into minor, major, or critical injuries. Minor injuries are limited to minor parenchymal damage, contusions, and superficial lacerations to the kidney. These are the most common and constitute 85% of renal trauma. Major injuries are considered to be deep lacerations involving the pelvicalyceal system and/or tears of the capsule. They result in major parenchymal damage and constitute 10% of renal injuries. Critical injuries include renal fragmentation and pedicle injuries (renal artery thrombosis, pelviureteric rupture, or avulsion of renal vessels) and occur in 5% of renal trauma. Major blood loss can occur in these patients with consequent hypovolaemic shock.

The patient sustaining a direct blow to the flank may elicit signs of bruising or swelling over the lower thoracic, loin, or upper abdominal areas. The patient will often complain of loin pain, and the anterior abdominal wall may be rigid on the affected side. Haematuria may be present and painful ureteric colic may occur if blood clots are passed through the ureter.

The initial management of the patient will depend on his/her clinical state. The airway, breathing, and circulation must be stabilized before attention is directed to a specific diagnosis of renal injury or lengthy X-ray investigations are carried out. Renal trauma alone rarely causes severe hypovolaemic shock or threatens life. If hypovolaemia is present other injuries must be considered beforehand as the prime cause. Once the patient's oxygen requirements and circulation are stabilized, diagnostic X-ray procedures can be undertaken. Intravenous urography is usually carried out in all patients with haematuria and a systolic blood pressure less than 90 mmHg. Renal ultrasonography is used on patients who are clinically stable but require evaluation of renal damage. Occasionally, a retrograde ureterogram may be required in patients with suspected disruption of the pelviureteric junction, and selective renal arteriography may be performed in patients with persistent haematuria (longer than 1 week), or those with vascular pedicle injuries.

Patients with critical renal injuries or penetrating trauma will require surgical exploration. Lacerations to the renal vessels may then be repaired and partial or total nephrectomy will be required for patients with fragmented kidneys. Patients with a renal artery thrombosis that has been identified within 10 hours of the trauma may be considered for thrombectomy.

All patients with renal injuries, however minor, must be observed closely. Vital signs should be recorded frequently and urine output monitored and observed for haematuria. Pain must be assessed and adequate analgesia administered. Any loin swelling should be observed for change in size and prophylactic antibiotics are usually given. Strict bedrest is enforced until the vital signs are stable, haematuria has ceased, and any perirenal swelling has clinically resolved.

Lower genitourinary injuries (bladder, urethra, genitalia)

Injuries to the bladder, urethra, and genitalia can be caused by penetrating trauma (particularly gunshot), but are more common from blunt trauma. In patients with suspected lower genitourinary trauma injuries the urethral meatus must be inspected for blood, the abdomen examined for signs of peritonism, and the perineum for signs of bruising. A urethral catheter must not be inserted in patients with suspected trauma or major pelvic fractures until advised by a urologist. If blood is present in the meatus, intravenous urography (antegrade or retrograde) will be required to detect a perforated or displaced bladder before suprapubic catheterization. Pelvic fractures are a common cause of injury to the bladder and urethra due to perforation from a bony segment. Signs of urethral injury are blood in the urethral meatus, inability to void, and perineal bruising. If these are present a urethral catheter must not be passed as the urethra is often traumatized and devascularized when torn and may be eroded by the catheter, disintegrate around it, or the catheter may be passed through the tear. The catheter would also prevent haematoma drainage and may introduce infection. A suprapubic catheter must therefore be inserted.

In patients with pelvic fractures, but no evidence of blood in the meatus, a urethral catheter may be passed and a cystogram used to exclude bladder rupture. Patients who are shocked, have peritonism (a rigid, painful abdomen), and in whom cystography shows bladder rupture will require laparotomy. In women, the urethra is rarely damaged from pelvic fractures and a urethral catheter can usually be passed, following which cystography may be performed to exclude bladder injuries.

Bulbar injuries are usually caused by direct trauma (e.g. a straddle impact) and such patients will have blood in the urethral meatus and perineal bruising. A urethral catheter must never be passed as this will introduce infection and aggravate the injury. The patient should be allowed to pass urine naturally, but if retention occurs a suprapubic catheter should be inserted. Prophylactic antibiotics should be given. Injuries to the scrotum and penis can also occur. Scrotal tears heal very well and do not normally require suturing but direct blows to the scrotum can cause large scrotal haematomas and damage to the testes, which may require surgical repair.

Specific nursing management

The nursing management of the patient with abdominal trauma (including pelvic fractures) will depend on the patient's specific injuries. Those patients with severe abdominal injuries will probably undergo explorative laparotomy and definitive surgery before they are admitted to the critical care unit. Care will then be directed towards anticipating potential problems relating to the specific surgery performed.

All patients will require careful monitoring of vital signs, urine output, wound drainage, and blood gas analysis. It is essential to always be aware of potential haemorrhage, even after surgery, as coagulation defects are common after major trauma and large blood transfusions. Anticipate complications arising from the hypoperfusion of major organs if large blood losses have occurred. Management must always be directed to re-

stabilizing vital functions and optimizing oxygenation and tissue perfusion. Blood glucose levels must be monitored, particularly after surgery to the pancreas or liver, and the need for parenteral nutrition considered if the enteral route cannot be used for some time.

Patients with pelvic fractures may pose particular problems in the care of pressure areas. Clear instructions must be obtained from the surgeons as to the degree of mobility that the patient is allowed. Nursing is made considerably easier if the fracture is stable or externally/internally fixed. However, some type of pressure-relieving mattress will be required as movement will still be considerably limited.

Patients with abdominal and pelvic injuries are more susceptible to infection, particularly if the injury results from penetrating trauma. Contamination may occur from foreign material (such as clothing in missile injuries) and if the gastrointestinal tract is disrupted the bowel contents may be distributed into the peritoneal cavity. Such patients are at risk from local infection (abscess formation), septicaemia, and multiorgan failure. Patients who have undergone total splenectomy are at risk from overwhelming bacterial sepsis due to diminished humoral immunity and operative measures now attempt to preserve some splenic tissue. Pro-

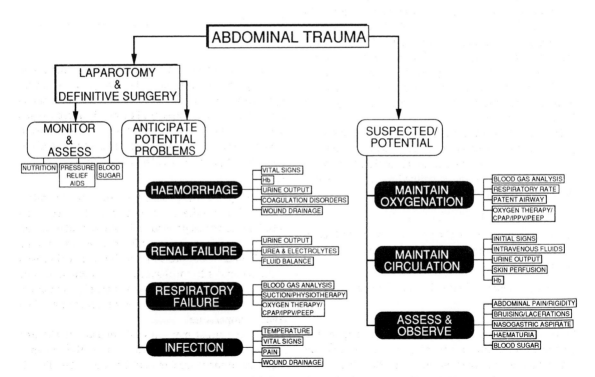

Fig. 13.6 Shows a schema summarizing the management of abdominal trauma.

phylactic antibiotics should be administered to patients with penetrating trauma and the patient must be monitored for potential infection (e.g. temperature, signs of peritonism, presence of purulent discharge from wounds or drains).

The immobile patient is also at risk of deep vein thrombosis and pulmonary embolus. Unless contraindicated (e.g. ongoing bleeding), prophylactic heparinization should be commenced.

The abdominal cavity is capable of containing a significant amount of blood without distension and large blood losses can occur retroperitoneally. An increase in girth, may therefore be a late sign of haemorrhage. It can also be due to the presence of excess air and/or fluid either inside or outside the bowel, or to oedematous bowel (see table). Girth measurements are generally inaccurate, particularly if wounds are padded. Intraabdominal pressure measurement is a more useful guide.

Fig. 13.6 shows a schema summarizing the management of abdominal trauma.

Intra-abdominal hypertension and abdominal compartment syndrome

Intra-abdominal hypertension (IAH) can occur as a result of medical and surgical pathologies, and may be acute or chronic. As the abdomen distends and abdominal wall compliance decreases there is a rise in intra-abdominal pressure (IAP), which may result in abdominal compartment syndrome (ACS). ACS is associated with a high incidence of morbidity and mortality because of the effects of high intra-abdominal pressure on the respiratory, cardiovascular, hepatic, renal, alimentary, and central nervous systems, and may result in multiorgan failure.

The critical level at which this occurs varies between patients but intra-abdominal hypertension is said to be present when the IAP rises to 10–15 mmHg. Abdominal compartment syndrome is defined as an IAP greater than 20 mmHg (Webber 2002).

Causes of intra-abdominal hypertension

The pressure inside the abdomen can increase following trauma or as a result of the accumulation of blood, gas, fluid or oedema (see Table 13.3).

Pathophysiological effects of intra-abdominal hypertension
Respiratory

Respiratory failure may be instigated or aggravated by the raised intra-abdominal pressure pushing the diaphragm higher than normal into the chest, thus increasing intrathoracic pressure, and reducing func-

TABLE 13.3   Causes of intra-abdominal hypertension

Cause	Additional risk factors
Trauma	Massive fluid resuscitation
	Coagulopathies
	Continued abdominal bleeding
	Intra-abdominal trauma
	Intra-abdominal haematomas
	Capillary leak due to release of vasoactive substances
Abdominal surgery	Presence of intra-abdominal packs
	Wound closed under tension
	Continued bleeding
	Extensive handling of the bowel
	Development of an ileus
	Massive fluid resuscitation
Gaseous distension (caused by an ileus, obstruction or post laparoscopy)	
Cirrhosis (ascities)	
Bowel ischaemia/infarction (causes oedema and distension)	
Gastrointestinal haemorrhage	
Pancreatitis	
Pregnancy	

tional capacity and compliance. This causes high peak airway pressures, reduced tidal volume, and atelectasis. Hypoxaemia and hypercapnia result, causing a respiratory acidosis. High levels of PEEP and inspired oxygen may be required to maintain oxygenation; however, PEEP has been shown to exacerbate the cardiac and respiratory complications of IAH (Lozen, 1999).

Cardiovascular

As the diaphragm is pushed upwards, the abdominal pressure is transmitted to the heart and the major vessels. This decreases preload and increases afterload on the left ventricle, reducing cardiac output and elevating SVR. Central venous pressure and PAWP may rise, even if the patient is hypovolaemic. The patient should be observed for any impaired distal extremity circulation secondary to pressure on the aorta (pedal pulses, limb colour, temperature).

Since the usual measures of preload are elevated in IAH it may be difficult to monitor the patient's response to intravascular fluid boluses unless flow is measured.

Gastrointestinal

As the IAP increases, blood flow to virtually every abdominal organ is decreased. Visceral perfusion may start to fall with an IAP as low as 10 mmHg, while an IAP > 15 mmHg reduces intramucosal gastric pH and mesenteric flow (Diebal *et al.* 1992, Webber and Mills 2002). At pressures greater than 40 mmHg the intestinal mucosa shows a severe degree of acidosis (Caldwell and Ricotta 1987) and a decrease in hepatic and microcirculatory flow (Diebal *et al.* 1992). These changes in splanchnic flow occur despite maintenance of mean arterial pressure, cardiac output, and volume loading.

Patients with ACS should be monitored for gastrointestinal bleeding due to ischaemia of the bowel.

Renal

Direct compression on the kidneys and renal veins cause the glomerular filtration rate to fall. The raised IAP reduces renal perfusion causing oliguria or anuria, and ultimately leads to renal failure. Glucose reabsorption is also decreased (Lozen 1999).

Neurological

IAH increases intracranial pressure (ICP) and cerebral perfusion pressure (CPP). The elevated intrathoracic and central venous pressures cause increased resistance to cerebral venous drainage, and CPP decreases as ICP rises. Volume expansion and any fall in mean arterial pressure further reduces CPP.

Table 13.4 summarizes the effects of IAH.

Management of intra-abdominal hypertension and abdominal compartment syndrome

Prevention and early detection of IAH in the high-risk patient is essential if the physiological consequences are to be prevented. In patients with oedema or swelling of the intestines, wound closure may be delayed following laparotomy, or alternative closures employed such as prosthetic mesh followed by staged abdominal reconstruction.

Supportive therapies include pressure-controlled ventilation with paralysis, PEEP and inverse I:E ratios, and inotropic and renal support.

Non-operative treatments include the use of prokinetic drugs if the condition is secondary to an ileus and diuretics and/or haemofiltration if due to bowel oedema. Neostigmine can be used for severe ileus but carries a risk of bowel ischaemia.

Definitive treatment of ACS is by abdominal decompression but there is no clear consensus on optimal timing. Burch *et al* (1996) have devised a grading system for ACS (see Table 13.5).

TABLE 13.4   Summary of effects of IAH

System	Increased	Decreased
Cardiovascular	CVP	Stroke volume
	Heart rate	Cardiac output
	SVR	Preload
	PAWP	Venous return
	Afterload	
Respiratory	Intrathoracic pressure	Functional capacity
	Peak inspiratory pressure	Tidal volume
	P_aCO_2	P_aO_2
		Compliance
Gastrointestinal		Intramucosal gastric pH (pH_i)
		Blood flow to all abdominal organs
		Mesenteric and mucosal blood flow
Renal		Oliguria or anuria
		Glomerular filtration rate
		Renal perfusion
		Glucose reabsorption
Neurological	Intracranial pressure	Cerebral perfusion pressure

TABLE 13.5   Burch's grading system for abdominal compartment syndrome

Grade	Bladder pressure (cmH_2O)	Equivalent pressure (mmHg)	Treatment strategy
I	10–15	7–11	Monitor only
II	15–25	11–18	Treatment based on clinical condition
III	25–30	18–26	Most will require decompression
IV	>35	>26	All require decompression

Patients undergoing surgical decompression are at risk of sudden and severe hypotension and asystolic cardiac arrest when the abdomen is opened. This may be due in part to hypovolaemia and also to reperfusion injury where mediators and free radicals are released following reperfusion of the splanchnic bed. It is therefore recommended that volume administration be given prior to decompression.

Measurement of intra-abdominal pressure

IAP can be measured indirectly by placement of trans-femoral catheters into the inferior vena cava, via intraperitoneal catheters, through gastrostomy or naso-gastric tubes and intrarectally. In addition, tonometry (gastric mucosal pH monitoring) is useful to assess local ischaemia, and may provide an earlier indication of gut ischaemia than abdominal pressure monitoring alone.

However, a quick and simple method is to use an existing Foley catheter to measure bladder pressure. At intravesical volumes of less than 100 ml the bladder acts as a passive reservoir and reflects the intra-abdominal pressure reasonably accurately within a range of 5–70 mmHg (Lozen 1999). It should be recorded 2–4-hourly according to clinical need, and the pressure trend can then provide information regarding the clinical progression.

Whilst abdominal pressure monitoring via the bladder may provide valuable information, abdominal compartment syndrome cannot be ruled out in the presence of normal pressures if organ dysfunction exists. It is also possible that bladder pressure may not capture an elevation of the abdominal pressure within a loculated area.

Measuring abdominal pressure via a urinary catheter

The procedure is relatively straightforward and involves instilling normal saline into the bladder, clamping the tubing, and connecting a transducer to measure the pressure (Fig. 13.7).

Though the bladder needs to be filled in order to transmit pressure to the transducer, there is no clear agreement regarding how much fluid should be instilled. Many of the studies correlating intracystic pressure to IAP have been carried out using animals, and human studies are lacking to date. Generally, 50–100 ml is used; when the bladder volume exceeds 100 ml the intrinsic contraction of the distended bladder wall causes pressure to increase thus intra-abdominal pressure is not accurately reflected (Lozen 1999, Gudmundsson et al, 2002).

Positioning of the patient is important in order to make accurate measurements. The patient should be placed supine so that the weight of the abdominal contents does not press on the bladder. If the patient is unable to lie supine, the position at which the first measurement is taken should be recorded, and all subsequent recordings made in the same position. Although the individual reading may not be the 'true' pressure, trends can still be assessed.

The transducer should be level with the pubic symphysis bone (this is approximates to the mid-axillary line).

There are several methods of measuring IAP using a Foley urinary catheter. Either a two- or three-way Foley

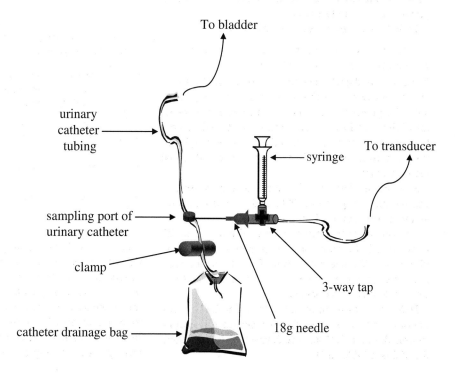

To bladder

urinary catheter tubing

syringe

To transducer

sampling port of urinary catheter

clamp

3-way tap

18g needle

catheter drainage bag

Fig. 13.7 Measurement of intra-abdominal pressure.

bladder catheter can be used. Most patients will have a two-way catheter *in situ* as a three-way catheter is used for bladder irrigation. The benefit of using a three-way catheter is that the saline can be instilled into the irrigation limb, thus avoiding the need to access a closed system.

◆ Equipment
  1 × transducer primed with normal saline (this does not need to be under pressure)
  1 × clamp
  1 × 18 gauge needle
  1 × 60 ml syringe
  1 × urinary drainage bag with a sampling port close to the catheter connection

◆ Method. The procedure must be carried out aseptically, using sterile gloves and placing a sterile towel beneath the catheter connection:
  1. Place the patient supine.
  2. Zero the transducer at the pubic symphysis pubis bone.
  3. Clamp the drainage bag distal to the sampling port.
  4. Draw up 50 ml of sterile saline into the catheter syringe.
  5. Disconnect the drainage bag, inject the saline and reconnect.
  6. Insert the 18-gauge needle (with the transducer attached) into the sampling port of the Foley catheter.
  7. Release the clamp momentarily until fluid fills the tubing, and then reclamp.
  8. Allow the transducer to equilibriate and then record the pressure.

An alternative method is to insert a three-way tap between the needle and transducer. The saline can be injected via this tap instead of disconnecting the catheter drainage bag, thus reducing the risk of infection.

A similar method is used when measuring abdominal pressure via a nasogastric tube.

Musculoskeletal injuries

Musculoskeletal injuries themselves are rarely life-threatening but any associated injuries can be. Up to 70% of multiply injured patients will have injured limbs, fractures, or dislocations. The management of limb trauma is always secondary to resuscitation and control of the airway, breathing, and circulation. Only when the multiply injured patient is stable should attention be directed to the definitive care of the limb injury. At this point a thorough head-to-toe examination is carried out and limb X-rays are taken. Certain musculoskeletal conditions are considered life-threatening. These include traumatic amputations (particularly of a whole limb), major haemorrhage from vascular injuries or open fractures, severe crush injuries to the pelvis and abdomen, and multiple long bone fractures.

Blood loss from open wounds is obvious, though often underestimated, but large amounts of blood can also be lost in closed fractures. Major haemorrhage can occur in closed fractures of the humerus and tibia (up to 1.5 litres each) and femur (up to 2.5 litres). Rapid resuscitation is vital to replace lost circulatory volume; however, the cause of haemorrhagic shock must never be presumed to originate solely from skeletal injury—other potential injuries must be considered. Open wounds or fractures may have bled extensively from the time of the injury and blood loss may be difficult to assess. Generally, for open fractures the blood loss is two to three times greater than that of closed fractures. Direct pressure should be applied to any open wounds that are bleeding by compression bandage or hand pressure, until definitive treatment can be carried out.

A fracture also produces damage to the muscles surrounding the injured bone and to the blood vessels and nerves in its vicinity. Penetrating trauma and local contusions may disrupt blood flow; furthermore, peripheral circulation may be poor in the hypovolaemic patient. Vascular impairment and neurovascular bundle injury may therefore compromise the survival of a limb and must be identified without delay. Bleeding or thrombosis in a blood vessel can impair the distal circulation and cause limb ischaemia. Vascular injury should be identified promptly by close and regular observation before ischaemia develops. Peripheral limb pulses must therefore be evaluated regularly to assess circulation, and an absent or diminished pulse reported without delay. Skin perfusion should be assessed by the capillary return, temperature, and colour of the limb distal to the injury. A low skin temperature indicates inadequate perfusion. Check that plaster casts, traction, and compression bandages are not impairing circulation.

If nerve damage has occurred sensation will be impaired. This sensation is lost early if ischaemia is present. Direct severing of nerve fibres by penetrating trauma or by stretching or compression of the nerve fibres causing variable degrees of paralysis may cause nerve injury.

Dislocations may produce neurovascular injury by stretching nerves and compressing blood vessels causing muscle injury. They should be reduced promptly,

MUSCULOSKELETAL INJURIES

Check limbs for:

- Colour
- Temperature
- Pulses
- Sensation/pain
- Local compression (plaster-of-Paris, splints, bandages)

TABLE 13.6 Types of dislocations and associated complications

Dislocation	Associated complication
Knee	Popliteal artery/nerve injuries
Ankle	Skin pressure and necrosis
Elbow	Ulnar and median nerve damage
Shoulder	Brachial plexus injury
Hip	Aseptic necrosis of femoral head

particularly at the knee, elbow, and ankle. Angiography may be required if vascular injury is suspected. Obvious and complete arterial occlusion will, however, require prompt surgical exploration.

Compartment syndrome and rhabdomyolysis are specific complications following musculoskeletal injuries and are discussed fully later.

Specific management

Open fractures

In this type of fracture a wound in the skin communicates directly with the broken bone. The most important factor in management is to prevent infection, thus ideally open fractures should be definitively treated within 8 hours of the injury. The fracture should be aligned and splinted and the wound covered with a sterile dry dressing. Antibiotic therapy should be instituted and tetanus prophylaxis administered. Surgery will include thorough cleaning of the wound and debridement of non-viable tissue. Wounds are often left open for 5–7 days to prevent a rise in tissue pressure, which contributes to wound hypoxia and infection. Open fractures are often unstable; rigid stabilization will promote tissue healing and a variety of methods can be used.

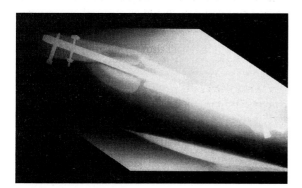

Fig. 13.8 Repair of compound femoral structure (intramedullary nail).

Closed fractures

In this type of fracture there is no open wound (Fig. 13.8). In the multiply injured patient early fixation of fractures (within 24 hours) can reduce mortality and morbidity from ARDS, fat embolism, and systemic sepsis. Nursing of the patient is made considerably easier and analgesia requirements can be reduced.

Dislocations

Dislocations must be reduced promptly to prevent potentially irreversible damage to neurovascular bundles and plexus injuries (Table 13.6).

All dislocations are extremely painful. Adequate analgesia must be given but caution may be needed in the presence of other injuries. The limb should be supported on a pillow or immobilized with traction whilst awaiting definitive treatment.

Specific nursing management of musculoskeletal injuries

The extent of the patient's injuries and his/her degree of immobility will dictate specific nursing care. Several methods can be used to maintain reduction of fractures depending on the nature of the fracture; for example, plaster casts, splints, continuous traction, pin and plaster techniques, and internal fixation devices (nails, plates, wires, screws, and rods). Continuous traction can be by means of skin traction or skeletal traction using wires, pins, or tongs placed through the bone with a system of ropes, pulleys, and weights. Space does not permit a comprehensive explanation of the nursing management of orthopaedic injuries. However, the patient in the ICU frequently has multiple injuries or has some other serious injury as well as a fracture that necessitates his/her stay on the unit. The following are basic points to remember:

For the patient in traction:

- Check the skin around the traction device for evidence of circulatory impairment.

- Give frequent and meticulous attention to pressure areas. Use a pressure-relieving mattress.

- Inspect pin sites daily and keep clean and dry.

- Passive/active exercises to non-immobilized joints.

- The knots on the traction rope should be secure and the supporting apparatus free of the pulleys.

- Check that the ropes are in the wheel groove and the weights hang free.

- The weights should not be removed when the patient is moved. One nurse must support the weights without relieving the traction if a patient is moved up the bed.

For the patient with a plaster cast:

- Constriction due to swelling may cause circulatory impairment, pain, and pressure on healthy tissue. Therefore, check skin temperature, colour, pulses, and sensation in the affected limb.

- Check the skin integrity around the edge of the cast. Pressure points may need extra padding.

- Pain under the cast may be due to pressure on a bony prominence, nerve, or blood vessel.

- Supracondylar fractures of the elbow are often accompanied by considerable swelling which may impair circulation in the forearm and hand. The radial pulse must be checked frequently in the first 24 hours. Elevating the limb on a pillow may alleviate swelling, but if severe, the plaster may need to be split.

Anticipate complications:

- *Haemorrhage*. Monitor vital signs, observe wounds and drains for bleeding, monitor haemoglobin.

- *Compartment syndrome*. Observe the limb frequently for tense swelling, pain, decreased temperature, and diminished sensation.

- *Infection*. Monitor temperature, inspect wounds, cannulae, and pin sites. Swab and culture if necessary.

- *Deep vein thrombosis*. Inspect calves for pain and swelling. Consider anti-embolic stockings and prophylactic anticoagulation. Passive/active limb movements may help prevent thrombosis.

- *Rhabdomyolysis*. Monitor urine output, daily urinalysis, observe urine for myoglobinuria, measure plasma creatinine kinase (CPK). Keep patient well hydrated and maintain a good diuresis. Monitor urea and electrolytes, including magnesium, calcium, and phosphate.

Flaps

The patient with severe musculoskeletal injuries may require reconstruction using free or pedicled flaps in order to correct an anatomical defect. A free flap is where a section of tissue (which can include a combination of skin, muscle, fascia, or bone) is detached from the body and microsurgically reattached elsewhere. A pedicled flap is where the tissue is transposed elsewhere while still attached to its original blood supply.

The post-operative survival of the flap is dependent on good perfusion. Close and frequent observation is needed to promptly detect arterial insufficiency or venous congestion, particularly in the first 72 hours.

Factors that may be detrimental to flap survival include:

- hypotension (decreases arterial flow through the flap),

- vasopressors (may decrease flow due to vasoconstriction),

- hypovolaemia,

- poor positioning.

A typical flap observation chart

Date and time	Temperature (°C)			Colour	Capillary refill	Turgidity	Pulse	Comments/seen by Dr.
	Core	Peripheral	Flap					

Recordings of core, flap, and peripheral temperature should be made. Ideally, the core–flap temperature difference should be less than 1.5°C. In order to achieve this, and to optimize blood flow, the patient and flap both need to be kept warm and the vessels dilated. Vasodilators such as glycerol trinitrate are often used intravenously, and the haemoglobin level is kept below 10 g/dl to reduce blood viscosity. Some protocols also use dextran infusions to reduce viscosity. A body-warming device, such as a Bair Hugger, should be used as necessary, and mean arterial blood pressure and CVP must be kept within set parameters.

The flap must be inspected regularly and an assessment made of its colour, temperature, capillary refill, turgidity, and the presence of a pulse (using Doppler). The frequency of these observations should be dictated by the surgeon's instructions and/or unit policy. Many critical care areas will have dedicated flap observation charts and an example is shown here.

Any changes in observation must be reported immediately as the salvage rate of a failing flap is dependent on rapid intervention.

Flap observations should include:

- *Colour*. The flap should be normal skin colour. A mottled or purple flap indicates venous congestion and a pale flap arterial insufficiency.

- *Capillary refill*. Normal capillary refill should be 2–3 s. Venous congestion is indicated if it is more than 3 s and arterial insufficiency if more than 6 s.

- *Turgidity*. The flap should feel soft to the touch. Arterial insufficiency causes the flap to feel flaccid and if venous congestion is present it will feel turgid or tense.

- *Pulse and temperature*. The flap should feel warm and a pulse present. An absent pulse indicates arterial insufficiency.

Complications following trauma

Complications secondary to trauma can result from:

1. Shock causing hypoperfusion of vital organs (e.g. renal and circulatory failure). The origin of the shock may be: hypovolaemic (e.g. haemorrhage), septic, neurogenic (e.g. spinal injury), obstructive (e.g. pulmonary embolus), or cardiogenic (e.g. direct myocardial contusion).

2. Specific types of trauma causing rhabdomyolysis, compartment syndrome, air embolism, and fat embolism syndrome (e.g. long bone fractures, chest injuries, crush injuries).

3. Transfusion of large amounts of blood causing anaphylactic reactions, ARDS, multiorgan failure, coagulopathies, and hypocalcaemia.

4. Infection causing wound breakdown, anastomotic breakdown, or sepsis.

5. Immobility causing pressure sores, chest infection, deep vein thrombosis (DVT), and pulmonary embolism.

6. Respiratory failure from chest, head, and neck injuries.

Shock

Although shock is generally described as hypotension and tachycardia, a more accurate definition is inadequate tissue oxygen utilization due to hypoperfusion or cellular poisoning. Hypotension need not necessarily be present to indicate organ hypoperfusion. At a cellular level, inadequately perfused cells compensate initially for the lack of oxygen supply by shifting to anaerobic metabolism. This results in lactic acid formation and thus development of a metabolic acidosis. If the lack of oxygen is both acute and severe, cell death (necrosis) ensues. Management is directed at reversing this phenomenon with adequate oxygenation, appropriate fluid resuscitation, and vasoactive drug support as necessary.

Hypovolaemic shock

All types of shock may be present in the trauma patient but the vast majority of injured patients in shock are hypovolaemic—usually due to haemorrhage.

Early haemodynamic responses to blood loss are compensatory (i.e. progressive vasoconstriction of cutaneous, visceral, and muscle regional circulations in order to preserve blood flow to the kidneys, heart, and brain). A young person can lose over 30% of circulating blood volume before showing any significant change in heart rate and blood pressure, especially if supine. Only when intravascular depletion is so great as to exhaust these compensatory mechanisms does hypotension ensue. The body also compensates for intravascular volume loss by redistributing fluid from the extravascular compartments into the bloodstream.

The direct effect of haemorrhage depends on the percentage of acute blood volume lost and can be considered in four classes:

1. *Class 1: loss of up to 15% of blood*. Clinical signs are lacking. Minimal tachycardia, no measurable changes in blood pressure, pulse pressure, respiratory rate, or capillary refill test. Replacement of the primary fluid losses will correct the circulatory state.

2. *Class 2: 15–30% blood loss.* This would represent 800–1500 ml of blood loss in a 70 kg adult. Clinical symptoms may include tachycardia, tachypnoea, a decrease in pulse pressure (the difference between the systolic and diastolic pressures), and a minimal change in systolic pressure. Other changes include subtle central nervous system changes, such as anxiety, fright, or hostility. Normally urine output is only mildly affected—usually falling to 20–30 ml/hour in the 70 kg adult.

3. *Class 3: 30–40% blood loss.* This would represent about 2000 ml loss in an adult and its clinical effects can be devastating. Patients present with classical signs of inadequate perfusion—marked tachycardia, tachypnoea, significant changes in mental state, and a considerable fall in blood pressure.

4. *Class 4: more than 40% blood loss.* This degree of blood loss is immediately life-threatening. Symptoms include a marked tachycardia, significant fall in blood pressure, a very narrow pulse pressure, or an unobtainable diastolic pressure. Urinary output is negligible and mental status markedly depressed. The skin is cold and pale. Such patients require rapid transfusion and immediate surgical intervention. Blood loss of over 50% of the patient's blood volume results in loss of consciousness, pulse, and blood pressure.

Management of hypovolaemic shock

Hypovolaemia must be promptly diagnosed and treated. Vascular access must be obtained immediately using large-bore cannulae. In severe cases, the peripheral veins may be collapsed and cannulation may prove impossible. A 'cut-down' onto a peripheral vein (i.e. a surgical incision through the skin to directly identify and cannulate the vein) is occasionally needed. Usually, cannulation of a central vein is successful. Difficulty can sometimes be experienced with a jugular or subclavian approach in the presence of severe hypovolaemia with an increased risk of complication (e.g. pneumothorax). In these cases, the femoral vein is a safer site to cannulate first.

Baseline observations of vital signs and sequential monitoring are crucial. The central venous pressure may simply reflect the body's continuing ability to vasoconstrict rather than restoration of an adequate circulating blood volume. The central venous pressure will also be elevated while fluids are being rapidly infused; a10 min period of cessation will allow equilibration between intra- and extravascular compartments. Thus a very low CVP, e.g. <2 mmHg, is suggestive of hypovolaemia while a 'normal' (5–10 mmHg) or even high (>10 mmHg) CVP may coexist with either hypovolaemia or normovolaemia. In this situation a fluid challenge, looking at the effect on CVP, is mandatory (see Chapter 6).

Normalization of blood pressure, heart, and respiratory rate, cerebration, peripheral circulation, and core–toe temperature gradient indicate that organ perfusion is improving. In tandem, a good urine output and disappearance of metabolic acidosis are good markers of the adequacy of resuscitation.

It is important to treat the cause rather than the effects of hypoperfusion. Thus bicarbonate should not be blindly given to correct the metabolic acidosis nor furosemide (frusemide) to increase the urine output. Likewise, inotropes should be withheld until adequate fluid has been administered. The patient may respond to either pain or a metabolic acidosis by hyperventilating; attention should therefore be directed towards adequate analgesia and proper fluid management.

Fluid administered for resuscitation should be a combination of blood, blood products, and clear fluids such as colloid or crystalloid. Colloid (e.g. gelatin (Gelofusin, Haemaccel), starch (Hespan) or human albumin solution) is a better intravascular volume expander than crystalloid, though no studies have conclusively shown an improvement in outcome either way. Blood provides the necessary haemoglobin replacement to carry oxygen to the tissues while blood products correct coagulopathy due to consumption of endogenous clotting factors and platelets.

Ideally, blood should be fully cross-matched and this can be achieved within 30 min. In dire situations either O-negative (universal donor) or, preferably, ABO group-specific (though otherwise antibody-untested) blood can be given while awaiting a more formal cross-match. The blood should be transfused if possible through a warming device if large amounts are required. Calcium gluconate 10% may need to be given if large volumes of blood are transfused, but should be guided by the patient's ionized calcium level or symptoms. This is because the citrate used as an anticoagulant in stored blood may induce hypocalcaemia with resulting tetany and decreased muscle contractility. Stored blood contains few platelets or clotting factors; consideration should be given to separate administration of fresh frozen plasma, platelets, and cryoprecipitate if large volumes are needed. Although the blood potassium may rise following infusion of stored blood, this will rarely cause a significant hyperkalaemia.

Compartment syndrome

This is due to swelling, bleeding, or ischaemia within the fascial compartments of the arm and/or leg. As these compartments are unable to expand to any significant degree, interstitial tissue pressure will rise. When this pressure exceeds that of the capillary bed, local ischaemia of nerve and muscle occurs. Rhabdomyolysis, permanent paralysis, or gangrene may result. This typically occurs after crush injuries, closed or open fractures, or sustained compression of a limb in an immobile patient.

If able, the patient will complain of increasing pain in the affected limb, despite immobilization of fractures. Pain on passive stretching of muscles within the affected region may also be evident. There will be tense swelling of the involved fascial compartment(s) and possibly reduced sensation over the dermatomes supplied by the affected nerves. The absence of distal pulses does not identify the early stages of compartment syndrome as these may be intact until late in the progression of the syndrome after irreversible damage has been done. Restricting dressings should be released. Development of a compartment syndrome may not be an immediate complication and careful observation of limbs for swelling, abnormal perfusion, temperature differences, or pain should be performed.

If recovery is not rapid, urgent fasciotomy should be considered to relieve the pressure. Compartmental pressures can be monitored with needle manometry and pressures greater than 20 mmHg are considered abnormal. Fasciotomies should be performed when the intracompartmental pressure exceeds 30–40 mmHg (or the diastolic blood pressure minus 30 mmHg) and remains at that level for more than 8 hours. Considerable blood loss may occur following fasciotomy.

Fat embolism syndrome (FES)

Patients with FES have emboli of fat macroglobules in the pulmonary and systemic circulations. Organs with high blood flow, such as the heart, lungs, brain, and kidney, show evidence of capillary obstruction by fat or microaggregates of platelets, red cells and fibrin. The syndrome usually presents as respiratory insufficiency, cerebral dysfunction, and petechial skin haemorrhages.

FES is associated with bone fractures, particularly of the long bones and pelvis. These fractures result in fat and marrow entering the venous circulation. Massive trauma may also disrupt adipose tissue causing large fat globules to enter the bloodstream. The onset of signs and symptoms of the syndrome is generally at 24–48 hours post-injury.

Mechanical obstruction of the pulmonary capillaries rapidly causes dyspnoea and tachypnoea, hypoxaemia, and, occasionally, production of bloodstained frothy sputum. A petechial rash develops, classically over the upper thorax, neck, and soft palate, and is seen in up to 50% of patients. Petechiae can sometimes be seen in the retina. A fever of up to 39°C often develops, with an associated tachycardia. Occlusion of cerebral vessels causes confusion, drowsiness, decerebrate signs, convulsions, and coma. If these signs become apparent other causes must be excluded by appropriate investigations (e.g. delayed post-traumatic intracranial injury by CT scanning). Obstruction of renal vessels causes oliguria or anuria and there may be diagnostic presence of fat globules in pulmonary artery blood or urine. Coagulopathies are sometimes seen with increased fibrin degradation products, thrombocytopenia, and anaemia. There may be significant intrapulmonary haemorrhage. ECG changes may reveal right heart strain in fulminant FES. Biopsy of skin or kidneys may reveal microinfarcts associated with fat globules.

Treatment is largely supportive and the prognosis in fulminant FES is poor. Supplemental oxygen therapy is used to correct hypoxaemia but often mechanical ventilation ± PEEP is required. An adequate circulatory volume must be ensured, taking into account blood loss at fracture sites, and fluid loss from wounds. Careful monitoring of blood pressure, heart rate, CVP, and, if possible, pulmonary artery pressures should be instituted. There is often a fall in cardiac output and an increase in pulmonary vascular resistance as the syndrome develops. Inotropic support may be required to maintain arterial pressure.

Renal support will be required if the patient becomes anuric or oliguric with rapidly deteriorating renal function. Close monitoring of serum electrolytes is essential.

The prevention of hypoxaemia reduces the severity of the syndrome. Early institution of oxygen therapy and maintaining good blood gas exchange are important preventative factors in the first 48 hours of patients at risk of FES. Anticoagulation with heparin is

---

SIGNS OF FULMINANT FAT EMBOLISM SYNDROME (FES)

- Hypoxaemia
- Increased respiratory rate, heart rate, and temperature
- Decreased blood pressure, cardiac output, and urine output
- Poor cerebral perfusion
- Petechiae

sometimes used though strong evidence for this therapy is lacking.

Air embolism

This results from air leaking from the lungs directly into the pulmonary vein and hence into the left heart. Massive air embolism may occur when patients with severe lung injury are mechanically ventilated and is due to a bronchopulmonary vein fistula or direct penetrating injury to the pulmonary veins. Major circulatory collapse follows; the patient is hypoxaemic and arterial blood samples may appear 'frothy'. Diagnosis is difficult in the presence of severe chest injuries or where there may be other causes of sudden cardiovascular collapse and hypoxaemia. Air embolism is uncommon and other causes, such as tension pneumothorax, should be excluded first. Treatment is by turning the patient on to his/ her left side in a head-down, feet-up position so that air in the ventricle will not enter the systemic circulation. Air is then aspirated from the left ventricle followed by thoracotomy of the injured side.

Hypothermia

Hypothermia is defined as a sustained core temperature below 35°C. It may be further classified as mild (32–35°C), moderate (28–32°C), or severe (<28°C).

In the patient with normal thermoregulation, accidental hypothermia may occur when the body is exposed to a cold environment or immersed in cold water. However, in the patient with abnormal thermogenesis a mild exposure to cold can cause hypothermia. This may occur for the following reasons:

- A reduced metabolic rate (e.g. hypothyroidism, hypopituitarism, or malnutrition, where heat production is insufficient to maintain the body's temperature).

- Spinal injury where muscle activity cannot be increased.

- Hypothalamic injuries (e.g. CVA), self-poisoning, alcohol abuse, and sedative drugs, which cause cutaneous vasodilatation and increased heat loss.

- The elderly, as a consequence of a reduced shivering response, immobility, poor living conditions, reduced subcutaneous fat, and a low metabolic rate.

Core temperature should be measured in hypothermic patients, ideally with an oesophageal or rectal temperature probe. The clinical manifestations of hypothermia vary according to the core temperature, rate of cooling, and duration of hypothermia. Thermo-regulatory mechanisms usually remain intact above 33°C but below this there is progressive physiological deterioration. Loss of consciousness and pupillary dilatation occurs at 30°C. The shivering mechanism is replaced by muscular rigidity at 33°C and a rigor mortis-like appearance, with cessation of respiration, at 24°C.

The solubility of gases in plasma increases with hypothermia and the oxygen dissociation curve is shifted to the right (due to an increased affinity of haemoglobin for oxygen). It is debatable whether blood gas analysis should be corrected for temperature in the hypothermic patient.

Mortality varies from 6% to 85%, depending on the severity of hypothermia, duration, underlying disease conditions, and associated complications (see Table 13.7 for the physiological manifestations of hypothermia).

Rewarming

The rate of rewarming depends on the degree of hypothermia. Rapid rewarming up to 15°C per hour can be achieved by extracorporeal circuits but this is reserved for severe cases only who have life-threatening complications. Generally, rewarming is at a rate of 0.5–4°C per hour. Rapid rewarming may precipitate 'rewarming shock' where sudden surface peripheral vasodilatation causes hypotension, an increase in metabolic acidosis, and a drop in temperature of up to 4°C due to cool peripheral blood perfusing the central organs. Cool blood perfusing the myocardium may give rise to fatal arrhythmias, such as ventricular fibrillation, during rewarming. The elderly and those with underlying cardiac disease are particularly vulnerable so rewarming should he controlled and cautious.

Methods of rewarming

Passive rewarming   This is suitable for mild hypothermia. Rewarming takes place slowly (0.5–1.0°C/hour):

- warm environment (25–30°C),

- reflective space blanket/warm air blanket,

- extra blankets,

- cover skin areas through which heat loss may occur (e.g. scalp).

Active rewarming   This is used in moderate hypothermia, those with impaired thermoregulation, and inability to shiver:

- heated humidified respiratory gases,

- warmed intravenous fluids,

- electrically heated mattresses or pads/warm air blanket,

TABLE 13.7 Physiological manifestations of hypothermia

System	Problem	Cause	Treatment
Cardiovascular	Tachycardia/pripheral vasoconstriction/↑ cardiac output	Elevated levels of noradrenaline due to increased sympathetic activity	Monitor vital signs. Passive rewarming
	↓ cardiac output/↓ BP (moderate hypothermia)	Bradycardia	Active rewarming. Intravenous fluids. Monitor vital signs
	Dysrhythmias: bradycardia, conduction disturbances, AF + SVT (<30°C), VF (<28°C). (VF may also be precipitated by stimulation, e.g. CVP insertion, endotracheal intubation)	Decreased tissue perfusion, acidosis, underlying cardiac ischaemia, direct effect of cold on sinus node	Continuous ECG monitoring. Avoid unnecessary stimulation. Treat bradycardias with atropine/pacing (as necessary). DC cardioversion is needed for VF; however, this may be resistant to electrical or pharmacological interventions until the core temperature >28° C. (Note: In cardiac arrest situations, resuscitation must continue until the core temperature approaches normal. Hypothermia does have a cerebroprotective effect even though drugs and defibrillation may be ineffective)
Respiratory	Hypoventilation	Decreased rate and depth of respiration	Monitor blood gases
	Hypoxaemia	Decreased gaseous diffusion capacity	Ensure patent airway. Use supplemental oxygen and mechanical ventilation as necessary
	Respiratory acidosis	Increased levels of CO_2 due to hypoventilation	Monitor blood gases. Mechanical ventilation may be necessary
Renal	Polyuria. Electrolyte imbalance	Impaired tubular function due to inhibition of enzyme systems and reduced responsiveness to ADH	Measure urine output and fluid input. Monitor urine specific gravity and electrolytes, vital signs, blood urea, and electrolytes. Electrolyte replacement as necessary. Some patients develop renal failure (this is usually associated with hypotension). Renal support (e.g. dialysis may be required)
Neurological	Cerebral depression	Decreased cerebral blood flow (7% decrease per °C)	Neurological observations. Maintain patent airway
Metabolic	Metabolic acidosis	Peripheral vasoconstriction and hypotension causing poor tissue perfusion. Lactate and other metabolites increase. Lactate clearance by liver is decreased. Decreased H^+ ion secretion by kidneys	Monitor blood pH. Intravenous fluid therapy (± vasodilators) as patient warms up
	Hyperglycaemia	Impaired peripheral circulation of glucose, decreased insulin release, glucose metabolized from liver glycogen. (Note: Pancreatitis may occur secondary to hypothermia)	Monitor blood glucose. Insulin infusion if necessary. In prolonged hypothermia, glycogen stores may be depleted and hypoglycaemia may develop

- hot baths (40–45°C) with limbs out of the water to avoid rewarming shock. These are only suitable for young adults and are usually not practicable. Monitoring is difficult in this situation.

Core warming   This is for severe hypothermia:

- peritoneal/haemodialysis,

- extracorporeal circuits (as in heart bypass),

- intragastric or bladder irrigation with warm fluids.

Burn injuries

Burn injuries may have psychological, systemic, and local effects on the patient. They can range from superficial, where the injury extends only partly into the skin and healing is spontaneous, to full thickness where the burn extends through the dermis, damaging the underlying fat and muscle tissue. Scarring will occur when a certain critical depth of damage to the dermis has occurred; this is permanent, often causing disability and disfiguration. Morbidity and mortality increases with increased body surface area (BSA) percentage of burn, in the very young or old, and when pre-existing diseases are present such as cardiovascular, renal, or pulmonary disorders.

Assessment of the severity of the burn injury is traditionally by the percentage of the BSA involved. A major burn is considered to be >10% BSA in a child and 15% BSA in an adult. Patients with >20% BSA plus a severe smoke inhalation injury have a 50–80% mortality.

The depth of the burn can be classified as follows.

- Erythema: redness of the skin, pain but no blistering.

- 1st degree: the burn involves only the epithelial layer of the skin. The skin is red and blisters, blanches on pressure, and is painful. There is no residual scarring on healing.

- 2nd degree: the burn extends through the epithelial layer to the dermis. The skin appears red and blis-

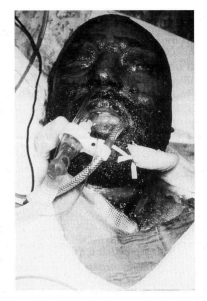

Fig. 13.9 Severe burn injury showing generalized swelling of face and upper airways.

tered. Pain and residual scarring will depend on the depth of dermis damaged.

- 3rd degree: involves full skin thickness. The skin is white. There is little or no pain as the sensory nerve endings are destroyed. Residual scarring usually occurs.

Areas of particular concern are burns to the face (especially around the nose and mouth which may indicate inhalational injury), circumferential burns of the limbs, and burns to the eyelids (Fig. 13.9). The cause of the burn should be taken into account when assessment is made. These may be from a dry source (e.g. flames), wet source (e.g. scalds), electrical (e.g. household appliances, pylons), or chemical (acid, alkali, radiation).

Initial management

If possible, the patient should be nursed in protective isolation and in an environment with humidity and temperature control. An air-fluidized bed may be required for severe burn injuries.

On arrival at the critical care unit, the patient must be assessed and vital signs recorded. A patent airway must be maintained and humidified oxygen therapy instituted. Patients with massive burns or inhalational injury may require urgent endotracheal intubation and mechanical ventilation. Intravenous access, preferably in a non-burned area, must be established. High fluid losses will occur from the burned area; CVP and, occa-

---

CALCULATION OF TOTAL PERCENTAGE OF BURNED SKIN: THE 'RULE OF 9'

- Head: 9%

- Arms: 9% each

- Front and back of trunk: 18% each

- Legs: 18% each

- Perineum: 1%

- Total: 100%

sionally, PAWP monitoring may be required. An arterial line should be inserted for systemic pressure monitoring and blood sampling. A nasogastric tube and urinary catheter will also be required in severe cases. Insertion of tubes and cannulae should be carried out at an early stage as the patient will become grossly oedematous within 24 hours due to massive capillary leakage, thus making instrumentation extremely difficult. For this reason, scrupulous attention should also be paid to the airway and endotracheal intubation performed on early signs of respiratory distress. Massive swelling may occur around the face and/or neck resulting in respiratory difficulties; an inhalational injury need not necessarily be present.

Various formulae exist for fluid replacement but these should only be used as guidelines. Fluid losses are commonly underestimated and frequent assessment of vital signs, urine output, haematocrit, and base deficit are vital. Care must be taken not to overload the patient with fluid. In the UK, the Muir Barclay (or Mount Vernon) formula is often used for guiding fluid resuscitation. The first 36 hours from the time of burn—not from the time of arrival in hospital—are divided into six periods of 4, 4, 4, 6, 6, and 12 hours. Over each period, 0.5 ml/g body weight/% burn of 5% human albumin solution is given with additional crystalloid as 5% dextrose at a rate of 1.5–2 ml/kg body weight/hour. Haemodynamic variables should be measured at the end of each period and the patient's intravascular fluid status reassessed and adjusted as necessary. A haematocrit of approximately 0.35 is considered satisfactory to ensure adequate oxygen carriage and a non-elevated blood viscosity. A high haematocrit may imply haemoconcentration and the need for more fluid. An increasing metabolic acidosis and a fall in urine output are signs of an inadequate intravascular volume. A low haematocrit is suggestive of fluid overload; however, blood loss should also be considered as a cause of a low haematocrit. This may either be from haemorrhage from non-burn injuries or from haemolysis of blood cells trapped in the burned areas. In general, blood transfusions are not needed in the first 24 hours unless escharatomies are performed.

Coagulation screens should be performed regularly as massive dilution may occur by the huge amount of fluid infused; clotting factors may also be consumed or production suppressed and replacement, usually as fresh frozen plasma, should be considered if significant derangement in coagulation occurs. Likewise, marked shifts may occur in electrolyte status; these should be measured regularly and corrected as necessary.

After 2–5 days the capillary leakage usually slows and the patient often enters a diuretic phase. Excessive tissue fluid is reabsorbed back into the intravascular compartment and thence excreted via the kidney. This diuresis is spontaneous and may be massive; although fluid and sodium input should be reduced at this stage, care must be taken not to allow intravascular depletion and electrolyte imbalance.

Subsequent management

Cardiovascular

The circulation of a burned patient after resuscitation is usually hyperdynamic with an elevated cardiac output. Shock can occur rapidly within the first 48 hours of the injury or later. Hypotension and a fall in cardiac output causes hypoperfusion of vital organs which may lead to single or multiple organ failure. Vascular permeability in the area of the burn increases and large amounts of fluid, similar in composition to plasma, leak out and are lost through the burnt tissue. Oedema is related to vasoactive substances released as a consequence of the injury. This is not just limited to the affected areas; there is widespread generalized swelling, indicative of the whole-body inflammatory response to the burn. The circulating intravascular volume is thus depleted resulting in hypoperfusion. The released inflammatory mediators may also cause progression to multi-organ failure with cardiovascular collapse. The first step in management is to ensure adequate fluid resuscitation, although vasoactive drugs, such as norepinephrine (noradrenaline), may occasionally be required to maintain an adequate blood pressure.

Respiratory

Pulmonary injury may result from inhalation of irritant or noxious gases such as carbon monoxide and cyanide. Heat may cause damage to the upper and lower airways and lung tissue. Smoke inhalation causes thermal injury only to the larynx and pharynx, as hot gases have a low specific heat content. Steam has a much higher heat content and causes injury to the whole respiratory tract. ARDS and pneumonia may be secondary complications of the primary burn injury.

Water-soluble gases found in smoke from burning plastics or rubber react with water in mucous membranes to produce strong acids and alkalis. These may cause bronchospasm, ulceration, oedema, and damage to the ciliary mechanism. Lipid-soluble compounds can be transported to the lower airways on carbon particles and produce cell membrane damage and alveolar flooding.

There should be a very low threshold for endotracheal intubation in patients with inhalational injuries as these patients can quickly progress to complete airway obstruction as oedema develops. Oedema with impaired upper airway patency may develop over 12–18 hours and is progressive for the first 18–24 hours.

Indications for intubation are:

◆ Failure to maintain an adequate airway.

◆ Respiratory failure.

◆ Severe cyanide or carbon monoxide poisoning.

◆ Convulsions.

◆ Stridor, lip swelling, or hoarseness .

◆ Circumferential chest burns.

◆ Severe facial burns or full thickness burns of nose or lips.

◆ Deep burns to the neck which may cause external compression of the airway.

◆ Evidence of pharyngeal or laryngeal oedema/ blistering/ erythema, soot.

When intubating, remember not to cut the endotracheal tube too short—leave several inches of endotracheal tube beyond the mouth to allow for facial and lip swelling, which can be extensive. Depolarizing muscle relaxants (such as suxemethonium) are contraindicated after the first few hours because they may worsen hyperkalemia; non-depolarizing agents (such as vecuronium) should be used instead.

Several factors can increase chest wall compliance. These are:

◆ Full thickness burns to the thorax due to loss of elasticity of the skin.

◆ Full thickness burns to the abdomen as they may cause abdominal compartment syndrome.

◆ Increased CVP, secondary to raised intrathoracic pressure, can accelerate the rate of protein and fluid loss into the burn tissue and thus increases chest wall oedema.

◆ Increased chest wall resistance from burned skin can lead to laboured breathing and rapid respiratory deterioration.

In such cases urgent escharotomy (surgical release of scar tissue) is usually required soon after admission and should extend into the fat and, possibly, through the fascia.

Arterial blood gas tensions must be monitored regularly, as pulse oximetry may be inaccurate (see later).

Soot in the airways should be promptly removed by aggressive per-endoscopic saline lavage to minimize local inflammation. Samples should be taken for bacteriological analysis and antibiotics (e.g. benzyl penicillin) commenced. Difficulty with the clearance of secretions increases the risk for secretion retention, and PEEP, bronchodilators, frequent suctioning, and physiotherapy are thus important therapies to minimize lung injury and deterioration in gas exchange.

Carbon monoxide (CO) poisoning should be considered in any patient burned in an enclosed space such as a building or vehicle. Confusion, drowsiness, or coma may be present as may the characteristic cherry-red appearance. Carbon monoxide levels in the blood may be rapidly measured as carboxyhaemoglobin (COHb) using a co-oximeter. Both arterial blood gas tensions and pulse oximetry will be unreliable as neither will recognize the percentage of haemoglobin molecules being occupied by carbon monoxide rather than oxygen. Carbon monoxide has 200–250 times the affinity for haemoglobin as oxygen, therefore, oxygen transport to the tissues may be severely compromised. High-flow, high-concentration oxygen should be administered immediately and continued until COHb levels fall below 10%. The half-life of carboxyhaemoglobin is 4 hours when breathing air, and only 45 min on 100% oxygen. Carbon monoxide toxicity may also cause a metabolic acidosis by poisoning the mitochondria, the ATP-generating organelles within cells.

Hydrogen cyanide poisoning may also occur from fires in enclosed spaces. This will also poison the mitochondria. Treatment is to administer 100% oxygen as soon as possible. Antidotes, such as sodium thiosulphate or dicobalt edetate, have particular dangers in themselves and should be reserved for cases where cyanide poisoning is known to have occurred or is strongly suspected and the patient's condition is deteriorating. Clues to making the diagnosis include increasing drowsiness and a progressive metabolic acidosis despite adequate fluid resuscitation. Confirmation by measuring plasma cyanide levels will take several days and there may be insufficient time to wait in life-threatening situations.

Renal

Renal failure can develop for several reasons. Most commonly, it results from hypoperfusion of the kidneys. Compartment syndrome can develop as a result of loss of tissue elasticity and requires early escharotomy to preserve tissue perfusion (note: late escharotomy can result in the release of lactic acid, potassium, and other metabolites from dead tissue with subsequent cardiovascular collapse). Rhabdomyolysis can occur as a result of compartment syndrome or burn injury and is diagnosed by an elevated serum creatinine kinase and myoglobinuria. To prevent renal failure in the presence of rhabdomyolysis, increased fluid resuscitation, urinary alkalinization, and aggressive diuresis is required. Urine output, urea, and creatinine must be closely monitored. Renal support in the form of dialysis or haemofiltration may be required.

Metabolic

Hyperkalaemia can develop early in the burn patient as a result of both the metabolic acidosis and release of potassium from damaged tissue. This will usually resolve with fluid resuscitation and correction of the acidosis. Hypokalaemia is also common during resuscitation and can be exaggerated by nasogastric loss and diarrhoea. Hyponatraemia can occur due to loss of sodium through the burn wound and dilution during fluid administration. Inflammatory mediators may generate a systemic inflammatory response syndrome (SIRS) and increases the potential for circulatory failure.

Burn injuries cause an increase in metabolic rate. This begins at about day 5 and gradually increases, until, by day 10, the metabolic rate is about 2.5 times normal. The hypermetabolic state is characterized by increased oxygen consumption, heat production, body temperature, hyperglycaemia, and protein catabolism. Cardiac output and carbon dioxide production can double.

Malnutrition may cause poor wound healing and an increase in mortality. Adequate and early institution of nutritional support is therefore vital (ideally within 24 hours of the burn injury). If enteral feeding is required, a fine-bore, polyurethane nasogastric tube should be passed as soon as possible after admission. Vitamin and mineral requirements, particularly zinc, iron, and vitamins B and C, increase in burn injuries and these may need to be supplemented. If the gut is inaccessible or non-functioning, total parenteral nutrition must be considered.

Pain

Pain can be considerable in all but full thickness burns. Continuous intravenous opiate infusions are necessary and can be supplemented by benzodiazepines. There is often an increased need with dressing changes and physiotherapy and Entonox (oxygen/nitrous oxide) or Ketamine can be administered if the patient is conscious.

Infection

Sepsis accounts for 50% of deaths from burn injuries. The immune system is generally depressed in severe injuries but prophylactic administration of antibiotics is not recommended unless there is evidence of an inhalation injury. In this case penicillin should be used as the main threat comes from pneumococcal infection.

Wounds should be swabbed and cultured regularly and antibiotics only begun when a specific pathogen has been isolated. Strict aseptic technique during wound redressing, protective isolation, good nutritional support, and avoidance of unnecessary instrumentation will help reduce the incidence of infection.

Thermoregulation

With a deep burn the barrier to evaporative heat loss is impaired, promoting heat loss. This can lead to an increased metabolic rate as the burn victim attempts to maintain body temperature. Covering the wounds and maintaining a high room temperature can decrease heat loss.

Gastrointestinal

Gastric dilation and ileus are common in the patient with a burn greater than 20% of BSA. A nasogastric tube will minimize gastric distension and the risk of aspiration. Increased stress hormone output increases the risk of gastric ulceration and the patient should be monitored for evidence of gastrointestinal bleeding (malaena, coffee ground aspirate, $\downarrow$Hb). Some units will use prophylactic H_2 blockers, proton pump inhibitors or sucralfate.

Haematological

Anaemia may follow either haemolysis or blood loss. The plasma concentration of clotting factors may be diluted by the massive fluid replacement needed and DIC can occur as part of the multiorgan failure syndrome. Treatment is by appropriate replacement of blood products.

Surgical

Urgent escharotomy (or limb amputation) may be required soon after admission. Escharotomy is the surgical release of a constricting area or circumferential burn by incising down to the fatty layer. Anaesthesia is not normally required as the skin area affected is usually dead. Debridement and grafting (using cadaveric tissue or the patient's own split skin from an unburnt site) will be indicated for full thickness burns. If this area is large, debridement may be advisable in the first few days with tangential excision of the necrotic area. Massive bleeding can occasionally occur both during and following this procedure.

Wound care

Dressing procedures will vary considerably from unit to unit. The following notes are thus intended as guidelines only.

Prior to any dressing procedure ensure that analgesia is adequate. Dressings should be changed every 24 hours except for recipient graft sites, which remain intact for 5 days post-operatively. Clean burned areas with normal saline using a strict aseptic procedure and keep wounds covered to minimize infection. Flamazine cream (a topical antibiotic) can be applied directly to full thickness burns of the limbs, trunk, hands, feet, and ears. Hands and feet can then be lightly secured in plastic bags. This will allow passive exercises and physiotherapy to be carried out. Flamazine can be applied to a Lyofoam sheet for burns to the back. Partial thickness burns of the limbs and trunk can be dressed with paraffin gauze. Following the application of Flamazine or paraffin gauze, the area is covered with Lyofoam, then gauze or absorbent dressing, and then a light bandage. Burns to the perineum may be dressed with Flamazine or paraffin gauze and nursed exposed with the legs abducted. Eyes should be cleansed hourly with sterile water, chloramphenicol eye ointment applied, and moistened gauze swabs or Geliperm applied. Limbs should be elevated to reduce oedema. Following escharotomy the wound should be dressed with tullegras (or any non-adherent dressing), gauze, and crêpe bandages.

Aggressive wound debridement is essential for the removal of potential sources of infection such as bacteria and necrotic tissue. Dead tissue (eschar) must be removed with scissors and forceps or scalpels; small areas can be debrided during routine dressing changes. Scrubbing of wounds during dressing changes can enhance mechanical debridement and enzymatic debriding agents may be used to loosen eschar and promote removal. Frequent surgical debridement is optimal to remove non-viable tissue, but bleeding and fluid losses can be significant post-operatively.

Grafts

Deep partial thickness and very small full thickness burns will heal spontaneously but large, full thickness burns will require grafting. Autografts (from an uninjured area of the patient's own skin or an identical twin) provide the only permanent graft material. Grafting shortens healing time, improves the cosmetic appearance of deep partial burns and is mandatory for the healing of full thickness burns. The decision to graft may be based on the total percentage BSA of the burn and the need to conserve donor sites for full thickness injuries.

In large area burns, the same graft donor site may need to be used repeatedly as the only source for graft material therefore protection of this donor site from infection is critical. When autograft sites are sparse, donor skin can be minced and placed in a growth medium to increase the number of epithelial cells, or small pieces of donor skin can be dropped across a large burn in an attempt to increase the benefit from a small donor site.

Cadaver skin (allograft or homograft) can be used as a temporary dressing. Allografts will promote vascular ingrowth to seal the wound against bacterial invasion; however, they will be rejected within about 2 weeks. Xenografts or heterografts (from another species) such as porcine grafts can also provide temporary wound dressings but should be removed in 3–4 days or if a purulent discharge is noted (porcine grafts may be digested by the wound, becoming a source of infection).

Tubular support dressings are applied 5–7 days after grafting and provide a pressure of 10–20 mmHg in order to minimize contracture formation.

Physiotherapy

This is important in all burn patients in order to maintain joint mobility, muscle strength, and functional joint positions. Chest physiotherapy is probably useful for inhalational injuries, trunk burns (especially circumferential), bed-bound patients, and before and after surgery. Limbs may need to be splinted in order to minimize contractures and maintain the functional position of joints Passive exercises should be carried out frequently to maintain a full range of movement of joints and to maintain muscle power. Prior to physiotherapy, ensure that pain control is adequate. Try to coordinate physiotherapy with dressing changes to avoid excessive use of analgesia.

Psychological aspects

Psychological problems following the injury pose a major challenge. The patient and family need help in coming to terms with disfigurement or disablement. Considerable psychological support will be required over a prolonged period. Many ICUs have access to specially trained counsellors who should be involved at an early stage.

Near-drowning

Near-drowning is usually the result of submersion in fresh or salt water. However, aspiration of fluid is not always necessary to 'drown'—the so-called 'dry drowning' (see later).

Alcohol and epilepsy are sometimes major contributing factors. Deliberate hyperventilation prior to prolonged underwater swimming is also a common cause. Hyperventilation causes hypocarbia and the low levels of PCO_2 suppresses respiratory effort, even in the presence of severe hypoxaemia, thus consciousness is lost while under water.

'Dry drowning' occurs when little or no fluid is aspirated into the lungs while under water. It is thought that reflex laryngospasm is caused by the presence of water in the larynx and this prevents fluid entry into the lungs. This glottic spasm persists until death from asphyxiation occurs. The prognosis for near-drowning victims who have not aspirated fluid is fairly good, provided they are promptly resuscitated, since they are not then subject to the secondary complications of fluid inhalation.

The diving reflex and hypothermia are potential protective mechanisms in submersion victims. The diving reflex is initiated by cold water on the face and consists of apnoea, bradycardia, and intense peripheral vasoconstriction. Blood flow is preferentially diverted to essential organs such as heart and brain. Hypothermia decreases cardiac output, cellular metabolism, and oxygen consumption. It is especially protective if it precedes anoxia. Survival without neurological damage has been reported after periods of submersion of longer than 20 min—the longest reported to date is 66 min. Neither a long submersion time nor the death-like appearance of the victim are reasons for not resuscitating. It is thus recommended to commence resuscitation in every victim who has been under water for less than 1 hour, and to stop on the basis of objective diagnostic criteria only when the patient has reached hospital and has been warmed to normothermia. Cervical spine injuries are frequently associated with diving accidents and these must be considered during resuscitation.

Submersion is primarily a ventilatory disturbance with hypoxaemia the cause of cardiac arrest. The nature of the inhaled fluid will cause different physiological effects. In freshwater drowning, fluid in the lungs is quickly absorbed into the circulation causing dilutional effects that may lead to haemolysis. Pulmonary surfactant is denatured and widespread atelectasis can result. Electrolyte disturbances are usually mild and transient. Salt water contains higher levels of sodium and chloride and this causes mucosal injury and loss of surfactant. This fluid is hypertonic and thus water and plasma proteins move rapidly into the alveoli and interstitium, resulting in an osmotic pulmonary oedema.

In most drowning victims, the stomach also fills with water and there is a high risk of inhalation of gastric contents. This is particularly likely during resuscitation and cardiac compression. Inhalation of gastric contents will produce further inflammatory reactions in the alveolar-capillary membrane.

Management

There is little difference in management between saltwater and freshwater drowning. Therapy is directed at restoring the circulation and oxygenation, correcting electrolyte imbalance, and maintaining cerebral perfusion.

Problems

Hypoxaemia

Full cardiopulmonary resuscitation will usually be required initially and comatose patients will require endotracheal intubation. The presence of severe hypoxaemia and, possibly, pulmonary oedema mean that mechanical ventilation, high inspired oxygen concentrations, and PEEP are usually needed. CPAP via a facemask may be used if the patient is conscious and able to maintain a patent airway and an adequate arterial oxygen saturation. Hypoxaemia and intrapulmonary shunting can occur with the inhalation of as little as 2.5 ml fluid/kg body weight. Hypoxaemia is usually the major problem in submersion victims. Pulmonary oedema may occur soon after endotracheal intubation following relief of the larygoscopy and the very high intrathoracic pressures. Therapy with high levels of PEEP is usually effective. Secondary pulmonary oedema can occur after 24 hours and patients should therefore be closely observed for at least this period of time. Denaturation of surfactant can continue even after resuscitation and ARDS and pulmonary infection are common. The type of immersion liquid may influence the type of inhaled organism and, in many instances, mud, sand, and particulate matter are aspirated. Multiple abscess formation may ensue.

High inflation pressures may be required during ventilation due to bronchospasm caused by water aspiration and altered surfactant activity, atelectasis, and pulmonary oedema which cause a decrease in lung compliance.

Circulatory failure

Positive inotropic agents may be required if the patient is hypotensive and not responding to adequate fluid replacement (see Chapter 6). In theory, salt water should cause hypovolaemia and fresh water should increase the circulatory volume. However, in practice, such small amounts of fluid are aspirated that significant changes in blood volume are not seen.

Dysrhythmias may result from acidosis, hypoxaemia, hypothermia, and electrolyte imbalance. These should revert to a normal rhythm once these abnormalities have been corrected.

Hypothermia

Hypothermia is common in submersion victims. Core temperature must be maintained and passive/active rewarming instituted (see hypothermia section). (Note: Dysrhythmias may occur during rewarming.)

Electrolyte imbalance

Plasma levels of sodium and chloride may be elevated in saltwater drowning but serious disturbances are unusual. Electrolyte abnormalities may be associated with acute renal failure and magnesium levels may be elevated in saltwater drowning.

Renal failure

In freshwater drowning haemolysis may cause haemoglobinuria and consequent acute renal failure. Urine output must be closely monitored.

Neurological damage

Ischaemic cerebral damage can follow prolonged hypoxaemia and some patients will develop cerebral oedema. Attempts should be made to reduce raised intracranial pressure and maintain cerebral perfusion. Pyrexia must be reduced, oxygenation and circulation maintained, and blood glucose monitored (see Chapter 9). The patient must be observed for seizures and frequent neurological assessments made.

Gastric dilatation

Submersion victims often swallow large amounts of water. A nasogastric tube should be inserted to prevent inhalation.

Metabolic acidosis

This may develop following intense peripheral vasoconstriction and hypoxaemia. Lactate levels rise as oxygen delivery to the tissues falls. The acidosis should improve as the patient is rewarmed and hypoxaemia corrected.

The success rate of resuscitation in submersion victims is relatively high but a multitude of fatal complications may develop, in particular, ARDS and multiorgan failure, septicaemia, and pneumonia. Prognosis is poor if the patient is comatose following resuscitation.

Diving injuries

Too rapid an ascent from depth will result in nitrogen bubbles coming out of solution. This can result in neurological consequences including coma and seizures, and excruciating abdominal and joint pains ('the bends'). Treatment is by placing the patient in a hyperbaric chamber where a slow and gradual decompression from the raised pressure experienced at depth to the lower atmospheric pressure of sea level can be performed. This may take several days.

Trauma scoring

Trauma scoring is a means of classifying the severity of injury. Various scoring systems have been devised and these usually combine both anatomical and physiological variables. Some are simple and specific for a particular type of injury such as the Glasgow Coma Scale (GCS) for head injuries. Others are complex and may even combine several individual scoring systems (see below).

Trauma scoring will allow an evaluation of trauma care provided and a means of comparing outcome, either over time or between different hospitals. It can aid the planning and provision of resources in special units and identify those patients who will benefit most from the specialized care that can be provided in these areas. Scoring is helpful in triage where patients are categorized into treatment hierarchies, enabling identification of the most severely injured patients who may require immediate transfer to specialized units or priority treatment. It may also distinguish those with a poor chance of survival and when resources are overwhelmed (e.g. following disasters, where treatment could be directed initially at those critically ill patients with a better prognosis).

TRISS

One method of trauma scoring called TRISS (Trauma Score—Injury Severity Score) has a world-wide reputation for consistency and reasonable predictions of outcome. It combines two scoring systems: the Revised Trauma Score (RTS), and the Injury Severity Score (ISS).

The threat to life can be measured by the extent of the anatomical injury and the degree of physiological derangement. However, the age of the patient and the method of wounding also influence mortality. The TRISS method of scoring takes into account the patient's age and if the injury was blunt or penetrating. TRISS combines four elements:

1. Revised Trauma Score (RTS).

2. Injury Severity Score (ISS).

3. Patient's age.

4. Penetrating or blunt injury.

The score provides a measure of predicted outcome— the probability of survival (P_s).

The RTS (Table 11.8) is composed of the GCS (see Chapter 10) and measurements of cardiopulmonary function. Each variable is given a number and multiplied by a weighting factor (see Table 11.9) derived from regression analysis of a large US database. This

TABLE 13.8 The Revised Trauma Score (RTS)

Variable	Score					Weighting factor
	4	3	2	1	0	
Systolic BP (mmHg)	>89	76–89	50–75	1–49	Pulseless	×0.7326
Respiratory rate	10–29	>29	6–9	1–5	0	×0.2908
GCS	13–15	9–12	6–8	4–5	3	×0.9368

Note. Add the combined scores for each variable to obtain the RTS.

TABLE 13.9 Weighted coefficient values

Injury	Constant	RTS	ISS	Age
Blunt	−1.2470	0.9544	−0.0768	−1.9052
Penetrating	−0.6029	1.1430	−0.1516	−2.6676

reflects the relative value of that variable in determining survival. The numbers are then totalled to provide the patient's RTS, which should be recorded on arrival in hospital.

The ISS provides a numerical measure of the injury severity in patients with multiple injuries. Every injury is given an AIS-85 code and classified into one of seven regions: head and neck, face, thorax, abdomen and pelvic contents, extremities, pelvic girdle, external and burns. The AIS-85 code is an abbreviated injury scale last revised in 1985 by the American Association for Automotive Medicine. It incorporates codes for assessment of blunt and penetrating injuries. Each injury is assigned a six-digit code based on anatomical site, nature, and severity. The ISS is the sum of the squares of the highest AIS scores from three of the seven body regions. There is a significant correlation of ISS with mortality, morbidity and length of hospital stay.

Calculation of probability of survival (P_s) is as follows:

$$P_s = \frac{1}{1 + e^{-b}}$$

where P_s is probability of survival, e (natural logarithm) = 2.718282 and b is the RTS + ISS + age coefficient (age coefficient = 0 if age =54 yr, or +1 if age =54 yr).

Although this scoring method appears complicated, a TRISS chart has been devised to allow rapid determination of the probability of survival.

Despite being able to predict outcome reasonably well, the quality of life of survivours can vary considerably. At present, there are no methods that measure the quality of life after major trauma. However, trauma scoring will allow audit and, one hopes, improvement in the quality of care and outcome for trauma patients.

Test yourself

Questions

1. At which abdominal pressure is abdominal compartment syndrome said to exist?

2. Name four complications that may occur in the patient with multiple trauma?

3. Which dysrhythmias may occur in a patient with hypothermia?

4. What are the clinical signs of hypovolaemic shock?

5. What is a tension pneumothorax and how can it be identified?

Answers

1. Abdominal compartment syndrome is defined as an intra-abdominal pressure of >20mmHg (Webber 2002).

2. Shock (hypovolaemic, septic, neurogenic, obstructive or cardiogenic).
   Compartment syndrome.
   Fat embolism syndrome.
   Air embolism.
   Infection.

3. Bradycardias, atrial fibrillation, supraventricular tachycardias, ventricular fibrillation, and conduction disturbances.

4. Tachycardia, hypotension, low CVP and PCWP, pale skin with poor peripheral perfusion.

5. A tension pneumothorax exists when air is drawn into the pleural space from a lacerated lung or through a hole in the chest wall. Air that enters with each inspiration is trapped, and cannot be expelled, therefore tension builds up. The lung is compressed and collapses, pushing the mediastinal structures (heart, trachea, and great vessels) towards the unaffected side of the chest (mediastinal shift), thus impairing ventilation in the other lung. Cardiovascular collapse and electromechanical dissociation may rapidly result if

not treated. The diagnosis is made clinically as there is usually no time to take an X-ray before treatment is instituted. The clinical signs are: hypoxia, tachycardia, hypotension, absent air entry over affected side, deviated trachea with distended neck veins.

References and bibliography

AAAM (American Association for Automotive Medicine) (1985). *The Abbreviated Injury Scale*, revised edn. AAAM, Arlington Heights, IL.

ACS (American College of Surgeons) (1984). *Committee on Trauma. Advanced Trauma Life Support Course*, student manual. ACS, Chicago, IL.

Bickerstaff, E.R. (ed.) (1977). *Neurology for Nurses*, 2nd edn. Hodder & Stoughton., London.

Bierens, J.J., van Zanten, J.J., van Berkel, M. (1991). Resuscitation of submersion victims; wet CPR. In: *Update in Intensive Care and Emergency Medicine*, Vol. 14 (ed. J.L. Vincent), pp. 11–17. Springer, Berlin.

Bloomfield, G.L., Ridings, P.C., Blocher, C.R., *et al.* (1996). Effects of increased intra-abdominal pressure upon intracranial and cerebral perfusion pressure before and after volume expansion. *Journal of Trauma* **40** 936–43.

Borel, C., Hanley, D., Diringer, M., *et al.* (1990). Intensive management of severe head injury. *Chest* **98**, 180–6.

Boyd, C.R., Tolsen, M.A., Copes, W.S. (1987). Evaluating trauma care; the TRISS method. *Journal of Trauma* **27**, 370–8.

Brunner, L., Suddarth, D. (ed.) (1975). *Textbook of Medical–Surgical Nursing*, 3rd edn. Lippincott, Philadelphia, PA.

Bullock, R., Teasdale, G. (1990). Head injuries: I. *British Medical Journal* **300**, 1515–18.

Bullock, R., Teasdale, G. (1990). Head injuries: II. *British Medical Journal* **300**, 1576–9.

Burch, J.M, Moore, E.E, Moore, F.A, *et al.* (1996). The abdominal compartment syndrome. *Surgical Clinics of North America* **76**, 833–42.

Burch, J.M., Ortiz, V.B., Richardson, R.J., *et al.* (1991). Abbreviated laparotomy and planned reoperation for critically injured patients. *Annals of Surgery* **215**, 476–84.

Caldwell, C.B., Ricotta, J.J. (1987). Changes in visceral blood flow with elevated intra-abdominal pressure. *Journal of Surgical Research* **43**, 14–20.

Champion, H.R., Sacco, W.T., Carnazzo, A.T. *et al.* (1981). Trauma score. *Critical Care Medicine* **91**, 672–6.

Cope, A., Stebbings, W. (1990). Abdominal trauma. *British Medical Journal* **301**, 172–6.

Copes, W.S. (1988). *Major Trauma Outcome Study (MTOS)*, Report of the American College of Surgeons. ACS, Chicago, IL.

Deane, A. (1990). Trauma of the lower urinary tract. *British Medical Journal* **301**, 545–7.

Diebal, L.N., Dulchavsky, S.A., Wilson, R.F. (1992). Effect of increased abdominal pressure on mesenteric and intestinal mucosal blood flow. *Journal of Trauma* **33**, 45–9.

Diebal, L.N., Wilson, R.F., Dulchavsky, S.A., *et al.* (1992). Effect of increased abdominal pressure on hepatic arterial, portal venous and hepatic microcirculatory blood flow. *J Trauma* **33**, 279–83.

Gibson, R.M., Stephenson, G.C. (1989). Aggressive management of severe closed head trauma; time for reappraisal. *Lancet* **ii**, 369–70.

Gudmundsson, F.F., Gislason, H.G., Dicke, A., *et al.* (2001). The effect of prolonged increased intra-abdominal pressure on gastrointestinal organs in pigs. *Surgical Endoscopy* **15**, 854–60.

Gudmundsson, F.F., Viste, A., Gislason, H., *et al.* (2002). Comparison of different methods for measuring intra-abdominal pressure. *Intensive Care Medicine* **28**, 509–14s.

Hutchinson, I., Lawlor, M., Skinner, D. (1990). Major maxillofacial injuries. *British Medical Journal* **301**, 595–9.

Johna, S., Taylor, E., Brown, C., *et al.* (1999). Abdominal compartment syndrome: does intra-cystic pressure reflect actual intra-abdominal pressure? A prospective study in surgical patients. *Critical Care* **3**, 135–8.

Johnston, R.A. (1989). Management of old people with neck trauma. *British Medical Journal* **299**, 633–4.

Lozen, Y. (1999). Intraabdominal hypertension and abdominal compartment syndrome in trauma: pathophysiology and interventions. *AACN Clinical Issues* **10**, 1.

Mendelow, A.D. (1990). Management of head injury. *Hospital Update* **10**, 195–206.

Oh, T.E. (ed.) (1990). *Intensive Care Manual*, 3rd edn. Butterworth, Sydney.

Price, A.M., Collins, T.J., Gallagher, A. (2003). Nursing care of the acute head injury; a review of the evidence. *Nursing in Critical Care* **8**(3), 126–31.

Smith, E.J., Ward, J., Smith, D. (1991). Trauma scoring methods. *British Journal of Hospital Medicine* **44**, 114–18.

Swaine, A., Dave, J., Baker, H. (1990). Trauma of the spine and spinal cord: I. *British Medical Journal* **301**, 595–9.

Terry, T. (1990). Trauma of the upper urinary tract. *British Medical Journal* **301**, 485–7.

Trevor-Roper, P.D. (1978). *Lecture Notes on Ophthalmology*, 5th edn. Blackwell, Oxford.

Van Niekerk, J., Goris, R.J.A. (1990). Management of the trauma patient. *Clinical Intensive Care* 1, 32–5.

Webber, S.J., Mills, G.H. (2002). The abdominal compartment syndrome: an under-recognised and inadequately treated condition. *Care of the Critically Ill* **18**(4), 115–17.

Westaby, S., Brayley, N. (1990). Thoracic trauma: 1. *British Medical Journal* **300**, 1639–43.

Westaby, S., Brayley, N. (1990). Thoracic trauma: II. *British Medical Journal* **300**, 1710–12.

Willett, K.M., Darrell, H., Kelly, P. (1990). Management of limb injuries. *British Medical Journal* **301**, 229–33.

Wong, F. (2000). Prevention of secondary brain injury. *Critical Care Nurse* **5**, 18–27.

Woodrow, P. (2000). *Intensive Care Nursing: a Framework for Practice*. Routledge, London.

Wright, M. (1999). Resuscitation in the multitrauma patient with a head injury. *AACN Clinical Issues* **1**, 32–45.

Yates, D.W. (1990). Scoring systems for trauma. *British Medical Journal* **301**, 1090A.

Haematological problems

Physiology of the blood cells

The basic cellular components of the blood are:

- erythrocytes (red cells)
- leucocytes (white cells)
- thrombocytes (platelets).

Table 14.1 summarizes of types of blood cells.

Erythrocytes (red cells)

These cells have no nucleus and consist mostly of cytoplasm and haemoglobin. Haemoglobin constitutes about 34% of the erythrocyte cell mass but may fall to 20% when its formation in the bone marrow is deficient. Each cell is biconcave in shape with a cell membrane considerably larger than is required; this surplus allows the cell to change shape as it passes through narrow capillaries.

TABLE 14.1 Types of blood cells		
Cell type	Normal adult value	Function
Erythrocyte	Male $(3.8–5.6) \times 10^{12}$/litre Female $(3.4–5.2) \times 10^{12}$/litre	Oxygen transport
Leucocytes:	$(4–11) \times 10^9$/litre	Resistance to infection and antibody production
neutrophil	$(2.0–8.0) \times 10^9$/litre	
eosinophil	$(0.1–0.5) \times 10^9$/litre	
basophil	$(0.01–0.1) \times 10^9$/litre	
monocyte	$(0.1–0.8) \times 10^9$/litre	
lymphocyte	$(1.0–4.0) \times 10^9$/litre	
Thrombocyte	$(150–400) \times 10^9$/litre	Blood clotting

TERMS ASSOCIATED WITH ERYTHROCYTES

Anaemia: this is defined as a haemoglobin level of less than 11.5 g/dl in the adult female or less than 13.0 g/dl in the adult male.

Erythrocyte sedimentation rate (ESR): this is the rate at which red cells will settle under gravity in a sample of blood. A blood sample is placed in a standard 100 mm long test tube, and after 1 hour the rate of sedimentation should be no more than 10 mm. Diseases involving inflammation, tissue destruction, or blood hyperviscosity will increase the sedimentation rate and this can serve as a useful guide to disease progression.

All blood cells are derived from a single cell type in the bone marrow, known as a pluripotent stem cell. The pluripotent stem cell gives rise to a myeloid stem cell and a lymphoid stem cell from which erythrocytes, leucocytes, and thrombocytes develop (Fig. 14.1).

Red cell formation is stimulated by the hormone erythropoietin, which is produced in the kidneys. The release of erythropoietin is thought to be influenced by the presence of renal hypoxia, but the maximum rate of red cell production is only seen 5 days after its release and is therefore a long-term rather than an immediate response. Lack of erythropoietin, as seen in patients with renal failure, can cause severe anaemia.

Several vitamins and elements are vital for the maturation of red cells. Vitamin B_{12} is essential for nuclear maturation and cell division while folic acid is required for the formation of DNA. Vitamin B_6, thiamine, riboflavin, manganese, and, cobalt are also important. Iron is vital for the formation of haemoglobin and is obtained either by absorption from the gastrointestinal tract or from the breakdown of old red blood cells by the reticuloendothelial system.

The prime function of erythrocytes is that of oxygen transport. Haemoglobin has a great affinity for oxygen with 1 g of haemoglobin capable of combining with 1.34 ml of oxygen. Oxygen combines with haemoglobin in the lungs to form oxyhaemoglobin and readily dissociates from it in the tissues where the cellular oxygen concentrations are lower than that of the blood (for full details of oxygen transport see Chapter 4).

Red blood cells also have high levels of the organic phosphate 2,3-diphosphoglyceric acid (2,3-DPG) which plays an important part in oxygen transfer. In the middle range of oxygen tensions this compound combines with reduced haemoglobin and decreases the affinity of haemoglobin for oxygen. The more 2,3-DPG present, the more oxygen will be released at a given oxygen tension; the oxyhaemoglobin dissociation curve is thus shifted to the right. Anoxia increases the amount of 2,3-DPG in the red cell thus increasing the amount of oxygen given off when blood reaches the tissues (see Chapter 4).

Erythrocyte disorders

Table 14.2 summarizes medical conditions associated with red blood cell disorders. Only those disorders relevant to treatment in the ICU are described in detail in the text (i.e. polycythaemia and sickle-cell anaemia).

Polycythaemia

This is an increase in the red cell count to $>6 \times 10^{12}$/litre or Hb > 18 g/dl. Primary polycythaemia is where the blood cell mass is increased due to excessive production;

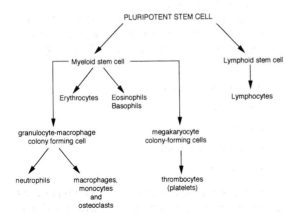

Fig. 14.1 Differentiation from the pluripotent stem cell.

TABLE 14.2 Erythrocyte disorders	
Disorder of:	**Result**
Production	Increased (polycythaemia): primary, secondary (e.g. altitude)
	Decreased due to: iron deficiency, folate deficiency, vitamin B_{12} deficiency, erythropoietin (non-production), bone marrow failure
Membrane	Hereditary spherocytosis
Enzyme	Glucose-6-phosphate dehydrogenase deficiency
Haemoglobin	Sickle-cell anaemia, thalassaemia

its aetiology is unknown. Secondary polycythaemia occurs when the red cell count is increased in response to chronic hypoxaemia and results from increased erythropoietin production. Conditions such as chronic obstructive pulmonary disease, cyanotic congenital heart disease, or adaptation to high altitudes cause secondary polycythaemia.

Primary polycythaemia (polycythaemia rubra vera)
In this condition, the bone marrow becomes more proliferative and all cellular factors—red cells, white cells, and platelets—are increased. There is a consequent increase in cell mass and thus blood volume. The resulting increase in viscosity of the blood and vascular occlusion causes cardiovascular, neurological, and vascular complications. Immediate treatment is aimed at reducing the blood viscosity, and this can be achieved by venesection to keep the haematocrit below 0.5. Concurrent volume replacement is given using crystalloids or colloids. Aspirin is also given to reduce platelet function.

More definitive treatments include cytarabine (to reduce platelet production), radioactive phosphorus, or chemotherapy to depress bone marrow production. Occasionally, such a condition may transform into acute myeloid leukaemia.

Sickle-cell anaemia

Normal adult haemoglobin (HbA) contains two alpha and two beta chains. There are two genes for the synthesis of each chain. Sickle-cell haemoglobin (HbS) has two alpha chains and two abnormal beta chains. The defect in the beta chain involves a single amino acid substitution and is inherited as an autosomal dominant gene. This defect leads to a chronic, haemolytic anaemia.

Patients with sickle-cell trait have mainly HbA and less than 50 per cent HbS. Sickle cell disease is predominantly found in individuals of African, Turkish, Indian, Greek, and Caribbean origin. The prevalence of the gene in these areas is probably because HbS protects against the serious effects of *Falciparum* malaria.

Sickle-cell anaemia occurs in homozygotes (HbS/HbS) and the consequence of this abnormal haemoglobin is that, when exposed to a low oxygen tension, the red cells become deformed, rigid and long in shape (sickle-shaped). These cells then became lodged and aggregate in small blood vessels in any part of the body, causing ischaemia or infarction. Abnormal red cells are also prematurely destroyed resulting in a haemolytic anaemia. Patients with sickle-cell anaemia suffer chronic ill health, thrombotic crises, leg ulcers, and infections. Many do not survive beyond 40 years of age. Those with sickle-cell trait are usually symptom-free unless the oxygen tension is very low since the HbA prevents the cells from 'sickling'.

Acute haemolytic crises (sickle-cell crisis) occur from 6 months of age. Haemolysis of the sickled cells produces anaemia and jaundice causing tachycardia and cardiomegaly; heart failure and arrhythmias may develop in older patients.

Vaso-occlusion causes infarction of tissues resulting in bone, pulmonary, or splenic infarcts, cerebrovascular accidents, haematuria, swelling (particularly of the toes and fingers), fever, and abdominal pain.

Acute splenic sequestration can occur and is a life-threatening complication in young patients. The spleen enlarges acutely and deformed red cells cannot be filtered and move back into the circulation. Anaemia rapidly develops, and as splenic function deteriorates the patient is at risk of overwhelming infection.

Pulmonary sequestration can also occur and can lead to rapid deterioration and death. Oxygen transfer in the alveoli is impaired leading to hypoxia that promotes further sickling. In combination with pulmonary infarction, consolidation and infection this is termed 'acute chest syndrome'.

Patients may be admitted to the ICU for management during these crises. Dehydration and hypoxia promotes sickling but the crises are unpredictable. Management is aimed at:

♦ adequate oxygenation

♦ rehydration

♦ pain relief

♦ prevention of infection

♦ exchange transfusion.

Correction/prevention of hypoxaemia   Blood gases and continuous pulse oximetry must be monitored closely; however, the normal values of haemoglobin and saturation when the patient is clinically well (the steady state) should be used as a guide for treatment. Many patients have steady state haemoglobin levels of only 5–9 g/dl. Those with low levels have HbS within the red cells that has a low affinity for oxygen, and maintain normal oxygen delivery because more oxygen can be unloaded per gram of haemoglobin. A higher level is therefore unnecessary. Oxygen saturations may also be lower than 90% in the steady state, therefore changes in saturation are more important than absolute values.

In order to maintain adequate oxygenation non-invasive or invasive mechanical ventilation may be required; however, there appears to be no benefit in attaining supranormal arterial oxygen tensions or saturations (Serjeant and Singer, 1999).

Rehydration   Increasing the plasma volume dilutes the blood and decreases the agglutination of sickled cells in small vessels. However, care must be taken not to overload these patients who usually have a cardiomyopathy and can thus be pushed into acute heart failure. CVP monitoring is usually necessary and occasionally pulmonary artery catheterization may be required.

Analgesia   Thrombotic episodes may cause severe pain in any part of the body. Oral analgesia or anti-inflammatory drugs such as codeine or diclofenac may be sufficient, but intravenous opiates such as pethidine or morphine may be required. Patient-controlled administration will give more sustained blood levels than intermittent injections and will benefit the patient psychologically.

Infection   The patient may often present with a fever and a raised white cell count during a crisis. Attempts must be made to rule out an underlying infection which, if found, requires appropriate treatment.

Patients with splenic dysfunction are prone to capsulate organisms such as pneumococcus and long-term prophylactic penicillin may be advocated.

Blood transfusion   If a crisis is severe, exchange blood transfusions may be carried out in order to reduce the levels of HbS. This is usually reserved for patients who have a rapid drop in haemoglobin, those who develop chest or cerebral crises, a severe painful crisis not responding to other therapy, or pre-operatively if elective surgery is required.

Leucocytes (white cells)

The function of the leucocyte is to resist infection by phagocytosis or by forming antibodies against foreign material or agents. Phagocytosis is the process by which white cells engulf a foreign agent and then destroy it by the release of digesting enzymes within the cell.

Most of the white cells are formed in the bone marrow. There are five types:

- neutrophils
- eosinophils
- basophils
- monocytes
- lymphocytes.

Neutrophils, eosinophils, and basophils are collectively known as granulocytes.

Neutrophils

Neutrophils are an essential part of the defence against infection and account for 40–75% of the white cell count.

When an area of tissue becomes inflamed it releases inflammatory mediators such as cytokines, for example interleukin-1 (IL-1), tumour necrosis factor (TNF), and histamine. These increase the number of neutrophils in the blood by up to four-fold. Neutrophils respond to chemotactic stimuli due to receptors on their cell wall and are directed into the area of infection. They engulf foreign matter by phagocytosis, and bacteriocidal enzymes, contained in granules within the cytoplasm, degrade the microorganism.

The normal concentration of neutrophils is influenced by age, gender, and ethnic origin. Females have a higher normal range than males and some non-Caucasian populations have lower ranges.

'Neutrophilia' is a term used to describe an increase in the number of circulating neutrophils in the blood. Leucocytosis is also often used in this context although it strictly means an increase in the number of circulating white cells of all varieties, not just neutrophils. Neutrophilia will occur following infection, trauma, burn injury, or tissue necrosis.

Eosinophils

These are weak phagocytes but collect at sites of antigen–antibody reactions in the tissues where they can phagocytose the antigen–antibody complex. They increase in number in allergic conditions (e.g. asthma and drug allergies) and parasitic infections, collecting around areas where histamine is released.

Basophils

These resemble the mast cells, which are found just outside the capillaries and are responsible for liberating heparin into the blood. It is possible that basophils may, in fact, be cells that are transported to the tissues where they then become mast cells. However, basophils provide a similar function as mast cells in that they release heparin into the blood, which prevents coagulation, and also produce small quantities of bradykinin and serotonin.

Monocytes

These are very active phagocytes and large numbers will infiltrate areas of inflammation The rate of monocyte production in the bone marrow increases with chronic infections (e.g. tuberculosis, endocarditis).

Lymphocytes

These are produced mainly in the lymph organs and nodes. B lymphocytes play an important part in the formation of antibodies and T lymphocytes are necessary for cellular immunity (e.g. in the non-rejection of transplant organs). The inflammatory reaction is very complex and is discussed in more detail in Chapter 15.

Tissue injury causes a local sympathetic reflex which results in an increased blood flow, a consequent increase in blood cells, and redness in the area of injury. Macrophage monocytes release cytokines such as IL-l, TNF, serotonin, and histamine. Histamine causes local swelling. IL-1 and TNF stimulate an increase in basophils, eosinophils, and lymphocytes and cause an

---

CAUSES OF NEUTROPENIA INCLUDE:

- Infection (bacterial and viral)
- Drug related (e.g. adriomycin, phenytoin, carbimazole, thiazides)
- Systemic lupus erythematosus
- Rheumatoid arthritis
- Crohn's disease
- Vitamin B_{12} and folate deficiency
- Lymphomas, Hodgkin's disease, carcinoma
- Autoimmune hepatitis

---

increase in production of granulocyte macrophage colony-stimulating factor (GM-CSF), which, with histamine, results in increased neutrophil and eosinophil chemotaxia. The Gram-negative bacteria cell wall also contains endotoxin. This stimulates inflammatory mediators (e.g. macrophages to release cytokines) and activates complement (catalysts which in turn stimulate other inflammatory mechanisms such as helping white cells to bind to bacteria).

Leucocyte disorders

Neutropenia

Neutropenia is defined as a neutrophil count below the normal range, taking into account the gender, age, and ethnic origin of the patient. It occurs when neutrophil survival in the circulation is decreased due to sepsis or immune destruction, or their production in the bone marrow is insufficient. The most common causes are viral infections and drug related.

Patients with neutropenia are at considerable risk from infection, and if severely neutropenic (below 0.2×10^9/litre) they are unable to mount an inflammatory response to infection. In such patients the normal signs of infection may be absent and they may deteriorate rapidly if not closely monitored. Pyrexia may be the only indication that infection is present and early treatment with broad-spectrum antibiotics is essential. If serial blood cultures are negative, fungal infection should be considered, particularly if the patient has been receiving high-dose corticosteroid therapy or has undergone organ transplantation.

The leukaemias

The leukaemias are neoplastic disorders of the blood-forming tissues (bone marrow, spleen, and lymphatic system). Commonly, there is unregulated and prolific accumulation of white cells in the bone marrow, liver,

---

TERMS ASSOCIATED WITH LEUCOCYTES

Leucopenia: the white cell count is $<4 \times 10^9$/litre. This may be due to a generalized bone marrow disorder (e.g. megaloblastic anaemia, aplasia, acute leukaemia, or metastatic tumour), viral or bacterial infections, or drug toxicity.

Leucocytosis: the white cell count is $>11 \times 10^9$/litre.

Neutropenia: the neutrophil count is $<1.0 \times 10^9$/litre (severe neutropenia is $<0.5 \times 10^9$/litre).

Eosinophilia: the eosinophil count is $>0.4 \times 10^9$/litre.

Lymphocytosis: the lymphocyte count is $>3.5 \times 10^9$/litre.

Monocytosis: the monocyte count is $>0.8 \times 10^9$/litre.

Agranulocytosis: a condition where the bone marrow stops producing white cells leaving the body open to overwhelming infection. It is often caused by irradiation or drug toxicity (e.g. carbimazole).

spleen, and lymph nodes with invasion of the gastro-intestinal tract, meninges, skin, and kidneys. They are classified according to the cell line involved and are either acute or chronic. Leukaemia may be caused by irradiation but the cause is often unknown.

The symptoms of acute leukaemias reflect the infiltration of organs by white cells and/or bone marrow failure. Infiltration can cause local pain in the liver, spleen, and lymph nodes as well as bone pain due to expansion of the marrow.

Bone marrow failure results in:

* anaemia causing lethargy and pallor,
* granulocytopenia causing increased risk of infection,
* thrombocytopenia causing increased risk of bleeding.

Summary of the types of leukaemia

Acute lymphatic leukaemia (ALL)   This type is more common in children. It is a severe disease where lymph nodes, bone, and nervous tissue can become infiltrated. Therapy aims to induce a remission by cytotoxic agents and irradiation of the central nervous system. Fifty per cent of children between the ages of 2 and 11 years survive for 5 years.

Chronic lymphatic leukaemia (CLL)   This occurs mainly in adults over 50 years of age, and it is often discovered at a routine medical examination or blood test, as the patients are usually symptom-free. Occasionally, pleural or peritoneal effusions develop. If asymptomatic, no treatment is required but combined chemo- and radiotherapy can reduce the size of glands. Fifty per cent of patients survive for 5 years.

Acute myeloid leukaemia (AML)   This affects people of any age, but is more common in adults. Until almost a decade ago the outcome was extremely poor. However, with intensive chemotherapy regimens and bone marrow transplantation, 30–50 per cent of patients may now have long-term survival.

Chronic myeloid leukaemia (CML)   This often occurs in the 30- to 50-year age group. The onset is insidious with fever and weight loss. Splenomegaly, hepatomegaly, and thrombocytopenia may develop later in the disease. The white blood cell count is often very high. Treatment is with chemotherapy. Overall survival is about 3 years. However, with the use of allogenic bone marrow transplantation, particularly in younger patients, 50 per cent may have greater than 5 years' survival (see later for the care and management of malignant haematological disease).

Thrombocytes (platelets)

Thrombocytes are actually fragments of a large type of white cell called a megakaryocyte. Megakaryocytes are formed in the bone marrow and the tips of the cells are thought to extend into the blood sinusoid. These tips are then nipped off and circulate in the blood as non-nucleated platelets. Platelets are essential for blood clotting, the mechanism of which is complex and is discussed later.

Thrombocyte disorders
Thrombocytopenia

A platelet count of 150×10^9/litre is the lower limit of the normal range but bleeding due to thrombocytopenia is unlikely to occur unless the count is below 50×10^9/litre. However, bleeding can occur at higher levels if generalized infection is present.

Thrombocytopenia can result from an increased destruction or decreased production of platelets.

Idiopathic thrombocytopenic purpura

Idiopathic thrombocytopenic purpura (ITP) is a rare, autoimmune disorder where autoantibodies are directed against the platelets so that their lifespan is considerably shortened. It can affect any age group but is more common in young adults, particularly following respiratory or gastrointestinal viral infections. Symptoms usually begin suddenly with petechiae and mu-

---

CONDITIONS CAUSING INCREASED DESTRUCTION OF PLATELETS INCLUDE:

* Idiopathic thrombocytopenic purpura
* Thrombotic thrombocytopenic purpura
* Disseminated intravascular coagulation
* Drugs (e.g. heparin)
* Sepsis
* Extra-corporeal circulation (e.g. dialysis)
* Autoimmune disorders (e.g. AIDS, malaria)

CONDITIONS CAUSING DECREASED PRODUCTION OF PLATELETS INCLUDE:

* Drugs (e.g. chemotherapy)
* Uraemia
* Megoblastic anaemia
* Leukemia, carcinoma, lymphoma

cosal bleeding. The platelet count is low, bleeding time prolonged, but coagulation times are normal. The acute form is usually post-infectious and recovery can take from weeks to months. The chronic form has a variable course and often does not recover.

There is no definitive treatment. Steroids are often tried with variable effect. In the acute form, steroids tend not to increase the platelet count but may have a role in reducing the incidence of bleeding. High-dose gamma-globulin has also been advocated, particularly in patients with bleeding complications.

In the chronic form, a rise in platelets is usually seen within a week or so of commencing steroid therapy. Platelet transfusions may be required to control severe bleeding. In some patients unresponsive to medical management splenectomy may be required.

Thrombotic thrombocytopenic purpura

Thrombotic thrombocytopenic purpura (TTP) is a rare condition and the aetiology is unknown. The mechanism may involve the vascular endothelium, which becomes unable to produce a prostaglandin platelet inhibitor that normally prevents platelet aggregation. Haemolysis, widespread intravascular thrombosis, and thrombocytopenia occur, affecting, in particular, the gut and cerebral circulation but also the liver, kidney, and lung.

TTP usually affects young adults. The presenting features include abdominal pain, purpura, and fever. There may be hypertension and fluctuating (or permanent) neurological signs. Haematuria may develop and progress to renal failure. Mortality is high. The mainstay of treatment is plasma exchange (using fresh frozen plasma) in conjunction with steroids. However, once relapses occur treatment can be very difficult. If cerebral TTP occurs with renal failure, prostacyclin may be given but this therapy is controversial.

Drug-induced thrombocytopenia

Some drugs may cause thrombocytopenia, in particular quinine, heparin, antituberculous drugs, thiazide diuretics, penicillins, sulphonamides, and anticonvulsants.

Heparin can sometimes cause heparin-induced thrombocytopenia syndrome (HITS). This is where an immune reaction occurs to the heparin, usually after 7–10 days of use. Thrombocytopenia will develop and platelet aggregation can cause venous and arterial thrombosis. Treatment is supportive, with platelet transfusions as necessary, and avoidance of all types of heparin administration, including the flushing of arterial lines. Low molecular weight heparin can occasionally be successfully substituted for heparin if anticoagulation is required.

Uraemia

Uraemia can cause defects in platelet function and bleeding can be a serious consequence of renal failure. These patients may have a prolonged bleeding time and develop gastrointestinal bleeding, nosebleeds, purpura, pericarditis, and cerebral haemorrhage. A prolonged bleeding time may be reduced by blood transfusion, DDAVP (l-deamino-8-D-arginine vasopressin) or dialysis. Low-dose heparin or prostacyclin should be used to maintain the patency of the circuit if haemodialysis is required.

The clotting mechanism and fibrinolysis

Rupture of a blood vessel leads to exposure of collagen fibres in the vessel wall. Platelets adhere to the collagen and roughened areas of the tear, forming a platelet plug. The platelets can then produce up to 40 substances, including catecholamines and coagulation factors; these initiate the cascade of reactions that will eventually form a fibrin clot. The damaged vessel vasoconstricts in response to the trauma and the release of noradrenaline, adrenaline, and serotonin by the platelets. Blood flow to the area is therefore reduced and a more durable effort to seal the tear begins. There are two pathways which may be activated, the intrinsic and extrinsic. These merge to form a common pathway (see Fig. 14.2).

Intrinsic pathway

When the endothelium of the blood vessel is damaged a cascade of reactions involving factors V, VIII, IX, X, XI, and XII, in the presence of calcium ions, produces prothrombin activator. Prothrombin activator (also known as prothrombinase complex) is formed by factors Xa, V, and platelet factor III (PF3). PF3 is a reaction surface, or template, for the clotting factors.

Extrinsic pathway

This is initiated by the release of tissue thromboplastin into the blood from damaged tissue outside the circulation. A series of reactions, involving factors VII and X, in the presence of calcium ions, produces prothrombin activator.

Common pathway

This pathway then begins, with prothrombin activator catalysing the conversion of prothrombin to thrombin.

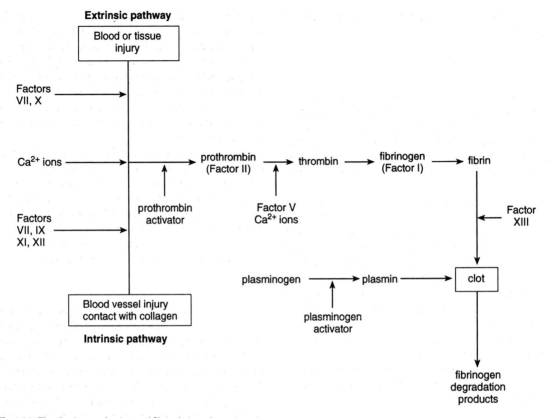

Fig. 14.2 The clotting mechanism and fibrinolytic pathway.

Thrombin acts as an enzyme to convert fibrinogen into fibrin threads, which forms the clot itself. Table 14.3 shows the blood-clotting factors.

There must, however, be a balancing mechanism to control clotting within the body so that the clot can be

TABLE 14.3	Blood-clotting factors
Factor	**Name**
I	Fibrinogen
II	Prothrombin
III	Tissue thromboplastin
IV	Calcium ions
V	Labile factor
VII	Stable factor
VIII	Antihaemophilic factor
IX	Christmas factor
X	Stuart–Prower factor
XI	Plasma thromboplastin antecedent
XII	Hageman factor
XIII	Fibrin stabilizing factor

dissolved when the injury is healed, and extensive clot formation prevented. The fibrinolytic system is responsible for the degradation of the clot and runs alongside the coagulation pathways. Its activation occurs immediately whenever the clotting cascade is triggered. Plasminogen may be activated intrinsically by the contact system via Factor XII, or extrinsically by tissue plasminogen activator found in many cells including endothelial cells. The activation of plasminogen produces the enzyme plasmin, which dissolves both fibrin and fibrinogen, thus lysing the clot.

The normal mechanisms of coagulation and fibrinolysis will complement each other until an underlying condition disturbs the body's homeostasis.

This traditional coagulation cascade is, however, inconsistent with clinical observations and is inadequate to explain the pathways leading to haemostasis *in vivo*. An updated, cell-based model has been proposed with the major initiating event being the action of Factor VIIa and tissue factor at the site of injury. In this model there is a continuous flow of reactants through the pathways, which are organized into three distinct steps. Haemostasis takes place on the surfaces of two cells: the tisssue factor-bearing cell and the activated platelet.

Clotting factor defects

Haemophilia

This is a sex-linked genetic disorder affecting men but carried by women. Haemophilia A is caused by deficiency of Factor VIII and haemophilia B (Christmas disease) by a deficiency of Factor IX. Clinically, they are indistinguishable. Haemophilia can cause severe bleeding from minor trauma and disabling muscle and joint haemorrhages.

Treatment is by administering purified Factor VIII or IX concentrate as soon as possible after the bleeding has started, or prophylactically before dental extractions or surgery. The aim is to raise the factor to above 30 per cent of normal. Repeated infusions may be necessary every 8–12 hours.

Fresh frozen plasma (FFP) contains both factors but vast quantities are usually required. This is usually given only if the single factor concentrates are unavailable. Patients with haemophilia should never be given aspirin as this impairs platelet function and may cause gastric erosions. Intramuscular injections must be avoided and dental hygiene is important since dental extraction can be so hazardous.

Von Willebrand's disease

This is an autosomal dominant disease affecting both males and females (these have different types of von Willebrand's disease). It is due to a mild deficiency of Factor VIII (15–50% of normal). There is a prolonged bleeding time and poor platelet adhesion resulting in variable degrees of bleeding. Commonly, patients have nose bleeds, post-operative bleeding, and bleeding from cuts, but do not suffer from the massive soft tissue or joint haemorrhages seen in haemophilia. Treatment is by the transfusion of cryoprecipitate (which contains Factor VIII) or by a purified concentrate of Factor VIII. Mild von Willebrand's disease may be treated by DDAVP infusion and this can also be used for prophylaxis prior to surgery.

Liver disease

The liver produces nearly all the factors involved in the formation and control of coagulation (except Factor VIII). Bleeding associated with liver disease can be devastating and difficult to manage. Liver disease may result in the reduced synthesis of all of the coagulation factors. Fat-soluble vitamin K, which is necessary for the precursors of factors II, VII, IX, and X, may not be absorbed if there is concomitant cholestasis. Disseminated intravascular coagulation (DIC) can be initiated or exacerbated by the release of tissue thromboplastin from damaged liver cells. The prothrombin time (PT) and partial thromboplastin time (PTT) are both prolonged in liver failure and the platelet count is low if there is splenomegaly. Fibrin degradation products (FDPs) may be elevated as a result of excessive fibrinolysis or because the liver fails to clear them from the blood.

Bleeding due to vitamin K deficiency may be reversed by the administration of vitamin K. Treatment of bleeding episodes associated with abnormal laboratory tests is by transfusions of FFP and platelets to maintain the platelet count $>50 \times 10^9$/litre and to normalize the prothrombin time. Low fibrinogen levels usually indicate severe liver disease or the presence of DIC. Cryoprecipitate can be used to increase fibrinogen.

Anticoagulant therapy

Anticoagulants are used to prevent thrombus formation or the extension of an existing thrombus. Such therapy is commonly used in the ICU, but always carries the potential complication of haemorrhage. Patients having anticoagulant therapy must be observed closely for signs of bleeding. This may be overt, with active bleeding from cannulae sites, drains, and wounds, or may be more occult (e.g. from the gastrointestinal tract: haematemesis, melaena).

Urine should be tested daily for blood and nasogastric aspirate also regularly observed or tested for blood. The skin should be observed for bruising, petechia, or purpuric haemorrhages. Purpura is the extravasation of blood into the skin causing purple areas, which may be variable in size. Pinhead sized spots are termed petechiae and larger areas ecchymoses (bruises). Purpura result from the increased fragility of the capillary due to a deficiency in the number or function of platelets, or damage to the capillary wall due to antibodies (allergic purpura) or metabolic/bacterial toxins (bacterial endocarditis and uraemia).

In order to prevent haemorrhage the effect of the anticoagulant must be monitored carefully and regular laboratory coagulation screens will be required.

Anticoagulation is kept within a specific therapeutic range of values depending on the drug used. It is possible to measure activated clotting times (ACTs) at the bedside and this is a simple and quick procedure. ACTs are commonly recorded in the ICU in patients undergoing renal replacement therapy as such patients are frequently anticoagulated with heparin. The dose of heparin can then be titrated according to the ACT level.

TABLE 14.4 Coagulation tests

Test	Abbreviation	Normal value	Use
Prothrombin time	PT	12.3–16.1 s	Assesses the extrinsic pathway. Used as a guide to warfarin dosage. Prolonged levels indicate deficiency of factors V, VII and/or X, I, II
Activated, partial thromboplastin time	APTT	27.4–40.3 s	Evaluates the intrinsic and common pathways. Prolonged level indicates deficiency of factors VII, IX, XI, or XII in the intrinsic pathway or factors II, V or X in the common pathway
Kaolin partial thromboplastin time	KPTT	<7 s above control	Assesses the intrinsic and common pathway as for APTT. The only difference between APTT and KPTT is the type of activator used
Thrombin time	TT	Control ±3 s	Assesses the conversion of fibrinogen to fibrin. Prolonged levels due to inhibition of fibrin formation and is an indication of the presence of FDPs
Fibrinogen degradation products	FDPs	<10 mg/ml	FDP's result from the breakdown of fibrin
Bleeding time		<8 min	Measures the effectiveness of platelet clots and their interaction with the vessel wall
Fibrinogen level		1.7–3.1 g/litre	Reduced levels found in deficiency of fibrinogen or with inappropriate activation of fibrinolysis

The value of the ACT aimed for will, however, vary according to the patient's clinical state and the purpose of the anticoagulation. Patients with extracorporeal circuits for renal replacement therapy usually require an ACT in the region of 170–200 s whilst those on cardiopulmonary bypass will need 400–600 s. The ACT cannot be used for determining the anticoagulant action of prostacyclin. (See Table 14.4 for coagulation tests.)

Anticoagulants commonly used in the ICU
Heparin

This is commonly used, for example, in patients with pulmonary embolus, deep vein thrombosis, and those undergoing heart surgery or renal replacement therapy. Heparin is administered intravenously, acts rapidly, but has a short half-life of about 90 min. Heparin may prolong the clotting time if heparin-induced antibodies block platelet aggregation. Heparin overdose may be corrected by stopping the heparin and, if necessary, by the intravenous administration of protamine sulphate. When used alone, protamine sulphate has an anticoagulant effect but when given in the presence of heparin, a stable salt is formed and the anticoagulant activity of both is lost: 1 mg of protamine sulphate will neutralize 100 IU of heparin, and is usually given in small doses with laboratory monitoring to assess the effect.

Warfarin

This is given orally and takes 36–48 hours' loading to achieve full anticoagulation. It is commonly used, for

example, in patients with poorly controlled atrial fibrillation or prosthetic heart valves to prevent thrombus formation. Warfarin antagonizes the effects of vitamin K, which is a co-factor for an enzyme essential for the synthesis of prothrombin and factors VII, IX, and X. It thus depresses the formation of the coagulation factors.

Warfarin readily combines with plasma proteins in the blood and can be displaced by some drugs (such as aspirin, chloral hydrate, and naladixic acid), so that levels of free warfarin in the blood rise. Other drugs, such as quinine, quinidine, and large doses of salicylates, further depress prothrombin formation in the liver. Patients receiving such drugs in combination with warfarin, are subject to increased sensitivity and must be monitored carefully.

The dosage of warfarin is controlled by regular estimations of the international normalized ratio (INR) which is derived from the prothrombin time. The INR is a ratio that relates the sensitivity of the thromboplastin reagent used in the PT test to that of a World Health Organization standard. The INR should be kept between 2.0 and 4.5, depending on the reason for anticoagulation. Warfarin overdose can be treated by the administration of vitamin K. This antagonizes the effect of warfarin in the liver cells and is necessary for the production of clotting factors. It, however, may take up to 24 hours to act and a dose greater than 10 mg will prevent oral anticoagulants from acting for up to several weeks. If the patient is bleeding, fresh frozen plasma (FFP) can be transfused to provide an immediate supply of the deficient clotting factors.

Streptokinose and tissue plasminogen activator

Both are fibrinolytic drugs that are used to break down a thrombus that has already formed (e.g. in acute myocardial infarction or pulmonary embolism). Tissue plasminogen activator (tPA) specifically activates fibrin-bound plasminogen while streptokinase can also activate circulating plasminogen.

Plasminogen is usually inactive until triggered. It is the precursor of plasmin, a proteolytic enzyme that dissolves fibrin. Allergic reactions to streptokinase can occur but are rare with tPA. Bleeding can be a major problem in fibrinolytic therapy and fibrinolysis can be corrected by the intravenous administration of tranexamic acid (plus FFP, cryoprecipitate, and blood transfusion, as necessary).

Epoprostenol sodium (prostacyclin)

Epoprostenol is a naturally occurring prostaglandin. It is a potent inhibitor of platelet aggregation and the degree of inhibition is dose-related. The effect on the platelets usually disappears within 30 min of discontinuing the infusion.

It is used as an alternative to heparin in renal support therapy where a high risk of bleeding from heparin exists. It must be given as a continuous infusion either intravenously or into the extracorporeal circuit.

Epoprostenol is also a potent vasodilator; hypotension and tachycardia may occur. If hypotension occurs the dose should be reduced or the infusion discontinued and supportive measures, such as plasma volume expansion, instituted.

Aspirin

Aspirin inhibits the cyclo-oxygenase enzyme in the pathway for the formation of thromboxane. It therefore inhibits platelet aggregation and the ensuing coagulation.

Clotting disorders

Disseminated intravascular coagulation

Disseminated intravascular coagulation (DIC) is an inappropriate, accelerated, and systemic activation of the coagulation cascade leading to the formation of soluble or insoluble fibrin within the circulation. DIC never occurs as a primary disorder but always arises as a secondary complication of an underlying condition (Table 14.5). Often, the primary condition that has induced the DIC will dominate the clinical picture, and the development of the syndrome provides a diagnostic and management challenge. The mortality of patients with DIC can be extremely high.

The normal mechanism of coagulation and fibrinolysis complement each other until an underlying condition or trigger disturbs this fine balance. The pathogenesis of DIC is complex, and the trigger mechanisms can also be complicated by hypoxia, acidosis, and hyperpyrexia.

The normal intact endothelium has an anticoagulant effect due to the secretion of prostaglandins which prevent platelet aggregation. Vascular damage exposes collagen fibres, attracts platelets, and triggers the intrinsic pathway of coagulation. Damage to the endothelium (e.g. by burns, trauma, or severe head injury), cytokine release, and bacterial endotoxin cause the release of tissue factor from endothelial cells and macrophages. Via a specific pathway, tissue factor leads to the conversion of prothrombin to thrombin.

Thrombin causes the deposition of fibrin within the microvasculature and the release of plasmin and other

TABLE 14.5 Disorders that may trigger disseminated intravascular coagulation (DIC)

Infection	Viral disease (varicella, rubella)
	Bacterial infections
	Parasitic infections
Obstetric	Septic abortion
	Eclampsia
	Amniotic fluid embolism
	Placental abruption
Liver	Cirrhosis
	Cholestasis
	Acute hepatic necrosis
Malignant disease	Carcinoma
	Leukaemia
Others	Crush injuries
	Burns
	Hypovolaemic shock
	Pulmonary embolism
	Organ transplant rejection
	Heat stroke
	ARDS
	ABO incompatible blood transfusions
	Penetrating head injuries
	Extra corporeal circulatory bypass
	Acute pancreatitis
	Myocardial infarction
	Fat embolism
	Falciparum malaria
	Snake venoms

LABORATORY VALUES IN DIC

(For normal values see Table 14.4)

- Prolonged prothrombin time >15 s
- Prolonged partial thromboplastin time >60–90 s
- Prolonged thrombin time >15–20 s
- Low fibrinogen levels <75–100 mg/dl
- Low platelet count (<20–75) × 10^9/litre
- High FDPs >100 mg/ml
- Raised levels of D-dimers

proteolytic enzymes. Plasmin causes the degradation of coagulation factors and other substances that inhibit clot formation and platelet function. The result is the formation of obstructive thrombi throughout the small vessels of the body leading to multiple organ ischaemia, infarction, and necrosis, and the consumption of coagulation factors and platelets resulting in bleeding.

The natural defence against this widespread clotting is the fibrinolytic system. Activated Factor XII, thrombin, and endothelial cells all stimulate the fibrinolytic system to release plasminogen activators. These stimulate plas-

min to degrade fibrin into fibrin degradation products (FDPs). FDPs are potent anticoagulants and further potentiate the haemorrhagic cycle. Specific inhibitors of clot formation include acivated protein C, antithrombin, and tissue factor pathway inhibitor which control the formation of fibrin. Antithrombin also inhibits the production of thrombin and promotes the release of prostacyclin (PGI_2) from endothelial cells inhibiting platelet aggregation and white cell activation.

In the patient with DIC the reticuloendothelial system (which normally removes FDPs) is overwhelmed and the patient has a self-perpetuating combination of thrombotic and bleeding activity.

There is no single laboratory test that will confirm the diagnosis of DIC. In order to make a diagnosis, the interpretation of a variety of laboratory tests must be correlated with the clinical presentation of the patient and an awareness of the conditions that predispose to DIC. Serial measurements are required in order to monitor the progression of the disease and to administer the appropriate treatment.

Treatment of DIC

The treatment of an individual presenting with DIC secondary to another disorder presents a considerable challenge. There is no single universally accepted treatment

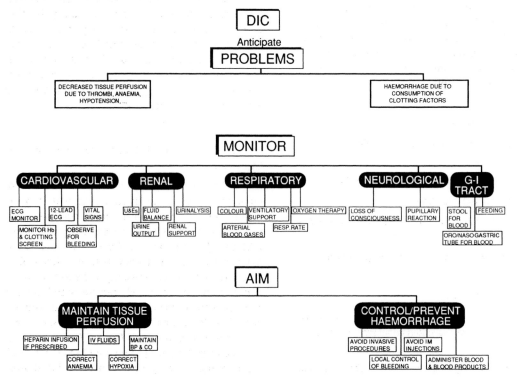

Fig. 14.3 The management of disseminated intravascular coagulation.

regimen and medical management is controversial (see Fig. 14.3). However, the agreed aims of therapy are:

- the elimination of the underlying cause;

- the restoration of haemostasis;

- the prevention of microemboli;

- the maintenance of blood volume and prevention of vascular stasis, hypoxia, and acidosis.

Transfusions of blood, FFP, platelets and cryoprecipitate are given in order to restore the blood volume and consumed coagulation factors while the underlying condition is brought under control. FFP is particularly useful as it provides all the clotting factors required; however, large volumes are needed. A platelet count below 50×10^9/litre in a patient who is actively bleeding would be an indication for platelet replacement therapy.

Heparin therapy may be indicated in situations of clear fibrin deposition in the form of dermal necrosis (e.g. venous thromboembolism), or when there is a retained dead fetus with decreased fibrinogen levels prior to induction of labour. However, mortality may be increased due to bleeding, and in 95% of cases of DIC there is no indication for heparin.

Protein C is activated and consumed in DIC process (Bianchi *et al.* 2001) and may prevent microthrombus formation and promote fibrinolysis. Infusions of plasma-derived protein C concentrate may protect against DIC and reduce the inflammatory response and consequent multiorgan failure associated with sepsis. At present, however, it is only licensed for use in patients with meningiococcal septicaemia.

Nursing management

The aims of management are:

- To identify the patient at risk of developing DIC (see trigger factors).

- Early detection and management of bleeding.

- To prevent further bleeding.

- To prevent the complications associated with decreased tissue perfusion or haemorrhage.

- To treat the underlying cause of DIC (if possible).

Problems associated with DIC
Cardiovascular disorders

- *Potential problems*: Hypovolaemia due to haemorrhage; skin necrosis due to decreased capillary refill or infarction.

- *Action*: Haemorrhage may be acute or chronic, insidious or massive. Some degree of hypotension is likely in DIC if there is a fluid volume deficit. Vital signs must be monitored closely in order to detect hypovolaemia and must be vigorously treated in order to prevent vascular stasis and maintain organ perfusion.

Cannulae sites, puncture sites, wounds, drains, and mucosal membranes must be observed for bleeding and the skin for petechiae and bruising. Observe for necrotic areas (particularly on the toes and fingers). Invasive procedures should be kept to a minimum in the patient with DIC. An arterial line *in situ* will avoid repeated puncturing of vessels for blood sampling and can be used to monitor blood pressure. If a blood pressure cuff is used it should be removed between recordings and alternate arms used if possible. Intramuscular injections should be avoided, but if essential, a small-gauge needle should be used. Mouth care must be gentle to avoid trauma to the gums. Local pressure or haemostatic dressings may be necessary if there is bleeding from cannulae sites.

Respiratory disorders

- *Potential problems*: Respiratory failure due to pulmonary haemorrhage, haemothorax, pulmonary embolus, adult respiratory distress syndrome.

- *Action*: Pulmonary bleeding will cause haemoptysis (in the self-ventilating patient) or blood-stained secretions on endotracheal suction. Respiratory function must be monitored closely (see Chapter 16). Oxygen therapy should be administered according to the arterial oxygen saturation but intubation and ventilation should not be delayed if the patient is hypoxaemic (despite the potential risk of bleeding associated with the procedure).

Renal disorders

- *Potential problem*: Renal failure due to microemboli or hypovolaemia.

- *Action*: The kidneys are a common site for microemboli and acute renal failure due to acute tubular necrosis often occurs. Urine output must be monitored and attempts made to maintain an output >0.5 ml/kg/hour in the adult. Oliguria can result from hypoperfusion of the kidney, therefore hypovolaemia must be treated aggressively and efforts made to maintain an adequate blood pressure (with inotropic support if the cause of hypotension is not volume depletion). If renal failure becomes established renal support will be required (see Chapter 9). Urine should be tested regularly for protein and blood and renal function monitored by measurements of blood urea, creatinine, and electrolytes.

Neurological disorders

◆ *Potential problem*: Cerebral ischaemia due to intercranial haemorrhage or thrombosis.

◆ *Action*: The patient must be observed for changes in conscious level, restlessness, agitation, visual disturbances, headaches, and sensory or motor function. Monitor pupillary reaction (see Chapter 10).

Gastrointestinal disorders

◆ *Potential problem*: Bleeding from the gastrointestinal tract.

◆ *Action*: Observe nasogastric aspirate, emesis, and stool for blood. Stools should be tested for occult blood. A mesenteric embolus may cause small bowel infarction and severe abdominal pain. Bleeding into the retroperitoneal space can result in varying degrees of pain, tingling, or numbness due to secondary nerve compression.

Blood transfusion and blood component products

Transfusions of blood and blood products are common in the ICU, both for the management of acute haemorrhage, where circulating volume and oxygen transport need to be restored, and in the treatment of a range of haematological disorders where specific components of the blood are needed.

Donated blood is collected and stored in closed plastic packs which can then be kept for up to 35 days at 4°C. Whole blood can be separated into its component parts after donation and stored separately. This is an economical way of using a valuable resource as several different patients can benefit from a single unit of blood. Specific blood components, once separated, have different uses and storage needs and these are detailed later.

Blood screening

All donated blood is screened for infectious risk and cross-matched with the recipient's blood for immunological compatibility. The purpose of cross-matching blood before transfusion is to ensure that there is no antibody present in the recipient's plasma that will react with any antigen on the donor's cells. The most frequent cause of giving incompatible blood is incorrect labelling of samples, confusion between patients of the same name, or failing to check from the label on the blood pack that the blood being transfused is the blood that has been cross-matched with the patient. Scrupulous and rigid checking procedures must be carried out at the bedside before any unit of blood or blood product is transfused. The patient identification details on the blood pack must be checked against those on the patient's wristband before the infusion is connected, no matter how urgent their need for the blood, as the consequences of giving mismatched blood can be dire (see transfusion hazards).

Blood and blood products

Fresh whole blood

This is blood that must used within 24 hours of donation. It contains functional platelets and coagulation factors. The use of fresh whole blood is now obsolete because testing to exclude viral infections takes 24 hours.

Stored whole blood

Donated blood is stored at 4°C in a special blood refrigerator from where it should not be removed for more than 30 min prior to the transfusion. Depending on the anticoagulant used in the blood pack, the red cells may remain viable for up to 5 weeks. The main use of stored whole blood is for the restoration of red cells and circulating blood volume in acute haemorrhage. It contains no therapeutic amounts of clotting factors, apart from fibrinogen, and no viable platelets or granulocytes. Whole blood is usually separated within a few hours of donation so that plasma, platelets and concentrated red cells can be stored under optimal conditions. The consequences of giving large volumes of whole stored blood are discussed later.

Packed red cells (red cell concentrate)

Much of the plasma is removed from whole blood leaving a concentrated solution of red cells to which 80 ml of anticoagulant nutrient solution is added. It is not given where volume replacement is needed but is used for chronic, persistent blood loss or bone marrow failure (e.g. anaemia, leukaemia). In the past it was thought necessary to maintain haemoglobin levels above 10 g/dl but there are no data to support this. Recent studies have shown that a level of above 8 g/dl is adequate, although some critical care patients such those who have cardiac disease, are elderly, or have COPD or cerebrovascular disease may need a higher threshold for transfusion.

Generally, in the anaemic patient, the transfusion of 4 ml/kg of packed cells should raise the haemoglobin by approximately 1 g/dl.

Leucocyte-depleted red cells

This contains concentrated red cells with no neutrophil-specific antigens. Alternatively, red cell concentrate can be used with a specific leucocyte-depleting filter attached to the giving set. It is used to prevent non-haemolytic transfusion reactions demonstrated to be due to leucocyte antibodies in the recipient. It must be stored at 4°C until its use and should be used within 12 hours of preparation. Check the pack carefully for expiry time and date.

Frozen red cells

These contain red cells, uncontaminated by other cells or plasma, in a suspending medium (usually saline). It is used in patients who have a rare blood group as a supply of blood; they donate blood and then the red cells are frozen for future use. Once frozen, these can be stored for an indefinite time but when thawed should be used within 12 hours.

Red cell concentrates can also be specifically CMV-negative or irradiated. CMV-negative products are from donors who have been screened for cytomegalovirus (CMV) and are found to be seronegative. They are used in patients who are recipients of bone marrow transplants or who may require one. Irradiation is actually used to destroy lymphocytes which can cause third-party graft verses host disease in the immunosuppressed patient. The CMV load can be reduced in leucocyte-depleted blood by using a filter.

Platelets

These are obtained by passing blood through a cell separator and may be from a single donor or random donors. A pack of random donor platelets contains platelet concentrate in 30–50 ml of donor plasma and is usually issued in pools of six packs. A single donor pack may contain up to 300 ml of platelets in plasma.

Platelet transfusions are used in:

- Patients with thrombocytopenia due to chemotherapy, radiotherapy, bone marrow failure, or congenital platelet defects.

- Cardiopulmonary bypass surgery if the patient is bleeding or has taken aspirin in the previous 10 days.

- Disseminated intravascular coagulation (DIC).

- Following massive blood transfusion.

- Platelet dysfunction disorders prior to surgery or invasive procedures.

- Prior to invasive procedures such as lumbar puncture, liver biopsy, CVP line insertion, epidural if platelet count is $<50 \times 10^9$/litre.

Platelet packs contain contaminating leucocytes, which may cause non-haemolytic febrile transfusion reactions. ABO ± RhD group-compatible platelets should ideally be given if possible, but in practice, any ABO group can be given if there is a shortage of ABO-compatible platelets. Rhesus-compatible platelets should be given to female patients of child-bearing age. If this is not possible, anti-D immunoglobulin should be given (50 IU per adult bag of platelets).

Once prepared, platelet function is best preserved at room temperature and must usually be used within 72 hours (check the expiry time carefully on the pack). Each pack of platelets should be transfused via a 170 mm in-line filter and specific platelet giving sets are available which have small filter surfaces and drip chambers to reduce the loss of platelets from volume left in the infusion line. Platelets can be infused as rapidly as the patient tolerates but should be completed within 30 minutes.

Fresh frozen plasma (FFP)

FFP is prepared in blood banks as a by-product of red cell concentrate preparation. The plasma is separated in a low-temperature centrifuge at 4°C and is then deep frozen within 30 minutes to –50°C. It is stored at –20°C and when needed can be prepared in about 15 min by immersion in a water bath at 37°C.

After thawing, the potency of the replacement factors deteriorate and therefore should be given as soon as possible and at least within 4 hours.

FFP contains normal amounts of all clotting factors, plasma proteins, and some contaminating red cell fragments. The ABO group of the FFP must be compatible with that of the recipient. Rhesus D compatible FFP should be given to women of child-bearing age. If this is not possible anti-D immunoglobulin should be given (50 IU per 200ml FFP).

FFP is used as a source of clotting factors for the treatment of DIC, the reversal of the effects of warfarin, and following rapid, large volume blood transfusions (1 unit of FFP is usually given per 5–6 units of stored blood, although replacement should be guided by clotting studies). FFP is also given to treat clotting factor deficiencies either when the deficient factor is not known or the specific factor is unavailable.

FFP is also useful in the treatment of liver disease where there is defective synthesis of coagulation factors, and is also beneficial in the treatment of thrombotic thrombocytopenic purpura (TTP) and haemolytic uraemic syndrome.

A pack of FFP is usually about 150–250 ml in volume. It should be given through an infusion set with a 170 mm filter. There is no added benefit in using microaggregate filters. It can be transfused as fast as the patient can tolerate.

Cryoprecipitate

Cryoprecipitate is prepared from FFP by collecting the precipitate that forms during controlled thawing and resuspending it in10–20 ml of plasma. It contains Factor VIII, fibrinectin, and fibrinogen. Cryoprecipitate is used to provide these replacement factors in haemophilia and von Willebrand's disease, or in patients with bleeding associated with hypofibrinogenaemia (<0.8 g/dl) or uraemia. It is usually prepared in pools of 6 units, each unit containing approximately 20 ml of donor plasma with Factor VIII, fibrinogen, and red cell fragments. ABO + RhD groups should be compatible between donor and recipient. Since six or more donors are usually involved in a single transfusion the likelihood of transmission of viral or bacterial infection is increased and anaphylactic reactions can occur to the plasma antigens.

Cryoprecipitate must be filtered because it contains cellular material from leucocytes, red cells, platelets, and fibrin. Transfuse through a 170 mm filter as rapidly as the patient's condition allows.

Notes on administering blood transfusions

1. If there are *any* discrepancies found when checking the identification details between the blood pack and the patient, do *not* connect the transfusion. Inform the haematology department immediately.

2. Gloves should be worn when handling blood or blood products in order to avoid skin contact.

3. Blood and component products should be administered through a 170 mm filter in order to remove particulate material. A fine 40 mm filter should be used in patients who are neutropenic as these will also remove leucocytes and leucocyte debris.

4. Do not use if the pack is perforated.

5. Do not mix any drugs or calcium-containing infusion fluids with whole blood or red cell concentrate transfusions.

6. If a unit of blood is out of the storage refrigerator or cooled transport box for more than 30 min it should be returned to the laboratory.

7. Do not store blood in the ward or kitchen refrigerator, even temporarily. It must be stored at 4°C (± 2°C) in a specified blood fridge.

8. When the transfusion is in progress be alert for transfusion reactions (see later).

Adverse reactions to blood transfusions

Blood transfusions are so common that it is easy to overlook the associated hazards. Unfavourable reactions usually occur within 20 min of starting the transfusion and it is during this time that particular attention must be paid. However, careful, continuous monitoring is vital throughout the transfusion, particularly in the ICU where circulatory overload can easily occur in patients with renal or cardiac impairment. Immediate transfusion reactions are usually due to pyrogens, allergens, bacteria, or incompatible blood, but delayed reactions can occur over a period of weeks or months. The acute reactions are:

- febrile non-haemolytic (due to cytokines released from transfused white cells)

- acute haemolytic (due to incompatible blood)

- allergic/urticarial

- anaphylactic.

Febrile non-heamolytic reactions

Monitoring of temperature is vital whilst a transfusion is in progress. Pyrexia may be due to pyrogens, leucocytes, or platelet antibodies. Pyrogens are polysaccharides produced by bacteria and can be present in distilled water, citrate, dextrose, and saline. Strict infection control procedures means that contamination has now been reduced, but febrile reactions may be caused by the presence of anti-HLA (human lymphocyte antibodies), granulocyte-specific, and platelet-specific antibodies in the recipient as a result of sensitization during pregnancy or from previous transfusions. Since pyrexia due to pyrogens is now rare, if it occurs it should be presumed to be due to incompatibility of the red cells, white cells, or platelets that have been transfused or to plasma proteins. Plasma proteins are the main cause of transfusion reactions. Urticaria and pruritis often develop in these reactions.

The fever should respond to antipyretics, such as aspirin or paracetamol. Antihistamines such as piriton (10 mg IV) in addition to hydrocortisone (100 mg IV) should also be administered. If mild the transfusion may continue slowly. However, if accompanied by rigors and a temperature exceeding 38°C, the transfusion should be stopped.

Acute haemolytic reactions

These occur when the red cells are destroyed in the circulation (haemolysed) following the transfusion. As the red cells break down, haemoglobin is released, and complement activation causes smooth muscle contraction, platelet aggregation, and the release of vasoactive substances. The reaction may be delayed or immediate and the consequences can be fatal. Most delayed haemolytic reactions are immune related and severity will depend on the red cell antibody involved. Most immediate reactions have an avoidable and identifiable cause and these can be the most dangerous. Immediate haemolysis can be caused by incompatible ABO blood groups, usually as a result of identification error (there is a10% mortality associated with this). Other immediate causes are incorrectly stored or out-of-date blood, over-heated, frozen, or infected blood, mechanical destruction of the red cells by administering the infusion under pressure, and the mixing of the blood with hypotonic infusion fluids.

The signs and symptoms of haemolysis can be immediate and severe. The patient may complain of pain at the infusion site, facial flushing, dyspnoea, headache, chest, abdominal, and loin pain. Nausea, vomiting, pyrexia, and rigors usually develop. Tachycardia and hypotension are common and may lead to complete circulatory collapse. Oliguria and consequent renal failure may follow. Other features of the reaction include the development of disseminated intravascular coagulation (DIC).

When a haemolytic reaction is suspected the blood transfusion must be stopped immediately. The blood bag must be retained and returned to the laboratory, together with samples of blood from the patient for checking the blood group and cross-match, full blood count, coagulation screen, fibrinogen, urea and electrolytes, and direct antiglobulin test. Blood cultures should be taken if sepsis is suspected. The full blood count, urea and electrolytes, and coagulation screen should be repeated 2–4 hourly. Full resuscitative measures may be required in order to restore cardiovascular stability. An ECG should be performed and urine output maintained at >1 ml/hour. A urine sample should be taken to test for haemoglobinuria. If DIC develops, replacement of clotting factors will be required.

Delayed haemolytic reactions are less severe and may occur over a period of days following the transfusion; symptoms include anaemia and jaundice.

Close monitoring of vital signs is essential for the early detection of immediate haemolytic reaction in any patients undergoing a blood transfusion. The sooner it can be identified, the transfusion stopped, and supportive treatment begun, the better the prognosis. Careful and rigorous attention to the correct procedures of storing and checking may prevent many such reactions.

Circulatory overload

This is not usually a problem in patients with normal cardiac and renal function. However, those with impaired function, the elderly, or the pregnant patient may not tolerate the fluid load associated with blood transfusions, and this may lead to the development of pulmonary oedema and heart failure. Careful monitoring of vital signs is again essential if this is to be recognized early. Dyspnoea and tachypnoea, elevated blood pressure, CVP, and heart rate may indicate fluid overload. In patients at risk, this complication may be avoided by the administration of a diuretic at the time the transfusion begins, and by the use of red cell concentrate instead of whole blood, when volume replacement is not required.

Transfusion-associated graft versus host disease

This is a rare, but usually fatal, complication of transfusion. It is due to engraftment of viable T lymphocytes, which cause widespread tissue damage. Patients who are immunosuppressed, such as those with Hodgkin's disease, bone marrow transplant recipients, and those with congenital immunodeficiency, are particularly at risk. Transfusion-associated graft versus host disease can be prevented by irradiating blood products (red cell, platelet and white cell transfusions) prior to transfusion.

Hazards of blood transfusion

Bacterial contamination

Contamination of the blood by bacteria is rare but may be lethal. Contaminants from the donor's skin may enter the blood while it is being donated. Usually, the bacteria responsible are staphylococci, which do not grow at 4°C and are killed during storage. However, any Gram-negative bacteria entering the blood will grow slowly at 4°C (their number doubling in 8 hours), and over several weeks of storage may be sufficient to cause a lethal septicaemia. It is essential that blood is stored at 4°C in order to minimize this risk as bacterial growth accelerates considerably at room temperature. The onset of pyrexia and circulatory collapse can be rapid if transfused blood is infected.

Transmission of disease

Donor selection criteria and the testing of donor blood for infectious agents have decreased the transmission of disease but can never completely eradicate it. Many of the organisms responsible far transmitting infection have a long incubation period and are stable in blood and blood products.

In 1983, the first deaths associated with transfusion-related HIV were reported. From 1986, those in high-risk groups were excluded from giving blood and all donor blood was tested for the presence of anti-HIV antibodies. However, the average delay in appearance of the antibody after the time of infection is 2–3 months, with 95% of infected people having seroconverted by 6 months. Thus donors giving blood within about 6 months of infection may not be detected. Factor VIII and IX concentrates used today in the UK carry a negligible risk of HIV transmission because of the use of anti-HIV screened plasma for their preparation. Furthermore, HIV appears to be inactivated by the heat treatment that such concentrates are now subjected to. Certain populations have a high incidence of viral carriers of hepatitis and post-transfusion hepatitis remains one of the mast common hazards of blood transfusion. Screening tests have been devised for hepatitis B surface antigen and the incidence of such carriers in the UK is fairly low. Transmission of hepatitis C is the cause of the majority of cases of post-transfusion hepatitis and there is now a serological test to diagnose this.

Cytomegalovirus (CMV) is a herpes virus present in white cells and found free in the plasma. The virus can persist latently after infection and it is possible that up to 3.5% of units of blood have the potential for transmission of the virus. The main danger of transmission of CMV is to infants and immunocompromised patients, and the only way to avoid transfusion transmission is by using anti-CMV-negative blood.

Malaria can be transmitted via transfused blood or products that contain red cells as the parasites can remain viable for a week at 4°C. Careful vetting of potential donors and screening for malarial antibodies is necessary now that travel to tropical countries is more widespread.

All donated blood in the UK is tested for syphilis and transmission by blood transfusion is now very rare.

Hazards associated with massive blood transfusion

A massive transfusion is defined as the transfusion of the patients' own volume of blood within 24 hours. Stored blood is deficient in platelets and coagulation factors. It is cold (4°C), acidic (pH 6.6–6.8), and contains citrate anticoagulant. Transfusions of large volumes of blood can therefore lead to metabolic and cardiac disturbances.

Hypothermia

A thermostatically controlled blood warmer should always be used when giving more than several units of blood to a normothermic patient as blood transfused at 4°C can rapidly cool the patient. If the patient is pyrexial, and the blood is not transfused rapidly, it may not be necessary to warm the blood until the patient is normothermic. Hypothermia increases the risk of cardiac arrhythmias, reduces metabolism, and shifts the oxygen dissociation curve to the left. Citrate toxicity (see below) is also more likely to occur when the patient is hypothermic.

Acid–base and electrolyte disturbances

Stored blood is acidic mainly due to the citric acid used as an anticoagulant and the lactic acid generated during storage. In the well-perfused patient, lactic and citric acid are rapidly metabolized by the liver, However, with hypoperfusion metabolism will be depressed and lactic acid production may continue increasing the metabolic acidosis. Frequent acid–base measurements are necessary to monitor this.

The sodium content of whole blood and FFP is higher than the normal blood level due to the sodium citrate anticoagulant (FFP contains approximately 35 mmol per unit and whole blood 49–53 mmol per unit, depending on the number of the days it has been stored). This should be remembered when giving such products to patients with renal failure or hypernatraemia.

Hypocalcaemia

Stored blood contains anticoagulants which cause calcium depletion. Following massive transfusions hypocalcaemia may occur, although physical manifestations are rare.

A fall in ionized calcium may cause tetany, muscle tremors, and cardiac dysfunction. Prolongation of the Q-T interval is seen on the ECG.

The routine use of intravenous calcium supplements during large-volume blood transfusion is controversial. Some authorities recommend that 2.2 mmol of calcium gluconate should be given for every 4 units of blood transfused. Others recommend that plasma ionized calcium levels should be monitored in the laboratory and supplements given as appropriate.

Haemostatic failure

Transfusion of the total body blood volume can lead to dilutional thrombocytopenia and haemostatic failure. Since stored blood contains no viable platelets and few of the clotting factors VIII and V, in these patients the platelet count will be reduced and the PT and KPTT increased. Laboratory monitoring is necessary to guide therapy; however, if it is unavailable, it is recommended that 2 units of FFP should be given per 10 units of blood transfused and platelet administration should be given according to the platelet count.

The ICU patient with haematological malignancy

Advances in supportive and antimicrobial therapy have meant that for many patients with malignant disease the long-term prognosis has improved. Although for some diseases mortality remains high, despite aggressive treatment, selected patients with life-threatening but potentially reversible complications can benefit from intensive care. Many of the reasons for their transfer to the ICU result from complications of the malignancy itself or from its treatment. These include:

- infection
- haemorrhage
- cardiac disturbances
- graft versus host reactions
- tumour lysis syndrome
- hypercalcaemia
- fluid overload/renal failure
- following extensive surgical procedures
- respiratory failure.

Infection

The most important cause of an increased susceptibility to infection is neutropenia. If the neutrophil count falls below $0.5 \times 10^9/1$ there is a very high risk of overwhelming infection and many critical care areas will advocate reverse barrier nursing for such patients. Scrupulous attention to hand-washing and hygiene is vital to minimize exogenous infection. Patients with neutropenia are susceptible to infection by bacteria (including atypicals such as mycobacteria), viruses, protozoa, and fungi. Most often the infection originates endogenously from the patient's own gut, airways, or skin. Broad-spectrum antibiotics suppress the normal bacterial flora; in the gut this can promote the overgrowth of pathogenic Gram-negative organisms. Chemotherapy can also cause areas of ulceration in the gastrointestinal tract and tracheobronchial mucosa. These areas can act as a focus for local colonization by organisms and may lead to invasion into deep tissues and septicaemia. There is a high incidence of fungal infection causing septicaemia and pneumonia (commonly *Candida* and *Aspergillus*). Herpes simplex and CMV are common viral infections and pneumocystis the most common protozoan infection.

Invasive procedures should be kept to a minimum and performed when the patient requires them rather than by virtue of being in ICU. Large-bore, soft Teflon catheters (such as Hickman lines) are often used for intravenous drug administration and are tunnelled subcutaneously to minimize infection from skin flora. Scrupulous attention must be paid to cannula insertion sites to keep them free of infection, and lines must be dated and changed according to hospital policy. Consider non-invasive methods of monitoring where possible (e.g. pulse oximetry, see Chapter 5).

Decontamination of the gastrointestinal tract by the use of oral, non-absorbable antibiotics to reduce the endogenous flora has been advocated. However, this may promote the emergence of resistant organisms. Selective decontamination, where the antibiotics reduce only the aerobic organisms but leave anaerobes to confer colonization resistance, has proved more successful but is costly, labour-intensive, and does not suppress all aerobic activity. Prophylactic antifungal drugs (such as 5-flucytosine) and antiviral drugs (such as acyclovir) have also been used with success in recipients of bone marrow transplants. In general, whatever antimicrobial therapy has been started on the ward is usually continued in the ICU.

Fungal infections (e.g. *Candida*) are common in warm, moist areas such as the groin, vagina, axilla, and in the mouth. Skin must be kept clean and dry and local antifungal cream applied as appropriate.

Mouth care is very important and a variety of antifungal preparations are available (such as lozenges, suspensions, and mouthwashes) and should be used at least five times a day.

Haemorrhage

Thrombocytopenia is the most common cause of haemorrhage and can result from bone marrow suppression by cytotoxic drugs, bone marrow infiltration by tumour, or sequestration of platelets in the spleen (in patients with chronic lymphatic leukaemia). DIC is common and may be a complication of septicaemia or the malignancy itself. Patients with leukaemia often have reduced levels of factors V, VII, and X and, in patients with liver metastases, production of clotting factors by the liver may be impaired.

Most patients with bone marrow failure will require multiple transfusions, particularly of red cells, platelets, and clotting factors. If DIC is present, FFP and cryoprecipitate may also be required.

Cardiac disturbances

Cytotoxic drugs can cause serious cardiac disturbances. Adriamycin in large doses is particularly cardiotoxic causing congestive cardiac failure, direct endothelial damage with myocardial necrosis, and cardiomyopathy. Some drugs cause a variety of acute dysrhythmias, particularly if the patient has existing cardiac disease. Cardiac tamponade can result from metastatic tumour, particularly those originating in the bronchus or breast. If the tumour extends around the heart a constrictive pericarditis can develop (this can also be caused by radiotherapy).

Graft versus host disease

This is an autoimmune reaction that can occur in allogenic bone marrow transplants. Immunocompetent donor T lymphocytes recognize the host histocompatability antigens as 'foreign' and produce a cell-mediated reaction against sensitive tissue, particularly the skin, gastrointestinal tract, liver, and bone marrow. It causes fever, diarrhoea, severe skin rashes, and hepatitis. Mortality is high and management is with steroids and appropriate supportive care. Mortality rates are approximately 25%.

Tumour lysis syndrome

The rapid lysis of malignant cells by cytotoxic drugs can cause hyperkalaemia, hyperuricaemia, hyperphosphataemia, and acute renal failure. This usually occurs in patients who present with a high white cell count (>100 × 10^9/litre). The patient must be kept well hydrated and is usually given allopurinol prophylactically prior to commencing cytotoxic therapy. Allopurinol prevents tissue urate deposition and renal calculi, which can occur secondary to elevated serum uric acid levels during cytotoxic therapy.

Hypercalcaemia

This is common in patients with malignant disease, particularly those with multiple myeloma. This can be due to invasion of the bone by tumour cells or stimulation of osteoclastic activity by mediators, such as osteoclastic-activating factor which causes bone reabsorption. Immediate treatment is aimed at reducing the calcium level by rehydration (3–6 litres/24 hours), furosemide (frusemide) (which prevents calcium reabsorption in the loop of Henle), calcitonin (which inhibits osteoclastic bone reabsorption), and sodium etidronate. Steroids are useful in reducing calcium reabsorption but this may take up to a week to show effect. Oral sodium phosphate is also effective but should be administered after hydration. For the long-term treatment of hypercalcaemia the cause must be removed by specific therapy (surgery, radiotherapy, or chemotherapy)

Hypercalcaemia is discussed in more detail in Chapter 16.

Fluid overload/renal failure

This is discussed in detail in Chapter 9.

Following extensive surgical procedures

Intensive care can benefit many patients undergoing lengthy, radical surgery to remove tumours. Such surgery (e.g. pelvic exoneration) can involve considerable blood loss and patients are often hypovolaemic on transfer from theatre. Continuous haemodynamic monitoring can permit optimal fluid replacement and preserve renal function. Analgesia can also be administered by intravenous infusion and titrated to achieve adequate pain control. Patients at high risk of respiratory failure are often electively ventilated post-operatively, especially if surgery is prolonged or the patient has pre-existing pulmonary disease.

Respiratory failure

There are a variety of factors that may precipitate respiratory failure in the patient with malignant disease and these are shown in Table 14.6.

Patients with malignant disease may also develop respiratory failure secondary to pleural effusions, fluid

TABLE 14.6 Causes of respiratory failure in the patient with malignant disease

Infection:	
Bacteria	*Klebsiella, Escherichia coli, Proteus, Staphylococcus, Pseudomonas*
Pneumococcal	
Fungal	*Aspergillus, Candida*
Protozoan	*Pneumocystis carinii*
Viral	Cytomegalovirus
Drug-induced lung disease	A variety of cytotoxic drugs (e.g. bleomycin) can cause interstitial inflammation
Radiation pneumonitis	Occurs approximately 8 weeks following radiotherapy
Pulmonary haemorrhage	Usually occurs only in patients with thrombocytopenia
Malignant lung disease	Metastatic spread of lymphoma or carcinoma
Tracheobronchial compression	Due to airway compression by tumour or haematoma formation
Adult respiratory distress syndrome (ARDS)	Secondary to sepsis, DIC, pulmonary aspiration, radiation pneumonitis or haemorrhage

overload, cardiac failure, pneumothorax, or may require endotracheal intubation following diagnostic surgical procedures such as mediastiotomy.

Mortality rates are high in critically ill cancer patients and those requiring prolonged ventilation and/or renal support have a particularly poor prognosis. Before such patients are admitted to the ICU the nature and progress of the underlying malignancy must be taken into account and the impact of ICU admission on the patient's quality of life must be considered. Invasive monitoring will limit mobility and intubation will prevent effective verbal communication. The requirements of life-sustaining therapy may simply prolong the patient's suffering. The admission of any of these patient's will almost certainly produce difficult ethical decisions which must be addressed on an individual basis for each patient.

Test yourself

Questions

1. What is the definition of anaemia?

2. In which conditions would platelet transfusions be necessary?

3. Name five causes of neutropenia.

4. What is agranulocytosis?

5. Name the five types of white cells.

6. What is primary polycythemia?

Answers

1. Anaemia is defined as a haemoglobin level of less than 11.5 g/dl in the adult female or less than 13.0 g/ dl in the adult male.

2. Platelet transfusions are used in:
   Patients with thrombocytopenia due to chemotherapy, radiotherapy, bone marrow failure, or congenital platelet defects.
   Cardiopulmonary bypass surgery if the patient is bleeding or has taken aspirin in the previous 10 days.
   Disseminated intravascular coagulation (DIC).
   Following massive blood transfusion.
   Platelet dysfunction disorders prior to surgery or invasive procedures.
   Prior to invasive procedures such as lumbar puncture, liver biopsy, CVP line insertion, epidural if platelet count is <50 × 10^9/litre.

3. Causes of neutropenia include:
   infection (bacterial and viral)
   drug related (e.g. adriomycin, phenytoin, carbimazole, thiazides)
   systemic lupus erythematosus
   rheumatoid arthritis
   Crohn's disease
   vitamin B_{12} and folate deficiency
   lymphomas, Hodgkin's disease, carcinoma
   autoimmune hepatitis.

4. Agranulocytosis is a condition where the bone marrow stops producing white cells leaving the body open to overwhelming infection. It is often caused by irradiation or drug toxicity (e.g. carbimazole).

5. The five types of white cells are:
   neutrophils
   eosinophils
   basophils
   monocytes
   lymphocytes.

6. In primary polycythemia, the bone marrow becomes more proliferative and all cellular factors—red cells, white cells, and platelets—are increased. There is a consequent increase in cell mass and thus blood volume. The resulting increase in viscosity of the blood and vascular occlusion causes cardiovascular, neurological, and vascular complications.

References and bibliography

Baughan, A.S., Hughes, A.S.B., Patterson, K.G., et al. (1985). Manual of Haematology. Churchill Livingstone, Edinburgh.

Bianchi, S.M, Gilligan, O.M, Eddleston, J, et al. (2001). Disseminated intravascular coagulation: pathogenesis and treatment. British Journal of Intensive Care 11(1), 21–4.

Bradbury, M., Cruickshank, J. (1995). Blood and blood transfusion reactions: 1. British Journal of Nursing 4(14), 814–17.

Bradbury, M., Cruickshank, J. (1995). Blood and blood transfusion reactions: 2. British Journal of Nursing 4(15), 861–8.

Cummins, D. (1999). Disseminated intravascular coagulation. In: Oxford Textbook of Critical Care (ed. A.R. Webb, M.J. Shapiro, S. Singer, et al.), pp. 668–670. Oxford University Press, Oxford.

Epstein, C., Bakanauskas, A. (1991). Clinical management of DIC, early nursing interventions. Critical Care Nurse 11, 42–51.

Gray, P.A., Park, M.A. (1989). Anaesthesia and Intensive Care. Castle House, Tunbridge Wells.

Hewitt, P., Regan, F. (1999). Blood transfusion. In: Oxford Textbook of Critical Care (ed. A.R. Webb, M.J. Shapiro, S. Singer, et al.), pp. 691–5 Oxford University Press, Oxford.

Hoffman, M.R., Martinowitz, U., Tobias, J., *et al.* (2002). Excessive bleeding in surgery and trauma: new concepts in coagulation theory and an updated treatment paradigm. *Surgical Rounds* October (special suppl.), 12–13.

Hoffman, M., Monroe, D.M., Roberts, H.R. (1998). Activated factor VII activates factors IX and X on the surface of activated platelets: thoughts on the mechanism of action of high-dose activated factor VI. *Blood Coagulation and Fibrinolysis* **9**, S61–S65.

Hughe-Jones, N.C., Wichramasinghe, S.N. (1991). *Lecture Notes on Haematology*, 5th edn. Blackwell, Oxford.

Isbister, J. (1986). *Clinical Haematology*. Williams & Wilkins, Baltimore, MD.

Jones, J. (1987). Abuse of FFP. *British Medical Journal* **295**, 287.

Ludlam, C. (1990). *Clinical Haematology*. Churchill Livingstone, Edinburgh.

Oh, T.E. (ed.) (1990). *Intensive Care Manual*, 3rd edn. Butterworth, Sydney.

Serjeant, G.R., Singer, M. (1999). Sickle crisis—prevention and management of complications. In: *Oxford Textbook of Critical Care* (ed. A.R. Webb, M.J. Shapiro, S. Singer, *et al.*), pp. 702–4. Oxford University Press, Oxford..

Tinker, J., Zapol, W. (1993). *Care of the Critically Ill Patient*, 2nd edn. Springer, Berlin.

Young, L.M. (1990). DIC, the insidious killer. *Critical Care Nurse* **10**, 26–53.

CHAPTER 15

The immune system and the immunocompromised patient

An understanding of the immune system is essential in order to understand many of the disease processes in the critically ill patient. Since immunosuppressive therapy is commonly used in treatment strategies, it is also important to be aware of any side-effects, and its effects on patient care.

The immune system is extremely complex and limited space does not permit more than an overview. Chapter 12 contains additional information, which expands on the concept of the immunocompromised critical care patient, and should be read in conjunction with this chapter.

The immune system

The immune system consists of many different tissues and cell types that collectively protect the body against infection and the growth of tumour cells. At certain sites, the cells of the immune system are organized into specific structures. These can be classified as central lymphoid tissue (bone marrow and thymus) and peripheral lymphoid tissue (lymph nodes, spleen, Peyer's patches, appendix, tonsils, and adenoids).

The organs of the immune system

The lymph nodes

These are small bean-shaped structures lying along the course of the lymphatic network and are aggregated in particular locations.

Lymph is a fluid containing white cells, chiefly lymphocytes, which bathes the tissues of the body and is collected by the lymphatic vessels. This fluid is immunologically filtered by the lymph nodes before returning into the circulation.

The lymph nodes are composed of mostly T cells, B cells, dendritic cells, and macrophages. The B cells enter the lymph node and, if activated by antigenic stimulation, proliferate and remain in the node. If not stimulated, they pass out of the node to return to the general circulation. Various types of T cells enter the node and when activated they form lymphoblasts. These divide to produce a clone of T cells responding to a specific antigen. Activated T cells then pass into the circulation to reach peripheral sites.

The bone marrow

In addition to red blood cells and platelets, the bone marrow produces all of the cells of the immune system by a process known as haematopoiesis. Stem cells from the bone marrow differentiate into either mature cells of the immune system or precursors of cells that mature elsewhere. Some develop into myeloid cells, a group typified by the large, cell- and particle-devouring white cells known as phagocytes. These include monocytes, macrophages, and neutrophils. Other myeloid descendants become granule-containing inflammatory cells such as eosinophils and basophils. Lymphoid precursors develop into lymphocytes. The two major classes of lymphocytes are B and T cells. B cells mature in the bone marrow while T cells, which originate in the bone marrow as immature thymocytes, mature in the thymus.

The thymus

The function of the thymus is to produce mature T cells from immature thymocytes that have migrated from the bone marrow. Mature T cells are then released into the circulation.

The spleen

The spleen contains B cells, T cells, macrophages, dendritic cells, natural killer cells, and red blood cells. Its function is to act as an immunological filter and to destroy old red blood cells. In addition to capturing antigens as blood passes through the spleen, the migratory macrophages and dendritic cells also bring antigens to it. When these cells present the antigen to the appropriate B or T cell, an immune response is initiated. The B cells become activated in the spleen and produce large amounts of antibodies.

Cells of the immune system (Fig. 15.1)

B cells

B cells produce antibodies in response to the foreign proteins of bacteria, viruses, and tumour cells. These antibodies circulate in blood and lymph, specifically recognizing and binding to one particular protein, thus marking it for destruction by other cells. They are part of what is known as antibody-mediated or humoral immunity.

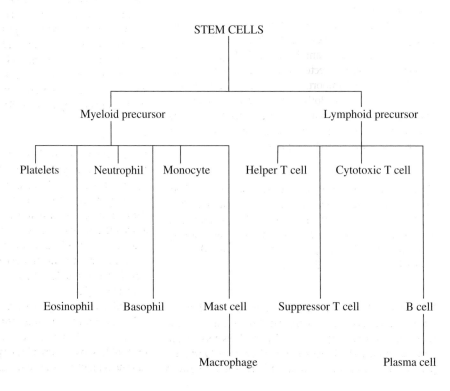

Fig. 15.1 Cells of the immune system.

The antibodies that B cells produce are basic templates with a special, highly specific region that can target a given antigen.

When some antibodies combine with antigens they activate a cascade of proteins, known as the complement system, that have been circulating in an inactive form in the blood. Complement forms a partnership with antibodies, once they have reacted with the antigen, to help destroy foreign invaders and remove them from the body. Other types of antibodies block viruses from entering cells.

T cells

T cells also circulate in blood and lymph. In addition to marking antigens for destruction, they can attack and destroy any diseased cells that they recognize as foreign. They depend on unique cell surface molecules called the major histocompatibility complex (MHC) to help them recognize antigen fragments.

T cells are usually divided into two subsets that are functionally different. The T helper subset, also called the CD4+ T cell, is a coordinator of immune regulation. The main function of the T helper cell is to augment or potentiate immune responses by the secretion of specialized factors that activate other white cells to fight off infection. They alert B cells to start making antibodies, activate macrophages, and influence what type of antibody is produced.

Another type of T cell is called the T killer (also known as suppressor or cytotoxic T cell) subset, or CD8+ T cell. These cells are important in direct killing of certain tumour cells, virally infected cells, and, sometimes, parasites. They are also important in the down-regulation of the immune response. Both types of T cell depend on the lymph nodes and spleen as sites where activation occurs, but are also found in other tissues such as the liver, lungs, and intestinal and reproductive tracts.

Natural killer cells (NK cells)

Natural killer cells are similar to the T killer cells. They directly kill certain tumours such as melanomas, lymphomas, and cell-infecting viruses such as cytomegalovirus and herpes. However, if they have been activated by secretions from the T helper cells (CD4+ T cells), they will kill their targets more effectively.

Dendritic cells

Dendritic cells originate in the bone marrow but are found particularly in the peripheral lymph nodes, thymus, and spleen. They are also found elsewhere in the body, including the bloodstream. They have long cytoplasmic processes that localize and present antigens to responsive T and B cells. They are more efficient antigen-presenting cells (APCs) than macrophages. Dendritic cells bind high amounts of HIV, and may be a reservoir of virus that is transmitted to CD4+ T cells during an activation event.

Phagocytes and granulocytes

Phagocytes are large white cells that can engulf and digest foreign invaders. They include monocytes (which circulate in the blood), macrophages (found in tissues throughout the body), and neutrophils (cells that circulate in the blood but move into tissues when needed). Macrophages are versatile cells; they act as scavengers, they can secrete a wide variety of powerful chemicals, and they play an essential role in activating T cells.

Neutrophils are both phagocytes and granulocytes; they contain granules filled with potent chemicals, which, in addition to destroying microorganisms, play a key role in acute inflammatory reactions. Other types of granulocytes are eosinophils and basophils. Mast cells are granule-containing cells in tissue. The release of these chemicals outside the cell is known as degranulation.

Cytokines

Cytokines are diverse and potent chemical messengers secreted by cells of the immune system. Lymphocytes, including B and T cells, secrete lymphokines, while monocytes and macrophages secrete monokines such as tumour necrosis factor and interleukin-1.

Cytokines recruit many other cells and substances by binding to specific receptors on target cells. They encourage cell growth, promote cell activation, direct cellular traffic, and destroy target cells including cancer cells.

Antibodies

Each antibody is made up of two identical heavy and light chains, shaped to form a Y. The sections that make up the tips of the Y's arms vary greatly from one antibody to another; this is called the variable region. It is these unique contours in the antigen-binding site that allows the antibody to recognize a matching antigen. The stem of the Y links the antibody to other participants in the immune defence system. This area is identical in all antibodies of the same class and is called the constant region.

Antibodies belong to a family of large protein molecules known as immunoglobulins. There are nine distinct classes of human immunoglobulins, namely four types of IgG, two types of IgA, plus IgM, IgE, and IgD. The immunoglobulins G, D, and E are similar in appearance.

IgG

This is the major immunoglobulin in blood and is able to enter tissue spaces. It coats the microorganisms and enhances their uptake by other cells in the immune system. It is antiviral, antibacterial, and can neutralize toxins. IgG can cross the placenta and is responsible for immunity in the newborn.

IgM

This is the first antibody to develop in response to an infection and is found only in serum. It is good at agglutinating and precipitating proteins, but its main function is to protect against bacteria in the blood. IgM is located on the B-cell wall and acts as a B-cell receptor for antigens.

IgE

This is found on the cell membranes of basophils and mast cells, where it acts as an antigen receptor. When it binds with an antigen it causes degranulation of basophils and mast cells. IgE levels rise during an allergic reaction. It can also fight parasitic infections.

IgD

This is almost exclusively found inserted into the membrane of immature B cells, where they regulate the cell's activation.

IgA

This is contained in secretions (tears, saliva, mucus, and breast milk) and in serum. It is important in preventing entry of bacteria into the body. IgA can cross membranes to get into the respiratory, gastrointestinal and genitourinary tracts and is particularly important in defending against respiratory infections.

Antigen receptors

B and T cells carry customized receptor molecules that allow them to recognize and respond to their specific targets. The B cell's antigen-specific receptor recognises antigen in its natural state.

Non-specific immunity (innate or natural immunity)

The non-specific immune response provides the first level of defence against organisms and is capable of being activated at all times. It does not require previous exposure or involve memory or recognition.

Examples of non-specific protection are:

- skin and mucous membranes
- the pH of body secretions
- antimicrobial enzymes
- complement proteins
- respiratory cilia.

The result of an activated non-specific immune response is inflammation and involves the actions of neutrophils, monocytes, mast cells, basophils and macrophages.

The inflammatory response

Chemical mediators

In response to injury, mast cells (histocytes if fixed in the body, or basophils if free flowing in blood) release the first chemical mediator, histamine. Histamine causes dilatation of local blood vessels, increased permeability, and contraction of smooth muscle. This causes fluid to move from the blood vessels into the tissues. Histamine also causes bronchoconstriction and mucus production, which becomes evident in allergic reactions.

When the injury releases clotting factors, a second mediator, bradykinin, is formed. This also causes increased permeability, vasodilatation, and smooth muscle contraction and is responsible for pain.

When tissue cells are injured, arachidonic acid is released from the cell membranes and is metabolized into a number of substances including prostaglandins, thromboxanes, and leucotrienes. These have a variety of often opposing actions such as vessel dilatation and constriction, or platelet aggregation and reduced adhesiveness. Some increase vessel permeability, whereas others act as a chemotactic factor to attract neutrophils to the site of injury.

Increased blood vessel permeability and vasodilatation allows plasma proteins, neutrophils, oxygen, and glucose to reach the site of injury more easily.

The classical signs of inflammation result. These are redness and heat (due to vasodilatation), oedema (due to increased permeability), and pain (due to pressure on the nerve endings).

Cellular actions

Neutrophils are attracted to the site of inflammation by chemotactic factors, which also stimulate more to be released from the bone marrow. They are highly phagocytic and engulf debris. Monocytes then arrive, again attracted by chemotaxins, to assist the neutrophils. Inside the neutrophils and monocytes are lysosomes, which contain lytic enzymes. These digest whatever the cell has engulfed, causing increased use of oxygen by the cell (the 'respiratory burst'). This, in turn causes the formation of reactive oxygen species such as peroxide and superoxide. The chemical reactions also decrease the pH within the cell because they produce hydrogen ions. Hydrogen ions, peroxide, and superoxide can also kill bacteria directly.

Healing

When debris has been removed the neutrophils self-destruct, and fibrin is laid down where capillaries have broken. This provides a framework for new tissue growth using collagen produced by fibroblasts. The monocytes release a substance that promotes the growth of endothelial cells and these become new capillaries. Gradually, fibrin is changed to granulation tissue. The fluid provides nutrition for the new tissue, but as the granulation tissue matures it dries and contracts to produce scar tissue. Scar tissue is white or pale in colour, and is dense with many collagen fibres. It has less flexibility and function than normal tissue and can become pathological depending on where it is formed (e.g. in the lungs, heart, or brain).

The specific immune response

The specific immune response is made up of two major categories—the cellular immune response (T cells) and the humoral immune response (B cells).

Microbes entering the body must first get past the skin and mucous membranes. These not only provide a physical barrier but are also rich in scavenger cells and IgA antibodies.

In order to initiate an immune response an antigen presenting cell (APC), usually a macrophage or dendritic cell, needs to be present in combination with a B or T cell. When an APC presents an antigen on its cell surface to a B cell, the B cell is signalled to proliferate and produce antibodies that specifically bind to that antigen. If the antibodies bind to antigens on bacteria or parasites it acts as a signal for polymorphonuclear leucocytes (PMNLs) or macrophages to phagocytose them. Antibodies also initiate the complement destruction cascade. When antibodies bind to foreign cells, serum proteins called complement bind to the immobilized antibodies and then destroy the bacteria by creating holes in them. Antibodies also signal natural killer cells and macrophages to kill virally or bacterially infected cells.

If the APC presents the antigen to T cells, the T cells become activated. Activated T cells then proliferate and become secretory if they are CD4+ T cells. If they are CD8+ T cells they become activated to kill target cells that specifically express the antigen presented by the APC. The production of antibodies and the activity of CD8+ killer T cells are regulated by the CD4+ helper T cell. The CD4+ T cells produce and secrete growth factors or cytokines signalling other cells to proliferate and function more efficiently. These CD4+ T cells are essential to ensure the activation of natural killer cells, macrophages, CD8+ T cells, and PMNLs.

The immunocompromised patient

An individual's resistance to infection may be reduced by many general factors such as extremes of age, nutritional state, and previous exposure to vaccination or infection. Profound impairment in immune response can be caused by autoimmune diseases, genetic disorders, immunosuppressive drug therapy, and certain infections such as the human immunodeficiency virus.

A person whose resistance to infection is reduced due to an abnormality in the immune response is said to be immunocompromised. Such patients are extremely vulnerable to infection, particularly in hospitals.

The immunocompromised critical care patient

Critical illness itself can cause depression of the protective immune mechanisms of the body, particularly in patients with burns or following trauma, major surgery, or massive haemorrhage.

Pro-inflammatory mediators and overproduction of endogenous anti-inflammatory agents (see Chapter 12), can cause detrimental effects when there is excessive immune cell stimulation. These mediators (e.g. tumour necrosis factor, interleukins, arachidonic acid metabolites) influence all immune cell functions, alter normal phagocytic function, and may lead to inappropriate inflammatory responses.

Following major surgery or trauma, for example, specific suppression of T-cell proliferation has been shown. Haemorrhage is associated with a reduction in IL-2 production while burn injury causes reduced natural killer cell function and reduced chemotaxis for neutrophils.

Activated macrophages can cause a rise in nitric oxide and prostaglandin E_2, both of which are immunosuppressive at high levels. They also release hydrogen peroxide, which, in addition to prostaglandin E_2, reduces B-cell responses. Hypoxia also stimulates prostaglandin E_2 and tumour necrosis factor-α production by the macrophages.

Many commonly used drugs have been implicated in immune suppression. These include H_2 blockers (e.g. ranitidine), some antibiotics (particularly chloramphenicol), cardiovascular drugs (e.g. propanolol), and nonsteroidal anti-inflammatory drugs (NSAIDs), which can all cause neutropenia. Heparin inhibits neutrophil adhesion, while propofol inhibits B-cell proliferation and reduces neutrophil chemotaxis.

Malnutrition also predisposes to infection and poor wound healing by reducing the number of T cells and depressing antibody responses. It can often be difficult to maintain sufficient calorific intake in catabolic patients, particularly those with burns or major trauma. Therefore, early nutritional replacement is very important. Additional supplements may be required; a deficiency of zinc, for example, is associated with lymphoid atrophy and poor wound healing.

Patients with renal and liver failure will also have impaired immune function. Acute or chronic renal failure causes reduced neutrophil bactericidal activity, inappropriate macrophage activation, impaired macrophage antigen presentation, and defective T-cell function. Uraemia also has a direct immunosuppressive effect. Acute and chronic alcohol consumption is associated with decreased phagocytic activity and depressed cellular immunity. Cirrhosis results in depression of antigen presentation and a decrease in the number of T cells.

Critically ill patients therefore have immune dysfunction for a multitude of reasons including their underlying illness, their drug therapy, nutritional factors, and the consequences of their illness such as organ failure. In addition, they are exposed to multiple invasive procedures and to other patients with nosocomial infections. They are at extreme risk of infection. The majority of deaths in patients who have been critically ill for more than 7 days are associated with sepsis (Bellingan 1999).

Specific immunosuppressive drug therapy

Immunosuppressive drug therapy can be extremely beneficial for a wide range of conditions within the critical care area. However, since the drugs are not specific to targeted cells, they can also have many deleterious effects.

Intentional immune suppression is used for:

• prevention of organ rejection following transplantation,

• treatment of malignant disease,

• management of asthma and inflammatory bowel disease,

• treatment of autoimmune connective tissue diseases (e.g. rheumatoid arthritis),

• treatment of some skin diseases (e.g. pemphigus),

• management of neurological diseases (e.g. multiple sclerosis),

• septic shock and anaphylactoid reactions.

The actions of different types of immunosuppressive drugs are complex and affect the immune processes in different ways. For example, steroids decrease the number of lymphocytes and block the production and release of a number of inflammatory cytokines such as prostaglandins and leucotrienes. They also increase the number of neutrophils. Ciclosporin is used to prevent the rejection of transplanted organs and acts primarily on T cells. It blocks the production of lymphokines and thus the response to new antigens, but not the response by old memory cells to previously encountered antigens. Cytotoxic drugs have profound effects on the bone marrow by non-specifically interfering in cell division. Monoclonal antibodies can specifically bind to the CD3 T cell causing cell death.

When nursing any immunosuppressed patient who may or may not be neutropenic, great care must be paid to infection control practices. Microbiological screening should be instituted if there is any deterioration in condition. Invasive procedures and manipulations should be kept to a minimum and non-invasive monitoring used where possible. Line insertion sites, wounds, and secretions must be observed carefully for signs of infection. Cannulae and catheters should be changed regularly according to unit policy.

Infective complications can be difficult to diagnose as a temperature rise may not be evident. Overuse of antibiotics should be avoided as these patients are predisposed to infection with fungal or resistant organisms. Protocols for prophylactic antibiotics should be followed and oral nystatin may be required as fungal infections are common. Protective isolation of the patient should be considered if the white blood count is less than 0.5×10^9/litre.

Altered immune response

Table 15.1 outlines a number of complications related to altered immune response.

Immunodeficiency disorders

Human immunodeficiency virus (HIV)

The human immunodeficiency virus is a retrovirus that causes AIDS, resulting in destruction of the immune system. Patients infected with HIV are at risk of illness and death from opportunistic infectious and neoplastic complications. The variant of HIV that causes almost all infections is known as HIV-1.

The virus primarily infects cells with CD4 cell-surface receptor molecules. In some cells that lack CD4 recep-

TABLE 15.1 Complications related to altered immune response

Type of reaction	Response
Type 1: Hypersensitivity reactions	Allergic responses
Type 2: Cytotoxic hypersensitivity	Incompatible blood transfusions
	Autoimmune haemolytic anaemia
	Drug induced reactions
Type 3: Immune complex hypersensitivity	Rheumatic heart disease
	Glomerular nephritis
	Goodpasture's disease
	Serum sickness
	Rheumatoid arthritis
Type 4: Cell-mediated delayed type hypersensitivity	Contact dermatitis
	Allograft rejection
	Graft versus host disease
Autoimmune disorders	Antibody mediated:
	Autoimmune haemolytic anaemia
	Myasthenia gravis
	Graves' disease
	Immune complex autoimmune disease:
	Systemic lupus erythematosus
	Rheumatoid arthritis
	Antibody- and T-cell mediated autoimmune disease:
	Primary immunodeficiency syndromes
	Secondary immune deficiency syndromes (HIV)
Unregulated immune excess disorders	Multiple myeloma

tors, such as macrophages and fibroblasts, an Fc receptor site or complement receptor site can be used instead. The primary targets for the HIV are blood monocytes, tissue macrophages, T, B, and natural killer lymphocytes, dendritic cells, haemopoietic stem cells, microglial cells in the brain, endothelial cells, and gastrointestinal epithelial cells.

After entry of the virus into the cells, replication may first occur within inflammatory cells at the site of infection or within peripheral blood mononuclear cells. However, the major site of replication then becomes the lymphoid tissues. Viral replication is stimulated by a variety of cytokines such as interleukins and tumour necrosis factor, which activate CD4 lymphocytes and make them more susceptible to HIV infection.

Viral replication actively continues following the initial infection and there is progressive destruction of the CD4 lymphocytes. The immune system is gradually destroyed but clinically, the HIV infection may appear 'latent' as this process may take some years. During this time, enough of the immune system remains intact to prevent most infections, but eventually the production of new CD4 cells cannot match their rate of destruction and the clinical picture of AIDS appears. This stage is marked by the appearance of one or more of the typical opportunistic infections or neoplasms that are diagnostic of AIDS.

Complications of HIV infection and admission to critical care

HIV patients may require critical care for a number of reasons. Acute respiratory failure is the most common reason for admission, but patients with neurological manifestations such as central nervous system (CNS) toxoplasmosis, primary CNS lymphoma, and cryptococcal meningitis, may require critical care for an altered level of consciousness or for intractable seizures. HIV-infected patients may also present to the critical care unit with medical or surgical issues unrelated to their HIV infection.

Infected individuals are susceptible to a diverse collection of bacteria, viruses, fungi, and protozoa that represent a major cause of death. However, as a result of effective antiretroviral therapies and the use of opportunistic infection prophylaxis, co-infections have emerged as important complications in HIV infection. Hepatitis B and C virus co-infections are becoming increasingly prevalent and chronic liver disease now represents a major cause of morbidity and mortality. Tuberculosis is also a key co-infection; world wide the numbers of TB cases are rising, driven largely by the HIV epidemic.

Respiratory complications: Pneumocystis carinii pneumonia (PCP)

PCP commonly occurs in patients infected by HIV, but can also affect immunocompromised patients in the following groups:

◆ patients receiving myelosuppressive chemotherapy,

◆ patients who have undergone organ transplantation,

◆ those with general immunosuppressive diseases such as Hodgkin's disease.

PCP is the leading cause of death in HIV-seropositive patients, and is the most common cause of admission to the critical care area in this group. These patients tend to have a prolonged prodromal illness of weeks or months before respiratory failure occurs, while those patients who are immunocompromised, but HIV-seronegative, tend to present acutely.

The causative agent, *Pneumocystis carinii*, is a fungus-like organism that is widespread in the environment and is transmitted through the air. When the organism is inhaled, it commonly infects both the upper and lower respiratory tract.

Clinical presentation   Typically, the patient presents with fever (usually >38.5°C), tachycardia, and a cough, which is usually non-productive in HIV-seropositive patients. There is exertional dyspnoea, followed by dyspnoea at rest as the disease progresses. As respiratory failure develops the patient becomes severely tachypnoeic and hypoxic.

The chest X-ray may be normal in the early stages. Later on, bilateral interstitial shadowing, most prominently in the midzones is commonly seen. This may resemble the radiological appearance of ARDS. Pneumatocoeles (thin walled cysts filled with air) may be present, or develop over the course of the disease. These can be multiple, large, and predispose the patient to pneumothoraces.

The diagnosis can be confirmed in most cases by Grogott's methenamine silver staining of alveolar lavage fluid taken at bronchoscopy.

Treatment   Antibiotic therapy is commenced, preferably using intravenous co-trimoxazole (alternatives are pentamidine, clindamycin plus primaquine, or trimetrexate plus folinic acid). Steroids are usually given concurrently.

The degree of respiratory support required will be dictated by blood gas analysis. Many will manage on oxygen by mask or CPAP. Some will need BiPAP whereas severe cases require intubation and mechanical ventilation.

Table 15.2 details some other causes of respiratory failure in HIV infection.

Neurological complications

HIV is a neurotrophic virus that can cause a variety of neurological insults including acute myelopathy, peripheral neuropathy, HIV encephalopathy, meningitis, dementia, and cerebral mass lesions.

AIDS related malignancies

AIDS is associated with a broad spectrum of neoplasms, including Karposi's sarcoma, lymphomas, cervical car-

TABLE 15.2   Other causes of respiratory failure in HIV disease

Bacterial pneumonia	*Streptococcus pneumoniae*
	Staphylococcus aureus
	Haemophilis influenzae
	Pseudomonas species (e.g. *Serratia marcescens*)
Atypical pneumonia	*Mycobacterium tuberculosis*
	Mycoplasma pneumoniae
Fungal pneumonia	*Cryptococcus neoformans*
	Histoplasma capsulatum
	Coccidioides immitus
	Aspergillus fumigatus
Cytomegalovirus pneumonia	
Lymphocytic interstitial pneumonia	
Toxoplasmosis gondii pneumonitis	
Non-Hodgkin's lymphoma and pulmonary Karposi's sarcoma	

cinomas related to the human papillomavirus, hepatitis B related carcinomas and non-Hodgkin's lymphoma.

Gastrointestinal

The most common cause of life-threatening abdominal pain in AIDS patients is CMV-related peritonitis from small bowel or colonic enteritis, with or without perforation. AIDS cholangiopathy, caused by a variety of infectious and neoplastic processes, can cause biliary sepsis.

Autoimmune diseases

In autoimmune disease the normal, protective mechanisms of the immune system are reversed. Antibodies are produced against the cells, organs, and tissues of the body causing chronic disease. The aetiology of autoimmune disease is not fully known though it is probably related to a combination of genetic and environmental factors.

Systemic lupus erythematosus (SLE)

SLE is a chronic, potentially fatal disease that is more common in women between the ages of 10 and 50 years. The disease may vary from a mild episodic illness to severe disease affecting multiple organs including joints, kidney, skin, brain, heart, lung, and gastrointestinal tract. It is a complex disorder but its aetiology remains unknown. Regardless of the trigger, it results in the production of antinuclear antibodies, the generation of circulating immune complexes, and activation of the complement system. The disease manifestations result from recurrent vascular injury due to immune complex deposition, white cell deposition, or thrombosis. In addition, the cytotoxic antibodies can mediate autoimmune haemolytic anaemia and thrombocytopenia while antibodies to specific cellular antigens can disrupt cellular function. The health of the patient is affected not only by the disease activity but also the consequences of recurrent episodes (e.g. deforming arthropathy, chronic renal failure) and the side-effects of treatment such as infection and avascular necrosis of bone.

The most frequent causes of mortality are progressive renal failure and sepsis.

Manifestations of SLE

Musculoskeletal   Almost all patients with SLE have joint pain and most develop arthritis. Frequently affected joints are the fingers, hands, wrists, and knees. Bone necrosis can occur in the hips and shoulders and is frequently a cause of pain in those areas.

Skin and mucosa   Approximately 80% of patients develop a photosensitive, malar flushing on the cheeks and bridge of the nose (called a 'butterfly rash'). Other parts of the body, particularly if exposed to the sun, may also develop rashes or skin lesions.

Alopecia occurs in approximately 50% of patients, particularly during an acute exacerbation of the disease.

Mucosal ulcers can occur on the soft and hard palate and the nasal septum. These are usually painless unless a secondary infection such as candidiasis develops.

Renal   Most patients will have some degree of renal impairment but lupus nephritis (persistent inflammation of the kidney) occurs in about 50%. They may eventually develop renal failure requiring dialysis or transplantation.

Haematological   Anaemia is a common feature of chronic SLE and autoimmune thrombocytopenic purpura may occur at any time during the course of the illness.

Venous or arterial blood clots can form and are associated with strokes and pulmonary embolism. However, platelets are often decreased, or antibodies are formed against clotting factors, which may result in significant bleeding.

Patients with SLE have an increased incidence of antiphospholipid antibody syndrome (also known as lupus anticoagulant). This is defined as the co-occurrence of thrombotic events and the presence of autoantibodies against negatively charged phospholipid. These patients are at risk of recurrent arterial and venous thrombosis and thrombocytopenia.

Serositis   Approximately 50% of patients develop inflammatory serositis of the pleura, pericardium, and peritoneum producing pleurisy, pericarditis, or peritonitis, respectively. Some patients develop large pleural effusions, pericardial effusions, and ascites.

Cardiac   Various parts of the heart may become inflamed, causing endocarditis, myocarditis, and/or pericarditis. Rarely, cardiac tamponade can result from pericardial effusions. Chest pain and arrhythmias may result from these conditions.

Lung   In addition to inflammatory serositis causing pleurisy, patients can also develop hypoxaemia due to sequestration of white cells, inflammatory pneumonitis, interstitial pulmonary fibrosis, pulmonary hypertension, pulmonary alveolar haemorrhage, diaphragmatic dysfunction, or phrenic nerve palsy.

Central nervous system   Neuropsychiatric complications can occur which may be acute or chronic. There are focal and diffuse manifestations. Focal manifestations include isolated nerve palsies. Diffuse cerebral dysfunction may manifest as psychosis, personality disorder, or coma. Recurrent involvement of the central nervous system may result in organic brain syndrome or dementia.

Cerebrovascular accidents can occur as a result of either inflammatory, non-inflammatory, or thrombotic vasculopathy. Seizures occur in 25% of patients.

Gastrointestinal   In addition to peritonitis with or without ascites and pancreatitis, mesenteric ischaemia can result from vasculitis. Inflammatory liver disease may occur but cirrhosis is rare.

Treatment

Systemic corticosteroid therapy is particularly useful in the treatment of pneumonitis, pleural effusion, and alveolar haemorrhage. Cytotoxic drugs have been used in patients refractory to corticosteroid therapy.

SLE may be induced by a number of drugs (e.g. procainamide and hydralazine) which commonly induce pulmonary and pleural problems. Cessation of these drugs usually leads to resolution of the symptoms.

Wegener's granulomatosis (WG)

This is a rare disease that can affect many organs of the body (classically the nose, eyes, lungs, and kidneys) and is characterized by necrotizing vasculitis affecting small and medium sized vessels. Necrotizing glomerulonephritis occurs in up to 80% of cases.

In WG, autoantibodies are directed against white blood cells. They bind to endothelial cells, forming clumps of immune complexes, which then accumulate in the tissues leading to granulomatous inflammation of the vessels. This reduces blood flow to the different organs and tissues, causing damage and resulting in the symptoms of WG.

Symptoms

These vary in severity from patient to patient. The most common features are cold-like symptoms that do not respond to conventional treatment, weight loss, fever, malaise, and myalgias. The majority of patients develop upper airway disease including sinusitis, a purulent or bloody nasal discharge, and epistaxis. The cartilage of the nasal septum may also be destroyed by the granulomatous process ('saddle-nose deformity'), and is a sign of chronic disease. Haemoptysis (caused by tracheal and laryngeal ulcers), pleurisy, and pneumonia can develop and pulmonary haemorrhage from necrotizing capillaries can be life-threatening. Granulomas in the lung may also coalesce into large masses, which cavitate. Subglottal stenosis can occur in a small proportion of patients.

Retro-orbital inflammation can cause a variety of ocular manifestations such as proptosis, conjunctival haemorrhage, keratitis, and ocular muscle paralysis.

Treatment

Drugs that suppress the immune system, such as corticosteroids and cyclophosphamide, are used to manage the disease. The prognosis is now much improved with 90% of patients achieving complete remission. Balloon dilatation and stent insertion can be used for tracheobronchial stenosis.

Polyarteritis nodosa

The aetiology of this disease is unknown, but some drugs (e.g. penicillin), bacterial infections (e.g. streptococcal, staphylococcal), vaccines, and viral infections (hepatitis B and C, HIV) have been associated with its onset.

The disease is characterized by segmental inflammation and necrosis of small and medium sized arteries and most commonly occurs at points of vessel bifurcation. Secondary thrombosis and occlusion of the vessels leads to ischaemia and infarction of multiple organs. Small aneurysms can develop in the weakened tissue wall and healing can result in fibrosis.

The kidney, liver, heart, and gastrointestinal tract are the most commonly affected organs, but it rarely affects the respiratory system.

Clinical manifestations

The course of the disease may be acute, resulting in death within a few months, or chronic, leading to debilitating illness. The severity of the disease is determined by the organs affected, but often multiorgan failure develops. Initial manifestations are fever, abdominal pain, weakness, weight loss, hypertension, oedema, and oliguria.

Gastrointestinal tract involvement may cause nausea, vomiting and bloody diarrhoea, and bleeding into the retroperitoneal space. Mesenteric artery thrombosis and bowel infarction may necessitate surgery.

The central and peripheral nervous system may be affected causing sensory changes (such as numbness and tingling) headaches, strokes, and seizures.

Cardiac involvement can result in myocardial infarction, pericarditis, and heart failure. The kidneys are often affected, and may result in renal failure.

Myalgia, with areas of focal ischaemia, and arthralgia are common. Occasionally, skin lesions occur with palpable nodules along the course of the affected blood vessel.

There is no specific laboratory test for polyarteritis nodosa. The diagnosis is made by clinical findings and the presence of necrotizing arteritis in a lesion biopsy.

Treatment

High doses of corticosteroids are given, but as these have to be taken for long periods the side-effects often cause further damage. Other immunosuppressive drugs may be needed, e.g. cyclophosphamide in patients who are unable to tolerate, or are refractory to, corticosteroids.

Rheumatoid arthritis

Rheumatoid arthritis is a chronic inflammatory disease of unclear aetiology. There is evidence of genetic predisposition to the disease and that it is immune mediated. However, it is not known if it is primarily an autoimmune disease or whether the initiating agent is infectious, a self-antigen, or both.

The disease usually presents with pain and signs of inflammation in small and/or large joints. If untreated, the inflammation can spread to additional joints with subsequent irreversible tissue damage causing deformity and instability. Other structures can be involved including tendons, ligaments, muscle, and fascia. The damage and displacement of tendons give rise to the typical deformities seen in patients (e.g. ulnar deviation of the fingers and 'z' deformity of the thumbs). The spine can also be affected and may lead to compression of the spinal cord. Instability of the cervical spine may preclude extension of the neck and is an important consideration when patients require tracheal intubation.

TABLE 15.3 Extra-articular complications of rheumatoid arthritis

Respiratory	Pleurisy and pleural effusion
	Fibrosing alveolitis
	Laryngeal nodules
	Pulmonary hypertension
	Bronchiectasis
	Pulmonary vasculitis
Cardiac	Pericarditis
	Conduction defects
	Mitral valve disease
Skin	Cutaneous vasculitis
	Palmar erythema
	Pyoderma gangrenosum
Neurological	Entrapment of peripheral nerves
	Peripheral neuropathy
	Compression of nerve roots
	Compression of cervical spinal cord

Rheumatoid arthritis may affect other body systems (Table 15.3) and most patients admitted to the critical care area do so as a result of pulmonary involvement or complications of their treatment (e.g. renal failure, bleeding disorders, immunosuppression).

Pulmonary and pleural involvement is common and respiratory failure may necessitate admission to critical care. Rheumatoid pleurisy, often with large pleural effusions that may be recurrent or chronic, occurs commonly. Another serious complication is diffuse interstitial pneumonitis and fibrosis, also known as rheumatoid lung. This causes restrictive lung dysfunction with reduced lung volumes.

The presence of laryngeal nodules, which may be asymptomatic, may also pose problems of tracheal intubation is required.

Treatment

The disease is primarily controlled using NSAIDs. Corticosteroids are used in rheumatic interstitial lung disease to reverses the inflammatory process and prevent the development of fibrotic lung disease. In chronic pulmonary disease, cytotoxic drugs such as methotrexate, gold, and cyclophosphamide can be used but their use may be limited by their side-effects. New treatments such as anti-TNF antibody, have produced some major improvement in some patients, though, again, the side-effect profile and cost may limit their use.

Goodpasture's disease (antiglomerular basement membrane disease)

This is a rare disease caused by antibodies formed against the glomerular basement membrane resulting in rapidly progressive global and diffuse glomerulonephritis. The antibodies also cross-react with the basement membrane in the lung, which can lead to pulmonary haemorrhage, particularly in patients who smoke.

Treatment

Daily plasma exchange may be used to remove the antiglomerular basement antibodies and corticosteroids combined with cyclophosphamide are given to treat the glomerular inflammation and prevent resynthesis of the antibodies. If left untreated, the disease is fatal.

Hypersensitivity reactions/drug allergy

These are immunologically mediated responses to pharmacological agents. They occur after exposure to a wide variety of chemicals, biological, and inert substances that are used in the formulation of drug products. Generally, the structural characteristics of the product determine the type of hypersensitivity reaction that results. Reactions to proteins and peptides, for example, are most often mediated by IgE antibodies or immune complex responses and topical exposure to fats and oils (e.g. lanolin, beeswax, camphor oil) can cause contact dematitis.

These reactions must be distinguished from anaphylactoid reactions which are caused by the direct release of mediators from mast cells and basophils.

The Coombs and Gell classification system of human hypersensitivity (Roitt 1988) can be used to categorize the clinical manifestations and mechanisms of drug allergy reactions (Table 15.4):

♦ Type 1: Immediate hypersensitivity reactions. Drug-specific IgE antibodies induce the immediate release of inflammatory mediators from mast cells and basophils. The reaction usually occurs within 1 hour of exposure and is typified by urticaria, angioedema (swelling, especially of face and neck), laryngeal oedema, wheezing, and cardiovascular collapse.

♦ Type 2: Cytotoxic antibody reactions. These are induced by complement-mediated, cytotoxic IgM or IgG antibodies, which are formed in response to drug-altered cell surface membranes.

♦ Type 3: Immune complex reactions. These are mediated by drug-specific IgG and IgM antibodies.

Type 2 and 3 reactions are late-occurring and generally cause urticaria, rash, fever, lymphadenopathy, and

TABLE 15.4 The Coombs and Gell classification of human hypersensitivity

Reaction	Classification	Examples of some causative drugs/agents	Examples of other conditions
Type 1	Immediate hypersensitivity reaction	Many drugs, e.g. penicillin	Anaphylaxis
			Atopic allergy
Type 2	Cytotoxic antibody reaction	Methyl dopa, penicillin, quinidine	Transfusion reaction
			Rhesus incompatibility
			Hashimoto's thyroiditis
			Goodpasture's syndrome
			Delayed transplant graft rejection
Type 3	Immune complex reaction	Penicillin, sulphonamides, thiouracil, phenytoin	Systemic lupus erythematosus
			Erythema nodosum
			Polyarteritis nodosa
			Rheumatoid arthritis
			Serum sickness
Type 4	Delayed-type hypersensitivity	Nickel	Mantoux test
			Allergic contact dematitis

arthralgias. Symptoms generally subside when the drug and its metabolites have been eliminated from the body.

- Type 4: Delayed-type hypersensitivity reactions. These are mediated by cellular immune mechanisms, which include CD4+ cells and/or CD8+ cells. The response may be limited to the skin (as in contact dermatitis) but may also be systemic affecting many tissues throughout the body.

TABLE 15.5 Some causes of anaphylactic and anaphylactoid reactions

Type of reaction	Cause
IgE-mediated reactions	Foods (e.g. nuts, shellfish, eggs)
	Venoms (insect stings and bites)
	Vaccines
	Latex
	Drugs (e.g. thiopental)
Complement activation	Blood products
	Immunoglobulins
Direct activation	Radiocontrast media
	Opiates
	Dextran
	Exercise
Cyclo-oxygenase inhibitors	Non-steroidal anti-inflammatory drugs
	Aspirin

Anaphylactic and anaphylactoid reactions

An anaphylactic reaction is a potentially life-threatening, systemic response that occurs after re-exposure to an antigen (Table 15.5). It is IgE mediated and causes the immediate release of potent mediators (e.g. histamine, kinins, leucotrienes, serotonin, tryptase) from tissue mast cells and peripheral blood basophils. These mediators cause the clinical manifestations of anaphylaxis by inducing mucus production. pruritus, increased vascular permeability, and smooth muscle constriction in various organs.

Anaphylactoid reactions are clinically indistinguishable from anaphylactic reactions but they are not IgE mediated and the mechanism of mediator release is different. In this type of reaction the mast cell can be induced to react:

- directly by exercise, stress, opiates, and, possibly radiocontrast agents,

- by some drugs, e.g. aspirin and other non-steroidals, which inhibit cyclo-oxygenase activity thus disturbing arachidonic acid metabolism,

- following complement activation by immune complexes (which may be caused by reactions to blood, blood products, and immunoglobulins).

Any drug can potentially cause anaphylactic and anaphylactoid reactions. The most frequent cause of severe reactions are antibiotic-related. Less commonly, enzymes (e.g.streptokinase), insulin, protamine sulphate, vaccines, blood products, and plasma expanders (e.g. dextrans, starches, and gelatins) are involved. Anaesthetic agents have also been implicated, in particular, thiopental, suxamethonium, and non-depolarizing muscle relaxants.

Clinical manifestations

Symptoms usually occur within 20 min of exposure to the stimulus but can occur within seconds (Table 15.6). The progression of the reaction can be variable. It often starts with a weak response that may cause nasal congestion, conjunctivitis, pruritus, and abdominal symptoms such as diarrhoea, nausea, and vomiting. However, in its severest form, cardiovascular collapse, myocardial depression, angioedema, laryngeal obstruction, and severe bronchospasm can lead to death within minutes of exposure to the allergen.

The response is initiated by the release of vasoactive mediators from the basophils and mast cells. Histamine binds to the H_1 receptors in the lung causing bronchospasm, and to the H_2 receptors in the upper respiratory tract causing vasodilation and inflammation. Leucotrienes induce the production of copious amounts of mucus in the lungs that then plug the constricted bronchioles and cause asphyxiation. Respiratory symptoms are further exacerbated by severe angioedema, pulmonary oedema and oedema of the tongue, larynx and glottis causing upper airway obstruction.

TABLE 15.6 Summary of potential clinical manifestations of anaphylactic and anaphylactoid reactions

Cutaneous	Flushing
	Urticaria/angioedema
	Pruritis
Respiratory	Bronchospasm, laryngospasm
	Pulmonary oedema
	Stridor
	Oedema of glottis , tongue, larynx
Cardiovascular	Vasodilation
	Hypotension and cardiovascular collapse
	Myocardial ischaemia
	Arrhythmias
	Cardiac arrest
Gastrointestinal	Abdominal cramps
	Nausea/vomiting
	Diarrhoea
Other	Rhinitis
	Conjunctivitis
	Coagulopathy

The systemic release of histamine and other vasodilating mediators causes shock due to generalized vasodilation of the arterioles and increased vascular permeability. A rapid fluid shift to the extravascular spaces results in a loss of blood volume and severe hypotension, although the patient initially tries to compensate for this by vasoconstriction due to the release of angiotensin and catecholamines. Hypotension can also cause myocardial ischaemia, arrhythmias, and cardiac arrest. Activation of the H_1 receptors in gastrointestinal tract causes contraction of the smooth muscle resulting in abdominal cramps, nausea, vomiting and diarrhoea.

Management of a severe reaction

Treatment is the same for both anaphylactic and anaphylactoid reactions and consists of immediate emergency management followed by less urgent secondary treatments. In a severe reaction, early intervention is critical for a favourable outcome. The ABC principles of resuscitation should be followed.

1. A: Airway and epinephrine

   ◆ Stop administration of the causal agent.

   ◆ Maintain an adequate airway and administer 100% oxygen.

   ◆ If possible, monitor oxygen saturation using pulse oximetry.

   ◆ Give epinephrine (adrenaline). This blocks the physiological effect of the mediators and should be given at the earliest opportunity. If no intravenous access is available it can be given intramuscularly in the thigh. Intravenously, 0.5–1.0 ml increments of 1:10 000 solution can be repeated as required. Intramuscularly, injections of 0.5–1.0 ml of 1:1000 solution can be repeated every 10 min as required. Intravenous epinephrine is preferable in life-threatening situations, but can cause myocardial ischaemia and arrhythmias and must therefore be given slowly in low doses. Patients with a history of anaphylaxis should carry a pre-filled syringe of epinephrine (e.g. Epipen, Ana-Guard) for immediate injection outside the hospital setting.

2. B: Breathing

   ◆ If breathing is inadequate, endotracheal intubation, cricothyroidotomy, or emergency tracheostomy may be required, depending on the extent of upper airway oedema.

   ◆ Nebulized bronchodilators (e.g. salbutamol 5 mg) or intravenous aminophylline may be required for bronchospasm (loading dose 6 mg/kg followed by

0.5 mg/kg/hour). In addition, nebulized epinephrine (adrenaline) may also be useful for laryngospasm, bronchospasm, and laryngeal oedema. Intratracheal epinephrine can be instilled in intubated patients with severe bronchospasm.

3. C: Circulation

- Assess the circulatory status and commence cardiopulmonary resuscitation if necessary.

- Establish intravenous access and rapidly infuse normal saline or colloid (unless it is the cause of the anaphylaxis).

- Continue to administer epinephrine (adrenaline) if hypotension persists. An epinephrine or norepinephrine (noradrenaline) infusion may be necessary, avoiding the dangerous surges in blood pressure seen with intravenous boluses.

- Monitor ECG and cardiac output if prolonged.

Secondary management

When the airway, breathing. and circulation have been stabilised, further management includes:

- Antihistamine agents to antagonise the effects of histamine. Chlorphenamine (chlorpheniramine) is an H_1 antagonist and is useful for urticaria and oedema while ranitidine, an H_2 antagonist, is gastro-protective.

- Corticosteroids (e.g. hydrocortisone 100 mg 4–6 hourly). They help dampen the inflammatory response and are also used to block the potential late phase response. This is where the physiological manifestations of anaphylaxis can reoccur several hours later, without additional exposure to the allergen.

- In patients already taking beta-blockers, anaphylaxis may be severe and refractory to treatment and additional therapy may be required. Beta-blockers act as competitive inhibitors of catecholamines and therefore high doses of β1 and/or β2 agonists may be needed.

- The patient should be transferred to a critical care area if not already there for full cardiovascular monitoring and respiratory support.

Test yourself

Questions

1. What is an anaphylactic reaction?

2. *Pneumocystis carinii* pneumonia commonly occurs in patients infected by the human immunodeficiency virus. What other groups of patients are also vulnerable to this condition?

3. What is IgG?

4. What are cytokines?

5. What is the function of B cells?

Answers

1. An anaphylactic reaction is a potentially life-threatening, systemic response that occurs after re-exposure to an antigen. It is IgE mediated and causes the immediate release of potent mediators (e.g. histamine, kinins, leucotrienes, serotonin, tryptase) from tissue mast cells and peripheral blood basophils. These mediators cause the clinical manifestations of anaphylaxis by inducing mucus production. pruritus, increased vascular permeability and smooth muscle constriction in various organs.

2. *Pneumocystis carinii* pneumonia can also affect immunocompromised patients in the following groups: patients receiving myelosuppressive chemotherapy patients who have undergone organ transplantation those with general immunosuppressive diseases such as Hodgkin's disease.

3. IgG is the major immunoglobulin in blood and is able to enter tissue spaces. It coats the microorganisms and enhances their uptake by other cells in the immune system. It is antiviral, antibacterial, and can neutralize toxins. IgG can cross the placenta and is responsible for immunity in the newborn.

4. Cytokines are diverse and potent chemical messengers secreted by cells of the immune system. Lymphocytes, including B and T cells, secrete lymphokines, while monocytes and macrophages secrete monokines such as tumour necrosis factor and interleukin-1. Cytokines recruit many other cells and substances by binding to specific receptors on target cells. They encourage cell growth, promote cell activation, direct cellular traffic, and destroy target cells including cancer cells.

5. B cells produce antibodies in response to the foreign proteins of bacteria, viruses, and tumour cells. These antibodies circulate in blood and lymph, specifically recognizing and binding to one particular protein, thus marking it for destruction by other cells. They are part of what is known as antibody-mediated or humoral immunity.

References and bibliography

Akil, M., Amos, R.S. (1995). ABC of rheumatology: rheumatoid arthritis—1: Clinical features and diagnosis. *British Medical Journal* **310**, 587–90.

Bellingan, G.L. (1999). Immune dysfunction associated with critical illness. In: *Oxford Textbook of Critical Care* (ed. A.R. Webb, M.J. Shapiro, S. Singer, *et al.*) pp. 898–902. Oxford University Press, Oxford.

Brook, M.G., Miller, R.F. (1999). Infections associated with HIV. In: *Oxford Textbook of Critical Care* (ed. A.R. Webb, M.J. Shapiro, S. Singer, *et al.*), pp. 903–6. Oxford University Press, Oxford.

Buckley, C.D. (1997). Science, medicine and the future: treatment of rheumatoid arthritis. *British Medical Journal* **315**, 236–8.

Chapman, M., Peake, S. (1999). Drug-induced depression of immunity. In: *Oxford Textbook of Critical Care* (ed. A.R. Webb, M.J. Shapiro, S. Singer, *et al.*), pp. 894–8. Oxford University Press, Oxford.

Christopher, M., Immanual, A., Cherian, V., Jacob, R. (2000). Anaphylaxis. *Update in Anaesthesia* **12**, 14.

Fisher, M. (1995). Treatment of acute anaphylaxis. *British Medical Journal* **311**, 731–3.

Hughes, G., Fitzharris, P. (1999). Managing acute anaphylaxis. *British Medical Journal* **319**, 1–2.

Linnemayer, P.A. (1993). *The Immune System- An Overview.* Seattle Treatment Education Project Factsheet. Seattle Treatment Education Project, Seattle, WA.

Mason, P.D., Pusey, C.D. (1994). Glomerulonephritis: diagnosis and treatment. *British Medical Journal* **309**, 1557–63.

Prakash, U.B.S. (1999). Systemic lupus erythematosus. In: *Oxford Textbook of Critical Care* (ed. A.R. Webb, M.J. Shapiro, S. Singer, *et al.*), pp. 940–3. Oxford University Press, Oxford.

Prakash, U.B.S. (1999) Rheumatoid arthritis. In: *Oxford Textbook of Critical Care* (ed. A.R. Webb, M.J. Shapiro, S. Singer, *et al.*), pp. 946–948. Oxford University Press, Oxford.

Roitt,A. (1988). *Essential Immunology*, pp. 193–214. Blackwell, Oxford.

Rusznak, C., Peebles, R.S. Jr (2002). Anaphylaxis and anaphylactoid reactions. A guide to prevention , recognition and emergent treatment. *Postgraduate Medicine* **111**(5), 101–14.

Savage, C.O., Harper, L., Cockwell, P., *et al.* (2000). Vasculitis. *British Medical Journal* **320**, 1325–8.

Shah, M.K., Hugghins, S.Y. (2002). Characteristics and outcomes of patients with Goodpasture's syndrome. *Southern Medical Journal* **95**, 1411–18.

Singer, M., Webb, A. (1999). *Oxford Handbook of Critical Care.* Oxford University Press, Oxford.

Wyatt, R. (1996). Anaphylaxis. How to recognise, treat and prevent potentially fatal attacks. *Postgraduate Medicine* **100**(2), 87–90, 96–9.

CHAPTER 16

Endocrine, obstetric, and drug overdose emergencies

Chapter contents

Endocrine disorders

Endocrine syndromes usually produce classical signs and symptoms but these may be difficult to identify in the severely ill patient. Appropriate investigations are essential in order to diagnose and treat these disorders promptly. Knowledge of the normal physiology of the endocrine glands is also vital in order to understand the systemic effects caused by their failure, the interactions between the glands and other body systems, and the effects of severe illness upon them.

Space does not permit a detailed account of the physiology of all the hormones produced by the endocrine glands or of every condition that may result from their dysfunction. Those discussed in detail are the endocrine emergencies and other conditions that require admission to the critical care area.

The adrenal glands

The adrenal glands can be divided into two independent areas: the medulla and the cortex. Each produces different hormones with different functions.

The adrenal medulla (the inner core of the gland)

The cells of the medulla are derived from the sympathetic nervous system and secrete the hormones adrenaline and noradrenaline in response to sympathetic stimuli. Noradrenaline is the transmitter substance of the sympathetic nervous system and pre-ganglionic sympathetic fibres innervate the medulla. Events that activate the sympathetic nervous system (e.g. fear, hypoxia, hypotension, anger, cold, pain, etc.) cause the release of noradrenaline and adrenaline (collectively known as catecholamines). The joint action of the two hormones is to prepare the body for action ('fight or flight'). The immediate energy needs of the body must be met and blood flow and volume increased to essential organs.

Adrenaline

This constricts blood vessels in the skin and mucosa but dilates those in the skeletal muscle and the eye. It relaxes the bronchioles, thereby increasing lung capacity, and increases heart rate and cardiac output. Adrenaline also dilates the blood vessels of the brain, muscles, and myocardium, ensuring that blood flow is maintained to these crucial areas. Liver glycogen is mobilized and converted to glucose, providing an immediate source of energy.

Noradrenaline

This raises the blood pressure by constricting arterioles and veins (except those in crucial areas where adrenaline counteracts this effect).

The adrenal cortex

The cortex secretes three categories of hormones: mineralocorticoids, glucocorticoids, and sex hormones. All are steroids and are similar in chemical composition to cholesterol.

Mineralocorticoids

These regulate sodium and potassium concentrations in the extracellular fluid. The most important is aldosterone, which accounts for 95% of mineralocorticoid secretion.

The effect of aldosterone is to increase extracellular fluid sodium and chloride ion concentration, and to decrease the potassium ion concentration. Aldosterone causes the reabsorption of sodium in the distal loops and collecting ducts of the kidney (see Chapter 9). Since sodium and potassium transport mechanisms in the epithelial cells are linked in a partial exchange process, potassium is also excreted at the same time. This sodium–potassium pump is stimulated by aldosterone. However, as the sodium–potassium ion exchange is unequal, this usually leads to more sodium being reabsorbed than potassium excreted.

A secondary effect of aldosterone is to decrease the number of chloride ions lost in the urine. As there is an increase in sodium and chloride ion reabsorption in the tubules, water is also reabsorbed by an osmotic effect.

Aldosterone secretion can be stimulated by:

- elevated levels of potassium ions in the plasma,
- a persistently low plasma sodium level,
- a prolonged decrease in extracellular fluid volume,
- angiotensin: the plasma level of angiotensin rises when renin production by the kidney is increased as a result of a low plasma sodium level or reduced renal blood flow.

Glucocorticoids

These regulate the metabolism of fat, protein, and carbohydrate and can enhance resistance to physical stress.

The most important glucocorticoid is cortisol. Cortisol production is stimulated by adrenocorticotrophic hormone (ACTH) secreted from the anterior pituitary via a negative feedback mechanism. It shows a diurnal variation in secretion, being highest in the morning and lowest at about midnight. The primary stimulus for secretion is physical stress (injury) which activates the hypothalamus via nerve impulses from the site of injury. Cortisol causes increased availability of fats, glucose, and amino acids to repair the damage.

Effects of cortisol

- Increases fat metabolism. Cortisol mobilizes fat from adipose tissue cells and this provides an important source of energy in starvation. Excessive fat breakdown, however, can cause ketosis.

- Increases the use of protein. Cortisol suppresses the rate of protein production in non-liver cells, thus amino acids in the blood increase and these are available in times of injury. Chronically, this causes weakening of capillaries and skin atrophy. The rate of protein formation in the liver cells is, however, increased (e.g. plasma proteins).

- Increases blood glucose. Cortisol increases the blood glucose level by two mechanisms:

  1. It decreases the utilization of glucose by tissue cells (i.e. antagonistic to insulin) thus raising glucose levels in the extracellular fluid.

  2. It stimulates liver cells to convert fat and protein into glucose (by gluconeogenesis). Gluconeogenesis is increased because cortisol causes amino acids to be mobilized from tissue protein and fat (in the form of glycerol) from adipose tissue. This provides the liver with material that can be converted into glucose. Excess cortisol can therefore cause insulin resistance and hyperglycaemia.

- Decreases the absorption of vitamin D from the intestine. With chronically high cortisol levels (e.g. in Cushing's disease or steroid treatment) it may cause osteoporosis and impedes the development of cartilage.

- Anti-inflammatory. It inhibits formation of pro-inflammatory mediators such as cytokines and nitric oxide. It also decreases the number of lymphocytes and eosinophils in the blood and thus suppresses allergic responses and the body's reactions to injury, inflammation, and infection.

- Can cause sodium (and water) retention and potassium depletion.

Sex hormones

Androgens, oestrogens, and progesterone are secreted by the adrenal cortex but are less important than those produced by the gonads. Occasionally, oestrogen-secreting tumours of the adrenal cortex develop.

Disorders of the adrenal medulla

Phaeochromocytoma

A phaeochromocytoma is a tumour of chromaffin cells usually involving the adrenal medulla where high levels of adrenaline and noradrenaline are secreted. In 90% of patients the tumour originates in the medulla, but in 10% it may occur anywhere along the sympathetic chain (aorta, bladder, pelvis, abdomen, thorax).

It can metastasize and behave like a malignant tumour. The secretion of catecholamines is usually inter-

> ### DIAGNOSIS OF A PHAEOCHROMOCYTOMA
>
> - Blood catecholamine levels and 24-hour urinary measurements of vanillylmandelic acid (VMA); a metabolic product of catecholamines (not useful in critical illness where levels are increased).
>
> - MIBG (*meta*-iodobenzylguanidine) radionuclide scan.
>
> - Computed tomography.

mittent and during acute attacks the patient develops pulsating headaches, tachycardia, hyperglycaemia, blurred vision, bowel disturbances, and very severe hypertension (systolic blood pressure up to 300 mmHg). Between attacks the blood pressure may be only slightly raised.

In up to 30% of patients the presenting features may be hypotension due to release of dilating catecholamines. It may thus mimic sepsis.

The treatment of a phaeochromocytoma is surgical removal but the blood pressure must be controlled well in advance of surgery using alpha- and beta-adrenergic blocking agents. Alpha blockade should begin before beta blockade or a severe hypertensive crisis can be precipitated. Phentolamine or phenoxybenzamine are commonly used for short-term, pre-operative alpha blockade and propanolol for beta blockade. Alternatively, labetolol can be used as it has both alpha- and beta-adrenergic blockade effects. During a severe hypertensive crisis an intravenous infusion of sodium nitroprusside can be used to control blood pressure.

Adrenoceptor blockade is usually withdrawn 12–36 hours pre-operatively. Post-operative care is as for any major abdominal surgery but continuous monitoring of blood pressure and heart rate is essential. Removal of the catecholamine source during surgery can cause hypovolaemic collapse unless the patient has been well prepared with alpha and beta blockade. If this occurs large volumes of fluid may need to be infused rapidly to restore blood pressure.

Disorders of the adrenal cortex

Addison's disease

This disease results from a chronic deficiency of cortical hormones. This can be due to absence, atrophy, or disease of the adrenal cortex or can occur secondary to hypopituitarism. The symptoms of Addison's disease reflect the lack of cortisol, aldosterone, and androgens.

Table 16.1 summarizes the tests used in the diagnosis of Addison's disease.

TABLE 16.1 Biochemical tests used for the diagnosis of Addison's disease

Test	Level
Serum electrolytes and urea	Low sodium. Raised potassium and urea
Serum ACTH levels: 24-hour urinary 17-oxogenic steroids. Serum cortisol (take at 08:00 hours)	High in adrenal disease. Low in pituitary disease. Both may be in normal range—additional dynamic stress tests are performed if the disease is suspected
Synacthen (tetracosactrin)	*Short test*: synacthen 250 mg is given IM and serum cortisol levels measured initially and then after 30 min. In normal patients the difference between the two levels should be least 200 nmol/litre. Longer tests can be performed where measurements are taken over 5 hours or 3 days

EFFECTS OF THE LACK OF ALDOSTERONE

- Polyuria, dehydration, thirst
- Hyponatraemia, hyperkalaemia
- Hypotension (often postural)
- Cardiac arrhythmias

EFFECTS OF THE LACK OF ANDROGENS

- Loss of body hair
- Loss of libido

EFFECTS OF THE LACK OF CORTISOL

- Muscle weakness and fatigue, weight loss
- Hypoglycaemia
- Gastrointestinal disturbances (nausea, vomiting, diarrhoea, abdominal pain)
- Emotional disturbances (irritability, depression)
- Low resistance to infection, inability to cope with any type of stress

Treatment of Addison's disease

The treatment of Addison's disease is by lifelong cortical hormone replacement therapy. Maintenance thera-

py consists of hydrocortisone, usually 20 mg in the morning and 10 mg in the evening. The difference in the 12-hourly dose reflects the normal diurnal variation in secretion of cortisol. Fludrocortisone may be added if a mineralocorticoid effect is required. This is a synthetic form of aldosterone and is given as a single dose in the morning (usually 0.05—0.3 mg). Dosages are prescribed according to plasma urea and electrolytes, and lying and standing blood pressure.

In a healthy subject, cortisol levels are increased in times of stress. However, a patient with Addison's disease is unable to increase secretion of cortisol and the maintenance therapy maintains adequate levels only under normal conditions. In times of 'stress' (e.g. surgery, trauma, infection) the oral dosage of hydrocortisone must therefore be increased.

Addisonian crisis

If an acute demand for cortisol cannot be met, an Addisonian crisis may develop. This is one of the most life-threatening of all the endocrine emergencies. The signs and symptoms of an Addisonian crisis result mainly from the deficiency of aldosterone. There may be severe hypotension and tachycardia due to dehydration and arrhythmias, such as atrial fibrillation, are common. Serum sodium levels will be low and potassium and urea high. Hypoglycaemia is common in advanced cases. The patient will be in shock and will progress to complete circulatory collapse unless immediate treatment is instituted.

Immediate management of an Addisonian crisis.

Urgent rehydration with colloid followed by 0.9% sodium chloride (3–4 litres will often be required over the first few hours). Central venous or flow monitoring is often necessary to monitor the response and to titrate fluid requirements optimally.

Hypoglycaemia should be corrected by infusions of hypertonic glucose ideally via a central venous catheter as these may irritate peripheral veins or cause cellulitis if they extravasate.

Cortisol must be administered without delay. The blood cortisol levels will not be known at the time but a blood sample should be taken, before treatment is instituted, for baseline cortisol levels. Hydrocortisone hemisuccinate 100–200 mg q.d.s. (or dexamethasone 4 mg q.d.s.) is given intravenously for the immediate crisis, followed, after stabilization, by an oral maintenance regimen of twice-daily hydrocortisone ± fludrocortisone.

The precipitating cause of the crisis must be identified and treated.

Nursing management

- **Problem**: Cardiovascular instability (hypotension, tachycardia, arrhythmias) due to dehydration.
  Management: Continuous ECG monitoring. 12-lead ECG. Correct hypokalaemia. Administer IV fluids according to monitored variables. If hypotension or low cardiac output persists after adequate rehydration, inotropic agents may be required (remember that the precipitating cause of the crisis may be sepsis).

- **Problem**: Oliguria due to hypotension and dehydration.
  Management: The patient should be catheterized and urine output measured hourly. Long periods of hypotension and hypovolaemia may precipitate renal failure. Oliguria should improve as the patient is rehydrated and becomes normotensive. Monitor blood urea and electrolytes.

- **Problem**: Respiratory failure.
  Management: Oxygen requirements and ventilatory support will be dictated by the patient's condition and blood gas analysis. Respiratory failure is not directly caused by an Addisonian crisis but may result from the underlying cause (e.g. chest infection, pulmonary embolus). There may be an increased sensitivity to opiates and sedatives in patients with Addison's disease and these should be used with caution in the spontaneously breathing patient.

- **Problem**: Hypoglycaemia.
  Management: Regular monitoring of blood glucose. Continuous infusions of 10 or 20% glucose may be required. Administer IV boluses of hypertonic glucose (20 or 50%) as required. Aim for blood glucose level of 5–8 mmol/litre.

- **Problem**: Pyrexia (if infection is the cause of the crisis).
  Management: Monitor core temperature. Identify source of infection by appropriate cultures. Give antibiotics as indicated. Cool the patient (e.g. fanning, tepid sponging, antipyretics) and aim for temperature <37.5°C.

Addisonian crisis is rare but should be considered in a shocked patient who is resistant to conventional treatment and where the cause cannot be identified.

The thyroid glands

The thyroid gland consists of two lobes, one each side of the larynx and trachea, joined at the midline by an isthmus. It produces three active hormones: thyroxine, triiodothyronine, and calcitonin.

The thyroid hormones

The thyroid gland actively removes iodide from the blood, concentrates it 40-fold and then stores it within the thyroid follicular cells. Thyroxine (T_4) and triiodothyronine (T_3) are synthesized from iodide and the amino acid tyrosine and stored as thyroglobulin. Thyroglobulin is released into the blood under the influence of thyroid-stimulating hormone (TSH) from the anterior pituitary. T_4 dissociates from the thyroglobulin, while T_3 is formed by cleavage of one iodide group from T_4 by a deiodinase enzyme. Most T_3 and T_4 is bound to circulating plasma proteins, mainly thyroxine-binding globulin (TBG); the remainder circulates free in the plasma. Free T_3 and T_4 can diffuse out of the vascular spaces and be metabolically effective. T_3 and T_4 are virtually identical but T_3 is much more potent, has a shorter duration and is present in smaller amounts than T_4. The normal level of plasma T_4 is 60–150 nmol/litre and T_3 is 1–3 nmol/litre.

Reverse T_3 is also produced by the deiodination of T_4 but only when there is excessive circulating thyroid hormone (hyperthyroid states). Reverse T_3 is not physiologically active and its production prevents excess catabolism. Levels of reverse T_3 are also elevated during severe illness (e.g. burns, sepsis).

Both T_3 and T_4 are responsible for the regulation of the metabolic rate in all tissues of the body. They direct growth, tissue differentiation, and mental and physical development. A third hormone, calcitonin, is also secreted by the gland. Calcitonin is not secreted by the same follicular cells that secrete T_3 and T_4 but by cells that lie between them. Calcitonin is responsible for lowering the serum calcium level. This is achieved by reducing the rate of calcium release from bone, removing calcium from the extracellular fluid by increasing deposition of calcium in the bones, and by reducing the rate of formation of new osteoclasts. Calcitonin can correct high serum calcium levels fairly quickly and its secretion is enhanced when blood calcium levels are elevated. Calcitonin is used by the body for the short-term control of hypercalcaemia, while parathormone is used for more long-term regulation (see parathyroid glands).

Regulation of T_3 and T_4

The hypothalamus and anterior pituitary control the release of T_3 and T_4 by a negative feedback mechanism (see Fig. 16.1).

The anterior pituitary is stimulated to synthesize and secrete TSH by thyrotrophin-releasing hormone (TRH) produced by the hypothalamus. TSH stimulates the thyroid gland to synthesize and secrete the thyroid hormones T_3 and T_4. The secretion of T_3 and T_4, in turn, inhibits the release of further TSH.

In hypothyroidism (where there is insufficient T_3 and T_4) the cause can be at the level of the hypothalamus, the anterior pituitary, or the thyroid gland itself.

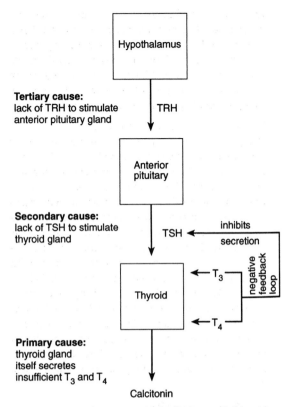

Fig. 16.1 Diagram showing negative feedback control of thyroid hormones.

> **CLASSIFICATION OF HYPOTHYROIDISM**
>
> ◆ Primary—due to disease of the thyroid gland.
>
> ◆ Secondary—where the anterior pituitary secretes insufficient TSH.
>
> ◆ Tertiary—where the hypothalamus does not secrete enough TRH.

Investigations of thyroid function determine at which level the cause of hypothyroidism is to be found.

Investigations of thyroid function

T₃ resin uptake

This test measures the unoccupied binding sites on TBG. The number of binding sites increases in hypothyroidism (where there is little thyroid hormone) and in pregnancy (where there is excess TBG), but decreases in hyperthyroidism.

Iodine-131 uptake

The patient is given radioactive iodine by mouth and this is taken up by the thyroid cells. The radioactivity of the gland is then measured after a set time. Uptake increases in hyperthyroidism and iodine deficiency and when taking certain drugs (e.g. phenothiazines).

Serum TSH

The serum TSH is increased in primary hypothyroidism (the pituitary gland is trying to stimulate the underactive thyroid), but decreased in secondary and tertiary hypothyroidism. In hyperthyroidism the serum TSH is decreased if there is primary thyroid overproduction, and increased if a pituitary tumour is responsible.

TRH test

TRH is given intravenously and the response of TSH release is measured. In pituitary hyperthyroidism there is a high basal level of TSH and a very marked increase in response to TRH. If hypothyroidism is caused by pituitary or hypothalamic disease there may be a reduction in response.

Disorders of the thyroid gland

Hypothyroidism (myxoedema)

This results from decreased thyroid hormone secretion.

Symptoms of hypothyroidism (myxoedema)

These reflect the lack of thyroid hormone and a hypometabolic state (see Table 16.2).

Once identified, hypothyroidism is treated by oral thyroxine (T₄) supplements but the cause of the disease must be ascertained by appropriate investigations. If the hypothyroid state continues myxoedema coma can result. Although rare, this would necessitate admission to the ICU.

Myxoedema coma

This arises when the patient with longstanding hypothyroidism encounters an additional stress that requires energy needs that cannot be met. Coma results from a

> **CAUSES OF HYPOTHYROIDISM (MYXOEDEMA)**
>
> ◆ Previous surgery to the thyroid gland (partial or complete thyroidectomy).
>
> ◆ Secondary to ¹³¹I therapy for hyperthyroidism.
>
> ◆ Spontaneous—the gland atrophies.
>
> ◆ Hashimoto's thyroiditis—destruction of thyroid hormone-producing tissues.
>
> ◆ Congenital absence of the thyroid gland.
>
> ◆ Disease (or surgery) of the anterior pituitary or hypothalamus.

TABLE 16.2	Signs and symptoms of hypothyroidism (myxoedema)
Cardiovascular	Bradycardia
	Decreased cardiac output
	Decreased cardiac contractility
Central nervous system	Slow mental function
	Dementia
	Slowed speech
	Hoarse voice
	Fatigue
	Excessive sleep
Gastro-intestinal tract	Constipation
	Weight increase
Other	Dry, scaly skin
	Oedema of hands and feet
	Face puffiness and periorbital oedema
	Coarse, easily broken hair
	Poor wound healing
	Night blindness

FACTORS PRECIPITATING MYXOEDEMA COMA

- Hypothermia
- Infection
- Trauma
- Cerebrovascular accident
- Myocardial infarction
- Drugs with an antithyroid action (e.g. lithium and amiodarone)

combination of metabolic derangement, hypothermia, hypercapnia, and hypoxia.

Treatment of myxoedema coma

The aims of treatment are to:

- support vital functions
- identify precipitating factors
- return to the euthyroid state.

Support of vital functions

- *Problem*: Hypoventilation (due to decreased conscious level) causing hypercapnia and a potential chest infection.
  Management: Ensure airway is protected. Endotracheal intubation may be required in deep coma. Ad-

minister humidified oxygen to maintain adequate oxygenation. If there is marked hypercapnia or hypoxaemia mechanical ventilation may be required. A respiratory acidosis is usually present and this should correct as efficient ventilation is restored. Aggressive physiotherapy to prevent/treat chest infection; culture sputum as appropriate (see Chapter 4).

- *Problem*: Hypotension and bradycardia.
  Management: Continuous ECG monitoring. No specific treatment is usually required for bradycardia, as the heart rate should increase as treatment is instituted. Perform 12-lead ECG to exclude myocardial infarction. Monitor blood pressure. Patients in myxoedema coma are often resistant to inotropes and hypotension is initially treated with IV fluid. These patients are usually elderly and may have compromised cardiac function, therefore fluids must be infused with caution and under appropriate monitoring. Sodium chloride 0.9% is used if the patient is hyponatraemic. Urinary retention can occur, therefore the bladder should be catheterized and urine output monitored. Oliguria should correct as the patient is rehydrated and normotensive. Pericardial effusion is a recognized problem and may progress to cardiac tamponade (see Chapter 8).

- *Problem*: Hypoglycaemia.
  Management: Monitor blood sugar regularly. Correct hypoglycaemia with glucose infusions or boluses of 50% glucose as required.

- *Problem*: Hypothermia.
  Management: Monitor core temperature. Rewarm patient (0.5–1°C/hour unless very hypothermic) using a rewarming blanket and, if necessary, warming IV infusion fluids. Nurse in a warm environment and warm humidified oxygen if administered. Observe ECG for potential arrhythmias while rewarming (see Chapter 13). A lactic acidosis is often present due to hypoperfusion of tissues. This should resolve as the patient is rehydrated, rewarmed, and adequately oxygenated.

- *Problem*: Convulsions due to hyponatraemia. Depressed level of consciousness due to cerebral hypoxia.
  Management: Assess level of consciousness. Observe and report seizures. Maintain patient safety at all times (cot sides on bed, ensure patent airway during seizures). Monitor serum sodium levels if symptomatic. Aim to correct hyponatraemia slowly by IV infusion of 0.9% sodium chloride. If having seizures and serum sodium is less than 120 mmol/litre more aggressive sodium replacement should be given using small, frequent volumes of hypertonic saline. The level of consciousness is

always depressed and some patients may be deeply comatose. Regular neurological assessments should be performed (see Chapter 10). Note that a cerebrovascular accident may be the precipitating factor of the coma.

◆ *Problem*: Paralytic ileus due to decreased gut motility. *Management*: A nasogastric tube should be inserted, regularly aspirated, and left to drain freely. Identification of precipitating factors. All potential sites of infection should be cultured (sputum, urine, blood, wounds, etc.). A 12-lead ECG should be recorded to exclude myocardial infarction and a full neurological examination performed to exclude a cerebrovascular accident, although this is difficult in the comatose patient. Other precipitating factors, such as hypothermia and trauma, will be obvious. The patient's own drug therapy should be considered as a potential precipitating factor (e.g. antithyroid medication).

Return to the euthyroid state

Thyroxine supplements will be required but the sudden introduction of high plasma levels of thyroxine are dangerous. The consequent abrupt increase in metabolism can cause angina, myocardial infarction, and arrhythmias. Many patients with long-term hypothyroidism have ischaemic heart disease to some degree. While oxygen demand to the heart is low in the hypothyroid state, a reduction in blood supply has little effect. However, when thyroid hormone is administered, oxygen demand is increased and requirements may not be met by increased delivery.

Most authorities recommend that small quantities of thyroxine be given initially and then gradually escalated.

If T_4 is administered it then has to be converted to T_3 by the body. This conversion is not efficient in the seriously ill (see later) and its half-life in the circulation can be more than 7 days. T_3 can be administered directly. Its onset of action is also not immediate and may take days to weeks to take effect. It can be given intravenously in slowly increasing dose.

Patients in myxoedema coma usually have an impaired glucocorticoid response to stress since the adrenals share the general hypometabolism of the body.

Myxoedema coma may also be secondary to hypopituitarism in which case there may also be an associated adrenal insufficiency. Corticosteroids (usually IV hydrocortisone 100 mg q.d.s.) are therefore given until adrenal sufficiency can be demonstrated.

Sick euthyroid syndrome

In critical illness the 'sick euthyroid syndrome' is commonly produced within hours to days. Instead of T_4 being metabolised to 'active' T_3, a different iodide is cleaved resulting in formation of the inactive 'reverse' T_3 (rT_3). TSH levels are often elevated, but on occasion may be depressed. The relevance of the sick euthyroid syndrome is its direct association with a poor prognosis. However, although limited studies have been performed, there does not seem to be any benefit from administering thyroid hormones; indeed this may even be harmful.

Hyperthyroidism (thyrotoxicosis)

Hyperthyroidism results from an excess of thyroid hormones (T_3 and T_4). It may be caused by primary disease of the thyroid gland or can be secondary to a pituitary tumour (where excess TSH is produced).

Effects of hyperthyroidism

These reflect the increase in metabolism caused by the thyroid hormones.

◆ Cardiovascular:
Increase in heart rate. Thyroid hormones are positive inotropes. They also increase sinoatrial firing and reduce the electrical threshold of atrial excitation. Atrial fibrillation or other tachyarrhythmias can develop and may further impair cardiac performance.
Blood pressure is often elevated, but also may be low if SVR is excessively decreased (see later).
Cardiac output is increased due to increased heart rate, preload, and myocardial contractility. This hyperdynamic circulation imposes an increase in cardiac work, which can lead to myocardial hypertrophy as the heart functions near to its limit. Heart failure can result from a combination of reduced myocardial contractile reserve, and tachyarrhythmias. 'High output' heart failure can also result from the failure of

---

CAUSES OF HYPERTHYROIDISM

◆ Autoimmune. Antibodies called thyroid-stimulating immunoglobulins are found in 50–80% of thyrotoxic patients. These cause structural and functional changes to the gland, the development of a goitre, and infiltration by lymphoid tissue. One of these antibodies is called long-acting thyroid stimulator (LATS) and causes prolonged stimulation of the thyroid cells.

◆ Thyroid adenoma. A tumour of the thyroid gland that secretes thyroxine independently of control by the anterior pituitary gland.

◆ Overtreated hyperthyroidism.

◆ Self-administered thyroxine.

the heart to meet the excessive metabolic demands of the body.

Management of heart failure in patients with hyperthyroidism is by reduction of volume overload (by venodilators and diuretics), control of heart rate (beta-blockers and/or amiodarone or digoxin for concurrent atrial fibrillation—often higher than normal doses are required), and treatment of the cause of the hyperthyroidism.

Systemic vascular resistance (SVR) may be decreased. Blood flow is not uniformly distributed in the body; it is greatly increased in the skin, skeletal muscle, and coronary arteries, although not to the cerebral, hepatic, or renal vessels. This may result in a fall in blood pressure.

Hyponatraemia may be present from excess fluid loss related to pyrexia, sweating, diarrhoea, etc.

Angina may be aggravated in patients with hyperthyroidism due to the increase in myocardial oxygen demand. The risk of thrombosis is also increased in patients with atrial fibrillation and prophylactic anticoagulation should be given.

◆ Gastrointestinal tract:
Nausea, vomiting, diarrhoea (due to increase in gut motility).
Weight loss.

◆ Central nervous system:
Nervousness, agitation, confusion.
Hyperactivity.
Tremors.

◆ Other effects of hyperthyroidism:
Frequent micturition.
Exophthalmus and corneal ulceration.
Increased body temperature, warm, moist skin.
Heat intolerance.
Goitre—may result in swallowing or breathing difficulties.

Exophthalmus This results from an excess growth of tissue and the formation of oedema behind the eye sockets causing the eyeballs to protrude. It is caused by the same autoimmune mechanism that causes the hyperthyroidism. The tissue growth cannot be eliminated once formed and even with adequate treatment of the hyperthyroidism the exophthalmus will remain throughout life. The eyelid retracts and the patient is unable to lubricate the cornea by blinking. The cornea is then prone to drying and ulceration. Specialist advice must be sought at an early stage if the eyes appear inflamed, as this is a serious complication and can cause blindness.

Goitre This is an enlargement of the thyroid gland, which becomes visible and palpable. This can be associated with hypothyroidism, hyperthyroidism, or a euthyroid state.

A non-toxic goitre occurs when the gland hypertrophies in response to an increase in secretion of TSH secondary to diminished output of thyroid hormones. In hypothyroidism the thyroid gland enlarges in an attempt to produce adequate quantities of thyroid hormone and in the euthyroid state a simple non-toxic goitre results from a dietary lack of iodine (also known as endemic goitre).

Some goitres became nodular and can cause hyperthyroidism (toxic goitre) or become malignant. The enlarged gland can also compress the larynx and trachea causing hoarseness of the voice and an inspiratory stridor.

Treatment of hyperthyroidism

Treatment is by:

◆ Propanolol or other beta-blockers to reduce sympathetic activity.

◆ Antithyroid drugs. Carbimazole is the drug of choice and acts by interfering with the synthesis of thyroid hormones. Iodine solution is also given as short-term treatment in thyrotoxic crisis or prior to surgery.

◆ Radioactive iodine (^{131}I). Thyroid cells take up the radioactive iodine and are then destroyed by it. This reduces the vascularity of the gland and hence its size. It is a long-term treatment and results may not be apparent for several months.

◆ Surgery to remove part of the gland. This is not done as an emergency procedure, but is delayed until the metabolic and cardiovascular status have stabilized.

Patients with hyperthyroidism will not usually require admission to the ICU unless symptoms are severe. Rapid atrial fibrillation may require synchronized cardioversion if this is unresponsive to anti-arrhythmics (beta blockade, digoxin, amiodarone, etc.). Severe heart failure will also require intensive monitoring. However, a thyroid crisis can develop in the untreated patient and, although rare, such patients will require management in the ICU.

Thyroid crisis

This is an exaggerated form of hyperthyroidism. It occurs acutely, in any age group, and is an extreme, life-threatening condition.

Advances in diagnostic methods have made this condition very uncommon and it is usually only seen in

PREDISPOSING FACTORS THAT MAY TRIGGER A THYROID CRISIS

- ◆ Infection
- ◆ Surgery, trauma
- ◆ Myocardial infarction
- ◆ Cerebrovascular accident
- ◆ Eclampsia, labour
- ◆ Uncontrolled diabetes mellitus
- ◆ Radioactive iodine if given to patients who are not euthyroid
- ◆ Palpation of the thyroid gland or inadequate beta-adrenergic blockade pre-operatively may be a cause (this is disputed by some authorities)

patients who have undiagnosed or inadequately treated hyperthyroidism. Even in these patients predisposing factors are usually required to trigger the acute crisis.

Whatever the predisposing factor the features and management of the crisis are the same and treatment must be rapid and aggressive.

Features of thyroid crisis

- ◆ *Hyperpyrexia*: This may be extreme (>40°C) and could be wrongly attributed to sepsis.
- ◆ *Cardiac failure*: This is often refractory to conventional treatment and may be fatal. Cardiomegaly and ECG changes of left ventricular hypertrophy may be apparent.
- ◆ *Tachycardia*: Can be sinus but frequently atrial fibrillation is seen in the middle-aged or elderly. Heart rate often exceeds 160 bpm and there may also be ventricular arrhythmias.
- ◆ *Neurological features*: Extreme agitation, tremors, and confusion which may lead to convulsions and coma.
- ◆ *Abdominal features*: Epigastric pain, vomiting and diarrhoea, and later, liver dysfunction and jaundice.
- ◆ *Skin*: Usually hot and moist with increased sweating.
- ◆ *Other symptoms* include those listed in Table 16.2.

Management of thyroid crisis

This is essentially aimed at reducing the effects of the thyroid hormones and supportive treatment until these effects can be bought under control. Before treatment begins blood samples are taken for measurement of TSH, free and total T_3, and T_4. Treatment, however,

should not be delayed to await the results as this test is merely to confirm the presence of thyroid overactivity.

Patients presenting in a thyroid crisis are extremely ill and mortality for this condition remains at 15–20%.

Drug therapy

Drugs are used to inhibit the catecholamine-like effects of the thyroid hormones and to inhibit their synthesis.

The large quantities of T_3 produced in a thyroid crisis have a similar effect to catecholamines; IV propanolol is the most commonly used beta-adrenergic receptor antagonist. Chlorpromazine or haloperidol are often used in combination with propanolol for its sedative effect.

Hydrocortisone should also be administered intravenously.

Iodine (in the form of Lugol's solution or potassium iodide) is given to inhibit the synthesis and release of thyroxine. This reduces the vascularity and size of the thyroid. It is usually given in milk, as it is unpalatable. Lugol's iodine must be drunk through a straw (or placed down a nasogastric tube) to prevent staining of the teeth. Potassium iodide can be given intravenously but requires dilution in 500 ml of 0.9% sodium chloride and if heart failure is present this must be administered with care.

Drugs, such as carbimazole (or propylthiouracil), are also used to inhibit the synthesis of T_3 and T_4, and work by blocking the reaction of tyrosine and iodine.

Support of vital functions

- ◆ *Problem*: Tachycardia.
  Management: Continuous ECG monitoring, 12-lead ECG. Observe for arrhythmias. Atrial fibrillation can be resistant even to large doses of digoxin and amiodarone. Serum potassium must be monitored and hypokalaemia corrected, particularly before antiarrhythmic drugs are given. Administer propanolol—orally or intravenously according to severity of illness.

- ◆ *Problem*: Heart failure.
  Management: Monitor pressure ± cardiac output. There may be considerable fluid loss from sweating and hyperpyrexia, and hypovolaemia should be corrected. Treatment depends on whether the heart failure is associated with 'high' or 'low' output. Low-output states are managed conventionally with intravenous nitrate infusions, CPAP, etc. For high-output states carefully monitored beta blockade may be indicated. Hypotension is not usually a problem if the cardiac filling pressures are maintained but continuous blood pressure monitoring should be carried out, particularly if intravenous propanolol is being given.

- *Problem*: Pyrexia.
  Management: Monitor core temperature. Actively reduce pyrexia by fanning, tepid sponging, and antipyretics. Salicylates should be avoided as they displace thyroid hormones from their binding proteins.

- *Problem*: Hypoglycaemia.
  Management: Monitor blood sugar levels. Give glucose infusions or boluses of 50% glucose as required. Early enteral nutrition should be encouraged but intestinal absorption is often impaired during a crisis.

- *Problem*: Agitation.
  Management: These patients can be very irritable and apprehensive. Chlorpromazine, haloperidol, or a benzodiazipine should be given as required for sedation. If untreated, convulsions may occur and progress to coma. Observe for seizures; maintain patient safety (cot sides, airway control). Protect patient from additional stresses and nurse in a quiet environment.

- *Problem*: Dyspnoea (secondary to heart failure).
  Management: Monitor respiratory rate and blood gases. Treat heart failure. Administer humidified oxygen therapy as required. CPAP or mechanical ventilation may be required to maintain adequate oxygenation.

- *Problem*: Corneal ulceration due to exophthalmia or lid retraction.
  Management: Protect the exposed cornea by frequent application of hypomellose eye drops. Local or systemic steroids may be required for exophthalmos with tarsorraphy (surgical closure of the eyelids) in severe cases. Lid retraction usually responds to treatment of the thyrotoxicosis.

The parathyroid glands

Four parathyroid glands are situated adjacent to the posterior and lateral aspects of the thyroid gland. They produce parathyroid hormone (PTH) which plays an essential part in the regulation of the plasma calcium level. Parathyroid hormone has several mechanisms by which it raises serum calcium and is itself regulated by a negative feedback mechanism so that calcium levels remain constant. The parathyroid glands can enlarge up to 10-fold if there is a long-term decrease in the plasma calcium level.

The parathyroid hormone

Calcitonin released from the thyroid gland and PTH have opposing effects; together, they maintain in adults a plasma calcium level of 2.3–2.8 mmol/l and an ionized calcium level (non-protein-bound) of 1.18–1.3 mmol/litre.

ACTIONS OF PARATHYROID HORMONE

PTH increases the plasma calcium level by:

- Increasing calcium reabsorption by the renal tubular cells.

- Causing phosphaturia, which promotes further release of calcium from the bone.

- Increasing osteoclastic activity in the bone which causes release of calcium and phosphate.

- Decreasing osteoblastic activity in the bone thus reducing bone matrix formation.

- Increasing calcium absorption from the gastrointestinal tract.

Functions of calcium

- Calcium decreases the permeability and increases the strength of capillary membranes. If the plasma calcium levels are low the membranes became very friable and there is increased permeability to fluid.

- At half the normal plasma calcium level the membranes of nerve fibres are more permeable to sodium ions and become partially depolarized. These fibres then transmit repetitive and uncontrolled impulses to the muscles resulting in spasm (tetany).

- Increased levels of calcium depress neuronal activity and the membranes will not depolarize easily.

- Calcium imbalances can have profound effects upon heart muscle. Low plasma levels cause the duration of systole to decrease and the heart dilates excessively during diastole. High calcium levels promote an overconstriction of the cardiac muscle causing it to contract too forcibly during systole and not relaxing satisfactorily during diastole. The reason for this is that when impulses pass through cardiac muscle small amounts of calcium ions are released into the sarcoplasm of the muscle fibres. These ions initiate the contractile process. If only small amounts are available in the extracellular fluid the intensity of the contraction is reduced, if excess is present there is overexcitation of the heart.

- Calcium is a vital component of the blood clotting process (see Chapter 14) and can occasionally be low enough to cause severe clotting abnormalities.

- There is no direct correlation between the severity of symptoms and the plasma calcium level in hypercalcaemia. Generally, symptoms appear at a level above 3.0 mmol/litre and can be fatal above 4–5 mmol/litre.

TABLE 16.3   Signs and symptoms of hypercalcaemia

ECG changes: short Q–T interval, prolonged P–R interval, AV block, VF

Hypertension

Ureteric stones may form and can lead to obstructive uropathy

Damage to the renal tubular mechanism causes polyuria with subsequent dehydration. Renal failure may develop later as glomeruli are damaged

Muscle weakness and general malaise due to neuropathy

Drowsiness, coma

Headaches, confusion, myalgia

Bone pain, joint effusions

Nausea and vomiting

Abdominal pain, pancreatitis

Anorexia, thirst, constipation, peptic ulceration

Conjunctivitis due to calcium deposits an the cornea

Psychiatric disorders

- Vitamin D is essential for the absorption of calcium through the gut wall (hence in childhood rickets, where there is a lack of vitamin D, the bone is soft and deforms).

Hypercalcaemia

See Table 16.3 for signs and symptoms of hypercalcaemia.

Management of hypercalcaemia

Symptomatic hypercalcaemia requires immediate treatment and, if severe, admission to the ICU will be necessary for monitoring purposes. The aims of treatment are to:

- Lower plasma calcium levels (see Table 16.4).
- Monitor and support vital functions.
- Identify the cause and treat where possible. e.g. malignancy, primary hyperparathyroidism, sarcoidosis.

Plasma calcium levels

Table 16.4 indicates methods of reducing plasma calcium levels.

Monitoring and support of vital functions

- *Problem*: Dehydration due to polyuria.
  Management: Monitor CVP or PCWP measurements. Rehydrate using colloid or 0.9% sodium chloride. Monitor urine output.
- *Problem*: Potential arrhythmias due to hypercalcaemia.
  Management: Continuous ECG monitoring. 12-lead ECG. Observe for and treat arrhythmias. Note that

TABLE 16.4   Methods of reducing plasma calcium levels

Treatment	Reason
Rehydration followed by low-dose intravenous furosemide (frusemide)	Patients with hypercalcaemia are often dehydrated due to polyuria. Following rehydration the administration of low-dose furosemide increases excretion of calcium by the kidneys
Glucocorticoid therapy (hydrocortisone or dexamethasone)	Reduces the intestinal absorption of calcium
Bisphosphonates (e.g. clodronate, pamidronate)	Compounds that are potent inhibitors of bone resorption and formation (i.e. inhibit osteoclastic activity)
Mithromycin (IV)	This inhibits mobilization of calcium from the skeleton. However, it cannot be given continuously for more than a few days, due to its bone marrow toxicity, and it can cause liver and renal failure
Calcitonin (IV or SC)	Inhibits osteoclastic activity. Not effective in all patients and may take several days to achieve effect
Peritoneal or haemodialysis	This effectively reduces the calcium level and avoids the dangerous side-effects of drug therapy. Note. use calcium-free dialysate

hypercalcaemia enhances the action of digoxin and can cause digoxin toxicity (particularly if there is concurrent renal impairment).

- *Problem*: Potential renal failure due to renal tubular damage or (long-term) stone formation/nephrocalcinosis.
  Management: Monitor urine output, plasma urea and electrolytes, arterial pH, and bicarbonate. Renal support therapy if required.
- *Problem*: Hypertension due to hypercalcaemia.
  Management: Correct hypercalcaemia. Monitor blood pressure. Antihypertensive therapy (e.g. calcium antagonists) if necessary.

Hypocalcaemia

See Table 16.5 for symptoms of hypocalcaemia.

Management of hypocalcaemia

Tetany is the major symptom of hypocalcaemia. The patient usually complains of numbness, stiffness, tremor, or tingling in the hands and feet. This progresses to

TABLE 16.5 Symptoms of hypocalcaemia

Tetany, muscle twitching, tremors, facial spasms

Paraesthesiae (tingling) of extremities and mouth

ECG changes: prolonged Q–T interval

Muscle weakness

Hypotension

Convulsions

(Long-term) cataracts, changes to teeth, nails, hair

generalized muscle hypertonia causing spasmodic and uncoordinated muscle contractions, particularly of the elbows, wrist, and carpophalangeal joints (carpopedal spasm). If untreated, this progresses to photophobia, bronchospasm, laryngeal spasm, cardiac arrhythmias, dysphagia, and, ultimately, convulsions. There may also be psychiatric disturbances such as anxiety, irritability, and neuroses.

Hypocalcaemia is generally better tolerated than hypercalcaemia; however, the onset of tetany or myocardial dysfunction requires rapid treatment.

This is relatively easy to correct by the administration of calcium salts. If hypocalcaemia is symptomatic this is given by intravenous infusion of 10–20 ml of 10% calcium chloride. If asymptomatic, calcium supplements can be given orally (calcium gluconate tablets, Sandocal).

Note that hypermagnesaemia (e.g. from excess diuretics, diarrhoea) may also cause hypocalcaemia which responds to magnesium replacement.

Nursing assessment

• *Problem*: Neuromuscular instability/anxiety.
  Management: Reassure patient and use calm manner. Nurse in an environment with minimum noise and avoid bright lights. Protect patient from injury (padded cot sides, remove articles that may cause harm). Anticonvulsive therapy may be required.

• *Problem*: Potential cardiac arrhythmias.
  Management: Continuous ECG monitoring. Note that calcium potentiates the effect of digoxin and both increase systolic contractions. Observe for arrhythmias and monitor blood pressure.

Disorders of the parathyroid glands

Hyperparathyroidism

Excess parathyroid hormone (PTH) is produced by the gland causing hypercalcaemia and hypophosphataemia (PTH causes increased excretion of phosphate ions by the kidney).

CAUSES OF HYPERPARATHYROIDISM

Primary hyperparathyroidism:

• parathyroid adenoma or hyperplasia

• carcinoma of the parathyroid

• multiple endocrine adenomatosis (may be produced by a tumour elsewhere, e.g. lungs, kidney).

Secondary hyperparathyroidism:

• can occur in response to hypocalcaemia resulting from another disease (usually chronic renal failure).

Tertiary hyperparathyroidism:

• longstanding secondary hyperparathyroidism can lead to autonomous function in one or more parathyroid adenomas.

Investigations for the diagnosis of primary hyperparathyroidism

Biochemical tests are shown in Table 16.6.

Hypoparathyroidism

This is caused by insufficient secretion of parathyroid hormone and may be due to primary idiopathic and autoimmune disease, or secondary to thyroid surgery.

TABLE 16.6 Biochemical tests for the diagnosis of primary hyperparathyroidism

Test	Level
Plasma ionized calcium	Raised
Plasma calcium[a]	Raised
Plasma phosphate	Low
Serum PTH	Raised
Serum alkaline phosphatase	Raised

[a]Corrected for serum albumin concentration.

For every 6 g/litre albumin below 42 g/litre add 0.1 mmol/litre to the calcium level.

TABLE 16.7 Biochemical tests for the diagnosis of hypoparathyroidism

Test	Level
Plasma ionized calcium	Low
Plasma calcium[a]	Low
Plasma phosphate	High
Serum alkaline phosphatase	Normal

[a]Corrected for serum protein or albumin concentration.

Investigations for the diagnosis of hypoparathyroidism are given in Table 16.7.

The pancreas

The pancreas secretes two hormones, insulin and glucagon, from the islets of Langerhans. The islets consist of two types of cell, alpha and beta. Insulin is secreted by the beta cells, and glucagon by the alpha cells. Both hormones have a profound effect upon metabolism.

Insulin

Functions of insulin

1. Promotes the transport of glucose into most cells of the body (particularly liver, fat, and muscle cells) by activating the carrier mechanism by which glucose is transported into the cells. Insulin therefore lowers the blood sugar. Lack of insulin causes hyperglycaemia.

2. Promotes glycogen storage in the liver and muscle. Insulin activates liver enzymes (glucokinase and glycogen synthetase) to enable storage of glucose either by combining glucose with phosphate ions, or combining many glucose molecules to form glycogen. When insulin is absent, phosphorylase activated within the liver depolymerizes glycogen, releasing glucose back into the circulation (glycogenolysis). Glycogen therefore provides a store of glucose for use when immediate energy requirements cannot be met by the body (e.g. during periods of starvation, increased exercise).

3. Converts glucose into fat. Excess glucose in the circulation is firstly stored as glycogen, but when these stores are filled it is then converted into fat. Most of the glucose is converted into fat by the liver and then released as lipoprotein for storage in fat tissues. However, some is synthesized directly by the fat cells.

4. Inhibits fat metabolism (except for the storage and synthesis of fat from glucose). Cells preferentially use glucose for energy rather than fat because of the nature of their enzyme systems. In times of insufficient circulating glucose, stored glycogen in the liver and muscle cells is broken down to release glucose. Insulin inhibits hormone-sensitive lipase, which is responsible for splitting fatty acids from stored fat before release into the blood. Therefore, once stored, fat is usually unavailable as a primary source of energy while there are sufficient levels of insulin, and energy requirements can be met from stored glycogen. However, when insulin is lacking, fat metabolism is greatly increased and large amounts of fatty acids are released into the blood. These fatty acids are used as an immediate energy source by the cells as they are unable to utilize glucose due to the lack of insulin.

5. Blood lipid levels greatly increase when insulin is lacking as the free fatty acids are transported to the liver and converted into cholesterol, triglycerides, and phospholipids (lipoproteins). This rapid and massive metabolism of fatty acids by the liver causes large amounts of acetoacetate acid and other ketones to be released into the blood. This causes a severe ketoacidosis.

6. Promotes protein deposition in cells. Insulin is an anabolic hormone which increases the formation of RNA in cells, the formation of protein by ribosomes and increases the rate that amino acids are transported into cells for the synthesis of protein. When insulin is lacking, protein as well as fat is used as a source of energy. Lack of insulin therefore affects growth as tissue formation (which utilizes protein) is inhibited.

Insulin secretion

Insulin is secreted from the pancreas as a direct effect of raised levels of glucose on the beta cells. As insulin facilitates transport of glucose into cells, the glucose level falls and secretion is inhibited (negative feedback mechanism).

Glucagon

Many of the actions of glucagon are opposite to those of insulin and its effect is to raise the blood glucose level. This is achieved by causing the breakdown of stored glycogen (glycogenolysis) and by converting proteins into glucose (gluconeogenesis).

Glucagon secretion is stimulated when the alpha cells detect subnormal blood glucose levels. Once released, glucagon causes blood glucose levels to rise within minutes as glucose is released from stored glycogen. As the blood glucose rises to normal, glucagon secretion is inhibited.

FUNCTIONS OF INSULIN

- Promotes transport of glucose into cells, hence lowers blood glucose level
- Promotes glycogen storage in liver and muscle cells
- Converts glucose into fat
- Inhibits fat metabolism
- Promotes tissue growth by protein deposition

FUNCTIONS OF GLUCAGON

- Raises blood glucose level
- Glycogenolysis
- Gluconeogenesis

By the opposing actions of insulin and glucagon, blood glucose levels can be kept within a fairly constant range.

Disorders of the pancreas

Diabetes mellitus

This is hyperglycaemia due to the deficiency, destruction (due to antibodies), or impaired effectiveness of insulin. There are two types.

- Type 1: insulin-dependent diabetes (IDDM). This accounts for approximately 20% of diabetes and usually has its onset in childhood or adolescence (also called juvenile onset diabetes). It results from destruction of the beta cells in the pancreas and there may be both a genetic disposition and a viral trigger (e.g. Coxsackie B, mumps). IDDM often presents acutely as hyperglycaemic ketoacidosis. Lifelong insulin therapy will be required.

- Type 2: non-insulin-dependent diabetes (NIDDM). This usually affects those over 40 years of age (also called maturity onset diabetes) and tends to occur in the overweight. Patients are often asymptomatic and may first present with related complications (see later). This type of diabetes is usually controlled by a combination of diet, weight loss (if appropriate), and oral hypoglycaemic drugs.

Secondary diabetes

This occurs secondary to drug therapy metabolic/ endocrine disease or critical illness. The term 'insulin resistance' is usually applied to these states and may be due

CAUSES OF SECONDARY DIABETES

- Drugs: glucocorticoids, adrenaline, thiazide diuretics, thyroid hormones, oral contraceptives.

- Metabolic/endocrine: Cushing's syndrome, Conn's syndrome (primary hyperaldosteronism), phaeochromocytoma.

- Other: acute or chronic pancreatitis, pancreatic cancer, pregnancy, 'stress', e.g. sepsis, major trauma, burns, head injury.

to problems of decreased secretion, decreased responsiveness of cellular insulin receptors, or modification of pathways further downstream. Increased release of hormones (e.g. cortisol, catecholamines, glucagon, growth hormone) in the acute response to stress will also antagonise insulin's metabolic actions.

Diabetic emergencies

There are three main diabetic emergencies:

1. Diabetic ketoacidosis (DKA) characterized by hyperglycaemia, ketosis, and acidosis, often with coma.

2. Hyperosmolar, hyperglycaemic states (HHS) usually characterized by hyperglycaemia but with minimal ketosis, often with profound coma.

3. Hypoglycaemic coma.

1. Diabetic ketoacidosis (DKA)

Approximately one-third of patients presenting with the symptoms of DKA are newly diagnosed diabetics. The causes of DKA in diabetics include infection, myocardial infarction, thromboembolic episodes, or noncompliance with treatment. Coma is not always a feature of the illness but the conscious level will vary according to the level of increased plasma osmolality. Hyperglycaemia and ketosis are always features of DKA though the blood sugar level does not have to be particularly elevated. This condition is life-threatening, even if the patient is not comatose.

Principal features of DKA

- *Hyperglycaemia.* Insulin facilitates the transfer of glucose into the cells; therefore lack of insulin means that the tissue cells are unable to utilize the glucose derived from carbohydrate metabolism. Other 'stress' hormones, such as adrenaline, noradrenaline, glucagon, cortisol, and growth hormone, are also released and their antagonistic action further exacerbates the hyperglycaemia.

- *Dehydration.* When the concentration of glucose in the blood is above the renal threshold (approximately 8.5–10.5 mmol/litre), the kidney does not reabsorb the excess glucose and this is excreted in the urine. An osmotic diuresis results and large volumes of water and electrolytes are lost. The patient experiences extreme thirst and becomes polydipsic but, nevertheless, still rapidly dehydrates. Dehydration initially depletes the intracellular compartment as this is the largest of the body's fluid spaces. At first there is little effect on intravascular volume but as the fluid loss becomes more severe, the intravascular volume falls and the patient progresses to hypovolaemic shock (hypotension, tachycardia). Fluid is not only lost through an osmotic diuresis but also via hyperventilation, nausea, vomiting, sweating fever, and decreased fluid intake due to coma.

- *Electrolyte loss.* This is associated with polyuria. In particular, sodium, potassium, phosphate, and magnesium ions are lost via the urine. Hypokalaemia can be a fatal complication of DKA and this results mainly from haemodilution following fluid resuscitation, the correction of hyperglycaemia by insulin infusion, and inadequate potassium replacement. Low serum concentrations of potassium, phosphate, and magnesium can cause cardiac arrhythmias or asystole, particularly if there is pre-existing cardiac disease. Hypophosphataemia can cause serious complications such as decreased level of consciousness, generalized muscle weakness, respiratory failure, and impaired myocardial contractility.

- *Ketoacidosis.* Although extremely hungry, the patient cannot utilize glucose derived from dietary carbohydrate due to insufficient insulin. Energy is provided by fat breakdown (lipolysis). Some of the free fatty acids released by lipolysis are converted into ketones by the liver and these can cause a profound metabolic acidosis. The patient compensates for this acidosis by hyperventilation (Kussmaul respiration—see Chapter 4).

Management of DKA

In the management of DKA there is no place for rigid regimens of fluid and insulin. Every patient will differ in their degree of hypovolaemia, blood glucose levels, and level of consciousness. They may also have an underlying condition, such as sepsis, which has triggered the illness or they may suffer from chronic disease such as renal failure or cardiac impairment. Resuscitation must be guided by measured cardiovascular variables and the response to treatment. The patient requires intensive monitoring (usually a central venous line and, if indicated by the precipitating condition or past medical history, cardiac output monitoring with frequent reassessment). Mortality is relatively low, of the order of 5–10%, and often depends on the precipitating condition and co-morbidities.

Nursing management

- *Problem*: Inadequate airway protection due to decreased level of consciousness.
  Management: Ensure patent and protected airway— endotracheal intubation may be necessary. Mechanical ventilation may be needed for deeply comatose patients or for concurrent lung pathology. A nasogastric tube should be inserted as gastric atony, which is

associated with DKA, increases the risk of aspiration. Observe the respiratory rate and pattern. Monitor blood gases and give oxygen therapy as indicated. Note that elderly patients may have underlying respiratory disease or may have been immobile at home prior to admission, thus increasing the risk of atelectasis or infection (this may also be a precipitating factor).

- *Problem*: Hypovolaemia due to dehydration
  Management: This must be promptly corrected, particularly in patients with pre-existing renal dysfunction where adequate organ perfusion must be maintained. Care should be taken not to overload the patient, especially if there is a pre-existing cardiac history.
  Average fluid requirements will be 5–10 litres in the first 24 hours but replacement must be governed by filling pressure or stroke volume measurements The choice of fluid used for replacement is controversial but should logically depend an the degree of hypovolaemia. Fluid is not lost equally from the three body spaces—intracellular (ICS), interstitial (ISS), and intravascular (IVS). Fluid is initially lost from the largest space (ICS) and least of all from the IVS. Therefore, it is logical to rehydrate using a fluid similar in sodium concentration to the fluid lost (i.e. hypotonic saline, 0.45%). If fluid loss is more severe and has caused hypovolaemia and shock (hypotension, tachycardia, low CVP or PAWP) then considerable fluid has also been lost from the IVS. The circulating fluid must be rapidly replaced; use of a colloid solution aids fluid retention in the IVS (only one-quarter to one-third of crystalloid will remain in the IVS, the remainder enters the ISS). Cardiovascular variables must be continuously monitored during rehydration. The rate of fluid infusion can be gauged by measuring the variables before and after 200 ml aliquots and assessing the response.
  Total body water losses are difficult to assess and will differ with each patient. If intravascular replacement needs are high then water loss will generally be high. A range of 50–200 ml/hour of 5% glucose is given for 48 hours or until the patient can take oral fluids. (Note: there is minimal extra glucose in 5% glucose and this will have a negligible effect on the blood glucose level.) Table 16.8 gives a summary of fluid replacement in DKA.
  Persisting hypotension and/or oliguria is not automatically due to hypovolaemia. Care should be taken to give adequate but not excessive fluid replacement.

- *Problem*: Hyperglycaemia.
  Management: Hourly blood glucose measurements initially. A continuous infusion of insulin should be titrated according to glucose levels, aiming for a smooth,

TABLE 16.8 A summary of fluid replacement in DKA

If hypovolaemic, rapidly restore intravascular volume using colloids

When dehydration is less severe (normal BP, heart rate, CVP) replace intracellular losses with normal saline (e.g. 100–200 ml/hour). Hypotonic saline may be needed if the plasma sodium level rises excessively

5% glucose (e.g. 100 ml/hour) when the blood sugar level is <10mmol/litre

Adjust rates and volumes of infusion according to cardiovascular variables and response

slow return to normal over the next 24–48 hours. A reduction in blood glucose of 2–4 mmol/hour is satisfactory. Rapid correction of hyperglycaemia should be avoided and an initial intravenous bolus of insulin is unnecessary. Insulin not only reduces the blood glucose level but also moves water and other ions into the cells. A rapid movement of water can increase CSF pressure and cause cerebral oedema. The movement of water out of the IVS into the ICS also exacerbates hypovolaemia.

Rigid regimens of insulin should be avoided as patients vary in their response. A low-rate infusion of 2–5 units/hour is commenced initially and can be increased as necessary to maintain a steady fall in blood sugar level. Initial insensitivity in some patients may be related to dehydration.

Insulin should be continued, even when normoglycaemia is eventually achieved, as the patient will need lifelong insulin. To prevent hypoglycaemia, more glucose can be introduced into the IV infusion. Alternatively, the patient may take oral fluids if able, or be fed enterally, if safe.

Some authorities recommend that insulin for infusions be mixed with a carrier solution, such as albumin, to prevent the absorption of insulin on to the plastic syringe. This is unnecessary, as it is not the amount of insulin given that matters but the patient's response to it.

Urine should be tested regularly for ketones and glucose.

- *Problem*: Electrolyte depletion due to polyuria.
Management: Continuous ECG monitoring, observe for arrhythmias. With the accompanying acidosis the patient is usually hyperkalaemic, though total body potassium is depleted. The potassium level may fall rapidly with insulin and fluid. Thus blood levels should be monitored 1–2 hourly. Give IV supplements accordingly (usually 5–20 mmol/hour are required).

Higher infusion rates are occasionally needed but there is an increased risk of rhythm disturbances. Serum phosphate and magnesium levels should be measured on admission and thereafter daily until normal. Supplements of both can be given IV until levels are normalized.

- *Problem*: Metabolic acidosis due to ketosis.
Management: Measure arterial pH, bicarbonate and base excess/deficit hourly initially. IV sodium bicarbonate is not currently recommended for routine use due to the dangers of paradoxical intracellular acidosis, sodium overload, and rebound alkalosis. However, if the blood pH is <6.9 then aliquots of bicarbonate (e.g. 50 ml of 8.4% solution) can be considered though the acidosis will usually correct naturally with insulin therapy and fluid replacement.

- *Problem*: Potential deep vein thrombosis due to dehydration and possible pre-existing vascular disease.
Management: Observe for thrombotic episodes (DVT, pulmonary embolus). Give prophylactic subcutaneous heparin.

- *Problem*: Precipitating factor.
Management: In the patient with DKA every attempt should be made to identify the cause of this illness. Potential sites of infection (urine, sputum, wounds, etc.) should be cultured. A 12-lead ECG should be taken to exclude a myocardial infarction.

2 Hyperosmolar, hyperglycaemic states (HHS)

HHS commonly occurs in undiagnosed patients with NIDDM and, typically, the patient is older. Often there is a predisposing factor that triggers the condition.

FACTORS PREDISPOSING TO HHS

- Elderly
- Infection
- Trauma (including burns)
- Myocardial infarction
- Pancreatitis, hepatitis
- Renal failure
- Hypothermia
- Carbohydrate overload (enteral feeding, dextrose solutions)
- Drugs: e.g. phenytoin, thiazides (may inhibit insulin release) glucocorticoids, growth hormone (stimulate gluconeogenesis)

HHS differs from DKA in that the level of free fatty acids and counter-regulatory hormones is lower. This is probably due to sufficient insulin still being secreted to prevent lipolysis but not hyperglycaemia. Ketosis may thus be absent or mild.

Mortality is higher at 40–70% and is often due to pulmonary embolus because the condition is usually slower in onset and the patient is often immobile. However, it is much less common than DKA.

Management of HHS

The management is similar to that for DKA (see Fig. 16.2); however, the principal differences are as follows:

1. *Level of consciousness.* The patient may stay in coma longer—up to a week—therefore active management is usually longer. The incidence of coma is higher than in DKA. Airway maintenance and prevention of pneumonia is paramount. Early endotracheal intubation is recommended for airway protection, tracheal toilet, and intensive physiotherapy. There may be a higher incidence of chest infection in these patients since they are usually elderly, have been immobile or semi-comatose prior to admission, and the coma may last longer. Whereas patients with DKA often do not require supplemental oxygen, these patients usually do and may benefit from mask CPAP or BiPAP if intubation is not required. Hyperventilation is not a major feature of HHS since the acidosis, if present, is usually mild.

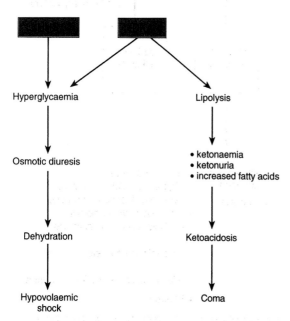

Fig. 16.2 Diagram showing the effects of HHS and DKA.

2. *Insulin therapy.* Patients with HHS are more sensitive to insulin than patients with DKA. Insulin infusions should therefore be commenced at a lower dose (e.g. 1–2 units/hour) and the dose altered according to response, aiming to reduce the blood glucose level by 2–4 mmol/litre/hour over 36–48 hours.

3. *Fluid replacement.* Dehydration is often more severe than in DKA and the patient is more likely to be hypovolaemic and shocked. However, the same principles of fluid replacement apply. Colloid is given to resuscitate the patient in shock. The rate of overall rehydration should be slower than for DKA because of the danger of rapid intracerebral fluid shifts precipitating cerebral oedema. The plasma sodium level is often elevated and, despite appropriate treatment, may even continue to rise for a few days, sometimes exceeding 170 mmol/litre. The total body sodium is, however, grossly depleted so the patient usually requires either 0.45% or 0.9% saline for electrolyte replacement. Potassium supplementation is also necessary to correct the large potassium deficit. Particular care must be paid to titrate fluid replacement against cardiovascular variables since these patients are often elderly and may have existing cardiac or renal dysfunction.

4. *Anticoagulation.* Pulmonary embolus is considered to be the major cause of mortality in these patients. It arises due to prolonged immobility and to the hyperviscosity of the circulating blood. Most authorities recommend anticoagulation with heparin, although whether this should be full intravenous heparinization or subcutaneous using low molecular weight heparin is still contentious.

3. Hypoglycaemic coma

Patients who develop hypoglycaemia are usually known diabetics controlled by insulin or oral sulphonylurea hypoglycaemics (e.g. glibenclamide). Occasionally, Addison's disease, liver failure or an insulinoma may also precipitate hypoglycaemia.

Hypoglycaemic symptoms (Table 16.9) result from a low blood glucose level. This may be caused by an insulin overdose (deliberate or accidental) or when the diabetic patient takes excessive exercise, has an inadequate food intake, or ingests excess alcohol.

The onset of coma is usually rapid, but most patients are aware of the onset of symptoms and can prevent an impending hypoglycaemic attack by taking sugar.

Hypoglycaemic patients admitted to the emergency department in coma can easily be diagnosed by bedside blood glucose analysis. Treatment must be rapid as hypoglycaemia can cause irreversible brain damage. Symp-

TABLE 16.9	Symptoms of hyperglycaemia and hypoglycaemia	
Hyperglycaemia	Restlessness
	Thirst
	Vomiting
	Abdominal pain
	Hot, dry, flushed skin
	Drowsiness
	Tachycardia
	Deep, sighing (Kussmaul) respirations
	Hypotension
	Coma
Hypoglycaemia	Headache
	Hunger
	Faintness
	Cool, moist skin
	Sweating
	Slurred speech
	Tachycardia/bradycardia
	Irrational behaviour, agitation
	Coma

toms can be reversed in minutes by the administration of aliquots of 20–50 ml IV of 50% glucose. If venous access proves impossible glucagon 1 mg IM can be given but is ineffective in hepatic dysfunction and alcohol ingestion and may exacerbate insulinoma-induced hypoglycaemia.

Such patients rarely require ICU care once the coma is reversed except those patients who have taken an insulin overdose (particularly if a long-acting insulin) where close monitoring of blood glucose levels will be required.

The pituitary gland

The hypothalamus and pituitary gland are anatomically and functionally closely linked. The hypothalamus lies below the third ventricle of the brain and extends down as the pituitary stalk to join the posterior pituitary gland. The anterior pituitary gland lies adjacent to the posterior pituitary but its secretions and functions are independent. The pituitary stalk contains nerves and capillaries through which hormones produced in the hypothalamus pass for storage in the posterior pituitary gland.

The anterior pituitary gland

Hormones produced by the anterior pituitary include:

◆ Growth hormone (GH)—affects fat, protein, and carbohydrate metabolism.

◆ Thyroid-stimulating hormone (TSH)—stimulates the thyroid gland to secrete thyroid hormones.

◆ Adrenocorticotrophic hormone (ACTH)—controls the secretion of adrenocortical hormones.

◆ Prolactin—produced during pregnancy and stimulates breast growth and secretory functions.

◆ Gonadotrophic hormones—involved in sexual functions: *in women* follicle-stimulating hormone (stimulates development of follicles in the ovaries) and luteinizing hormone (causes oestrogen and progesterone secretion by the ovaries and allows rupture of follicles); *in men* interstitial cell-stimulating hormone stimulates the testes to produce androgens.

The posterior pituitary gland

Two hormones are released from the posterior lobe. These are produced in the hypothalamus and stored in the posterior pituitary gland:

◆ Oxytocin—stimulates contraction of the uterus and the muscles of the milk ducts in the breast.

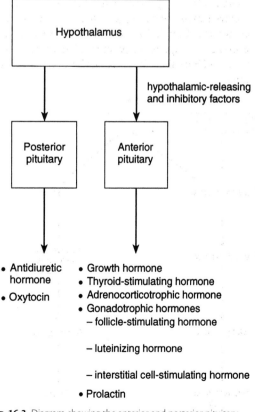

Fig. 16.3 Diagram showing the anterior and posterior pituitary hormones.

CAUSES OF DIABETES INSIPIDUS

- ◆ Neurosurgery
- ◆ Head injury
- ◆ Hypoxic brain injury
- ◆ Infarction of a pituitary tumour (pituitary apoplexy)
- ◆ Also, rarely, following meningococcal meningitis, penetrating thoracic trauma, coronary artery bypass surgery, amiodarone therapy

- ◆ Antidiuretic hormone (ADH)—stimulates the reabsorption of water from the distal tubules of the kidney.

Fig. 16.3 shows the hormones secreted by the pituitary gland.

Disorders of the posterior pituitary

Diabetes insipidus

Diabetes insipidus results from a lack of ADH causing polyuria and polydipsia.

Nephrogenic diabetes insipidus is a primary renal tubular defect of water reabsorption in which there is a poor response to ADH (a hereditary disorder). Water balance in the body is regulated by a complex negative feedback system involving thirst, ADH secretion, and responses by the kidney, which maintains the plasma osmolality at 275–295 mOsmol/kg. There are many factors that influence ADH secretion (see later). One of the most important is a change in plasma osmolality; above 280 mOsmol/kg there is a steady increase in ADH response.

Actions of ADH

- ◆ Induces reabsorption of water in renal tubules.
- ◆ Vasoconstriction, particularly of skin, mesenteric, and coronary vessels.
- ◆ Stimulates prostacyclin production and increases fibrinolytic activity.
- ◆ Increases Factor VIII coagulant activity.

Factors influencing ADH secretion

Table 16.10 shows factors that influence ADH secretion.

Effects of diabetes insipidus

Failure of adequate secretion of ADH in response to plasma hyperosmolality results in the passage of huge volumes of dilute urine (6–30 litre/day). If the thirst mechanism or water intake are impaired the plasma will become hyperosmotic and hypernatraemic. Total body sodium is, however, decreased due to renal losses

TABLE 16.10	Factors that influence ADH secretion
Increased by:	Hyperosmolality
	Hypotension
	Trauma, surgery
	Stress, pain
	Hyperthermia
	Positive pressure ventilation
	Exercise
	Drugs: cholinergic, beta-adrenergics, nicotine, barbiturates, chlorpropamide, angiotensin II
Inhibited by:	Causes of cranial diabetes insipidus (see earlier)
	Opioid antagonists
Potentiated by:	Drugs: thiazide diuretics, chlorpropamide, carbamazepine, clofibrate, prostaglandin, synthase inhibitors (e.g. indomethacin)
Antagonized by:	Hypokalaemia
	Hypercalcaemia
	Excess vasopressinase
	Prostaglandin (PGE_2)
	Drugs: amphoteracin B, lithium carbonate

and inadequate intake. Gross dehydration will cause hypovolaemic shock and death. Hypernatraemia will cause delirium, lethargy, convulsions, and coma.

Other causes of polyuria should be excluded by appropriate investigations; in particular hyperglycaemia, recovery from fluid overload, polyuric renal disease, and psychogenic polydipsia.

Investigations

See Table 16.11 for the investigations for the diagnosis of diabetes insipidus.

Management of diabetes insipidus

Mild polyuria (<250 ml/hour) may simply require fluid replacement with a crystalloid infusion. Plasma and urine osmolality must be measured frequently. If the

TABLE 16.11	Investigations for the diagnosis of diabetes insipidus	
Test	Normal value (mOsmol/kg)	Diabetes insipidus (mOsmol/kg)
Plasma osmolality[a]	275—295	<280
Urine osmolality	300–1300	<150

[a]Plasma osmolality can be also be calculated from serum sodium, potassium glucose, and urea (all values in mmol/litre): osmolality in mOsmol/kg = 1.86 ($Na^+ + K^+$) + glucose + urea.

urine output is persistent or more excessive, specific drug therapy will be required. In this case DDAVP, a specific synthetic antidiuretic hormone given intravenously or by nasal snuff, is the drug of choice. The dose and frequency depends on the clinical response and can be variable. When the urine volume has been lowered to about 2 ml/min an infusion of 0.9% sodium chloride should be used to maintain the plasma osmolality at 280–300 mOsmol/kg. Measurements of plasma and urine osmolality should be made every 8 hours.

Cardiovascular variables (CVP, BP, heart rate) and urine output must be monitored closely. Urine specific gravity should be measured regularly (aim for a value of 1005–1010). (See Chapters 10 and 13 for diabetes insipidus in head injury.)

Test yourself (Endocrine emergencies)

Questions

1. Which hormones are produced by the anterior pituitary gland?

2. List some causes of diabetes insipidus.

3. What are the signs and symptoms of hyperglycaemia?

4. Which factors predispose to a hyperosmolar, hyperglycaemic state (HHS)?

5. What are the functions of insulin?

6. What are the signs and symptoms of hypocalcaemia?

Answers

1. The hormones produced by the anterior pituitary are as follows:
Growth hormone (GH)—affects fat, protein, and carbohydrate metabolism.
Thyroid-stimulating hormone (TSH)—stimulates the thyroid gland to secrete thyroid hormones.
Adrenocorticotrophic hormone (ACTH)—controls the secretion of adrenocortical hormones.
Prolactin—produced during pregnancy and stimulates breast growth and secretory functions.
Gonadotrophic hormones—involved in sexual functions: *in women* follicle-stimulating hormone (stimulates development of follicles in the ovaries) and luteinizing hormone (causes oestrogen and progesterone secretion by the ovaries and allows rupture of follicles); *in men* interstitial cell-stimulating hormone stimulates the testes to produce androgens.

2. Causes of diabetes insipidus:
Neurosurgery.
Head injury.
Hypoxic brain injury.
Infarction of a pituitary tumour (pituitary apoplexy). Also, rarely, following meningococcal meningitis, penetrating thoracic trauma, coronary artery bypass surgery, amiodarone therapy.

3. The signs and symptoms of hyperglycaemia are:
thirst
vomiting
abdominal pain
hot, dry, flushed skin
drowsiness
tachycardia
deep sighing (Kussmaul) respirations
hypotension
coma.

4. Factors that predispose to HHS are:
elderly
myocardial infarction
trauma (including burns)
infection
pancreatitis, hepatitis
renal failure
hypothermia
carbohydrate overload (enteral feeding, dextrose solutions)
drugs: phenytoin, thiazides (all inhibit insulin release), glucocorticoids, growth hormone (stimulate gluconeogenesis)

5. The functions of insulin are to:
Promote transport of glucose into cells, hence lowering the blood glucose level.
Promote glycogen storage in liver and muscle cells.
Convert glucose into fat.
Inhibit fat metabolism.
Promote tissue growth by protein deposition.

6. The signs and symptoms of hypocalcaemia are:
tetany, muscle twitching, tremors, facial spasms
paraesthesiae (tingling) of extremities and mouth
ECG changes: prolonged Q–T interva
muscle weakness
hypotension
convulsions
(long-term) cataracts, changes to teeth, nails, hair.

Obstetric emergencies

The pregnant patient near term is unique because the feto-placental unit has radical effects on maternal physiological function. When treating the critically ill preterm women, the welfare of the fetus must always be considered. Pregnancy-associated emergencies that require admission to the ICU are uncommon but an understanding of the pathological mechanisms underlying the disorders is essential.

Major pathological changes that occur during pregnancy

Respiratory

◆ A decrease in functional residual capacity (FRC) in the second half of pregnancy. This is due to elevation of the diaphragm by the developing fetus. In late pregnancy, airway closure occurs above or closer to the FRC than in the non-pregnant state and may adversely affect gas exchange.

◆ Minute ventilation can be increased by up to 50% by term due to hyperventilation and an increase in tidal volume caused by the central respiratory stimulant effects of progesterone. This decreases the P_aCO_2 to approximately 4 kPa and results in a respiratory alkalosis with a pH of 7.4–7.5 and HCO_3 to 20 mmol.

◆ Oxygen consumption increases by up to 15% by term due to demands from the developing fetus, uterus, placenta, and breasts. This is met by an increase in minute ventilation, an increase in cardiac output and a shift of the maternal oxyhaemoglobin dissociation curve to the right.

Cardiovascular

◆ Maternal blood volume increases from the first trimester and reaches its maximum by weeks 24–34. This increase is necessary to compensate for blood lost at delivery and for the placenta. About one-third of the extra blood fills the sinuses of the placenta and the remainder stays in the circulation. The volume of increase varies with the number of fetuses and can be up to 50% greater than in the non-pregnant state. The increase in plasma volume exceeds that of red cell volume creating a physiological anaemia.

◆ Cardiac output rises gradually from the first trimester due to the increase in blood volume and an increase in heart rate (up by 20%) and stroke volume. By 30 weeks it can be 30–50% above non-pregnant values. During labour, cardiac output is further increased by each uterine contraction.

◆ Systemic vascular resistance decreases. This is induced by oestrogen and progesterone, which cause smooth muscle relaxation and ensure oxygen and nutrient needs are met for the developing fetus.

◆ Immediately after delivery, cardiac output rises due to autotransfusion by uterine contractions and the relief of venocaval obstruction.

◆ Within 3 weeks of delivery the expanded blood volume has been reabsorbed and cardiac output is restored to normal values.

Utero-placental perfusion

◆ The utero-placental circulation is a pressure-dependent system without its own regulatory mechanism. Any factor that decreases venous return or cardiac output in the mother will impair uterine flow (e.g. mechanical ventilation or venocaval compression).

◆ Hypotension can develop due to compression of the iliac vessels, inferior vena cava, and aorta due to the enlarging uterus. This is evident during the second half of pregnancy and is maximal when the patient is supine (up to a 30% reduction in blood volume). Hypotension can critically impair utero-placental blood flow and patients beyond approximately 20 weeks' gestation should not be nursed in a supine position. Such patients must be nursed in the left lateral position in order relieve compression, or a pillow or wedge can be placed under the right hip in order to tilt the uterus. This is the position in which cardiopulmonary resuscitation is performed since an adequate cardiac output cannot be achieved if the patient is left supine.

◆ Hypoxaemia, acidosis, and vasopressors all cause utero-placental constriction and impair perfusion.

◆ Utero-placental perfusion can be increased by correct positioning, volume infusion, and leg raising.

Obstetric disorders

Pre-eclampsia

Pre-eclampsia is one of the most serious complications of pregnancy, and is a leading cause of maternal and perinatal mortality in the UK. It is more common in the first pregnancy and 10% of all pregnancies are affected; the incidence of severe pre-eclampsia is about 1%.

The 'classic' signs of pre-eclampsia are hypertension and proteinuria, but pre-eclampsia is a multiorgan disorder and their absence does not exclude the diagnosis. Manifestations of pre-eclampsia present during the latter half of pregnancy, intrapartum, or post-partum.

The precise aetiology is still unclear. It is postulated that trophoblast invasion is defective and the spiral arteries (which supply the placenta) fail to undergo the physiological dilatation in the first trimester. Therefore the utero-placental circulation remains in a state of high resistance, leading to placental ischaemia as the pregnancy progresses. Persistent placental underperfusion is thought to stimulate the release of pre-eclamptic factors (possibly free radicals) that lead to endothelial cell damage. The normal homeostatic function of the endothelium is disrupted and there is a decrease in endothelial prostacyclin synthesis (a vasodilator and inhibitor of platelet aggregation). Defective production of nitric oxide (a vasodilator) and an increase in thromboxane synthesis (a vasoconstrictor and platelet aggregator) contribute to the platelet activation and vasoconstriction seen in pre-eclampsia. There is an increased vascular response to vasoconstrictor agents, greater cell permeability, reduced plasma volume, clotting cascade activation, and fibrin deposition in the systemic vascular beds. Thrombosis and vasospasm develop, exacerbate the ischaemia and endothelial cell dysfunction, and lead to multiorgan involvement.

Clinical features of pre-eclampsia (Table 16.12)

Pre-eclampsia is a progressive disorder, which can only be arrested by the delivery of the fetus. Many women develop the signs of pre-eclampsia (hypertension and proteinuria) but can remain unsymptomatic and deliver at term. However, pre-eclampsia has various modes of presentation and severity. A small proportion of women (1%) progress rapidly through the phases of pre-eclampsia and develop the clinical features of severe pre-eclampsia, increasing their risk of developing the numerous complications. If this occurs before term,

TABLE 16.12	Clinical features of pre-eclampsia
Cardiovascular	Hypertension (diastolic >15–25 mmHg from early pregnancy)
	Thrombocytopenia
	Prolonged clotting time
	Increased packed cell volume and haemoglobin
Renal	Hyperuricaemia
	Proteinuria (>300 mg in 24 hours)
	Oedema (including laryngeal oedema)
	Rise in creatinine and urea
	Oliguria
Neurological	Headaches
	Visual disturbances
	Hyperreflexia
Hepatic	Elevated liver function tests, particularly transaminases
	Epigastric pain
	Nausea and vomiting
Utero-placental	Reduced fetal growth
	Possible intrauterine death

there is the risk of neonatal prematurity to consider. Attempts will be made to prolong the pregnancy by close maternal and fetal surveillance, but it is rarely possible for more than a few weeks, and for some women only a matter of hours, before delivery is necessary.

Complications of pre-eclampsia

Complications of pre-eclampsia include:

- eclampsia
- renal failure
- HELLP syndrome (Haemolysis, Elevated Liver enzymes, Low Platelets)
- hepatic rupture
- cerebral haemorrhage
- cerebral oedema
- disseminated intravascular coagulation
- pulmonary oedema
- ARDS
- placental abruption.

Nursing management

Women with severe pre-eclampsia will require admission to the ICU if they require more intensive monitoring or the deterioration in their clinical condition is rapid. The majority will have delivered before admission to ICU but still require close monitoring as there is likely to be further clinical deterioration for at least 48 hours after delivery.

Hypertension

The single largest cause of death is cerebral haemorrhage. This reflects a failure of effective antihypertensive treatment. The blood pressure must be monitored but automated blood pressure recording systems can underestimate blood pressure in pre-eclampsia to a serious degree. Arterial monitoring should therefore be considered.

Administer antihypertensive drug therapy. There is no clear consensus on the drug of choice but intravenous hydralazine (a peripheral vasodilator) or labetolol (an alpha- and beta-adrenergic blocker) are commonly used. Severe pre-eclampsia may be accompanied by a reduced intravascular volume and requires pre-treatment with colloid before parenteral treatment commences. This optimizes cardiac preload, reduces the vascular resistance, and improves renal and utero-placental blood flow.

Intravenous nitrates are useful if there is evidence of pulmonary oedema. Sodium nitroprusside is useful for acute hypertensive crises complicated by pulmonary oedema and left ventricular failure. However, this should be avoided in the antenatal period due to the risk of fetal toxicity from cyanide poisoning.

Sudden falls in mean blood pressure or hypotension must be avoided, as this will be detrimental to utero-placental and cerebral perfusion. Diastolic blood pressure should not be reduced below 90 mmHg. The mean arterial pressure should be maintained below 125 mmHg.

Potential haemorrhage due to DIC

Observe for evidence of bleeding. Correct the coagulopathy using fresh frozen plasma and cryoprecipitate. Significant thrombocytopenia will require platelet transfusion.

Cerebral haemorrhage can occur if coagulopathy and blood pressure are not controlled. Thromboembolism remains a risk in pre-eclampsia.

Potential eclampsia

Eclampsia is a grand-mal convulsion occurring in association with features of pre-eclampsia. It occurs in 1–2% of women with pre-eclampsia. Forty-four per cent of convulsions occur post-natally, the remainder being antepartum (38%) and intrapartum (18%).

Eclampsia is thought to be attributed to cerebral vasospasm, ischaemia, cerebral oedema, disruption of the blood–brain barrier, or microemboli in the cerebral circulation. Cerebral haemorrhage can occur irrespective of an elevated blood pressure.

Intravenous magnesium sulphate is the drug of choice for primary prophylaxis in severe pre-eclampsia (Magpie Trial Collaborative Group 2002), especially those with continued signs of cerebral irritation. Magnesium probably acts as a cerebral vasodilator and relieves vasospasm.

If a convulsion occurs, the priorities of care are maintenance of the airway, oxygenation, and control of the seizures (usually by IV magnesium). Endotracheal intubation and ventilation may be required. The neurological management of these patients includes maintenance of cerebral perfusion and control of intracranial pressure. If the patient remains in coma, cerebral oedema or haemorrhage must be suspected.

The results of the Eclampsia Trial Collaborative Group (1995) show that if women who have had a seizure are treated with magnesium sulphate they have fewer recurrent seizures compared with women treated with phenytoin or diazepam. Each hospital should have a protocol for the dosage and administration of magnesium sulphate. This comprises a loading dose, followed by a maintenance infusion for at least 24 hours after the last convulsion.

Magnesium acts as a central nervous system depressor. Therapeutic maternal blood levels are 2–3.5 mmol/litre but respiratory paralysis can occur when levels are greater than 5 mmol/litre. Careful observation of respiratory rate and depth will be required to avoid respiratory arrest. Magnesium also increases patient sensitivity to all neuromuscular blocking agents.

Liver disturbances

Twenty to fifty per cent of all pre-eclamptic women have mild abnormalities of hepatic enzymes. However, 5–20% develop HELLP syndrome (Haemolysis, Elevated Liver enzymes and Low Platelets). Most cases arise antenatally and 40% of cases are multigravid. It is one of the possible crises of pre-eclampsia, although pre-eclampsia does not have to occur for HELLP to be present. It involves endothelial cell injury and microangiopathic platelet activation and consumption. The clinical signs and symptoms of patients are classically related to the impact of vasospasm on the maternal liver. These include epigastric or right upper quadrant pain, malaise, and nausea. Any woman presenting with these symptoms should have platelet and liver function tests performed irrespective of her blood pressure. Liver disturbance is of a major concern since encephalopathy, liver haemorrhage, necrosis, or rupture can occur. Prognosis is unpredictable and immediate delivery is usually indicated. Patients given high-dose corticosteroid therapy seem to recover from the disease process more quickly (Magann et al. 1994). There may be particular problems with haemorrhage and transfusions of red cells, fresh frozen plasma, cryoprecipitate, and platelets may be required.

Thromboembolism

Thromboembolism is the leading cause of maternal mortality in the UK, and pulmonary embolism in pregnancy and the puerperium kills 8–10 women each year. Pregnancy increases the risk of thromboembolism six-fold and Caesarean section further increases the risk approximately 10- to 20-fold. The risk of a deep vein thrombosis following Caesarean section is around 1–2% and persists for at least 6 weeks post-partum.

Additional risk factors are:

◆ age (risk 10 times greater if >40 years)

◆ obesity

◆ increased parity (4 or more)

◆ operative delivery

◆ previous thromboembolism

◆ prolonged bedrest

- pre-eclampsia

- gross varicose veins.

Pregnancy is a hypercoagulable state in which there exists an increased potential for coagulation and thrombosis. This is due primarily to changes in clotting factors (an increase in factors V, VII, VIII, IX, X, and XII) and an increase of 50% in fibrinogen levels. Plasma fibrinolytic activity also decreases as a result of placental inhibitors, but can return to normal 1 hour after delivery. When the placenta separates, tissue thromboplastin is released in the circulation, increasing the chance of thrombosis. These physiological changes serve to control blood loss at delivery.

Pulmonary embolism (PE)

The size, number and location of the emboli determine the clinical features of pulmonary embolism.

Management

A correct diagnosis is vital because of the major implications in pregnancy of long-term anticoagulation, the potential need for prophylaxis in any future pregnancy, and the concerns regarding the future use of contraceptives and hormone replacement therapy. In addition to the clinical findings further investigations such as ECG, CXR, and V/Q scan will be required to confirm the diagnosis.

Routine haemodynamic and respiratory monitoring will be instituted according to the severity of the condition.

The aims of treatment are to maintain adequate oxygenation according to blood gas analysis and promote the resolution of the thrombus by intravenous anticoagulation. A heparin infusion should be administered according to blood clotting analysis and maintained for 7–10 days. Anticoagulation should continue for 6 weeks post-partum using subcutaneous heparin (antepartum or post-partum) or oral warfarin (only if post-partum).

Institute bedrest, use elastic stockings, and monitor any swelling, pain, or redness in limbs if a deep vein thrombosis was the source of the embolus.

Massive obstetric haemorrhage

Life threatening haemorrhage occurs in approximately 0.1% of deliveries.

Any disruption in the integrity of the maternal vascular system during pregnancy has the potential for massive blood loss. Usually, the myometrial fibres contract causing an occlusive action that stops bleeding. Most serious haemorrhage occurs in the post-partum period when the uterus is unable to contract and may be further exacerbated by the onset of DIC. DIC may occur as a consequence of the haemorrhage or secondary to severe pre-eclampsia, amniotic fluid embolism, placental abruption, or intrauterine death.

Risk factors for massive obstetric haemorrhage are:

- Antepartum haemorrhage (due to likelihood of DIC).

- Grand multiparous.

- Pre-eclampsia.

- Previous post-partum haemorrhage.

- Multiple pregnancy.

- Previous Caesarean section.

- Large baby.

- Fibroids.

- Placental site disorders, i.e. praevia, accreta, increta, percreta. With placenta praevia haemorrhage is due to the inability of the lower segment to contract effectively. With the remaining abnormalities it is the fact that the placenta cannot be fully removed, which prevents contraction of the uterus and therefore bleeding persists.

The normal expected blood loss at delivery is 600 ml for a vaginal delivery and 1000 ml for a Caesarean section. Hypotension below 80 mmHg usually indicates a blood loss >1500 ml. Catecholamine-induced vasoconstriction will maintain maternal blood pressure at the expense of the fetus, therefore fetal distress is an important sign.

SIGNS AND SYMPTOMS OF PULMONARY EMBOLISM

- Dyspnoea and tachypnoea

- Hypoxia/cyanosis

- Pleuritic chest pain (sudden onset)

- Haemoptysis

CAUSES OF MASSIVE OBSTETRIC HAEMORRHAGE

- Tears of uterus, cervix, or vaginal wall.

- Uterine anatomy (inability to contract).

- Retained placenta or placental fragments.

- Coagulation defects.

Management

The essentials of management are to identify the cause of the bleeding, stop it, and replace the circulating blood volume. The contents of the uterus must be emptied. This is achieved in the third stage by early clamping and cutting of the cord, prophylactic administration of an oxytocic drug, and controlled cord traction. If bleeding persists further techniques include:

◆ vaginal packing

◆ B-Lynch suture

◆ Foley catheter or Sengstaken–Blackmore tube (used as a tamponade)

◆ direct ligation of the uterine vessels (requires a laparotomy)

◆ radiographic embolization

◆ hysterectomy.

Intensive haemodynamic monitoring will be required whilst the patient is resuscitated and blood volume rapidly replaced. Some conditions such as uterine rupture and placenta praevia may cause massive blood loss (4–5 litres). Coagulopathy must be corrected using fresh frozen plasma, platelets, and cryoprecipitate.

If the airway is not patent or oxygenation inadequate endotracheal intubation and ventilation will be required.

Monitor for the effects of massive loss such as renal failure, ARDS, and DIC.

Amniotic fluid embolism (AFE)

This is an uncommon disorder with an estimated incidence of 1:80 000 pregnancies. However, it has become one of the top three causes of maternal death in industrialized countries with a mortality rate of 26–86%.

There are no clear risk factors associated with the condition and it is not preventable.

The pathophysiology of AFE remains unclear, but it is no longer thought to be caused by an embolic episode. The basis of the mechanism appears to be immunological, and it is recommended that the name amniotic fluid embolism should be changed to 'anaphylactoid syndrome of pregnancy'.

AFE can be described as the entrance of amniotic fluid, containing fetal cells and debris, into the maternal circulation. However, it is suggested that it is not the amniotic fluid *per se*, but the woman's individual response to amniotic fluid that is the crucial factor in the development of AFE.

The release of soluble mediators into the maternal circulation results in a syndrome of haemotological and cardiovascular manifestations. Metabolites of arachidonic acid can produce many of the haemodynamic and haemotological effects found in AFE. Such metabolites, including prostaglandins and leucotrienes, are found in the amniotic fluid in increasing concentrations during labour. The prostaglandins thromboxane and prostaglandin F2 cause pulmonary vasoconstriction. Leucotrienes may also be responsible for coronary vasoconstriction, a reduction in cardiac output, and vascular permeability.

Clark *et al.* (1996) proposed that there are two phases to the syndrome. In the first phase, there is pulmonary artery spasm with pulmonary hypertension leading to right heart failure causing hypoxia. Hypoxia causes myocardial and pulmonary damage, the left ventricle fails due to possible coronary artery spasm, and myocardial ischaemia and ARDS develop. This initial period of hypoxia might account for 50% of patients who succumb in the first hour.

The second phase consists of non-cardiogenic pulmonary oedema, due to increased alveolar capillary permeability (incidence 75%), and a haemorrhagic phase (incidence 43–83%) characterized by massive haemorrhage with uterine atony (lack of contracting ability) and DIC. DIC may be caused by the action of amniotic fluid on platelets, causing the release of clotting Factor III. Amniotic fluid also contains large amounts of thromboplastin 3, which activates the clotting cascade to form fibrin.

Invasive monitoring demonstrates LVF, moderate or severe elevations in PCWP, and depressed left ventricular contractility.

Signs and symptoms of AFE

◆ Sudden dyspnoea in late stages of labour or shortly after birth.

◆ Hypotension (shock).

◆ Hypoxia/cyanosis.

◆ Cardiorespiratory arrest.

◆ Seizures.

◆ Pulmonary oedema/ARDS.

◆ DIC causing massive haemorrhage.

AFE is diagnosed on clinical grounds only as there is no definitive diagnostic test. Differential diagnoses include pulmonary embolism, septic shock, myocardial infarction, anaphylaxis, aspiration pneumonia, air embolism, and abruption.

Management of AFE

Management is entirely supportive:

◆ Initiate cardiopulmonary resuscitation.

◆ Maintain oxygenation. Direct therapy according to ABGs. Endotracheal intubation and ventilation are usually necessary.

- Restore normal pressure directed by full haemo-dynamic monitoring. Rapid volume infusion and ino-tropic support may be necessary. Use appropriate intravenous fluid. This may include blood transfusion in the presence of haemorrhage.

- Correct coagulopathy using blood component thera-py (fresh frozen plasma, cryoprecipitate, platelets).

- Expedite delivery, if undelivered, and perform cor-rective surgery to control haemorrhage.

- Renal support may be required.

Acute fatty liver of pregnancy (AFLP)

This is a rare condition that usually occurs in the third trimester and never has its onset after delivery. The aetiology of AFLP is unknown and the relationship between pre-eclampsia and AFLP has not been clearly established. The diagnosis of AFLP is made primarily on history, physical examination, laboratory data, and in some cases liver biopsy.

Symptoms include nausea, vomiting, anorexia, and right upper quadrant pain. There may be jaundice, encephalopathy and fulminant hepatic failure, increased transaminase levels, decreased platelet count, increased prothrombin time, and renal failure. There may be associated hypertension, oedema, and ascities. Maternal and fetal death may occur if treatment is delayed.

Treatment is aimed at early delivery and supportive care. AFLP is usually a reversible condition and sur-vivors rarely have any long-term sequalae.

Peripartum cardiomyopathy

This disorder presents in the last month of pregnancy or the first 6 months after delivery. It is a dilated car-diomyopathy that is more common in older, multi-parous, Black women. The aetiology is uncertain but several mechanisms have been proposed including hor-monal changes of pregnancy, nutritional deficiencies, and autoimmune or viral processes.

The patient usually presents with classic signs of left or biventricular failure. There is severe reduction in left ventricular performance and gross dilatation of the left ventricle.

A major complication is pulmonary or cerebral em-boli. Mortality is 25–50% and death can be caused by ventricular arrhythmias, diminished cardiac output, or the consequences of emboli.

There is a tendency for this condition to recur with subsequent pregnancies, particularly in patients whose heart size does not return to normal within 6 months of delivery.

Management is by systemic anticoagulation and the conventional treatment for congestive cardiac failure.

Breastfeeding in the ICU

Many mothers are keen to commence breastfeeding in the ICU but this must be balanced against their level of illness and the drugs that are administered to them.

Breastfeeding works on a supply and demand basis, i.e. the more the baby feeds, or the mother expresses, the more milk is produced.

Mothers should be encouraged to rest, and if they wish to express milk this should be done during the day (two to four times) in order to promote sleep at night. However, in order to feel comfortable, they may need to express during the night, especially on the third day post-delivery when full milk production occurs. If the mother has been sedated for several days she can be reassured that she will be able to breastfeed, but it will take several attempts to obtain milk. There may be a decrease in milk supply following a massive haemorrhage.

Breast pump kits can be used but they must be sterile if the milk is to be used by the baby. The milk can be kept in sterile plastic bottles for 24 hours if refrigerated.

The drugs that are being administered to the mother must be taken into account as many can be transferred into the milk. Always check the drug prescribing infor-mation or consult the pharmacist for advice. Medical staff should be encouraged to use drugs that are safe for breastfeeding, particularly if these will be required long-term such as antihypertensive therapy.

Many obstetric departments will have a breastfeed-ing advisor who can offer advice and practical support.

Test yourself (Obstetric emergencies)

Questions

1. Which are the three leading causes of maternal death in the UK?

2. What are the essential characteristics of HELLP syn-drome?

3. What are the causes of massive maternal haemor-rhage?

Answers

1. Pre-eclampsia, thromboembolism, and massive maternal haemorrhage.

2. Haemolysis, Elevated Liver function tests, and Low Platelet count.

3. Tears of the uterus, cervix or vaginal wall.
   Uterine atony.
   Retained placenta or placenta fragments.
   Coagulation defects.

Drug overdose and toxic substance ingestion

Poisoning may follow deliberate or accidental exposure or ingestion and may be acute or chronic. Substances include therapeutic drugs, plant or animal toxins, industrial or agricultural chemicals, and substances found in the home such as cleaning materials.

Self-administered drug poisoning accounts for over 10% of acute medical admissions to hospital. Death from acute poisoning is relatively uncommon except in children under 4 years of age where accidental poisoning remains an important cause of death.

In deliberate drug overdose, often more than one drug will be ingested and alcohol is a common co-agent. Complications can be unexpected and require prompt action and specific treatments. Supportive therapy in the critical care unit can be life-saving.

General principles

The consequences of a drug overdose depend on a variety of factors including:

- the patient's size, age, health,
- the drug,
- the route,
- how long ago the drug was taken and over what period of time,
- the quantity taken,

CONDITIONS THAT REQUIRE ADMISSION TO THE CRITICAL CARE AREA

Admission will be required if the patient is or may become:

- cardiovascularly unstable (hypotensive, hypertensive cardiac arrhythmias),
- unconscious,
- requires endotracheal intubation or mechanical ventilation,
- requires specialist therapy (e.g. haemodialysis/ filtration, temporary pacing),
- suffers convulsions.

- other drugs that may have been taken at the same time (e.g. alcohol).

For some drugs that require specific treatment (e.g. antidotes) recovery is dependent on the time interval between ingestion and the time that treatment begins. Definitive treatment must therefore begin as soon as resuscitation is completed.

Resuscitation

- Vital functions must be assessed and the principles of resuscitation applied in order to stabilize the patient before a general assessment is made:
- The airway must be kept patent. If the patient is comatose with no cough or gag reflex then endotracheal intubation will be required.
- Establish intravenous access.
- Give oxygen by mask or, if spontaneous respiration is inadequate, mechanical ventilatory support will be required.
- Take baseline measurements of heart rate, rhythm, blood pressure, and core temperature. Assess peripheral perfusion and skin colour.
- Correct hypovolaemia.
- Carry out a bedside blood glucose test.
- Assess conscious level.
- Take blood samples for glucose, urea, creatinine, and electrolytes, liver function tests, full blood count, coagulation screen, arterial blood gases, and drug assays.
- Take urine sample for drug screen.
- Chest X-ray and ECG (if indicated).
- Continually reassess the patient for impaired vital functions.

Physical examination

Self-poisoning is the cause of undiagnosed coma in 15% of patients aged between 15 and 55 years. Although other causes of coma must be excluded, this should always be suspected.

A careful history must be obtained from the patient (if conscious), ambulance personnel, and relatives or friends. Empty bottles, drugs, or a suicide note may have been found with the patient. The patient's general practitioner can provide details of recently prescribed medication or any history of depressive illness.

The physical examination can provide important evidence and assessment should be made of:

- The central and autonomic nervous system.

- The appearance of the skin and mucous membranes, e.g. colour (jaundice, cyanosed, cherry red) blisters, lesions, venepuncture marks.

- Odours. Particular toxic substances cause specific odours, e.g. cyanide causes a bitter almond odour, isopropyl alcohol, phenol, and salicylates an acetone odour, and heavy metals and organophosphates a garlic odour.

Urine, blood, and gastric contents should be sent for analysis but urgent laboratory drug screening is usually limited to paracetamol and salicylate screening. Bedside kits will detect the presence of recreational drugs including opiates and cannabis. A more comprehensive drug screen can be carried out by a specialized Poisons Unit. When the cause of coma is unknown a blood sugar should always be performed urgently. Appropriate measures should be taken if meningitis is suspected (see Chapter 10).

Some examples of the clinical manifestations of toxic substances are given in Table 16.13, but the list is by no means exhaustive.

The clinical manifestations of some substances show characteristic signs and symptoms and are termed toxidromes. The toxidromes of specific groups of toxins may help in determining the substance that has been taken. Some examples of common toxidromes are:

- Amphetamine/ecstasy/cocaine: fever, tachycardia, hypertension, hyperactive/delirious, tremor, convulsions, sweating.

- Opiates/clonidine: bradycardia, slow, depressed respirations, hypotension, hypothermia, pinpoint pupils, hyporeflexia, reduced level of consciousness, coma.

- Barbiturates/benzodiazipines: hypotension, bradypnoea, confusion, coma, ataxia, hypothermia, skin vesicles and bullae.

- Salicylates: tachypnoea, pyrexia, lethargy/coma, vomiting.

Management

After basic resuscitation, treatment is aimed at:

1. Decreasing further drug absorption.

2. Increasing drug excretion.

3. Administration of specific antidotes.

4. Supportive therapy.

1. Decreasing further drug absorption

The traditional techniques of gastric lavage and emesis using emetic drugs such as ipecacuanha syrup are now

TABLE 16.13 Clinical manifestations of toxic substances

Clinical manifestation	Toxic substance
Bradycardia	Digoxin, opiates, cyanide, carbon monoxide, clonidine, organophosphates, calcium-channel blockers, beta-blockers
Tachycardia	Alcohol, amphetamines, tricyclic antidepressants, theophylline, salicylates, cocaine
Hypotension	Nitrates, cyanide, carbon monoxide, tricyclic antidepressants, barbiturates, iron, theophylline, opiates, clonidine, beta-blockers, calcium-channel blockers, phenothiazines
Arrhythmias, heartblock	Chloroquine, tricyclic antidepressants, class 1 anti-arryhthmics
Atrioventricular block	Beta-blockers, digoxin
Hypertension	Amphetamines, monoamine (MAO) inhibitors, antihistamines, clonidine, cocaine
Respiratory depression	Opiates, alcohol, benzodiazipines, barbiturates
Hypothermia	Ethanol, amphetamines, barbiturates, opiates, clonidine, carbamazepine, sedatives
Hyperpyrexia	Quinine, salicylates, amphetamines, tricyclic antidepressants, MAO inhibitors, theophylline, cocaine
Hypoglycaemia	Insulin, oral hypoglycaemic drugs
Hyperkalaemia	Digoxin, potassium supplements, excess liquorice
Hypokalaemia	Theophylline, chloroquine, diuretics
Coma	Opiates, anticholinergics, alcohol, anticonvulsants, carbon monoxide, salicylates, organophosphates
Convulsions, agitation	Alcohol, lead, organophosphates, salicylates, antihistamines, tricyclic antidepressants, cocaine, ecstasy, amphetamines
Paralysis	Botulism, alcohol, carbon monoxide, barbiturates, heavy metals, hydrocarbons, organic solvents

declining in popularity as doubts exist over their efficacy and the fact that they carry a recognized complication rate, particularly in obtunded patients.

Complications of lavage include oesophageal perforation, gastric rupture, hyponatraemia, water intoxication, and aspiration pneumonia.

- *Activated charcoal* is the treatment of choice for adsorption of drugs to prevent absorption from the stomach into the bloodstream. It should ideally be given as early as possible following ingestion of a substantial amount of toxin but it may still be effective for up to 24 hours, especially with drugs such as aspirin that are slowly absorbed. Repeated doses are given for some drugs, which may help reduce their toxicity. It is an effective adsorbent of many kinds of substances such as phenobarbital, theophylline, and phenytoin, but is ineffective for others such as alcohol, heavy metals, lithium, and petroleum solvents. The airway must be protected as there is a risk of pulmonary aspiration, but other side-effects are relatively rare. It should not be given to patients with an ileus.

♦ *Whole bowel irrigation.* A solution of polyethylene glycol is given orally or via a nasogastric tube at 2 litre/hour in the adult until the rectal effluent becomes clear. It is used when patients have ingested a potentially serious substance, such as enteric coated preparations, or those for which activated charcoal are ineffective (such as iron). It is also sometimes used for the intact elimination of 'body packer' packets of cocaine and heroin. It cannot be used in patients who have unprotected airways, bowel obstruction, ileus, or perforation.

2.　Increasing excretion of the drug

♦ *Forced diuresis.* Large volumes of intravenous fluid are infused, often in combination with diuretics, in order to promote urinary excretion of the drug.

♦ *Alkalinization.* An infusion of sodium bicarbonate is given to alkalinize the urine and prevent reabsorption of the drug in the kidney. It is useful in salicylate and barbiturate overdose. This can be potentially hazardous in patients with cardiac or renal dysfunction, and can cause electrolyte imbalance and cerebral oedema so vigilant monitoring of vital signs, electrolytes, and arterial blood pH is essential. Urinary pH should be monitored and maintained at about 8.0.

♦ *Extracorporeal elimination.* This includes haemodialysis, haemofiltration, haemodiafiltration, and haemoperfusion using a charcoal filter.

In order for these methods to be effective the toxin must have limited protein binding, small volumes of distribution and a plasma concentration that relates to toxicity.

3.　Antidotes/alteration of drug metabolism

Specific antidotes can be given for certain overdose/poisons. These can either compete for the same receptors (e.g. naloxone for opiates, flumazanil for benzodiazipines), block metabolism by using the same enzyme (e.g.

ethanol for methanol) or protect body tissues (e.g. *N*-acetylcysteine providing sulphudryl groups to prevent liver damage by paracetamol).

4.　Supportive therapy

The action and side-effects of the drug taken (if known) should be documented in order to anticipate and observe any problems that may occur. Specific supportive treatments will vary according to the drug taken (see Table 16.14). The basic principles are:

♦ *Respiratory*

Maintain airway (depends on level of consciousness): oropharyngeal (Guedel) airway, endotracheal intubation, patient positioning.

Monitor blood gases, acid–base status, and oxygen saturation. Give oxygen therapy or ventilatory support as indicated.

Hypoxaemia may indicate additional pulmonary pathology such as aspiration, infection, oedema, atelectasis.

♦ *Cardiovascular*

Monitor cardiovascular status: continuous ECG recording, observe for arrhythmias, perform 12-lead ECG, monitor vital signs.

Circulatory failure can result from a variety of causes (hypovolaemia, myocardial insufficiency, vasodilatation, or reduced cardiac output due to negative inotropy or cardiac arrhythmias). The mechanism of shock must be ascertained by appropriate monitoring of cardiovascular variables and acid–base status in order to institute effective treatment.

♦ *Neurological*

Assess neurological status. Perform full neurological assessment, document regular neurological observations until fully conscious. Observe for and report convulsions.

Convulsions may occur as an effect of the poison taken or following a hypoxic episode.

Exclude hypoglycaemia or other metabolic causes. Ensure protected airway and consider hypercapnoea as a cause of obtunded level of consciousness.

♦ *Renal*

If unable to take oral fluids an IV infusion will be required. Monitor urine output, blood urea, electrolytes, and creatinine. Perform urinalysis.

Rhabdomyolysis can be a complication of some poisonings, particularly when the patient is comatose but also with drugs that cause 'hyper-exercise' (strychnine, cocaine, amphetamines including Ecstasy). Diagnosis is usually confirmed by a grossly elevated

TABLE 16.14	Specific management strategies for drug overdose and poisons	
Poison	**Features**	**Management**
Antidepressants:		
Tricyclics	Dilated pupils, dry mouth, urinary retention, ileus, agitation, convulsions, hyperpyrexia. Cardiotoxic effects may appear after up to 3 days: AV conduction disturbances, sinus tachycardia, VF, VT	Supportive. Maintain pH >7.5 with bicarbonate if cardiotoxic
Monoamine oxidase inhibitors (MAOIs)	Hypertensive crisis when taken with tyramine-containing foods (e.g. cheese, red wine, Marmite) and sympathomimetic agents (e.g. dopamine, epinephrine (adrenaline))	Phentolamine, sodium nitroprusside, or diazoxide to control hypertension
Amphetamines	Tachycardia, hypertension, fatal arrhythmias. Confusion, psychosis, convulsions	Supportive
Anticholinergics and antihistamines	As for tricyclics. Cardiotoxic effects after 48 hours	Antidote: physostigmine (target competitor)
Barbiturates	CNS depression—coma. Respiratory depression. Skin blisters and red wheals on pressure points of limbs. Hypothermia. CVS depression—hypotension, peripheral vasodilation. Dilated pupils	Supportive. Correct hypovolaemia. Alkalinization of urine hastens elimination of phenobarbital
Benzodiazipines	CNS depression, potentiated by alcohol. Respiratory depression	Supportive therapy. Antidote: flumazenil (receptor antagonist). Note: this is short-acting and may also precipitate convulsions. It is predominantly used diagnostically
Beta-blockers	Cardiotoxic effects within 48 hours: sinus bradycardia, AV conduction disturbances. Circulatory failure. Occasional bronchospasm	Supportive. Temporary ventricular pacing may be required. Inotropes and/or glucagon may be needed
Carbon monoxide	Displaces oxygen from Hb, producing carboxyhaemoglobin and hypoxaemia. It also blocks cellular mitochondrial respiration. Hypertonicity, pulmonary oedema, coma, agitation. May have cherry pink skin and mucosae	100% oxygen. Mechanical ventilation often necessary. Hyperbaric oxygen (if readily available) should be considered at levels of >20% COHb or if the patient is symptomatic
Cocaine	Chest pain, hypertension, hypermetabolic state (hyperpyrexia, rhabdomyolysis), arrhythmias, seizures, agitation	Rapid cooling. Sedation with benzodiazepines. Supportive therapy
Cyanide	Prevents mitochondrial cellular respiration—circulatory failure due to cellular hypoxia even though P_aO_2 normal. Convulsions and respiratory failure. Death often rapid	100% oxygen. Antidotes: dicobalt edetate or sodium nitrite when diagnosis certain. If uncertain, sodium thiosulphate
Chloroquine	Cardiotoxic effects after 2–6 hours: AV conduction disturbances, VF. Negative inotropic effect, vasodilation, hypotension. Sudden cardiac arrest	Supportive. Epinephrine (adrenaline) for hypotension
Digoxin	May take 24–76 hours for toxic effects. Sinus bradycardia, VT, VF, and AV conduction problems. Vomiting	Antidotes: antidigoxin Fab (receptor antagonist). Phenytoin can also be given. Temporary pacing if necessary
Ethylene glycol (antifreeze)	Severe metabolic acidosis due to oxalic acid. Acute renal failure. Inebriation	Antidote: ethanol (metabolic competitor) or 4-methylpyrazole. Haemodialysis
Heavy metals:		
Iron	Corrosive to gastrointestinal tract. Nausea, haematemasis, abdominal pain, malaena. Gastric perforation may occur	Antidote: desferrioxamine mesylate
Lead	Liver and renal failure. Diarrhoea, vomiting, abdominal pain, convulsions, coma	Antidote: EDTA (calcium disodium edetate)

TABLE 16.14 Specific management strategies for drug overdose and poisons – *continued*		
Poison	**Features**	**Management**
Mercury	Burns to skin if local contamination. CNS damage—tremor, ataxia, dysarthria	Antidote: acetyl penicillamine
Arsenic	Causes increased permeability of blood vessels and vasodilation. Abdominal pain, nausea, vomiting, profuse diarrhoea, profound electrolyte disturbances (hypokalaemia, hyponatraemia). Circulatory collapse, cellular enzyme disturbances	Antidote: *N*-acetyl penicillamine
Methanol	Methanol is metabolized to formaldehyde and then formic acid which causes blindness and metabolic acidosis	Antidote: ethanol (metabolic competitor)
Opiates	CNS depression. Pin-point pupils. Respiratory depression—hypoxaemia and hypercarbia	Antidote: naloxone (receptor antagonist). Supportive treatment including IPPV
Organophosphates	CNS depression—hypoxia. Muscular paralysis/fasciculations. Bradycardia, asystole. Hypothermia, abdominal pain, diarrhoea. Bronchospasm, salivation	Antidote: atropine to control parasympathetic activity. Supportive—mechanical ventilation
Paracetamol	Hepatocellular necrosis with ingestion >7.5 g. Nausea, vomiting, anorexia, and right upper quadrant pain in first 24 hours, liver failure 3–6 days after ingestion. Lactic acidosis, hypoglycaemia and renal failure may occur	Gastric lavage and activated charcoal. Supportive therapy. Antidote: *N*-acetylcysteine (or oral methionine if given within 10–12 hours of ingestion). Its protective effect is time-dependent but it can still be given up to 36 hours after overdose with some benefit. Toxicity can be assessed by referring to a graph of plasma paracetamol levels against time after ingestion
Paraquat	Causes local irritation to mucosal membranes—vomiting, abdominal pain, diarrhoea, difficulty swallowing, and oesophageal ulceration. Multiorgan failure. Pulmonary fibrosis develops within 10–14 days. Death usually ensues within 24–48 hours. 10 ml can be fatal	No antidote. Supportive treatment. After gastric lavage instillation of Fuller's Earth or betonite with magnesium sulphate can lessen absorption. Haemodialysis or haemoperfusion should be instituted if within about 6 hours of ingestion
Phenothiazines	As for tricyclics	Supportive. May require diazepam for seizures
Salicylates	Flushing, sweating, tinitus, deafness, hyperventilation. Cellular hypoxia. Acid–base disturbances. Hypokalaemia, pulmonary oedema	Alkalinization of urine increases elimination. Haemodialysis in severe poisoning

creatine phosphokinase (CPK), a high creatinine, and myoglobinuria. Circulatory and renal failure can develop (for further details see Chapter 9) as can compartment syndrome (see Chapter 13).

◆ *Other*
Monitor blood glucose regularly.
Monitor body temperature. Hypothermia is a common manifestation of many poisonings (often accompanied by hypotension and oliguria). Such patients must be rewarmed with close monitoring of volaemic status. If plasma expanders are vigorously overinfused they may cause circulatory overload and

pulmonary oedema. Caution is required, especially when the core temperature is <32°C. (See Chapter 13 for further details on hypothermia.)

Specific management of common drug overdoses

Table 16.14 details the management of drug overdose. During the recovery period patients who have made a deliberate suicide attempt may become withdrawn and uncommunicative, or aggressive and uncooperative. Skill and understanding is needed by the nurse during this difficult period. A psychiatric referral should be arranged as soon as possible so that the acute problem can be alleviated and further suicide attempts prevented. Assistance from other support agencies may be required (e.g. social workers, ministers of religion).

Test yourself (Drug overdose)

Questions

1. Following resuscitation of a patient who has taken a drug overdose, or has been exposed to poisons, a physical assessment is performed. What essential features should this include?

2. What is a toxidrome?

3. What are the effects of and treatment for an overdose of paracetamol?

Answers

1. The physical examination can provide important evidence and assessment should be made of:
   Airway, breathing and circulation.
   The central and autonomic nervous system.
   The appearance of the skin and mucous membranes, e.g. colour (jaundice, cyanosed, cherry red) blisters, lesions, venepuncture marks.
   Odours. Particular toxic substances cause specific odours e.g. cyanide causes bitter almond odour, isopropyl alcohol, phenol and salicylates an acetone odour and heavy metals and organophosphates a garlic odour.

2. A toxidrome is a collection of signs and symptoms that are characteristic of a drug or group of drugs that have been taken in excess.

3. If more than 7.5 g of paracetamol is ingested hepatocellular necrosis develops, proceeding to liver failure over the next 3–6 days. Early signs and symptoms include anorexia, nausea, vomiting, and right upper quadrant pain. Hypoglycaemia, lactic acidosis and renal failure may also occur.
   Treatment consists of initial gastric lavage (if within 1 hour of ingestion) and instillation of activated charcoal. The antidote N-acetylcysteine should be given intravenously as soon as possible. This has a protective effect but is time-dependent and can be given up to 36 hours after the overdose. Toxicity can be assessed by referring to a graph of plasma paracetamol levels against time after ingestion. Oral methionine can be given if within 10–12 hours of paracetamol ingestion. Full supportive care should be given with early referral for a liver transplant should this become necessary.

References and bibliography

Behi, R. (1989). Treatment and care of thyroid problems. *Nursing* **3**, 4–6.

Bhattarai, M.D., Dacruz, D., Chaudhry, M., *et al.* (2000). Managing self poisoning. *British Medical Journal* **320**, 711.

Bird, J. (1997). Intensive care problems in obstetric patients. *Care of the Critically Ill* **13**(6), 241–4.

Borron, S.W., Bismuth, C. (1999). Elimination techniques. In: *Oxford Textbook of Critical Care* (ed. A.R. Webb, M.J. Shapiro, S. Singer, *et al.*), pp. 622–5. Oxford University Press, Oxford.

Byth, P.L. (1990). Obstetrical emergencies. In: *Intensive Care Surgical Nursing,* 3rd edn (ed. T.E. Oh), pp. 355–7. Butterworth, London.

Clark, S.L, Hankins, G.D, Dudley, D.A, *et al.* (1996). Amniotic fluid embolism: analysis of the National Registry. *American Journal of Obstetrics and Gynecology* **172**(4, Part 1), 1158–67.

Confidential Enquiry into Maternal Deaths (2002). *Why Mothers Die 1997–1999.* Royal College of Obstetricians and Gynaecologists, London.

Dugernier, T., Reynaert, M. (1991). Cardiocirculatory emergencies related to pregnancy. *Clinical Intensive Care* **2**, 163–71.

Eclampsia Trial Collaborative Group (1995). Which anticonvulsant for women with eclampsia? Evidence from the Collaborative Eclampsia Trial. *Lancet* **345**, 1455–63.

Evangelisti, J., Thorpe, C.J. (1983). Thyroid storm—a nursing crisis. *Heart and Lung* **12**, 184–93.

Fahy, K.M. (2001). Amniotic fluid embolism: a review of the research literature. *Australian Journal of Midwifery* **14**(1), 9–13.

Hardcastle, W. (1989). Management of Addison's disease. *Nursing* **3**, 7–9.

Hillman, K. (1991). Management of acute diabetic emergencies. *Clinical Intensive Care* **2**, 154–61.

Hurtando, J., Esbrit, P. (2002). Treatment of malignant hypercalcaemia. *Expert Opinion in Pharmacotherapy* **3**(5), 521–7.

Jones, A.L., Volans, G. (1999). Management of self poisoning. *British Medical Journal* **319**, 1414–17.

Koh, L.K. (2003). The diagnosis and management of hypercalcaemia. *Annals of the Academy of Medicine Singapore* **32**(1), 129–39.

Magann, E. *et al.* (1994). Postpartum corticosteroids: accelerated recovery from the syndrome of HELLP. *American Journal of Obstetrics and Gynecology* **171**(4), 1154–8.

Magpie Trial Collaborative Group (2002). Do women with pre-eclampsia, and their babies, benefit from magnesium sulphate? The Magpie Trial: a randomised placebo controlled trial. *Lancet* **359**, 1877.

Mokhlesi, B., Leiken, J.B., Murray, P., *et al.* (2003). Adult toxicology in critical care. Part I: General approach to the intoxicated patient. *Chest* **123**, 577–92.

Mokhlesi, B., Leiken, J.B., Murray, P., *et al.* (2003). Adult toxicology in critical care. Part II: Specific poisonings. *Chest* **123**, 897–922.

Smallridge, R.C. (1992). Metabolic and anatomic thyroid emergencies: a review. *Critical Care Medicine* **20**, 276–91.

Shulbam, C. (1985). Diabetic ketoacidosis—an endocrine emergency. *Nursing* **2**, 246–9.

Stayer Leske, J. (1985). Hyperglycaemic hyperosmolar nonketotic coma: a nursing care plan. *Critical Care Nurse* **5**, 49–56.

Tinker, J., Zapol, W.M. (1992). *Care of the Critically Ill Patient*, 2nd edn, pp. 546–9, 761–92. Springer, Berlin.

Vedig, A. (1990). Adrenocortical insufficiency. In: *Intensive Care Manual*, 3rd edn (ed. T.E. Oh), pp. 345–7. Butterworth, London.

Weekes, J. (1990). Drug overdose. In: *Intensive Care Manual*, 3rd edn (ed. T.E. Oh), pp. 480–6. Butterworth, London.

(1997) Critical Care Obstetrics, 3rd edn, pp. 369–419. Blackwell Science, Oxford.

CHAPTER 17

Evaluating the effects of care in the critical care unit

Introduction

Critical care is expensive and labour-intensive, it carries a high cost for the patient in terms of physical and mental distress and may offer only limited benefit. In spite of this, little work has been carried out evaluating the cost–benefit implications and the value for money offered by critical care. As early as 1989, the King's Fund report recommended that:

1. Those responsible for critical care should collect and evaluate data on the clinical outcome and costs, in general and of the care of individual patients.

2. Research should focus on the data required to allow proper audit and the evaluation of specific practices in critical care.

However, by 1999, The Audit Commission of the NHS reported that little seemed to have changed.

Currently, no guidelines exist as to who should be admitted to critical care, what treatment is considered appropriate in what circumstances, and to what lengths that treatment should extend. These are some of the most difficult ethical dilemmas faced by critical care staff. The problem is intensified as technology progresses offering more intervention at greater cost while resources remain static or dwindle.

One of the most important responsibilities of those working in this area is evaluation of the effectiveness and value of the care they offer. This applies to all types of care offered by the multidisciplinary team.

This chapter will address the following issues:

◆ evidence-based practice

◆ auditing care and assuring clinical quality (clinical governance)

◆ costing and monitoring outcomes in critical care

◆ ethical issues.

Evidence-based care

The introduction of an evidence component in the way nursing and medical care is delivered has been a major influence in recent years. The need to critically evaluate the research carried out and to test the generalizability of studies to other groups of critical care patients has become paramount.

Evidenced-based care is defined as 'an approach to practice and teaching that is based on knowledge of the evidence upon which practice is based, and the strength of that evidence' (Cook *et al.* 1996). It was described by Sackett *et al.* (1996) as the 'conscientious and judicious use of current best evidence in making decisions about the care of individual patients'. Although there is a strong emphasis on randomized controlled trials as the 'gold standard' of evidence, there is also great stress on a cautionary approach to the validity and applicability of these studies that is both important and relevant to extrapolating their results to nursing practice. French (1999) feels that the emphasis on randomized controlled trials and the quantitative aspect of research is disadvantageous to nursing research which has relied heavily on the more qualitative research methods such as phenomenology, grounded theory, and action research to establish a nursing evidence base. Although these more subjective approaches bring limitations in terms of generalizability and application across different groups of patients, the generation of theoretical constructs and frameworks (based on observational data) ensure that a body of evidence can be developed which is equally rigorous and can be tested and applied in local context.

Application of research to practice

Use of published research can provide a trigger for introducing new methods of care delivery. French (1999) suggests that the combination of tacit knowledge (the knowledge of local context and application as well as unpublished but generally accepted knowledge) with empirical knowledge allows the practitioner to validate research within his or her local context. However, there is an implicit assumption that the practitioner is equipped with the skills of research appraisal as well as the resources to pilot work within the local context, which may not always be present.

The key features of any research appraisal is to be familiar with the methodology, to understand the limitations of the study data, recommendations, and conclusions and to consider carefully the applicability of the results to one's practice.

Outcome measurement and prediction

Outcome measurement is the process of collecting and analysing data specific to outcomes that reflect the effects of interventions. In order to critically appraise the ability of a study to prognosticate outcome, Randolph *et al.* (1998) suggest that the following points should be considered:

1. Is the sample of patients representative?

2. Are patients homogeneous with respect to prognostic risk?

3. Is follow-up sufficient to minimize the possibility that the missing patients could alter the interpretation of the results?

4. Are health outcomes evaluated, using objective and unbiased criteria?

Risk adjustment

Risk adjustment is a method of comparing the outcomes of patients with varied levels of illness severity. Risk adjustment 'levels the playing field' by providing clinicians with meaningful comparisons of outcomes such as mortality or length of stay across critical care units (CCU), different hospitals, and diagnoses (Cook *et al.* 1996). The predicted risk of mortality based on severity scores such as APACHE II (see Table 17.2) are used as a comparison between two groups of patients. Risk adjustment can be used for comparing outcomes between different units and to ensure patient groups are similar when comparing the effect of interventions.

Use of statistical tools for evaluating the ability to predict accurately

Clinical researchers often use a receiver operating characteristic (ROC) curve to describe the discriminating ability of a predictive tool. An example is shown in Fig. 17.1. The ROC plots true-positive predictions (sensitivity) against the false-positive predictions (specificity) (Cook *et al.* 1996). The closer to 1.0 the area under the curve is, the more accurate the tested predictive model. Pure chance will result in a ROC area of 0.50. The minimal clinically acceptable ROC area typically is ≥0.704.

Quality of care, audit, standards of care, and benchmarking

The measurement or monitoring of the quality of care delivered has become a central part of the delivery of 21st-century healthcare. The original professional (and often medical) focus of what should and should not be done has been replaced by a partnership approach between healthcare users (patients) and their relatives and the staff within the system. This change means that the views of users and relatives on the critical care service must be actively sought in order to provide

feedback to the staff so that healthcare delivery is more responsive to the patient's and their family's needs.

Audit

Audit has been defined as the systematic and public examination of factors which affect the delivery of good care. Quality assurance has been defined as a planned system of activities which, if carried out correctly, should provide a product or service satisfying agreed standards within agreed resources and timescales (Five Regions Consortium 1991).

Management of quality can be controlled on three levels (Macfarlane 1989):

- ◆ 'pre-action control' (setting the standards or goals of care);
- ◆ 'concurrent control' (monitoring the care given);
- ◆ 'feedback control' (evaluating the level of practice).

Maxwell's dimensions of quality (cited in Redfern and Norman 1990) allow one method of reviewing quality issues in healthcare. There are six dimensions: (1) access, (2) equity, (3) relevance to need, (4) social acceptability, (5) efficiency, and (6) effectiveness.

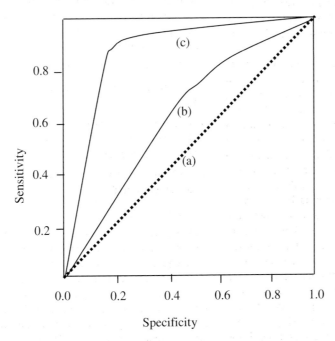

(a) = area under the curve of 0.5 and a discrimination that is no better than chance
(b) = small area under the curve and a poor discrimination
(c) = large area under the curve and a good discrimination

Fig. 17.1 The receiver operating characteristic (ROC) curve.

This approach allows far more input from the consumer and is specific to formulating the service to their needs. It does, however, produce problems in application to the intensive care area because many of the criteria involved may have different standards in differing circumstances. For example, desired outcomes of the consumer may alter from recovery when the patient is first admitted, to a peaceful and dignified death when recovery is no longer possible.

Measurement of quality is a complex and difficult task. This is particularly so in nursing where many of the skills are problematic to quantify, and quality almost always carries value judgments based on socialization (Norman *et al.* 1992) (see Fig. 17.2).

Measurement of quality in nursing is associated with two approaches:

1. The objective quantitative measurement of care criteria.

2. The qualitative analysis of caring.

The first approach is by far the easiest to measure, but the second may be a truer reflection of real quality in terms of nursing care. If these factors can be measured then comparison can be made between levels of quality and cost between different units, wards, and hospitals.

Redfern and Norman (1990) suggest that quality incorporates not just consumer satisfaction, but also all the considerations of equity, accessibility, acceptability, efficiency, effectiveness, and appropriateness of the

> ### QUANTITATIVE INDICATORS OF QUALITY
>
> ◆ Rates of nosocomial infection: cannulae, urinary tract infection, wound infection, chest infection.
>
> ◆ Incidence of pressure sores evaluated against severity of illness and chronic health problems.
>
> ◆ Patients' or relatives' complaints and/or satisfaction.
>
> ◆ Achievement of pain relief using visual analogue scoring.
>
> ◆ Amount of time spent on non-nursing duties.
>
> ◆ Number of drug errors.
>
> ◆ Incidence of sharps injuries, back injuries, etc.
>
> ◆ Critical incident analysis.

care offered. They believe that 'these considerations highlight the point that high-quality health care or, more specifically, high-quality nursing care is influenced predominantly by social values'.

Quantitative audit

Areas that can be assessed quantitatively are useful objective measures for audit of practice. They are most frequently markers of outcome or structure rather than of process.

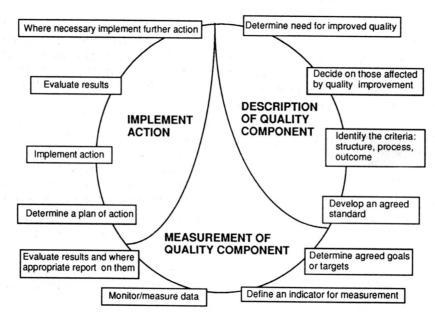

Fig. 17.2 The quality assurance cycle.

Standard of care

This is a professionally agreed level of performance appropriate to the population addressed which is achievable and desirable. Donabedian (1966), in a seminal paper on evaluating quality in medical care, divided standard setting and markers of quality into three categories: structure, process, and outcome. Structure includes the fabric and facilities of the environment, the staffing and organization, and the resources. Process includes the delivery of care, the values and philosophy of the caregivers, and the way care is organized. Outcome includes survival, the quality of life of survivors, and relative satisfaction with care. This has come to be regarded as an appropriate framework for developing standards in all areas of care.

The increasing emphasis on an evidence base of quality studies has meant that most standards will incorporate a systematic review of published papers from which support for the standard proposed can be drawn.

Outcome is probably the easiest and most frequently audited area but depends heavily on factors involved in both structure and process.

Process can be examined using established standards against which comparisons of practice can be made. This is the area the generic nursing quality assessment tools are designed to cover based on expert professional opinion.

Critical care has some specific disadvantages which make audit more complex. These are the lack of a satisfactory definition of what constitutes critical care, the heterogeneity of the patients involved, and the difficulty of establishing a link between particular therapies and survival.

There are, however, considerable data available in critical care on all aspects of the patient's illness and response to interventions. In fact, recording of observations about the patient can occupy up to 20% of the nurses' time (Price and Mason 1986). This wealth of information would provide considerable insight into many aspects of patient care if it could be collated and analysed in a structured format. The use of computerized clinical information systems for the future may well allow such complex data analysis to be performed regularly providing a clearer view of the effects of therapeutic interventions.

Benchmarking

Benchmarking refers to the comparison of audited processes of care to an agreed optimum standard based on published evidence and expert opinion. Ellis (2000) identifies it as 'professional consensus of best possible achievable practice; rather than comparison with actual best practice, clinical practice benchmarking ensures utilization of all levels of evidence in the identification of standards of excellence, with benchmarking activity supporting structured comparison and sharing'.

The concept of benchmarking allows comparison of care delivery between different critical care units and the possibility of publication of these results. While it remains a laudable method of reviewing care practice, the lack of research data to support one practice as opposed to another makes the development of the benchmarking standard very difficult and in many cases it is based purely on local expert opinion which may differ across the country (see Table 17.1).

Critical incident reporting and risk management

Adverse events can occur in any critical care area but the rate of occurrence of iatrogenic (occurring as a result of medical/nursing intervention) complications can reflect the quality of care provided. The Quality in Australian Health Care Study (Wilson et al. 1995) has

---

SOURCES OF DATA FOR QUALITY CRITERIA

- Patient observation
- Patient interview
- Environmental observation
- Nurse interview
- Patient record review
- Ancillary staff interview
- Family and relatives interview

EXAMPLES OF RISK MANAGEMENT RESPONSES TO CRITICAL INCIDENTS

1. The incidence of contamination through eye splashes from ventilator tubing disconnections may be reduced by instigating mandatory safety goggles when approaching the patient.

2. The likelihood of drug error may be reduced by altering the number of drugs given as IV boluses at the same time.

3. The education of staff about specific drug interactions may reduce the incidence of adverse interactions.

TABLE 17.1 Perceived impact of benchmarking over other quality initiatives (from Ellis 2000)

Quality initiatives	Benchmarking
Fit for purpose	Best possible practice
Traditional practice	Evidence-based practice
Internal focus	External focus
Professional fragmentation	Patient-focused care
Internal efficiency	Recognized excellence
Management led	Practitioner led with management support
Pockets of good practice	Dissemination of good practice
Outcome measurement	Process improvement to outcome improvement
What is done	How it is done
Achieving agreed standards	Continuous improvement
Repetition of effort	Sharing
Competitive protectionism	Open comparison and sharing

provided a huge amount of data into the types of errors that occur. The cause is human error in up to 70% of occasions. In a retrospective study of patient records in the UK, Vincent *et al.* (2001) found a rate of adverse incident events of almost 11%, a third of which led to greater disability or death. In both these studies about half of the events were thought to be preventable. More detailed examination of critical incidents will enable identification of educational needs, additional safety processes, or extra resources to reduce the risk of reoccurrence.

Some studies suggest (Pronovost *et al.* 1999, Baggs 1999) that organizational issues such as a dedicated intensivist, daily critical care unit rounds by the consultant, nurse:patient ratios of 1:2 or more, and limited collaboration between staff have a strong influence on outcomes in critical care. Pronovost (2001) also emphasizes the need for a systems approach to reducing clinical risk rather than the older style of individual liability so that likelihood of reoccurrence is reduced and reporting of possible adverse incidents is encouraged.

Illness severity scoring systems in critical care

The scoring system was introduced in the 1980s to allow an objective assessment of illness severity which can then be used to compare a wide range of disorders or disease states. Most scoring systems are designed to define the extent of deviation from normal of acute and chronic disease variables. These include physiological, functional, and psychosocial variables. Mourouga

et al. (2000) state, 'the purpose of scoring systems in critical care, as for many other areas of health care, is to take into account the characteristics of patients that could affect their risk of a particular outcome, irrespective of the effect of the care they receive'. However, recently they have been subjected to some criticism based on the lack of inclusion of pre-critical care variables and organizational variables within the critical care unit such as presence of an intensivist or nurse: patient ratios (Moreno and Matos 2001)

Outcome prediction

Some scoring systems are used to predict outcome. This outcome applies only to a patient population and cannot be applied to the individual. The aim is to reduce prognostic uncertainty by giving the probability of an outcome. The scoring system cannot therefore be used as the basis for withholding or withdrawing treatment from a patient. It is valuable for comparison of the predicted outcome with the actual outcome and can be used to assess the efficacy of therapeutic intervention or other factors such as the environment, organization, staffing, etc.

A variety of scoring systems have evolved in critical care to provide:

- An index of disease severity—either general (e.g. APACHE II, SAPS II) or specific (e.g. Glasgow Coma Scale, Trauma Score).

- An index of workload and consumption of resources (e.g. TISS).

- A means of comparison for: (i) audit of performance (either in the same unit over time or between units) and (ii) research (e.g. evaluation of new products and treatment regimens).

- Patient management objectives (e.g. sedation, pressure area care).

Severity scoring systems

These have been devised either for specific conditions, e.g. trauma (Trauma Score, Injury Severity Score), sepsis (Sepsis Score), pancreatitis (Ransom Score), and head injury (Glasgow Coma Score), or for the general CCU patient (e.g. APACHE II , SAPS II). Most systems rely to a great extent on physiological and clinical assessment though are often complemented by readily obtainable laboratory measurements such as haematocrit and white blood cell count.

APACHE

The APACHE (Acute Physiology And Chronic Health Evaluation) classification was devised by Knaus *et al.*

TABLE 17.2 APACHE II score

Variable	+4	+3	+2	+1	0	+1	+2	+3	+4
Temp (rectal) (°C)	≥41	39–40.9		38.2–38.9	36–38.4	34–35.9	32–33.9	30–31.9	≤29.9
Mean BP (mmHg)	≥160	130–159	110–129		70–109		50–69		≤49
Heart rate (bpm)	≥180	140–179	110–139		70–109		55–69	40–54	≤39
Respiratory rate (breaths per min)	≥50	35–49		25–34	12–24	10–11	6–9		≤5
If F_iO_2 ≥ 0.5: A–a DO_2 (mmHg)	≥500	350–499	200–349		<200				
If F_iO_2 < 0.5: PO_2 (mmHg)					>70	61–70		55–60	≤55
Arterial pH	≥7.7	7.6–7.69		7.5–7.59	7.33–7.49		7.25–7.32	7.15–7.24	≤7.15
Serum Na (mmol/litre)	≥180	160–179	155–159	150–154	130–149		120–129	111–119	≤110
Serum K (mmol/litre)	≥7	6–6.9		5.5–5.9	3.5–5.4	3–3.4	2.5–2.9		<2.5
Serum creatinine (μmol/litre) (double if acute renal failure)	≥300	171–299	121–170		50–120	<50			
Haematocrit (%)	≥60		50–59.9	46–49.9	30–45.9		20–29.9		<20
Leucocytes (per mm³)	≥40		20–39.9	15–19.9	3–14.9		1–2.9		<1
Neurological = Glasgow Coma Score									

Age points: patient's age ≤44 years, 0 points; 45–54 years, 2 points; 55–64 years, 3 points; 65–74 years, 5 points; ≤75 years, 6 points.

Chronic health points: 2 points for elective post-operative admission or 5 points if emergency operation or non-operative admission, if patient has either cirrhosis, heart failure (NYHA Grade 4), respiratory failure, dialysis-dependent renal disease, or is immunocompromised.

(1981). Now known as 'APACHE I', this was a score derived from the degree of abnormality of 34 physiological and biochemical variables, age, and chronic health status (e.g. severe heart failure, cirrhosis, immunosuppression). The amount of physiological scoring proved rather unwieldy so a simplified version, 'APACHE II', was developed and published in 1985. APACHE II uses the most extreme levels recorded in the first 24 hours following admission of the 12 most commonly measured physiological and biochemical variables in addition to age and chronic health grading (Table 17.2). The level of risk of subsequent death from a wide range of admission disorders was computed, although burns and cardiac surgery were specifically excluded from analysis. Validation of this risk stratification was performed in 6000 patients in 13 American critical care units. This validation study was repeated in 26 British CCUs to see whether the American model was applicable to British patients (Rowan et al. 1993). Although a generally good agreement was noted some significant differences were found. For example, the British study performed better in acute surgical conditions but worse in acute medical admissions. Age also had a greater impact on outcome in Britain.

The APACHE system has been refined still further with the introduction of 'APACHE III' in 1990. The APACHE III database contained an initial 17 457 patients from 40 American hospitals. However, it is being continually expanded and now includes a data set of non-US patients. APACHE III attempts to improve the statistical predictive power by: (1) adding five new physiological variables (albumin, bilirubin, glucose, urea, urine output), (2) changing the thresholds and weighting of existing variables, (3) comparing both admission and 24-hour scores, (4) incorporating the source of admission (e.g. casualty, ward, operating theatre), and (5) reassessing the effect of age, chronic health, and specific disease category. Comparative studies between APACHE II and III have yet to be published to confirm the superiority of the modified system. Furthermore, the APACHE III risk stratification is now proprietary and has to be purchased; this may limit its general acceptance.

SAPS

SAPS (Simplified Acute Physiology Score), devised by Le Gall et al. (1984), is very similar to the APACHE II system though it uses 14 readily measured clinical and biochemical variables. It too has been modified ('SAPS II') (Le Gall et al. 1993) (Table 17.3).

Chang (1989) developed the Riyadh Score—a computer model based on trends of daily APACHE II scores

TABLE 17.3 Simplified Acute Physiology Score (SAPS) II (point score in brackets)

Variable	Score
Age	<40 (0); 40–59 (7); 60–69 (12); 70–74 (15); 75–79 (16); ≥80 (18)
Heart rate (bpm)	<40 (11); 40–69 (2); 70–119 (0); 120–159 (4); ≥160 (7)
Systolic BP (mmHg)	<70 (13); 70–99 (5); 100–199 (0); ≥200 (2)
Body temp (°C)	<39 (0); =39 (3)
P_aO_2/F_iO_2 (kPa) (only if ventilated or CPAP)	<13.3 (11); 13.3–26.5 (9); ≥26.6 (6)
Urine output (litre/day)	<0.5 (11); 0.5–0.999 (4); ≥1 (0)
Serum urea (mmol/litre)	<10 (0); 10–29.9 (6); ≥30 (10)
White blood count (per mm³)	<1 (12); 1—19.9 (0); ≥20 (3)
Serum potassium (mmol/litre)	<3 (3); 3–4.9 (0); ≥5 (3)
Serum sodium (mmol/litre)	<125 (5); 125–144 (0); ≥145 (1)
Serum bicarbonate (mEq/litre)	<15 (6); 15–19 (3); ≥20 (0)
Serum bilirubin (μmol/litre)	<68.4 (0); 68.4–102.5 (4); ≥102.6 (9)
Glasgow Coma Score	<6 (26); 6–8 (13); 9–10 (7); 11–13 (5); 14–15 (0)
Chronic disease	Metastatic cancer (9); haematological malignancy (10), AIDS (17)
Type of admission	Scheduled surgical (0); medical (6); unscheduled surgical (8)

and organ system failures—to further refine outcome prediction.

However, none of the above systems (APACHE, SAPS, Riyadh) are totally infallible; the individual patient with very poor outcome may well defy the odds while the expected survivor may still die. For this, and other more emotive reasons, outcome prediction systems have yet to be used either to instigate early withdrawal or refusal of critical care treatment. Proponents, however, claim that progressive rationalization of healthcare resources will eventually force the institution of this decision-making process and a refined scoring system will be vital.

The Therapeutic Intervention Scoring System (TISS) provides an index of workload activity by attaching a score to procedures and techniques being performed on an individual patient (e.g. use and number of vasoac-

tive drug infusions, renal replacement therapy, administration of enteral nutrition). This system has been used by some CCUs to develop a means of costing individual patients by attaching a monetary value to each TISS point scored. A discharge TISS score can also be used to estimate the amount of nursing interventions required for a patient in step-down facilities (e.g. a high-dependency unit) or on the general ward. TISS does not accurately measure nursing workload activity as it fails to cater for tasks and duties such as coping with the irritable or confused patient or dealing with grieving relatives. A number of nursing workload scoring systems have been developed in order to assess nurse staffing requirements (e.g. GRASP). Although not developed specifically for critical care, GRASP determines the type and amount of care required for a patient rather than measure severity of illness or bed occupancy. The GRASP score indicates the sum of estimated time units needed to perform a variety of nursing duties, including the provision of emotional support to patient and/or family.

Unfortunately, other than the Glasgow Coma Score (see Chapter 10), there is no universally accepted system practised by every CCU. Competing systems have often been developed simultaneously. For example, APACHE and SAPS are both widely used for scoring disease severity—APACHE is the predominant system in America and Britain, while SAPS is more popular in mainland Europe. Each system has its devotees not prepared to shift allegiance and, due to considerable financial implications, a common system is unlikely to be agreed upon.

Specific scoring systems

Trauma

Trauma scoring systems have been utilized for a variety of purposes:

♦ performing rapid field triage to direct the patient to appropriate levels of care;

♦ quality assurance;

♦ developing and improving trauma care systems by categorizing patients and identifying problems within the systems;

♦ making comparisons between groups from different hospitals, in the same hospital over time, and/or undergoing different treatment strategies.

The Injury Severity Score (ISS) is a severity scoring system for trauma patients based on the anatomical injuries sustained. The Revised Trauma Score (RTS) uti-

TABLE 17.4 Revised Trauma Score. Score = coded value × weighting

	Coded value	Weighting
Respiratory rate (breaths/min)		
10–29	4	0.2908
>29	3	
6–9	2	
1–5	1	
0	0	
Systolic blood pressure (mmHg)		
>89	4	0.7326
76–89	3	
50–75	2	
1–49	1	
0	0	
Glasgow Coma Scale		
13–15	4	0.9368
9–12	3	
6–8	2	
4–5	1	
3	0	
Total = Revised Trauma Score		

lizes measures of physiological abnormality to predict survival (see Table 17.4). A combination of ISS and RTS, TRISS, was developed to overcome the shortcomings of anatomical or physiological scoring alone. The TRISS methodology uses ISS, RTS, patient age, and whether the injury was blunt or penetrating to provide a measure of the probability of survival. It is the current system of choice in Britain for auditing effectiveness of care in trauma patients admitted to hospital for more than 3 days, managed in a critical care area, referred for specialist care; or who die in hospital.

Head injury

The Glasgow Coma Scale, first described by Teasdale and Jennett (1974) utilizes eye opening, best motor response, and best verbal response to categorize the severity of head injury. It is probably the only system used universally in CCUs. Apart from its ability to prognosticate, it is also frequently used for therapeutic decision-making (e.g. elective ventilation in patients presenting with a GCS score of less than 8).

Sepsis, multiple organ failure, ARDS

A variety of definitions exist for ARDS and for multiple organ failure (MOF). Knaus produced his definitions for MOF which are frequently cited, though others are also quoted. Recent attempts to clarify the area have been made by Bone *et al.* (1992) who coined the terms systemic inflammatory response syndrome (SIRS) and multiple organ dysfunction syndrome (MODS) (see Chapter 12).

A more surgically oriented definition of sepsis, the Sepsis Score, was proposed by Elebute and Stoner (1983) for grading the severity of sepsis from the local effects of infection, pyrexia, secondary effects of sepsis, and laboratory data.

Sedation

A variety of scoring systems have been developed for gauging and recording the level of sedation of a mechanically ventilated patient. The aim is to enable the staff to titrate the dose of sedative agents to avoid either over- or undersedation. The Ramsay Sedation Score developed in 1974 consists of a six-point scoring system separated into three awake and three asleep levels where the patient responded to a tap or loud auditory stimulus with brisk, sluggish, or no response at all. The main problem lies in achieving reproducibility of the tap or loud auditory stimulus. Bion (1990) developed a more complex score by combining analogue scales representing sedation: from alert to unrousable; distress, from calm to agitated; and comprehension, from orientated to uncomprehending. A set of observations could be recorded and linked by three lines to form a triangle. Triangles can be produced from subsequent observations of the same patient to indicate whether or not the change in sedation was better or worse. Bion also included the APACHE II score as the need for sedation is naturally linked to the degree of disease. Combining these analogue scales with the APACHE II score makes the whole concept too complex to be used in daily CCU practice; however, it does provide a good illustration of changes in the quality of sedation in an individual patient.

The Cambridge Sedation Score allocates a number from 1 to 7 ranging from agitated to unresponsive. Level 3 describes a patient who is awakened when spoken to with a normal voice.

Injury severity score

This system has the following scoring system:

1. Use the A1S90 (Abbreviated Injury Score 1990) dictionary to score every injury.

2. Identify the highest abbreviated injury scale score for each of the following: head and neck, abdomen and pelvic contents, bony pelvis and limbs, face, chest, body surface.

3. Add together the squares of the three highest area scores.

Cost versus outcome

The escalation in costs for critical care has engendered a need to examine financial outlay in the light of outcome and effectiveness. The ultimate benefit of prolonging meaningful quality of life must be weighed against the huge cost of treatment. In particular, length of survival following discharge and the quality of life for survivors are key factors. Dragsted (1990) has stated that evaluation of critical care medicine may be expected to have the following consequences:

◆ An improvement of procedures which might lead to an improvement in the quality of CCU care.

◆ Modifications in teaching.

◆ Reduction of the economic costs for society.

◆ An increased efficiency as an effect of a better control of the organization.

Parno et al. (1982) investigated hospital charges and long-term survival in CCU and general hospital patients in the United States. The average total hospital charge was nearly five times greater for CCU patients compared with general patients and the mortality rate in hospital was 17.3% for CCU patients as opposed to 3.4% for general patients. Following discharge, the 2-year survival rate was 83% of CCU patients and 89% of non-CCU patients, suggesting that providing patients survive their hospital stay the likelihood of a reasonable extension of life is good. However, there was some difference in age and sex distribution between the two groups which casts doubt on the validity of the observation.

In a smaller study in the UK, Shiell et al. (1990) compared survival and long-term outcome in two CCU care units. Mortality rates at discharge were 15 and 25% in each unit, rising to 38 and 31% 6 months after admission. Thus, mortality post-discharge from the CCU in the short term was 23% for one unit and 6% for another. Mortality was positively associated with severity of illness and age. Cost was heavily weighted towards a small group of 10 patients who had significantly longer lengths of stay and who were responsible for over 45% of total expenditure.

In a study of 337 CCU patients following both emergency and elective admission, Sage et al. (1986) found that those patients who did not survive until follow-up incurred the greatest cost, in this instance, due to greater intensity of treatment.

FACTORS INFLUENCING OUTCOME FROM CRITICAL CARE
◆ Age
◆ Previous health status
◆ Severity of acute illness
◆ Diagnosis

Significant factors in outcome for emergency admissions were APACHE II scores and TISS scores indicating severity of illness and intensity of intervention. However, factors in outcome following discharge were age and chronic health suggesting that once critical care is successful then subsequent events may be determined by pre-existing factors.

High usage of resources and therefore high costs were associated with hospital mortalities of 30–45% and cumulative mortalities of 35–60%. There is an important obvious difference in outcome between emergency and elective admission to the CCU. The French multicentre study (French Multicenter Group of ICU Research 1989) showed that mortality in the emergency surgical admission group was 27% compared with a mortality of 5% in the elective group.

Cost therefore, is, usually related to severity of illness, length of stay, and intensity of treatment. It is unfortunate that this is frequently associated with the greatest mortality rate. Detsky et al. (1981) found that those patients attracting the highest cost were those with the least expected outcomes (i.e. survivors who had been expected to die and non-survivors who had been expected to live). They suggest that refining prognostic accuracy may reduce inappropriate treatment.

The cost per survivor may seem high, but if viewed as the cost per extended life-year the investment may seem a reasonable one.

Quality of life

Shiell et al. (1990) investigated quality of life in survivors assessed using the Nottingham Health Profile which shows how patients' current health is affecting their daily lives. One-third of the patients had problems with employment, carrying out housework, and sexual relations; almost one-half had difficulty pursuing personal interests, socializing, or going on holiday. In all, 22% of patients reported substantial levels of disability and 19% reported substantial levels of distress.

Sage et al. (1986) found quality of life was good in the 140 patients who responded to follow-up questionnaires 16–20 months after discharge from the CCU.

This was only 41% of the initial sample, with an 11% hospital mortality and a post-discharge mortality of 24.6%, and it is possible that some bias was introduced (only those patients satisfied with their outcome responded). Goldstein *et al.* (1986) studied functional outcomes in 2213 patients admitted to a CCU. Unlike other studies they grouped the patients according to their pre-admission functional status and found that mortality was clearly related to prior functional status. However, they found that activity level was reduced in 74% of those initially admitted with an active level functional status, although 60% of the previously employed returned to work. This is consistent with the results of Zaren and Hedstrand (1987) who found that 75% of those in employment prior to CCU admission were back at work within 1 year and concluded overall that there was no great deterioration in quality of life among long-term survivors of critical care.

Dragsted and Qvist (1989) followed up 1308 patients for 12 months following CCU admission and found that 44% of the survivors returned to their pre-hospital activity level within 1 year. Increasing age and chronic disease were found to influence functional outcome significantly.

Although there is some variation in the groups of patients studied and the criteria used to define quality of life, there are some fairly consistent results among several studies. Most interestingly, it would appear that quality of life as denoted by activity and return to employment is high, including up to three-quarters of those working prior to CCU admission.

However, there are clear indications that those whose life quality is limited prior to admission, either by chronic health problems or age, are less likely to regain an acceptable level of function and more likely not to survive the admission.

Recovery and follow-up

Until recently, little work had been undertaken in following up and identifying problems in post-intensive care patients. The need for justifying the benefits of CCU care has ensured that clinicians are starting to use the ultimate quality of life of the patient rather than

simply their condition at transfer to the ward as the end-point of their interventions.

Some CCUs now run follow-up clinics for ex-patients who have spent a period of time in critical care (Griffiths 1992). The purpose of these clinics is two-fold. One function is to allow assessment, diagnosis, treatment, counselling, and support of the individual patient and his or her family. The other purpose is to allow collection of data regarding specific problems, both short and long term, associated with the interventions used in the CCU and evaluation of the efficacy of treatment.

Long-term problems associated with prolonged CCU admission

The effect of critical care on the patient is overwhelming and there are few patients who spend longer than 2–3 days in critical care who do not continue to suffer mental and physical problems as a result.

Physical problems

- *Weight loss and muscle wasting.* Skeletal muscle loss during illness is due to inactivity, catabolism, and frequently inadequate nutrition. In many patients, this loss will take months to recover and other pathology may limit the patient's ability to exercise and rebuild muscle bulk.

- *Reduced respiratory function.* Diaphragmatic and intercostal muscle loss may contribute to this as well as residual pulmonary pathology from infection or other problems. Patients may remain short of breath on exertion due either to respiratory problems or cardiac insufficiency.

- *Complications of endotracheal intubation or tracheostomy.* Patients may experience vocal disturbance due to vocal cord damage or stridor and wheezing due to tracheal stenosis.

- *Neurological problems.* Sensory and motor neuropathies may occur and there may be disturbances of fine motor control. Same patients experience visual deficits and auditory problems such as tinnitus.

Psychological problems

These can be severe and are often associated with hallucinations and nightmares experienced during the period in critical care. Many patients continue to suffer nightmares and sleep disturbance for many years after their illness. Friedman *et al.* (1992) surveyed 46 patients following CCU discharge and found that 24% of patients contacted after a mean of 8 months had sleeping problems and CCU-related dreams. The adjustment of role

---

FACTORS INFLUENCING FUNCTIONAL OUTCOME FOLLOWING CCU ADMISSION

- Age
- Chronic disease/previous health status
- Previous functional level

from total dependence to relative independence can be traumatic and coming to terms with the nearness of their own mortality may also cause problems. Some patients have complete memory loss of the time spent in critical care and this may lead to false expectations of their ability to recover from their illness. Patients may also suffer loss of concentration, mental fatigue, and difficulty in following a line of reasoned thought. Short-term memory may also be affected. There may be abrupt mood swings and periods of severe depression.

Social factors

Relationships with family and friends may suffer as a result of the patient's experiences and the associated psychological problems. There may be personality changes and difficulty in relating to people.

General problems

Loss of appetite, alteration in taste sensation, altered body image, and sexual dysfunction can all cause problems in the long-term recovery period. Friedman *et al.* (1992) recorded that only 54% of patients had returned to their daily routine.

The extent of problems which may be experienced by these patients requires a broad range of professional expertise in providing advice and assistance. If a clinic is to function successfully it should involve a multidisciplinary approach to problems and assessment. Further details can be found in Chapter 1.

Follow-up service for bereaved relatives

Jackson (1992) found that only 12% of CCUs in the UK offered a formal follow-up service for bereaved relatives. They are often left to cope with sudden and traumatic death after a variable length of time spent in the CCU. Coming to terms with this sudden loss may prove difficult, especially after the period of hope (sometimes false) offered by admission to the CCU. There may be difficulty separating from what was a safe, supported environment (the CCU) to face the problems of home and its accompanying memories.

Most CCUs offer a high degree of support, advice, and information at the time of death but this is unlikely to be taken in or remembered.

Collins (1989) recommends that families receive a follow-up visit by a nurse or chaplain within 2 weeks of the death. This is not usually practical, and it may be more appropriate to ask the relative to visit the CCU or an area close by. The nurse or appropriate person can then discuss problems, answer questions, and supply information, as well as listen and express empathy for their grief. In units where primary nursing is carried

---

> ### SOURCES OF FURTHER HELP
>
> - Bereavement support groups
> - Chaplains or ministers of other religions
> - Bereavement counsellor (if available)
> - Citizen's Advice Bureau (for assistance with practical difficulties)

out, it may be most appropriate that the primary nurse follows-up the family.

Ideally, a trained bereavement counsellor would be available to support the family but this resource is not always available.

Jackson (1992) suggests a phone follow-up service where the responsible nurse rings the bereaved family and offers condolence and further support where necessary.

Ethics

The exact definition of 'ethics' is the philosophical study of the moral value of human conduct and the rules and principles that govern it. However, it has come to be regarded as the morals or code of conduct of particular social groups such as the professions.

Morals are the principles of behaviour actually held or followed by individuals or groups in accordance with standards of right and wrong.

Ethics in critical care are an important issue partly due to the increasing sophistication of medical science and technology balanced by a growing emphasis on the autonomy of the individual. The effect of financial constraints on resources have also led to an upsurge in ethical dilemmas in this expensive area of care.

Among the many ethical dilemmas facing staff in critical care a number are encountered with reasonable frequency. These are:

- determining the point of withdrawal of treatment;
- withholding resuscitation measures;
- deciding when the burdens of further therapeutic measures outweigh the benefits;
- when resources are limited, deciding which patient will receive critical care;
- evaluating when critical care is an appropriate measure.

Although the final decision in most cases will rest with the consultant involved, the situation will usually be discussed beforehand among the staff, with the patient's relatives, and, where appropriate, with the patient. The establishment of a consensus view is an important part of acceptance of the final decision. If those heavily involved in the patient's care have no opportunity to explore and express their feelings there may be a loss of trust in the validity of the decision and resentment about its outcome.

Ethical decision-making is complex, stressful, and extremely difficult. The same decision must be re-appraised for each case and guidelines can only be broad and non-specific. Ethical decisions depend on moral judgments and these will be based on personal values and social pressures.

Use of a decision-making process may help in clarifying the pros and cons of the situation. The unit philosophy will also provide a record of the attitudes and values that the staff generally hold and can be useful in providing some clear ideals with which to examine the ethical dilemma.

Knowledge of the basic principles of ethics may help to provide a foundation on which to base decisions.

Ethical theories

There are two major theories for determining whether an action is right or wrong. The first refers to the consequences of the action (consequentialist) and the second to the moral rules or guidelines governing that action (deontological).

Consequentialist theory

Moral or ethical dilemmas are resolved by calculating the good over harm expected to be produced by each alternative. Utilitarianism is the best known consequentialist philosophy (Mill 1867) and is based on the need for human beings to act in bringing about the best outcome for all concerned.

Deontologicol theory

Moral or ethical dilemmas are resolved by considering the action in its own right according to duties, rights, and justice. The act itself is judged right or wrong and the consequences of the action do not matter. The greatest proponent of this was the German philosopher, Immanuel Kant, who advocated using the individual's moral sense to judge each act.

Tschudin (1986) quotes the principles of ethics established by the philosopher Thiroux as a readily applicable formulation of ethical theory. The five principles are:

1. The value of life—humans should revere life and accept death.

2. Goodness or rightness—promote good over bad, cause no harm, prevent harm.

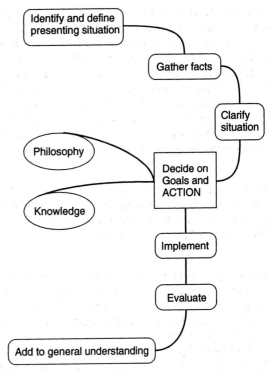

Fig. 17.3 The ethical decision-making process.

3. Justice or fairness—egalitarianism over scarce resources.

4. Truth-telling or honesty—there may be circumstances when this is not always best.

5. Individual freedom—freedom to choose and to choose what may not always be best.

These principles act as foundations for ethical decision-making and may help to clarify the decision although they cannot direct the choice itself (see also Fig. 17.3).

Withdrawing treatment

One of the most difficult decisions in critical care is deciding the point at which treatment is no longer likely to bring benefit to the patient either in terms of relief of symptoms or in terms of recovery. The emphasis of intervention must then be changed from cure to care and the goals redefined to allow death within a comfortable, humane, and peaceful environment:

> In the irreversible illness, LIFE is neither the absolute good nor DEATH the absolute evil.
>
> Hugh Casson

It is frequently difficult to accept that all the technological and pharmaceutical interventions and support that have been so important to the patient up till now are no longer going to benefit him or her. This may be more of a problem to the medical than nursing staff due to the values and ethos attached to each profession. In a convenience sample of readers the *Nursing Times* (1988) found that 91% would agree with removing life support in the case of prolonged and irreversible coma.

The Society of Critical Care Medicine consensus report on the ethics of foregoing treatment (ACCP/SCCM Consensus Panel. 1990) recommends discussion in the following situations:

1. When the patient has a diagnosis with a grave prognosis.

2. When the burdens of therapy outweigh the benefits.

3. When the quality of the patient's life is expected to be unacceptable to the patient.

Frequently, it is the nursing staff who will first bring up the possibility of withdrawing treatment. They are usually closest to both the patient and family and have a very clear view of the burden of treatment. In these circumstances, the nurse will act as advocate on the patient's behalf and these skills can be vital in limiting the length of unnecessary and unproductive treatment.

Advocacy is seen by Brown (1985) as a means of transferring power back to the patient to enable him/her to control his/her own affairs. It is not about taking over for the patient but about assisting patients so that their needs and rights are met.

Expanding critical care nursing

If critical care nursing is to continue to progress and improve there must be an expansion of knowledge and understanding of the effects of critical illness and the critical care environment on the patient. Alternative

methods of structuring care and of delivery must be explored and made known. This will only be achieved by a programme of structured research which is coordinated, repeated, and validated in a variety of settings and institutions. The multidisciplinary approach which is so important in the delivery of care must also encompass the approach to research. Currently, few institutions offer the facility for nursing involvement in research and the studies undertaken are usually performed by individuals with a commitment to research or as part of a thesis leading to a higher education award. There is an urgent need for a structure that will allow collaborative research looking at all angles of care in numerous situations and applying a logical approach to testing different methods of treatment and care.

References and bibliography

ACCP/SCCM Consensus Panel (1990). Ethical and moral guidelines for the initiation, continuation and withdrawal of critical care. *Chest* **97**, 949–50.

Baggs, J.G., Ryan, S.A., Phelps, C.E., *et al.* (1992). The association between interdisciplinary collaboration and patient outcomes in a medical intensive care unit. *Heart and Lung* **21**, 18–24.

Baker, S.P., O'Neill, B., Haddon, W., *et al.* (1974). The Injury Severity Score: a method of describing patients with multiple injuries and evaluating emergency care. *Journal of Trauma* **14**, 187–96.

Bion, J. (1990). Audit in intensive care. In: *Update in Intensive Care and Emergency Medicine*, Vol. 10 (ed. J.L. Vincent), pp. 851–6. Springer, Berlin.

Bone, R.C., Balk, R.A., Cerra, F.B. *et al.* (1992). Definitions for sepsis and organ failure and guidelines for the use of innovative therapies in sepsis. The ACCP, SCCM Consensus Conference Committee. American College of Chest Physicians/Society of Critical Care Medicine. *Chest* **101**, 1644–55.

Boyd, C.R. Tolson, M.A., Copes, W.S. (1987). Evaluating trauma care: the TRISS method. *Journal of Trauma* **27**, 370–8.

Brown, M. (1985). Matter of commitment. *Nursing Times* **81**, 26–7.

Champion, H.R., Sacco, W.J., Copes, W.S. *et al.* (1989). A revision of the Trauma Score. *Journal of Trauma* **29**, 623–9.

Chang, R.W.S. (1989). Individual outcome prediction models for intensive care units. *Lancet* **ii**, 143–6.

Collins, S. (1989). Sudden death counselling protocol. *Dimensions of Critical Care Nursing* **8**, 375–83.

Cook, D.J., Sibbald, W.J., Vincent, J.-L., *et al.* (1996). Evidence based critical care medicine: what is it and what can it do for us? *Critical Care Medicine* **24**, 334–7.

Cook, D.J., Hebert, P.C., Heyland, D.K., *et al.* (1997). How to use an article on therapy or prevention: pneumonia prevention using subglottic secretion drainage. *Critical Care Medicine* **25**, 1502–13.

CRITERIA TO BE CONSIDERED WHEN DISCUSSING WITHDRAWAL OF TREATMENT

- Prognosis

- Age

- Chronic health status

- Attainable quality of life

- Family

- Social support

- Cultural and religious background

Cullen, D.J., Civetta, J.M., Briggs, B.A., *et al.* (1974). Therapeutic intervention scoring system: a method for quantitative comparison of patient care. *Critical Care Medicine* **2**, 57–60.

Detsky, A.S., Stricker, S.C., Mulley, A.G., *et al.* (1981). Prognosis, survival and the expenditure of hospital resources for patients in an intensive care unit. *New England Journal of Medicine* **305**, 667–72.

Donabedian, A. (1966). Evaluating the quality of medical care. *Millbank Memorial Fund Quarterly* **44**, 166–206.

Dragsted, L. (1990). Long-term outcome from intensive care. In: *Update in Intensive Care and Emergency Medicine*, Vol. 10 (ed. J.L. Vincent), pp. 865–9. Springer, Berlin.

Dragsted, L., Qvist, J. (1989). Outcome from intensive care III. A 5 year study of 1308 patients activity level. *European Journal of Anaesthesiology* **6**, 385–96.

Elebute, E.A., Stoner, H.B. (1983). The grading of sepsis. *British Journal of Surgery* **70**, 29–31.

Ellis, J. (2000). Sharing the evidence: clinical practice benchmarking to improve continuously the quality of care. *Journal of Advanced Nursing* **32**, 215–25.

Five Regions Consortium with Greenhalgh and Co. Ltd (1991). Quality. In: *Using Information in Managing the Nursing Resource*. H. Charlesworth, Huddersfield.

French Multicenter Group of ICU Research (1989). Factors related to outcome in intensive care: French multicenter study. *Critical Care Medicine* **17**, 305–8.

French, P. (1999). The development of evidence-based nursing. *Journal of Advanced Nursing* **29**, 72–8.

Friedman, B.C. Boyce, W., Bekes, C.E. (1992). Long-term follow-up of ICU patients. *American Journal of Critical Care* **1**, 115–17.

Goldstein, R.L., Campion, E.W., Thibault, G.E., *et al.* (1986). Functional outcomes following medical intensive care. *Critical Care Medicine* **14**, 783–8.

Goldstone, L.A., Ball, J.A., Collier, M. (1983). *Monitor: An Index of the Quality of Nursing Care for Acute Medical and Surgical Wards*. Newcastle upon Tyne Polytechnic, Newcastle upon Tyne.

Griffiths, R.D. (1992). Development of normal indices of recovery from critical illness. In: *Intensive Care Britain* (ed. M. Rennie), pp 134–7. Greycoat, London.

Jackson, I. (1992). Bereavement follow-up service in intensive care. *Intensive and Critical Care Nursing* **8**, 163–8.

Keene, A.R., Cullen, D.J. (1983). Therapeutic intervention scoring system: update. *Critical Care Medium* **11**, 1–3.

King's Fund Report (1989). *Intensive Care in the United Kingdom: Report from the King's Fund*. King's Fund Centre, London.

Knaus, W.A., Zimmerman, J.E., Wagner, D.P., *et al.* (1981). APACHE—acute physiology and chronic health evaluation: a physiologically based classification system. *Critical Care Medicine* **9**, 591–7.

Knaus, W.A., Draper, E.A., Wagner, D.P., *et al.* (1985). APACHE II: a severity of disease classification system. *Critical Care Medicine* **13**, 818–29.

Knaus, W.A., Draper, E.A., Wagner, D.P., *et al.* (1986). An evaluation of outcome from intensive care in major medical centers. *Annals of Internal Medicine* **10**, 410–18.

Knaus, W.A., Wagner, D.P., Draper, E.A. *et al.* (1991). The APACHE III prognostic system. Risk prediction of hospital mortality for critically ill hospitalized adults. *Chest* **100**, 1619–36.

Le Gall, J., Brun-Buisson, C., Trunet, P., *et al.* (1982). Influence of age, previous health status, and severity of acute illness on outcome from intensive care. *Critical Care Medicine* **10**, 575–7.

Le Gall, J.R., Lemeshow, S., Saulnier, F. (1993). A new Simplified Acute Physiology Score (SAPS II) based on a European/North American multicenter study. *Journal of the American Medical Association* **270**, 2957–63.

Le Gall, J.R., Loirat, P., Alperovitch, A. *et al.* (1984). A simplified acute physiology score for ICU patients. *Critical Care Medicine* **12**, 975–7.

Maxwell, R. (1984). Quality assessment in health. *British Medical Journal* **288**, 1470—72.

Meyers, D. (1978). *GRASP, a Patient Information and Workload Management System*. MCSI, Morgantown, NC.

Moreno, R., Matos, R. (2001). New issues in severity scoring: interfacing the ICU and evaluating it. *Current Opinion in Critical Care* **7**, 469–74.

Norman, I., Redfern, S, Tomalin, D., *et al.* (1992). Applying triangulation to the assessment of quality of nursing. *Nursing Times* **88**, 43–6.

Mill, J.S. (1867). *Utilitarianism*. Longman, London.

Nursing Times (1988). Euthanasia, what *you* think? *Nursing Times* **84**, 38–9.

Parno, J.R., Teres, D., Lemeshow, S., *et al.* (1982). Hospital charges and long-term survival of ICU versus non-ICU patients. *Critical Care Medicine* **10**, 569–74.

Phaneuf, M. (1976). *The Nursing Audit*. Appleton Century Crofts, New York.

Price, D.J., Mason, J. (1986). Resolving the numerical chaos at the bedside. In: *Current Perspectives in Health Care* (ed. J. Bryan, T. Roberts, P. Windsor), pp. 147–57. British Journal of Health Care Computing, Weybridge.

Pronovost, P.J., Jenckes, M.W., Dorman T., *et al.* (1999). Organizational characteristics of intensive care units related to outcomes of abdominal aortic surgery. *Journal of the American Medical Association* **281**, 1310–17.

Randolph, A.G., Guyatt, G.H., Richardson, W.S. (1998). Prognosis in the intensive care unit: finding accurate and useful estimates for counselling patients. *Critical Care Medicine* **26**, 767–72.

Redfern, S., Norman, I. (1990). Measuring the quality of nursing care: a consideration of different approaches. *Journal of Advanced Nursing* **15**, 1260–71.

Ridley, S., Jackson, R., Findlay, J., *et al.* (1990). Long-term survival after intensive care. *British Medical Journal* **301**, 1127–30.

Rowan, K.M., Kerr, J.H., Major, E., *et al.* (1993). Intensive Care Society's APACHE II study in Britain and Ireland—II: Outcome comparisons of intensive care units after adjustment for case mix by the American APACHE II method. *British Medical Journal* **307**, 977–81.

Sackett, D.L., Rosenberg, W.M.C., Gray, J.A.M., *et al.* (1996) Evidence-based medicine: what it is and what it isn't. *British Medical Journal* **312**, 71–2.

Sage, W.M., Rosenthal, M.H., Silverman, J.F. (1986). Is intensive care worth it? An assessment of input and outcome for the critically ill. *Critical Care Medicine* **14**, 777–82.

Shiell, A.M., Griffiths, R.D., Short, A.I.K., *et al.* (1990). An evaluation of the costs and outcome of adult intensive care in two units in the UK. *Clinical Intensive Care* **1**, 256–62.

Teasdale, G., Jennett, B. (1974). Assessment of coma and impaired consciousness. *Lancet* **ii**, 81–4.

Tschudin, V. (1986). *Ethics in Nursing. The Caring Relationship.* Heinemann Nursing, Oxford.

Wandelt, M., Ager, J. (1974). *Quality Patient Care Scale.* Appleton Century Crofts, New York.

Vincent, C, Neale, G, Woloshynowych, M. (2001). Adverse events in British Hospitals :preliminary retrospective record review. *British Medical Journal* **322**, 517–19.

Zaren, B., Hedstrand, U. (1987). Quality of life among long-term survivors of intensive care. *Critical Care Medicine* **15**, 743–7.

Index